BUSINESS/SCIENCE/TECHNOLOGY DIVISION
CHICAGO PUBLIC LIBRARY
400 SOUTH STATE STREET
CHICAGO, IL 60605

CHICAGO PUBLIC LIBRARY

W9-BYM-740

NUTRITION in EXERCISE and SPORT
2nd Edition

NUTRITION in EXERCISE and SPORT
2nd Edition

Editors

Ira Wolinsky, Ph.D.
Professor of Nutrition
Department of Human Development
University of Houston
Houston, Texas

James F. Hickson, Jr., Ph.D., R.D.
Retired
Houston, Texas

CRC Press
Boca Raton   Ann Arbor   London   Tokyo

Library of Congress Cataloging-in-Publication Data

Nutrition in exercise and sport / editors, Ira Wolinsky and James F. Hickson, Jr.—2nd ed.
p. cm.
Includes bibliographical references and index.
ISBN 0-8493-7911-3
1. Athletes—Nutrition. 2. Exercise—Physiological aspects.
I. Wolinsky, Ira, 1938– . II. Hickson, James F., 1954– .
TX361.A8N88 1993
612'.044—dc20   93-17120
                                                 CIP

This book contains information obtained from authentic and highly regarded sources. Reprinted material is quoted with permission, and sources are indicated. A wide variety of references are listed. Reasonable efforts have been made to publish reliable data and information, but the author and the publisher cannot assume responsibility for the validity of all materials or for the consequences of their use.

Neither this book nor any part may be reproduced or transmitted in any form or by any means, electronic or mechanical, including photocopying, microfilming, and recording, or by any information storage or retrieval system, without prior permission in writing from the publisher.

All rights reserved. Authorization to photocopy items for internal or personal use, or the personal or internal use of specific clients, may be granted by CRC Press, Inc., provided that $.50 per page photocopied is paid directly to Copyright Clearance Center, 27 Congress Street, Salem, MA 01970 USA. The fee code for users of the Transactional Reporting Service is ISBN 0-8493-7911-3/94/$0.00+$.50. The fee is subject to change without notice. For organizations that have been granted a photocopy license by the CCC, a separate system of payment has been arranged.

CRC Press, Inc.'s consent does not extend to copying for general distribution, for promotion, for creating new works, or for resale. Specific permission must be obtained in writing from CRC Press for such copying.

Direct all inquiries to CRC Press, Inc., 2000 Corporate Blvd., N.W., Boca Raton, Florida 33431.

© 1994 by CRC Press, Inc.

No claim to original U.S. Government works
International Standard Book Number 0-8493-7911-3
Library of Congress Card Number 93-17120
Printed in the United States of America 1 2 3 4 5 6 7 8 9 0
Printed on acid-free paper

R00977 99006

BUSINESS/SCIENCE/TECHNOLOGY DIVISION
CHICAGO PUBLIC LIBRARY
400 SOUTH STATE STREET
CHICAGO, IL 60605

PREFACE

The CRC series *Nutrition in Exercise and Sport* is designed to provide the setting for in-depth exploration of the many and varied aspects of nutrition and exercise, including sport. The topic of sports nutrition gained real interest among physiologists in the 1960s, and since then, numerous scientific studies have been performed, many of which have focused on the healthful benefits of good nutrition and exercise. As we move forward to the next century, scientists will search evermore for the elusive "optimum" nutritional preparation. As they try to unlock nature's secrets, it will be necessary to remember that there must be a range of diets that will support excellent physical performance, there will inevitably be attempts by scientists and laymen alike to distill the diets to some common denominator — a formula for success. The CRC series in *Nutrition in Exercise and Sport* is dedicated to providing a stage upon which to explore these issues. Each volume seeks to provide a detailed and scholarly examination of some aspect of this topic. Ultimately, the series will comprise a set of authoritative volumes for consultation by scientists, physicians, and a broad range of health-care providers and individuals who participate in exercise and sport, whether for recreation or competition.

We respectfully submit the second edition of our volume, *Nutrition in Exercise and Sport,* to the series. The first edition of this volume was very well received and was praised in many quarters of the field of sport nutrition and by many health professionals. In several cases, it found use as a college textbook, which is high praise indeed. This second edition represents a newly updated and expanded contribution to keep pace with the latest developments in the rapidly burgeoning field of sport nutrition. The growth of the wellness movement and athletic competition, coupled with an increase in research in nutrition and physical activity, makes it possible for one to say today that sport nutrition has come of age. We hope this volume, as we aspired for the first edition, will be useful to the scientific, athletic, and lay communities in evaluating the existing body of knowledge on sport nutrition. We mean this volume to be a scholarly effort, well grounded in physiology and nutrition. As such, it differs from a popular, dietetics approach taken by other recent books of similar content. We trust that the expert information presented will facilitate the recommendation of appropriate food choices by both the competitive and recreational athlete.

Editors
Ira Wolinsky, Ph.D.
James F. Hickson, Jr., Ph.D., R.D.

Ira Wolinsky, Ph.D., is a Professor of Nutrition at the University of Houston. Dr. Wolinsky received his B.S. degree in chemistry from the City College of New York in 1960 and his M.S. (1965) and Ph.D. (1968) degrees in Biochemistry from Kansas University. He has served in research and teaching positions at the Hebrew University, the University of Missouri, and Pennsylvania State University.

Dr. Wolinsky is a member of the American Institute of Nutrition and the American Society for Clinical Nutrition, among other scientific organizations.

Dr. Wolinsky had contributed numerous nutrition papers and has also co-authored a book on the history of the science of nutrition. His current major research interests include the nutrition of bone and calcium and sports nutrition.

James F. Hickson, Jr., Ph.D., R.D., received his B.S. and Ph.D. (Human Nutrition) degrees from Virginia Polytechnic Institute and State University in 1976 and 1980, respectively. He was formerly a faculty member at Indiana University, the University of Texas, and the University of Houston (adjunct). He is presently retired from the University of Texas System.

Dr. Hickson is a member of, among others, the American Dietetics Association, the American Institute for Nutrition, the American Society of Clinical Nutrition, the Institute of Food Technologists, the Society for Experimental Biology and Medicine, and the honorary society Sigma Xi.

Dr. Hickson's specialties by training and experience are protein metabolism and exercise, computerized dietary analysis, and amino acid analysis. His primary research interest is the study of how strength- and endurance-building modes of exercise influence the efficiency of protein utilization in humans.

CONTRIBUTORS

John J. B. Anderson, Ph.D.
Department of Nutrition
University of North Carolina School of
    Public Health
Chapel Hill, North Carolina

Sara B. Arnaud, M.D.
Life Sciences Division
NASA
Moffett Field, California

Eldon W. Askew, Ph.D.
Military Nutrition Division
U.S. Army Research Institute of
    Environmental Medicine
Natick, Massachusetts

David R. Bassett, Jr., Ph.D.
Department of Human Performance and
    Sports Studies
University of Tennessee
Knoxville, Tennessee

Terry L. Bazzarre, Ph.D.
American Heart Association
National Center, Scientific Affairs
Dallas, Texas

Luke R. Bucci, Ph.D.
SpectraCell Laboratories, Inc.
    and
InnerPath Nutrition
Houston, Texas

Elsworth R. Buskirk, Ph.D.
Noll Laboratory for Human Performance
    Research
Pennsylvania State University
University Park, Pennsylvania

David S. Chance, M.S.
Department of Food and Nutrition—Food
    Service Management
University of North Carolina
Greensboro, North Carolina

Alexander N. Erin, Ph.D.
National Center for Mental Health
Moscow, Russia

Ann C. Grandjean, Ed.D.
International Center for Sports Nutrition
Omaha, Nebraska

G. Harley Hartung, Ph.D.
Department of Cardiac Rehabilitation
Tripler Medical Center
Honolulu, Hawaii

Emily Haymes, Ph.D.
Department of Nutrition, Food and
    Movement Science
Florida State University
Tallahassee, Florida

James F. Hickson, Jr., Ph.D., R.D.
Retired
Houston, Texas

Laurie Hoffman-Goetz, Ph.D.
Department of Health Studies and
    Gerontology
University of Waterloo
Waterloo, Ontario, Canada

Valerian E. Kagan, Ph.D., D.Sc.
Department of Environmental and
    Occupational Health
University of Pittsburgh
Pittsburgh, Pennsylvania

Robert E. Keith, Ph.D., R.D., F.A.C.S.M.
Department of Nutrition and Food Science
Auburn University
Auburn, Alabama

Donald K. Layman, Ph.D.
Divisions of Foods and Nutritional Sciences
University of Illinois
Urbana, Illinois

Michael Liebman, Ph.D.
Department of Home Economics (Nutrition)
University of Wyoming
Laramie, Wyoming

Robert G. McMurray, Ph.D.
Department of Nutrition and Physical
    Education
University of North Carolina
Chapel Hill, North Carolina

Gregory D. Miller, Ph.D., F.A.C.N.
Department of Nutrition Research
National Dairy Council
O'Hare International Center
Rosemont, Illinois

Tinker D. Murray, Ph.D.
Department of Health, Physical Education
    and Recreation
Southwest Texas State University
San Marcos, Texas

Francis J. Nagle, Ph.D.
Department of Physical Education
    and Dance
University of Wisconsin
Madison, Wisconsin

Melissa B. Olken, M.D., Ph.D.
University of Michigan
Ann Arbor Veterans Administration
    Medical Center
Ann Arbor, Michigan

Lester Packer, Ph.D.
Department of Molecular and
    Cell Biology
University of California
Berkeley, California

Robert A. Palmer, M.Ed.
Houston, Texas

Greg Paul, M.S.
Division of Nutritional Science
University of Illinois
Urbana, Illinois

James M. Pivarnik, Ph.D.
Department of Pediatrics
    (Section of Nutrition and GI)
Baylor College of Medicine
Houston, Texas

Susan M. Puhl, Ph.D.
Noll Laboratory for Human Performance
    Research
Pennsylvania State University
University Park, Pennsylvania

Jaime S. Ruud, M.S., R.D.
International Center for Sports Nutrition
Omaha, Nebraska

Anthony Scarpino, M.S.
Department of Food and Nutrition—Food
    Service Management
University of North Carolina
Greensboro, North Carolina

Elena A. Serbinova, Ph.D.
Department of Molecular and
    Cell Biology
University of California
Berkeley, California

Sarah H. Short, Ph.D., Ed.D., R.D.
Department of Human Nutrition
Syracuse University
Syracuse, New York

Vladimir B. Spirichev, M.D., Ph.D.
Institute of Nutrition
Russian Academy of Medical Sciences
Moscow, Russia

William G. Squires, Jr., Ph.D.
Department of Biology
Texas Lutheran College
Seguin, Texas

Ronald R. Watson, Ph.D.
Department of Family and Community
    Medicine
University of Texas College of Medicine
Health Sciences Center
Tucson, Arizona

John G. Wilkinson, Ph.D.
Human Energy Research Laboratory
University of Wyoming
Laramie, Wyoming

Eric Witt, Ph.D.
Department of Molecular and Cell Biology
University of California
Berkeley, California

Ira Wolinsky, Ph.D.
Department of Human Development
University of Houston
Houston, Texas

CONTENTS

*Dedicated to the many students we taught,
and from whom we learned far more.*

Chapter 1

INTRODUCTION TO NUTRITION IN EXERCISE AND SPORT

Robert G. McMurray
John J. B. Anderson

CONTENTS

0-8493-7911-3/94/$0.00+$.50
© 1994 by CRC Press, Inc.

I. INTRODUCTION

Nutrition is the total of the processes of the intake and conversion of food substances into nutrients that can be used to maintain bodily function. These processes involve nutrients that can be used for energy (carbohydrates, fats, proteins), to build and repair tissue (proteins, fats, minerals), to build and maintain the skeletal system (calcium, phosphorus, proteins), and to regulate body physiology (vitamins, minerals, fats, proteins, water).

When nutrients are present in optimal amounts, the health and well-being of the individual is maximized. The determinations of what nutrients are essential and the optimal amounts of the essential nutrients have been the focus of study for decades and the specific nutrient recommendations have been summarized in the Recommended Dietary Allowances.[1] However, these RDAs apply to the normal nonathletic population and may not meet the needs of athletes. Presently, sufficient data are not available to devise a separate set of "RDAs" for athletes. Yet, athletes and coaches need concrete recommendations in order to optimize performance and reduce the risk of injury.

Sport has reached the status in which the outcome can have both political and economic ramifications. Olympic gold medals can demonstrate a country's prowess, and concomitantly, success can transfer into major economic gains for the medalist. Obviously, genetics and training are two of the major contributors to such success. However, when the differences between fame and fortune is measured in hundredths of a second, any factor that optimizes performance can, and will, be tried.

Nutrition is one of the factors that can optimize athletic performance. Optimal nutrition can reduce fatigue, which allows the athlete to train for longer durations, or recover faster between exercise sessions. Nutrition can possibly reduce injuries, or speed injury repair, ultimately affecting training status.[2] Proper nutrition can also optimize energy stores for competition, which can make the difference between first and second place for both sprint[3] and endurance activities.[3,4] Finally, nutrition is important for the general health of the athlete. Adequate nutrition can reduce the possibilities of infirmities which can reduce training time or even shorten an athlete's career. With all these benefits it is easy to discern why nutrition receives much attention.

The present idolization of the importance of nutrition for the athlete has become overstated. Clearly, the data demonstrate that nutritional deficiencies can reduce the ability to perform exercise. However, minimal evidence exists to suggest that over-nutrition can improve exercise performance. Nutrition cannot replace the athlete's genetics, training, and psychological readiness. Although we would all like to believe there is a nutritional supplement that could cause an athletic metamorphosis, no such nutrient presently exists. Athletes have tried various protein, vitamin, mineral, and chemical supplements, but little or no physiological benefits have been documented.[5,6] Thus, good nutrition can only optimize the body's capacity to exercise, but will not insure peak exercise performance.

The literature on sports nutrition is filled with fallacies, misconceptions, and misinterpretations. These include the use of proteins and amino acids to stimulate and build muscle,[7] or the use of high-sugar substances immediately before exercise to provide immediate energy.[5] Other fads have included the use of bee pollen,[6] caffeine,[8] or phosphates[9] to improve endurance performance. In some cases the use of these substances is based on testimonials, in other cases the studies demonstrating significant effects have been flawed. In the zeal for finding the magic formula, the media have drawn conclusions from some research which surpass the results of the studies. For example, the use of electrolyte and carbohydrate solutions to improve performance has been frequently publicized. However, an examination of the literature indicates that such drinks are of benefit only if the exercise is prolonged, i.e., 2 to 4 h or more.[3] Thus, for the typical athlete whose event lasts less than 4 to 5 min (which represents over 90% of the athletes), such solutions may be of no benefit. This, and other related topics, will be discussed in greater depth later in the text.

The remainder of this chapter will provide an overview of general nutrition needs of healthy populations and the general needs of athletes. Specific topics addressed will include the Recommended Dietary Allowances, food groups, dietary guidelines, exceptions for athletes, special nutritional considerations of athletes, and potential nutritional problems of athletes. This information will serve the reader as an introduction to virtually all of the specific chapters that will follow.

II. GENERAL NUTRITION

A. Recommended Dietary Allowances

The Recommended Dietary Allowances (RDAs) were designed to serve as an aid to design nutrition education programs, establish standards for food assistance programs, develop new products, and to evaluate the adequacy of food supplies in meeting the general nutritional needs of the general population.[1] They are not intended to meet the needs of all individuals, and as such, serve as recommendations over and above requirements of a large percentage of the population. The RDAs are based on available scientific evidence indicating safe and adequate levels of nutrients and are routinely revised. Except for energy, the RDA levels are set reasonably high to meet the theoretical needs of 97.5% of the population, assuming an adequate selection of foods.

The 10th, most recent, edition of the RDAs, published in 1989, includes some significant changes.[1] The current RDAs are given in Table 1. The recommendations for thiamin, riboflavin, and niacin have been increased slightly for males and females in many of the age groups. The calcium allowances of young adult females and males (19 to 24 years) have been increased to 1200 mg/day. Conversely, the vitamin B_6, folacin, and B_{12} recommendations have been lowered. Iron allowances have been reduced for adolescent males and for females from 18 to 15 mg/day. In addition, selenium has been added to the list. The recent edition of the RDAs includes Safe and Adequate Daily Dietary Intake levels for five trace elements (copper, manganese, fluoride, chromium, and molybdenum) and two vitamins (biotin and pantothenic acid).[1] The authors of the RDAs do not recommend micronutrient supplementation and they have stated that habitually surpassing these safe intake levels can pose significant health risks because of potential toxicities. As with previous editions, no RDAs were set for fats and carbohydrates. Finally, the RDAs do not take into consideration the demands of an exercise program.

B. Basic Food Groups

The "Basic Four Food Groups" has served as the foundation for good nutrition since the 1940s.[10] The current recommendations of servings each day are two from the meats group, two to four of the milk group, five from the fruits and vegetables group, and four or more from the bread and cereal group.[11] While this approach to nutrition is easy to understand, considerable problems may occur in individuals following this basic food guide. Despite following these recommendations, deficiencies in vitamins B_6 and E, as well as iron, zinc, and magnesium, can occur. The nutrient deficiencies usually occur because of limited daily selection of specific foods, or the fact that not all foods in the same category contain the same nutritive value. For example, an orange contains about 70 mg of vitamin C, whereas a peach contains only 6 mg.[12] Likewise, a serving of whole grain bread contains four times the iron of unenriched Italian bread (13.6 vs. 3.2 mg/454 g).[12] Yet, the servings are interchangeable. Also, categorizing complex foods such as pizza, casseroles, or processed foods is difficult. Finally, no methodology is given to modify the scheme for individuals requiring low-calorie diets or increased energy, such as athletes might need.

TABLE 1. Nutrient Allowances for Children and Adults

A. Recommended Dietary Allowances

Age (years)	Energy (kcal)	Protein (g)	Fat-Soluble Vitamins			
			Vitamin A (µg RE)	Vitamin D (µg)	Vitamin E (mg α-TE)	Vitamin K (µg)
Males						
11–14	2500	45	1000	10	10	45
15–18	3000	59	1000	10	10	65
19–24	2900	58	1000	10	10	70
25–51	2900	63	1000	5	10	80
Females						
11–14	2200	46	800	10	8	45
15–18	2200	44	800	10	8	55
19–24	2200	46	800	10	8	60
25–51	2200	50	800	5	8	65

Age (years)	Water-Soluble Vitamins						
	Vitamin C (mg)	Thiamin (mg)	Riboflavin (mg)	Niacin (mg NE)	Vitamin B_6 (mg)	Folate (µg)	Vitamin B_{12} (µg)
Males							
11–14	50	1.3	1.5	17	1.7	150	2.0
15–18	60	1.5	1.8	20	2.0	200	2.0
19–24	60	1.5	1.7	19	2.0	200	2.0
25–51	60	1.5	1.7	19	2.0	200	2.0
Females							
11–14	50	1.1	1.3	15	1.4	150	2.0
15–18	60	1.1	1.3	15	1.5	180	2.0
19–24	60	1.1	1.3	15	1.6	180	2.0
25–51	60	1.1	1.3	15	1.6	180	2.0

Age (years)	Minerals						
	Calcium (mg)	Phosphorus (mg)	Magnesium (mg)	Iron (mg)	Zinc (mg)	Iodine (µg)	Selenium (µg)
Males							
11–14	1200	1200	270	12	15	150	40
15–18	1200	1200	400	12	15	150	50
19–24	1200	1200	350	10	15	150	70
25–51	800	800	350	10	15	150	70
Females							
11–14	1200	1200	280	15	12	150	45
15–18	1200	1200	300	15	12	150	50
19–24	1200	1200	280	15	12	150	55
25–51	800	800	280	15	12	150	55

B. Estimated Sodium, Chloride, and Potassium Minimum Requirements of Healthy Persons

Age (years) males and females	Weight (kg[a])	Sodium (mg[a,b])	Chloride (mg[a,b])	Potassium (mg[c])
10–18[d]	50.0	500	750	2000
18+[e]	70.0	500	750	2000

C. Estimated Safe and Adequate Daily Dietary Intakes

Age (years) males and females	Vitamins		Minerals				
	Biotin (μg)	Pantothenic acid (mg)	Copper (mg)	Manganese (mg)	Fluoride (mg)	Chromium (μg)	Molybdenum (μg)
11–18	30–100	4–7	1.5–2.5	2.0–5.0	1.5–2.5	50–200	75–250
Adults	30–100	4–7	1.5–3.0	2.0–5.0	1.5–4.0	50–200	75–250

[a] No allowance has been included for large, prolonged losses from the skin through sweat.
[b] There is no evidence that higher intakes confer any health benefit.
[c] Desirable intakes of potassium may considerably exceed these values (~3500 mg for adults).
[d] Values for those below 18 years assume a growth rate at the 50th percentile reported by the National Center for Health Statistics and averaged for males and females.
[e] For individuals greater than 18 years of age.

From The National Research Council, *Recommended Dietary Allowances*, 10th ed., National Academy Press, Washington, D.C., 1989.

C. Dietary Exchanges

Dietary exchange patterns may be an appropriate alternative for optimizing nutrition for a variety of individuals.[13] The system was originally developed for diabetics; however, other exchange systems have been developed for low-sodium, low-fat, or weight-loss diets. Although the exchange is somewhat confusing and time-consuming, once learned the system can avoid both under- and overnutrition, and it is easily modified for vegetarians. The appropriateness of this system for athletes may be questioned from a pragmatic viewpoint; however, sports nutritionists have suggested its use for athletes.[14] The exchange system divides foods into six categories, based on calories per portion: starches/breads, vegetables, fruits, milk, meats/meat substitutes, and fats. In this system one slice of bread equals a small potato and 30 g of meat equals 30 g of cheese. Contrary to the "Basic Four Food Groups", cheese is placed in the meat group (due to the high protein and fat content), corn is a starch rather than a vegetable, and bacon is a fat rather than a meat. Caloric intake becomes the focus and exchanges can be added or removed as required by the individual to meet goals.

Recently, the suggestion has been made to modify the exchange system into a "pyramid", which is actually a low-fat and low-cholesterol exchange system.[15] The original exchange was based on 30% fats while the new pyramid approach recommends approximately 20 to 25% fats.

D. General Dietary Guidelines for Americans

During the 1960s an awareness began to develop that overnutrition was contributing to the major chronic diseases, obesity, diabetes mellitus (type II), cardiovascular diseases, hypertension, and cancers. The U.S. Government, through its commitment to promoting health, has attempted to develop guidelines for all Americans.[16] The emphasis was to prevent overconsumption, particularly of fats, sugar, and salt. The seven, fairly nonquantitative recommendations follow.

Eat a wide variety of foods — No one food can provide all the necessary nutrients. For example, meats are considered one of the best sources of protein (and cholesterol); yet, most meats do not contain all eight essential amino acids in adequate amounts. Thus, in addition to meat, eggs, and fish, whole grains or legumes are needed in the diet to secure adequate amino acid status. Similar scenarios can be developed for vitamins or minerals.

Increase complex carbohydrate intake and decrease the intake of refined sugars — The increase in complex carbohydrates serves as a source of energy and simultaneously provides other nutrients not available in refined sugars. Refined sugars result in increased insulin levels which, if carbohydrate stores are filled, can cause fat deposition.

Reduce fat intake to 30% of the caloric intake with saturated fats comprising only 10% of the caloric intake — Lowering fat intake will not only affect low-density lipoprotein (LDL) cholesterol but can also cause weight loss. Replacing fats with a similar amount of carbohydrates can reduce caloric intake as fats have over twice the caloric density of carbohydrates. High-fat diets have also been shown to limit athletic performance.[17]

Reduce cholesterol intake to 300 mg or less per day — This goal is important for the reduction of cardiovascular disease risk. Since animal products which provide protein are also sources of cholesterol (and saturated fats), considerable attention must be paid to locating sources of protein that are low in cholesterol.

Increase fiber intake — The increase in fiber reduces the risk of certain cancers, heart disease, diabetes, diverticulosis, and hemorrhoids.[18] A high-fiber diet can aid in weight control by promoting satiety and lowering caloric intake; high-fiber foods are lower in caloric density than fats or sweets.[18]

Consume alcohol in moderation — The calories in alcohol can become the precursors for fatty acids and weight gain.[17] Alcohol can also suppress glucose utilization for energy.[6] Finally, alcohol is a diuretic which can have harmful effects for the athlete training in the heat without adequate fluid replenishment.

Reduce sodium or salty food intake — These can effect hypertension.

III. EXCEPTIONS TO THE GUIDELINES FOR ATHLETES

The nutritional recommendations and guidelines outlined above were developed without taking the athlete into consideration. Thus, although these guidelines provided the basis for optimal nutrition, modifications are needed for athletes. The general recommendations of a low-fat and high complex-carbohydrate diet benefits the athlete, as does the recommendation to eat a variety of foods. However, the other basic guidelines may not apply to athletes.

The development of diets based on percentages of macronutrients may not be in the best interest of the athlete who is exercising 3 to 5 h each day. Consider a 20-year-old, 80-kg male swimmer, who practices 4 to 5 h a day. This athlete may consume up to 6000 kilocalories (kcal) per day. Practitioners have suggested that the optimal diet consists of 15 to 20% protein, 50 to 55% carbohydrates, and 30% fats (of which no more than 1/3 should be saturated fats). Based on the recommended percentages, our swimmer should ingest 3000 to 3300 kcals from carbohydrates, 1800 kcals from fats, and 900 to 1200 kcals from proteins. The swimmer's protein intake would be approximately 3.4 g/kg body weight, four times the RDA! Although several sports nutritionists[7,17,19] suggest increasing protein intake up to double the RDA (1.6 g/kg), our swimmer would have a protein intake higher than recommended by any nutritional standards. Since high-protein diets have been associated with renal disease, osteoporosis, gall bladder disease, and hypercholesterolemia,[18] our athlete might increase his risk for one or more of these chronic diseases or disorders.

Fat intake of the swimmer would be approximately 196 g, with 65 g of saturated fat. In contrast, the iso-nutrient diet of a nonathlete of the same size and sex would contain only 78 g of fat, of which 26 g would be saturated. The athlete would be consuming almost as much saturated fat as the total fat intake for the nonathlete! The high-fat dietary pattern may have prolonged implications for cardiovascular disease and diabetes.[18] The athlete could use these extra fat calories as a source of energy for exercise. However, as shown in Chapters 3, 4, and 7, fats cannot be used as the major source of energy for high-intensity exercise; the body demands carbohydrates. Thus, the high-fat intake could compromise exercise performance.[17]

TABLE 2. Purposes of Pre-Event Meal

1. Maximize glycogen stores
2. Minimize digestion during competition
3. Avoid hunger
3. Provide fluids
5. Avoid gastric distress

Considering this swimmer may expend up to 4000 kcals with exercise, lowering the proportions of fats (particularly saturated fats) and proteins and increasing the carbohydrate is prudent. Thus, an athlete's diet may consist of only 10 to 15% proteins, 70% carbohydrates, and 15 to 20% fats (with no more than 1/4 from saturated fat). Such alterations in dietary pattern need to be defined on an athlete-by-athlete basis, considering the additional caloric and nutrient needs of the specific events and training regimen of the athlete.

The dietary sodium and mineral recommendations most likely need to be increased for athletes who are exercising for prolonged periods of time with considerable sweat loss.[14,19] This population includes such diverse athletes as football players, wrestlers, soccer players, long-distance runners, triathletes, and even swimmers. As indicated in later chapters in this book, these athletes may not only need additional amounts of sodium, but also of zinc, calcium, potassium, and possibly iron.[14,19,20] Once again, these additional needs should be individually evaluated.

IV. PRE- AND POST-GAME/EVENT MEALS

The pre-event meal can do more to hinder than to enhance competitive performance. Therefore, planning of the pre-event meal can be critical. Several important factors must be taken into consideration: (1) general dietary pattern and foods normally eaten by the athlete, (2) timing of the meal, (3) specific components of the meal, (4) fluids, and (5) foods to be avoided.

It is important that the pre-event meal should not be a drastic change from the normal dietary pattern of the athlete. For example, if the athlete normally does not eat sugars, switching to a high-carbohydrate and -sugar pre-event meal may cause diarrhea,[21] which would ultimately limit performance. Also, it is important that the athlete not fast before competition. Dohm et al.[22] and Loy et al.[23] have independently shown that 24 h of fasting result in considerable decrement in exercise performance, due to reduced glycogen stores.

The pre-event meal should be eaten approximately 4 h before competition. This timing will allow for any deficiency in the glycogen stores to be replenished or "topped off" and will allow the stomach to be relatively empty by the time of competition. The meal should consist of mainly complex carbohydrates with some protein and limited fat. Research has suggested about 75 to 150 g of carbohydrate.[24] Lesser amounts of carbohydrate may not adequately replenish glycogen stores, whereas larger amounts may result in insulin rebound or gastric distress and discomfort. The protein intake will assist in avoiding sensations of hunger. The low fat content of the meal is important because the digestion of fats is a prolonged process, lasting up to 8 h. If digestion continues during competition, some blood and energy stores that could be used by the exercising muscle will be redistributed to the gut for digestion. It has been hypothesized that high free fatty acids levels reduce carbohydrate oxidation, which, in turn, should spare glycogen stores during prolonged exercise,[21] i.e., a beneficial effect. However, research does not support this hypothesis.[25,26] Thus, a high fat intake may not be beneficial to the athlete. The meal should also provide ample fluids to insure proper hydration before competition.

Certain foods should be avoided as they may be hard to digest, produce gastric distress, flatulence, or add bulk to the colon which may stimulate a defecation response. Beans and spicy ingredients may cause heartburn and flatulence. Ingestion of cellulose, roughage, and seedy vegetables may produce gastric distress and add bulk. Greasy foods will slow gastric emptying and, thus, digestion. Additionally, intake of large quantities of simple sugars may cause diarrhea.

Several investigators have suggested that the ingestion of fructose 1 to 2 h before competition may be beneficial.[27-29] The use of fructose, rather than sucrose or glucose, to provide additional carbohydrate is based on the fact that fructose is largely insulin-independent[30] and is more slowly metabolized by the system. The slower conversion could provide a stable fuel source during prolonged activity. However, this procedure is still controversial as it may not result in the hypothesized effects[31] and may cause gastrointestinal distress.[21] Instead of fructose, practitioners have suggested the use of commercially available liquid meals 2 h before competition; however, no data are presently available.

The post-game/event meal should include more food than any other meal of the day. This recommendation, which is also applicable after workouts, should insure adequate total nutrient intakes over the 24-h period and sufficient fluid replacement to rehydrate the bodies of athletes. These practical guidelines should help athletes plan their meals for better performance.

V. SPECIAL NUTRITIONAL CONSIDERATIONS OF ATHLETES

Both female and male athletes may have special nutritional needs because of either physiological changes or sport specificity. In this section, the special consideration of females will be covered first, and then of males.

Young female athletes undergo significant physiological, reproductive, and psychological changes that can have potentially adverse impacts on both performance and injuries. Dietary practices often change as girls begin the path toward womanhood and concerns about body composition and conformation often become predominant. Among female athletes, weight control often emerges as a major reason for altering food habits, becoming a partial or total vegetarian, and in extreme cases skipping meals with sufficient frequency to develop eating disorders.[32-36]

In addition to disorders relating to general undernutrition, female athletes also commonly have marginal intakes of iron or calcium, and sometimes both, despite adequate consumption of total energy and protein from foods. The more marginal status of iron deficiency, not accompanied by anemia, is prevalent among female athletes, especially in menstruating athletes.[37-40] Inadequate intake of iron-rich animal products (except for milk which is iron-poor) are primarily responsible for iron deficiency. More severe inadequacy of iron consumption leads to iron-deficiency anemia. Women diagnosed with iron deficits will, in virtually all cases, require iron supplementation for a period of several months,[39] but not all female athletes will benefit from iron supplements.[41] Vegetarian athletes, or those who exclude red meats as a minimum, generally develop iron deficiency and often amenorrhea.[38-42]

Two major factors contribute to bone loss in otherwise healthy female athletes: too little calcium in the diet and amenorrhea. Low calcium consumption nearly always results from insufficient ingestion of dairy products, although other calcium-rich foods may also be neglected in the typical diets of female athletes. Although osteopenia, or too little bone mass, most commonly occurs because of diets inadequate in calcium-rich foods,[43-45] amenorrhea secondary to intensive physical training also may significantly contribute to low bone mass.[46,47] Use of oral contraceptive agents by amenorrheic adolescent athletes may actually improve their bone mass without any detraction from their athletic performance.[46,47] The potential adverse consequences of amenorrhea-induced osteopenia, complicated by low calcium intake, include leg injuries and stress fractures, which are especially common in distance runners and ballerinas.[48,49] Calcium supplements may help those young female athletes retain more skeletal mineral if milk and related foods cannot be consumed in adequate amounts.

Female athletes also have been reported to display deficiencies in other micronutrients besides iron and calcium that may place them in jeopardy of diminished performance levels and increased injury rates. In the latter regard, females seem to experience greater disability from these micronutrient deficits than do males because of lower total caloric intakes. Male athletes usually have little difficulty consuming enough energy and protein from foods, but unlike many weight-conscious females they generally have far too high consumption of fat.

In contrast to females, male athletes have had no known reports of problems of eating disorders and any associated undernutrition. Similarly, calcium and iron deficiencies have been rarely diagnosed in males, but iron deficits may be under-recognized, especially in rapidly growing adolescent athletes whose requirements for iron are increased for muscle growth.

In general, male athletes tend to have irregular eating habits, including much snacking. While such practices do not necessarily lead to inadequate intakes of macronutrients, they may contribute to micronutrient insufficiencies because of a limited number of food choices. In many cases, males have restricted consumptions of fruits and vegetables, except for fries and other forms of potatoes. Because fruits and vegetables provide many of the B vitamins, vitamin C, and many trace elements, males can develop marginal nutritional status with respect to several vitamins and other trace minerals. They can also become iron deficient if they do not consume enough meats and other high-iron foods.[40]

More than anything else, male athletes need to broaden their choice of foods and select more fruits and vegetables and whole-grain breads and cereals, which assure a greater percentage of complex carbohydrates of their total energy intake and also provide greater amounts of micronutrients and dietary fiber. Fruits and vegetables contain good amounts of potassium, the electrolyte critical for muscle function. Enough sodium is usually consumed from many of the other foods in a balanced diet, especially meats and dairy products, and most processed foods contain large amounts of added sodium. The high-fiber foods should, of course, be largely consumed in the bigger meal of the day after any daily sports activities have been concluded.

VI. POTENTIAL NUTRITIONAL PROBLEMS OF SPECIFIC TYPES OF ATHLETES

Several sports and related activities, including dance, contribute to less than satisfactory nutritional status. The suboptimal nutritional status not only affects performance but probably increases the likelihood of injuries related to these activities. The specific sports focused on here are gymnastics, wrestling, long-distance running, and ballet dancing. The contact and collision sports also contribute to both exertional dehydration and mineral losses in sweat, which can hasten the loss of mental concentration and thereby increase the chance of injury in these sports.

Performance in gymnastics and certain other sports requires physical attributes that are based on a low percentage of body fat and, conversely, a relatively high percentage of lean body mass, particularly skeletal muscle. Female gymnasts typically consume too little energy from foods, which translates into inadequate consumption of nearly all of the micronutrients.[50,51] Vitamin–mineral combination supplements can be recommended for these underconsuming female athletes,[52] but it is advisable first to have a physical examination by a physician and a nutritional assessment by a dietitian/nutritionist.[53]

Wrestlers typically reduce their energy consumption from foods to meet the upper limits of body weight for specific competitive classes. Although such underconsumption by wrestlers and female gymnasts will temporarily suspend physical growth by young athletes, later catch-up development and growth normally follows when energy and protein intakes are increased. The major problem of weight control among athletes, including wrestlers, is dehydration associated with both extreme water restriction and excessive sweating.[51,54,55] Since wrestlers generally have poor nutrition knowledge, they frequently make unhealthy food choices and have limited selections of fruits and vegetables. Thus, their unbalanced diets are most likely deficient in one or more micronutrients.[56] The unbalanced diet coupled with water deficits increase the potential for the wrestler to suffer from colds and other infections and to experience minor but nagging injuries. Thus, wrestlers are recommended to take a daily supplement of micronutrients at RDA levels throughout their competitive season as long as weight restrictions apply. The same suggestion holds for any other sport with rigid weight classifications.

Long-distance runners, especially females, typically have low-calorie diets despite their tremendous expenditure of energy in training and competitive events.[51,57,58] Like female gymnasts, they usually are amenorrheic (either secondary or primary), which places them at increased risk for stress fractures and other injuries. Female runners, whether or not they are taking oral contraceptive agents, should make certain that they consume calcium at or approaching the RDA level for their age. They may also benefit from a daily micronutrient supplement if their typical food patterns do not provide minimum servings from each of the basic food groups. Male long-distance runners should follow the same guidelines as for the females.

Female ballet dancers, and possibly other dancers, represent another class of athletes with generally inadequate nutrient intakes. Because of the physical demands of training and performance, ballerinas need to be light and lean. The notoriously poor intakes of ballerinas put them at high risk of injuries, including the legs, feet, and joints of the lower extremities. They tend to suffer from the same problem as female gymnasts and, thus, they should take a one-a-day type of micronutrient supplement and assure that they have adequate intakes of calcium from foods and/or supplements, i.e., RDA amounts.[32,51,59,60]

VII. NUTRITION AND THE PREVENTION OF ATHLETIC INJURIES

The most important nutrient deficit associated with athletic injuries is that of water. Dehydration contributes to injuries in all sports and dance, but it is especially important in football and wrestling because of the reduction in mental function. Water replacement during games/events and practices cannot be overemphasized as one of the most critical factors in preventing tissue sprains, muscle pulls, contusions, and even more serious injuries. Water replacement also helps to prevent problems such as heat cramps, heat exhaustion, and heat stroke. Under conditions of high temperature and high humidity, water replacement is absolutely essential if practices and games are to take place. Under certain conditions when excessive losses of electrolytes occur through sweat, electrolyte drinks may be needed to replace both fluids and the important electrolytes. A more in-depth discussion of this topic can be found in Chapter 13 of this text.

Severe deficiencies or even modest underconsumption of macro- or micronutrients remain more difficult to link directly to injuries in sports. Chronic low energy intakes, of course, have been shown to limit work output in various activities, but micronutrient deficits generally have to be greatly reduced to demonstrate an adverse effect on physical function. Nevertheless, poor nutritional status, as evidenced by low glycogen stores, iron deficiency, or depleted stores of other micronutrients, has been demonstrated experimentally to result in substandard performance. For example, injuries have been reported to be increased in female endurance athletes, dancers, and gymnasts who are amenorrheic[59-63] or anorexic.[64,65] Other specific nutrient deficits have also been reported among athletes with injuries.[66]

55. **Maughan, R. and Noakes, T.,** Fluid replacement and exercise stress: a brief review of studies on fluid replacement and some guidelines for the athlete, *Sports Med.,* 12, 16, 1991.
56. **Steen, S. and McKinney, S.,** Nutrition assessment of college wrestlers, *Phys. Sportsmed.,* 14, 100, 1986.
57. **Clark, N., Nelson, M., and Evans, W.,** Nutrition education for elite runners, *Phys. Sportsmed.,* 16, 124, 1988.
58. **Nelson, M., Fisher, E., Catsos, P., Meredith, C., Turksoy, R., and Evans, W.,** Diet and bone status in amenorrheic runners, *Am. J. Clin. Nutr.,* 43, 910, 1986.
59. **Warren, M., Brooks-Gunn, J., Hamilton, L., Warren, L., and Hamilton, W.,** Scoliosis and fractures in young adult ballet dancers: relation to delayed menarche and secondary amenorrhea, *N. Engl. J. Med.,* 314, 1348, 1986.
60. **Benson, J., Geiger, C., Eiserman, P., and Wardlaw, G.,** Relationship between nutrient intake, body mass index, menstrual function, and ballet injury, *J. Am. Diet. Assoc.,* 89, 58, 1989.
61. **Cann, C., Martin, M., Genant, H., and Jaffe, R.,** Decreased spinal mineral content in amenorrheic women, *JAMA,* 251, 626, 1984.
62. **Marcus, R., Cann, C., Madvig, P., Minkoff, J., Goddard, M., Bayer, M., Martin, M., Gaudiani, L., Haskell, W., and Genant, H.,** Menstrual function and bone mass in elite women distance runners: endocrine and metabolic features, *Ann. Int. Med.,* 102, 158, 1985.
63. **Drinkwater, B., Bruemner, B., and Chestnut, C., III,** Menstrual history as a determinant of current bone status in young athletes, *JAMA,* 263, 545, 1990.
64. **Rigotti, N., Nussbaum, S., Herzog, D., and Neer, R.,** Osteoporosis in women with anorexia nervosa, *N. Engl. J. Med.,* 311, 1601, 1984.
65. **Brooks-Gunn, J., Warren, M., and Hamilton, L.,** The relation of eating problems and amenorrhea in ballet dancers, *Med. Sci. Sports Exer.,* 19, 41, 1987.
66. **Anderson, J.,** Nutrition and injury prevention, in *Prevention of Athletic Injuries: The Role of the Sports Medicine Team,* Mueller, F. O. and Ryan, A. J., Eds., F. A. Davis, Philadelphia, 1991, 230.
67. **Parr, R. B., Porter, M. A., and Hodgson, S. C.,** Nutrition knowledge and practice of coaches, trainers, and athletes, *Phys. Sportsmed.,* 12, 127, 1984.
68. **Warblow, J. A.,** Nutritional knowledge, attitudes and food patterns of women athletes, *J. Am. Diet. Assoc.,* 73, 242, 1978.
69. **Short, S. H. and Short, W. R.,** Four-year study of university athletes' dietary intake, *J. Am. Diet. Assoc.,* 82, 632, 1983.
70. **Chen, J. D., Wang, J. F., Zhao, Y. W., Wang, S. W., Jaio, Y., and Hou, X. Y.,** Nutritional problems and measures in elite and amateur athletes, *Am. J. Clin. Nutr.,* 49, 1084, 1989.

Chapter 2

CARBOHYDRATE METABOLISM AND EXERCISE

Michael Liebman
John G. Wilkinson

CONTENTS

0-8493-7911-3/94/$0.00+$.50
© 1994 by CRC Press, Inc.

I. INTRODUCTION

Carbohydrates are an important energy source for human metabolism. Skeletal muscle glycogen and liver-derived blood glucose are readily available carbohydrates which are used as primary sources of fuel during both anaerobic and aerobic exercise. The breakdown of muscle glycogen or blood-borne glucose to lactic acid contributes to muscular fatigue during high-intensity exercise. The dietary manipulation of carbohydrate intake prior to, during, and after exercise can improve exercise performance largely through optimizing muscle and liver glycogen stores or through the maintenance of blood glucose homeostasis. Recent research on carbohydrate metabolism during exercise has established the following:

1. Blood glucose becomes an increasingly important energy source as prolonged moderate exercise continues beyond 2 h.
2. Carbohydrate metabolism during exercise is regulated by a complex interaction of hormonal and local control.
3. Glucose transport into muscle appears to regulate glucose utilization and glycogen synthesis during and following exercise, respectively.
4. The effectiveness of carbohydrate supplementation during exercise is dependent upon the rate of gastric emptying and the type, timing, and rate of carbohydrate ingestion.
5. Postexercise glycogen resynthesis is also dependent upon type, timing, and amount of carbohydrate ingested following exercise.

The purpose of this chapter is to review these topics related to carbohydrate metabolism and to provide practical guidelines for carbohydrate nutrition and optimal exercise performance. Additional information on carbohydrate metabolism and exercise is given Chapter 3.

II. CARBOHYDRATE INGESTION AND UTILIZATION
A. Dietary Carbohydrates, Digestion, and Storage

Carbohydrates are the most abundant and readily available source of energy for human nutrition. The 1989 Recommended Dietary Allowance (RDA) Subcommittee recommended that more than half the energy requirement beyond infancy be provided by carbohydrate.[1] Important dietary carbohydrates have a general formula of $(CH_2O)_n$ and include sugars and complex carbohydrates. Commonly consumed sugars can be subdivided into monosaccharides, such as glucose and fructose, and disaccharides, such as sucrose, maltose, and lactose (milk sugar). Dietary polysaccharides, or complex carbohydrates, include the glucose polymer, starch, and a number of indigestible plant cell wall materials (cellulose, hemicellulose, pectins) which are classified as components of dietary fiber. In terms of discussing the relationship between dietary carbohydrates and carbohydrate metabolism in exercise, this section will focus only on "available" carbohydrates — i.e., those that can be hydrolyzed by human digestive enzymes and absorbed in the small intestine.

In 1985, average daily carbohydrate intake in the U.S. was 287 g for males[2] and 177 g for females.[3] An average of 41% of daily carbohydrate intake came from grain products and 23% came from fruits and vegetables. Monosaccharides and disaccharides, found primarily in fruits, milk (lactose), and processed foods containing added sweeteners, account for about half of the total digestible carbohydrate intake in the U.S.[1]

Dietary carbohydrates are hydrolyzed in the stomach and small intestine to monosaccharides, with glucose typically predominating. Both glucose and galactose are absorbed by an active transport mechanism, whereas fructose is absorbed by facilitated diffusion.[4] The fact that rate of glucose absorption is more than twice that of fructose[5] has important implications with respect to the comparative value of ingesting these monosaccharides during exercise. Absorbed monosaccharides are transported to the liver via the hepatic portal vein. The maintenance of minimal plasma fructose and galactose levels even in the fed (postprandial) situation supports the role of the liver as a "sink" with respect to these monosaccharides. Both can be metabolized via the triose phosphate stage of the glycolytic pathway to pyruvate, thereby contributing to the hepatic pool of acetyl coenzyme A (CoA), or can serve as gluconeogenic precursors which ultimately provide substrate for glycogen synthesis.[6]

Glycogen is the major storage form of carbohydrate in animals. In addition to α-1,4 glycosidic linkages which produce the straight-chain polymer of glucose, glycogen has branch points produced by α-1,6 bonds. Thus, the structure of glycogen resembles that of the branched-chain component of starch (amylopectin) rather than the straight-chain component (amylose).

Overall storage of carbohydrate in the body as glycogen is small. Glycogen in liver and muscle, the two primary storage sites, accounts for about 1 to 2% of the total substrate reserves of the body. The greatest potential source of fuel is triglyceride, stored predominantly in adipose tissue, which accounts for about 80% of substrate reserves. The only other potentially significant source is body protein, accounting for about 17% of energy reserves.[7] However, amino acids derived from body protein will be used primarily for protein synthesis and other anabolic functions in the well-fed individual who has adequate stores of carbohydrate and lipid. Most estimates of the contribution of amino acids as a fuel during exercise have ranged from 1 to 15% of total energy expenditure.[7] Thus, it is clear that lipid and carbohydrate constitute the two most physiologically important energy substrates in individuals consuming normal diets. This generalization holds true not only during the fasting (postabsorptive) state when the body must rely totally on endogenous stores of energy, but also during the prolonged exercise situation in which glucose and fatty acids are oxidized to provide the fuel needed for contracting skeletal muscle.

There is a higher concentration of glycogen in liver (up to 6%) compared to skeletal muscle, where it typically contributes less than 1%. However, the average total amount of glycogen stored in muscle (300 to 400 g) is greater than that in liver (80 to 90 g), due to the substantially greater overall mass of skeletal muscle.[8] There appears to be an even distribution of glycogen within skeletal muscle fibers, although slightly more is stored in fast- than in slow-twitch fibers.[9] When taken together, hepatic and muscle glycogen stores combined with circulating blood glucose (approximately 20 g) represent only about 1800 kcal, an energy level which would not be sufficient to support the total daily caloric expenditure of most adults for even one 24-h period.

B. Carbohydrate Metabolism
1. Postabsorptive State

Muscle glycogen provides a readily available source of glucose for glycolysis only within the muscle itself because of the absence of the enzyme glucose-6-phosphatase. In contrast,

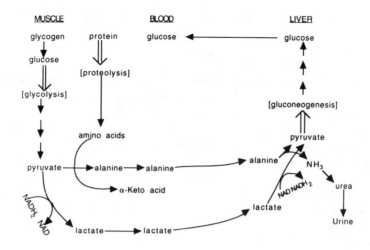

Cori Cycle: lactate generated in muscle is gluconeogenic precursor in liver

Alanine Cycle: alanine generated in muscle is gluconeogenic precursor in liver

FIGURE 1.   Use of lactate and alanine as gluconeogenic precursors in liver.

the presence of this enzyme in liver allows hepatocytes to play a predominant role in mobilizing stored glycogen for maintenance of the blood glucose level, particularly during the postabsorptive state. Via the stimulation of the glycogenolytic pathway and the pathway by which glucose is synthesized from noncarbohydrate precursors (gluconeogenesis), the liver is the sole contributor of glucose to maintain glucose homeostasis, except during prolonged fasting, when an enhancement of gluconeogenesis in the kidney also contributes to the maintenance of normal blood glucose levels.[10]

It should be noted that fasting will essentially deplete hepatic glycogen stores within 24 to 48 h post-meal ingestion.[11] Blood glucose homeostasis is achieved during fasting by the hepatic release of glucose at rates equal to those of tissue utilization. A continual supply of glucose is necessary to serve as the primary energy substrate for the nervous system and erythrocytes. Hypoglycemia can lead to brain dysfunction and severe hypoglycemia can result in coma and death.[10]

In the first few hours during the transition from the fed to the fasted state, release of glucose fom liver is largely met via glycogenolysis. After an overnight fast, approximately 65 to 75% of basal hepatic glucose release is derived from glycogenolysis and the remainder (25 to 35%) from gluconeogenesis.[11] As the fast continues, increased reliance on gluconeogenesis for blood glucose homeostasis parallels the decreased reliance on glycogenolysis as hepatic glycogen stores become progressively depleted.

Physiologically important gluconeogenic precursors in liver are lactate, alanine, pyruvate, glycerol, and a number of other amino acids.[10] Lactate, formed by the glycolytic catabolism of glucose in skeletal muscle and by erythrocytes, can be transported to the liver for glucose resynthesis. The use of lactate produced in extrahepatic tissues as a gluconeogenic precursor in liver is called the Cori (or lactic acid) cycle[10] (Figure 1). There is also evidence to support the existence of a glucose–alanine cycle analogous to the Cori cycle.[12,13] In skeletal muscle, glucose is oxidized to pyruvate, followed by transamination to alanine. The alanine is transported to liver and after removal of the amino group is converted to glucose via the gluconeogenic pathway (Figure 1). Figure 2 also indicates the reactions catalyzed by the key gluconeogenic enzymes in liver by highlighting the reactions which differ between glycolysis and gluconeogenesis. There are three irreversible reactions in glycolysis due to

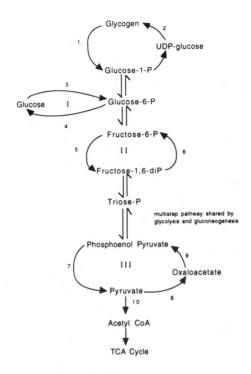

Points of divergence between glycolysis and gluconeogenesis (I, II, III) indicated
Key enzymes: 1 Phosphorylase, 2 Glycogen Synthase, 3 Hexokinase,
4 Glucose-6-phosphatase, 5 Phosphofructokinase,
6 Fructose-1,6-diphosphatase, 7 Pyruvate Kinase,
8 Pyruvate Carboxylase, 9 PEP Carboxykinase,
10 Pyruvate Dehydrogenase

FIGURE 2. Hepatic glucose metabolism indicating key glycolytic and gluconeogenic enzymes.

their highly exergonic nature — i.e., those catalyzed by hexokinase/glucokinase, phosphofructokinase, and pyruvate kinase. It is at these three points that specific gluconeogenic enzymes are required. For example, pyruvate carboxylase and phosphoenol pyruvate (PEP) carboxykinase are required to circumvent the pyruvate kinase reaction of glycolysis.

A summary of the predominant carbohydrate-related metabolic pathways during the postabsorptive state is given in Figure 3. These general metabolic alterations also occur during endurance exercise although there is a significantly greater dependence on glucose oxidation for energy production during exercise. During the fasting, resting state, fatty acids ultimately derived from triglycerides stored in adipose tissue would provide the major energy substrate for skeletal muscle, thus sparing glucose for tissues with obligatory glucose requirements.

In terms of carbohydrate utilization during the postabsorptive state for energy production, glycogen can be degraded to glucose-1-phosphate by action of the enzyme phosphorylase, after which it is converted to glucose-6-phosphate by the enzyme phosphoglucomutase. Although this degradative pathway also involves a debranching mechanism, the step catalyzed by phosphorylase is rate-limiting in glycogenolysis.

In skeletal tissue, glucose-6-phosphate can also be produced by the action of hexokinase on free glucose obtained from the blood. Thus, this compound constitutes a merge point for glucose units derived from glycogen and those transported across the cell membrane from the blood. Due to the inability of phosphorylated glucose molecules to diffuse out of tissues, glucose-6-phosphate produced in skeletal muscle will invariably be metabolized via the glycolytic pathway.

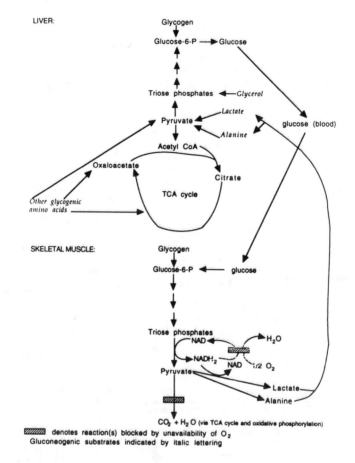

FIGURE 3. Carbohydrate-related metabolic pathways in liver and skeletal muscle during the postabsorptive state; similar metabolic alterations occur during endurance exercise.

2. Postprandial State

In the postprandial state, the absorbed macronutrients are used for energy, the structural repletion of tissues, and in the case of glucose and fatty acids, stored for use during the postabsorptive state, especially during the overnight fast. Thus, pathways ultimately dependent on the availability of glucose are activated in the fed state. These include glycogen synthesis (glycogenesis), glycolysis, and in adipose tissue, lipogenesis, where glucose is required to provide the α-glycerol phosphate backbone needed for triglyceride formation. It follows that glycogenolysis and lipolysis would be minimally active in this situation. After a few hours of fasting, there is essentially a total reversal as pathways activated in the fed state slow down and those depressed after food ingestion are stimulated. The production of glucose from glycogenolysis and from peripheral precursors (amino acids, lactate, glycerol) becomes an important function of the liver when dietary glucose is not available.

Until fairly recently, it was assumed that little gluconeogenic activity would occur during the fed state. The relative importance of the direct utilization of glucose for anabolic processes in hepatic tissue has recently been questioned, in light of convincing evidence that there is significant gluconeogenic flux even in the face of glucose loading. According to this construct, only a small fraction of dietary glucose is initially metabolized in the liver. Rather, much of the dietary glucose bypasses hepatic tissue, is metabolized to lactate in extrahepatic tissues such as skeletal muscle, and lactate recycles back to liver for conversion to glycogen via a still-active gluconeogenic pathway.[14,15] Radziuk[16] reported that two thirds of hepatic glycogen synthesized in fasted subjects given an oral glucose load was of gluconeogenic origin. McGarry et al.[15] suggested that glucose may not be used efficiently during the initial pass through the liver because glucose phosphorylating capacity may be insufficient to support glycogen synthesis directly from glucose.

A possible advantage of the so-called "indirect pathway" for glycogen synthesis in liver is that skeletal muscle and peripheral tissues with obligatory glucose requirements (e.g., the central nervous system, red blood cells, the kidney medulla) would be provided with substrate in the form of glucose for oxidation or for the restoration of glycogen reserves (in the case of skeletal muscle) prior to the repletion of glycogen reserves in liver. If only limited carbohydrate is provided by the diet, the higher priority of providing peripheral tissues with glucose can be met if this indirect pathway operates to the extent suggested in the literature.

The physiological significance of the indirect pathway is supported by the finding in humans of minimal glucose uptake by the liver after exercise in spite of blood glucose levels of approximately 8 mmol/l resulting from glucose ingestion.[17] Repletion of leg muscle glycogen after glucose feeding accounted for 50 to 66% of total splanchnic glucose release. These results further support the assertion that liver defers its glycogen restitution to that of other tissues, such as cardiac and skeletal muscle.

In the postprandial state, much of the fructose and galactose absorbed from the small intestine would be converted to glucose in the liver.[6] Fructose enters the glycolytic sequence at the triose phosphate stage and thus provides intermediates for glucose synthesis. Humans have been shown to deposit more than two times as much liver glycogen when given fructose as compared to glucose.[18]

3. Glycolysis

The ability of glycolysis to generate adenosine triphosphate (ATP) in the absence of oxygen is of physiological significance because it provides useful energy to working skeletal muscle even when aerobic oxidation is limited. This ATP production also enables tissues with significant glycolytic capacity to survive hypoxic episodes. Tissues with poor glycolytic ability (e.g., cardiac muscle) are characterized by poor survival under conditions of ischemia.[19]

Although glycolysis can be discussed in terms of anaerobic and aerobic phases, the relative availability of oxygen does not alter in any way the actual sequence of reactions in glycolysis, but rather is a primary determinant of the metabolic fate of pyruvate produced from glycolysis. Under normal conditions, with an adequate supply of oxygen, most pyruvate is transported into the mitochondria for terminal oxidation to carbon dioxide and water via the tricarboxylic acid cycle and respiratory chain. When oxygen is limited, reoxidation of NADH formed from NAD during glycolysis by transfer of reducing equivalents through the respiratory chain to oxygen is impaired. In this situation, the oxidation of NADH to NAD can be coupled to the reduction of pyruvate to lactate, a reaction catalyzed by lactate dehydrogenase (see Figure 3). Thus, glycolysis can proceed under anaerobic conditions but the amount of energy liberated per mole of glucose oxidized (2 or 3 ATP for glucose derived from blood or from glycogen, respectively) is severely limited compared to the amount generated when glucose is completely oxidized in the mitochondria to carbon dioxide and water (38 ATP).

It is an oversimplification to imply that oxygen status of the cell is the sole determinant of the metabolic fate of pyruvate. During periods when there is high glycogenolytic activity (e.g., during the early stages of aerobic exercise), pyruvate can be reduced to lactate even under conditions of adequate oxygen supply. This occurs via a mass action reaction of lactate dehydrogenase when excess pyruvate is produced in the cell.[20]

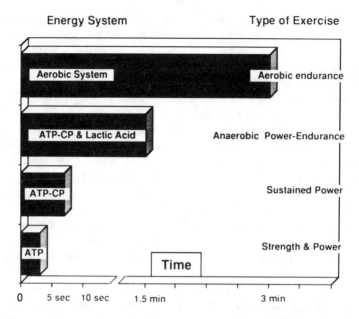

FIGURE 4. Energy systems used and performance times for different types of exercise. (Modified from McArdle, W. D., Katch, F. I., and Katch, V. I., *Exercise Physiology: Energy, Nutrition, and Human Performance,* Lea & Febiger, Philadelphia, 1991.)

III. ENERGY SYSTEMS FOR EXERCISE

Adenosine triphosphate is the common energy currency used for all biological work done within cells. Useful energy gained following the breakdown of ATP to adenosine diphosphate (ADP) and inorganic phosphate (Pi) is the energy used for skeletal muscle contraction during exercise. In addition to ATP, skeletal muscle has another high-energy phosphate, called creatine phosphate (CP), which can be used for the resynthesis of ATP. Physical activity in the form of muscular work or exercise demands large quantities of immediate energy. The energy demand of skeletal muscle during high-intensity sprint exercise may be 120 times greater than at rest.[21] Even prolonged endurance activity such as cross-country skiing may require ATP energy production 20 to 30 times above rest. Three energy systems are responsible for ATP supply and production during exercise: (1) the ATP–CP system, (2) the lactic acid system, and (3) the aerobic system.[21]

The *ATP–CP (phosphagen) system* involves the storage of both ATP and CP in skeletal muscle fibers. Depending upon the muscle fiber type and the state of training, the concentration of CP in skeletal muscle is three to five times greater than that of ATP. However, only a very small quantity of ATP is stored within the muscle, enough to perform maximal exercise for perhaps several seconds (Figure 4). Therefore, there is only enough stored high-energy phosphate (ATP and CP) for about 6 to 8 s of all-out exercise.[21] Performance of short-duration, high-intensity exercise such as 100-meter sprint, weight lifting, football, and field events in track is reliant upon this energy system. The ATP–CP system is nonaerobic in that ATP and CP breakdown take place whether or not oxygen is available. Creatine phosphate is considered the high-energy phosphate "reservoir" used for resynthesis of ATP. This system provides the most rapidly available source of ATP for muscular contraction.

The *lactic acid system* is an anaerobic system in which ATP is produced in skeletal muscle via glycolysis. It involves the incomplete breakdown of glucose to lactic acid (hence the name "lactic acid system"). ATP is generated from the breakdown of either glucose (glycolysis) or stored muscle glycogen (glycogenolysis) to two molecules of lactic acid. However, muscle glycogen is by far the most important substrate used during high-intensity anaerobic exercise. This system provides ATP energy for strenuous high-intensity exercise when oxygen supply is inadequate or the energy demands of the exercise are greater than the capacity of the aerobic system to provide ATP. The lactic acid system is operative with the onset of all-out exercise; however, it only becomes the predominant energy system when CP stores are depleted. Much like the ATP–CP system, it can provide energy for muscle contraction for a brief period of time. After 1.5 to 2 min of anaerobic exercise, the accumulation of lactate and its associated hydrogen ion (H^+) inhibits the reactions of glycolysis, thereby contributing to muscle fatigue.[20,22] Without this rapid anaerobic production of ATP, skeletal muscle fatigue would occur very quickly. Thus, the lactic acid system is critically important for high-intensity anaerobic power events which last 20 s to 2 min, such as 200-, 400-, and 800-meter sprinting and 100- and 200-meter swimming events (Figure 4).

The *aerobic system* requires oxygen for the breakdown of glucose to pyruvate and subsequent degradation to CO_2 and H_2O via the tricarboxylic acid cycle and the electron transport system. However, it should be reemphasized that in the first 2 h of exercise the most important source of glucose for aerobic energy production is stored muscle glycogen. As discussed previously, the aerobic system is far more efficient than the lactic acid system in terms of ATP production. When the energy requirements for exercise are not greater than the ability of the aerobic system to supply ATP, and when oxygen is available, complete catabolism of glucose occurs with little formation of lactic acid. Another difference between the lactic acid and the aerobic systems is the type of substrate catabolized. The lactic acid system only breaks down glucose and, preferentially, glucose subunits from glycogen. The aerobic system can degrade glycogen, fats (fatty acids), or proteins (amino acids) to CO_2 and H_2O.

Maximal oxygen consumption ($\dot{V}O_2$ max) or maximal aerobic power involves the full engagement of the aerobic system. This is the upper limit of an individual's ability to consume oxygen. It involves pulmonary ventilation and oxygenation of the blood, cardiovascular system blood circulation to exercising skeletal muscle, and oxygen utilization in skeletal muscle mitochondria, where the aerobic energy system is housed. The aerobic system is the predominant energy system used in exercise that lasts longer than 3 min (Figure 4). There are many examples of this so-called endurance or aerobic exercise, such as 1500-meter to marathon running, road cycling, soccer, and cross-country skiing. For additional information on the energy systems used for exercise, see McArdle et al.,[21] Katch and McArdle,[23] and Fox et al.[24]

IV. SUBSTRATE UTILIZATION DURING EXERCISE

Glucose stored as glycogen and fatty acids stored as triglycerides are the quantitatively important energy sources during exercise. Key factors dictating the relative contribution and absolute quantity of these substrates oxidized are intensity and duration of exercise, level of physical conditioning, and initial muscle glycogen levels. How the fuel mixture is affected by each of these factors will be discussed.

Skeletal muscle glycogen stores and circulating blood glucose originating in liver from glycogenolysis or gluconeogenesis represent the primary sources of carbohydrate used for energy production by exercising muscle. Triglycerides stored in adipose tissue and muscle provide most of the free fatty acids (FFA) oxidized during exercise. Fatty acid uptake by skeletal muscle is dependent on blood FFA concentration, which in turn is dependent on the relative activation of lipolysis in adipose tissue.

It is generally acknowledged that the oxidation of amino acids makes only a minor contribution to the total amount of ATP synthesized by exercising muscle.[7] The relative amount of carbohydrate to fat utilized by humans can be indirectly assessed from ventilatory exchange by computation of the nonnitrogen R-value or respiratory exchange ratio (RER). RER is the ratio of the volume of expired CO_2 to the volume of oxygen absorbed by the lungs per unit of time. The predominance of carbohydrate or fat as energy substrate is indicated by a RER near 1.00 or 0.7, respectively. The transition from resting to the exercise state is characterized by a shift from almost exclusive dependence on fatty acids to heavy dependence on glucose as an energy substrate for skeletal muscle.

A. Exercise Intensity

The relative contribution of carbohydrate oxidation to total metabolism increases as a curvilinear function of exercise intensity up until approximately the point of $\dot{V}O_2$ max, at which time glucose essentially becomes the sole energy substrate.[20] During light exercise, there is a gradual increase in the absolute amount of fat oxidized as aerobic endurance exercise progresses. In this situation, fatty acids can serve as the primary fuel source[25] which allows very prolonged activity, such as walking, even in the fasted state. Maximal utilization of fatty acids in the untrained individual may occur at about 50% $\dot{V}O_2$ max. With higher exercise intensities, reliance on fatty acids decreases such that there is a reciprocal relationship between the substrate contribution of fat and carbohydrate during exercise.[26] Even at relatively high exercise intensities, fatty acids serve as an important secondary fuel. This spares muscle glycogen, thereby prolonging the exercise time before glycogen depletion and exhaustion occur.[27] Depletion of muscle glycogen is invariably associated with reduced exercise output and eventual discontinuation of strenuous exercise.[28,29] Thus, muscle glycogen plays a primary role in determining exercise capacity, even when other energy substrates are available.

There is a direct relationship between exercise intensity and dependence on muscle glycogen as an energy substrate. During low-intensity exercise (i.e., <50% $\dot{V}O_2$ max), muscle glycogen is used slowly and sedentary individuals will not become exhausted at this exercise intensity.[20] A linear relationship between exercise intensity and reductions in muscle glycogen was documented by Hermansen and co-workers.[29] These investigators showed that muscle glycogen was reduced by only 20% after 2 h of cycling at low intensity, whereas glycogen was essentially depleted when subjects performed at near maximal effort. In addition, exercise intensities corresponding to 50, 75, and 100% $\dot{V}O_2$ max have been demonstrated to produce glycogenolysis rates of 0.7, 1.4, and 3.4 mmol/kg/min, respectively.[30]

At very high exercise intensities, oxygen transport to working muscle may not adequately meet the demands of oxidative metabolism, thus necessitating a greater reliance on carbohydrate for energy. At intensities above 90% $\dot{V}O_2$ max, exhaustion typically occurs before muscle glycogen depletion. Thus, the strong relationship between muscle glycogen depletion and exhaustion occurs only at exercise intensities corresponding to approximately 60 to 75% $\dot{V}O_2$ max.[31]

Exercise intensity is also directly related to glucose uptake from the circulation by muscle, as well as to liver glucose output.[32] Thus, a rise in RER with increased exercise intensity results from an augmented rate of both muscle and liver glycogenolysis.[33] The increased glucose uptake by contracting muscle can be attributed to increases in muscle blood flow and in the efficiency of muscle glucose extraction. The magnitude of blood flow to working muscle is linearly related to the intensity of exercise.[34] The approximately two- to threefold increase in fractional glucose extraction can be attributed to a greater demand for glucose by each active muscle fiber and/or an increase in the number of active muscle fibers.[35] Increased arteriovenous glucose difference has been suggested to play a relatively minor role compared to the dramatic rise in muscle blood flow in mediating the exercise-induced stimulation of glucose uptake.[36]

B. Exercise Duration

At the onset of exercise, muscle glycogen declines rapidly.[29,37,38] After the first 5 to 20 min of exercise, the use of muscle glycogen slows as the stores become partially depleted. This decrease in the use of muscle glycogen-derived glucose is associated with an increased utilization of blood glucose. The inverse relationship between glucose uptake by skeletal muscle and rate of glycogen utilization may be mediated by the smaller extracellular downhill gradient for glucose uptake when significant cellular glucose is being derived from glycogenolysis.[20] The accumulation of glucose-6-phosphate, which is likely to occur with rapid glycogenolysis, is negatively correlated with rate of plasma glucose uptake during exercise.[35]

Wahren et al.[32] demonstrated that during moderate to strenuous cycling exercise, net glucose uptake by leg muscles increases 10- to 20-fold above the resting value. With continuing exercise, there is an increase in plasma glucose utilization while total carbohydrate oxidation remains constant or decreases. Thus, the use of plasma glucose represents an increasing percentage of both total energy expenditure and total carbohydrate oxidation during prolonged exercise and can account for 70 to 100% of total carbohydrate oxidation after 2 to 3 h of exercise, provided that plasma glucose availability is maintained.[35]

Heavy reliance on blood glucose as an energy substrate is associated with a concomitant increase in hepatic glucose output, primarily by means of augmented glycogenolysis, in order to maintain euglycemia.[32] The markedly greater reliance on glycogenolysis compared to gluconeogenesis for hepatic glucose production is more pronounced during early phases of exercise and at higher exercise intensities. The relative contribution of gluconeogenesis to total liver glucose output increases with increased duration of exercise, and may provide between 20 and 50% of total glucose release at the end of prolonged exercise.[35]

In humans, blood glucose levels are typically maintained within a narrow range due to a close coupling between peripheral tissue utilization of blood-borne glucose and hepatic output of glucose.[20] However, glucose production from gluconeogenesis is relatively limited such that decreases in plasma glucose may occur once hepatic glycogen stores are severely depleted.[39,40] This can occur during prolonged exercise, with the rate of blood glucose decrease partially dictated by exercise intensity.[39-41] Decreases in blood glucose to approximately 2.5 mmol/l (45 mg/dl) can precipitate symptoms related to hypoglycemia-induced neuroglucopenia (lightheadedness, lethargy, nausea)[31] and can thus be an important contributing factor to the onset of fatigue during prolonged exercise. There is evidence that less than 50% of individuals exercising at 60 to 70% $\dot{V}O_2$ max for 2.5 to 3.5 h will exhibit symptoms of hypoglycemia.[40,42]

In summary, as prolonged exercise continues, RER typically decreases, indicating a shift from carbohydrate to fat oxidation, while at the same time the quantitative importance of blood glucose compared to endogenous muscle glycogen as an energy source for muscle oxidation increases. Plasma glucose is clearly an important energy substrate, as it can supply between 20 and 50% of the total oxidative energy production during submaximal exercise.[35] For additional information regarding the effects of exercise intensity and duration on carbohydrate utilization, see Saltin and Gollnick,[20] Coggan,[35] and Björkman and Wahren.[36]

C. Physical Conditioning

Endurance training enhances an individual's ability to perform more aerobically at the same absolute exercise intensity. This appears to be related to an increased mitochondrial volume density within the trained muscle and the corresponding increase in respiratory capacity.[20] After endurance training, the increased utilization of fat as an energy source during submaximal exercise may be attributed to the adaptive increase in mitochondrial enzymes required for fatty acid oxidation. In skeletal muscle, FFA oxidation appears to inhibit glucose uptake, glycolysis, and glycogenolysis.[43] This carbohydrate-sparing effect of increased fat oxidation results in slower depletion of muscle glycogen and decreased utilization of plasma glucose during exercise.[44]

Depletion of muscle glycogen is associated with cessation of exercise or a decrease in exercise intensity.[26] Thus, the glycogen sparing effect of increased lipid oxidation appears largely to account for the training-induced increase in endurance for prolonged exercise. Lower plasma FFA combined with evidence of decreased adipose tissue lipolysis has been reported in trained vs. untrained individuals during submaximal exercise of similar absolute intensity. This suggests that intramuscular triglyceride stores, rather than triglyceride stored in adipose cells, are the primary source of the additional fatty acids used.[27]

Increased capacity for glycogen storage in muscle also occurs as a result of endurance training. Thus, the trained athlete is likely to have higher glycogen stores at the onset of exercise which are depleted at a slower rate during exercise.[45]

D. Initial Glycogen Levels

It has been long appreciated that the relative proportion of carbohydrate and fat oxidized during an exercise session is markedly affected by the dietary carbohydrate and initial muscle glycogen content.[33] For example, a standard 30-min exercise test at 74% $\dot{V}O_2$ max was associated with less muscle glycogen oxidation when subjects consumed a fat–protein diet compared to a mixed or high-carbohydrate diet.[46]

The ability to sustain prolonged moderate to heavy exercise is largely dependent on the starting glycogen content in the skeletal muscles. Bergstrom et al.[28] demonstrated that an initial glycogen content of 1.75 g/100 g wet muscle allowed subjects to tolerate a standard work load for 114 min. When the carbohydrate content of the diet was altered to produce initial glycogen levels of 0.63 or 3.31 g/100 g, work times to exhaustion were 57 min and 167 min, respectively. Thus, high muscle glycogen levels allow exercise to continue longer at a given submaximal workload. The strong correlation between initial glycogen level and time to exhaustion has been consistently observed, even though there is a significant uptake of blood-borne metabolites (glucose and fatty acids) during exercise. Saltin and Gollnick[20] suggested that the importance of initial glycogen stores is related to the inability of glucose and fatty acids to cross the cell membrane rapidly enough to provide adequate substrate for mitochondrial respiration.

Coggan[35] recently summarized a number of studies which suggested that alterations in carbohydrate intake can affect the utilization of plasma glucose during exercise. Most work in this area has demonstrated that the contribution of plasma glucose as an energy substrate is inversely related to the utilization of FFA and directly related to the dietary carbohydrate level, at least when it is varied over the range of low to normal.

As stated previously, hepatic glucose production during exercise results from a combination of glycogenolysis and gluconeogenesis. With restricted carbohydrate intakes, liver glycogen is largely depleted, which necessitates a greater reliance on gluconeogenesis during exercise. Increased glucose production from gluconeogenesis, however, cannot totally compensate for reduced hepatic glycogenolysis, thus increasing the likelihood of hypoglycemia during prolonged exercise.[35] In contrast, exercise-induced reductions in plasma glucose are less likely after the ingestion of high-carbohydrate diets because of the relatively greater contribution of glycogenolysis to liver glucose production. This allows a closer coupling between the utilization of blood-borne glucose by exercising muscle and hepatic output of glucose.[28,47]

E. Lactate Production

As alluded to earlier, the breakdown of glycogen to lactate with production of some ATP is of physiological significance because it allows skeletal muscle to perform very high intensity exercise even when oxygen transport to muscle is limited. Lactate production occurs in muscle even under aerobic conditions and accelerates when oxygen supply is limited.[20] Lactate production under aerobic conditions results from a mismatch between rate of pyruvate production from glycolysis and the rate of pyruvate transport into the mithcondria for the terminal reactions of its oxidative metabolism. The lactate dehydrogenase reaction is an equilibrium reaction, and will thus favor the production of lactate whenever pyruvate and NADH are available to the enzyme.

During exercise, lactate production is directly related to the intensity of exercise. A minor fraction of the lactate produced appears to serve as a gluconeogenic precursor, thereby playing a role in the maintenance of blood glucose. More importantly, much of this lactate is shuttled via the interstitium and vasculature to areas of high cellular respiration. Thus, lactate provides the vehicle by which more glycolytic fibers within a working muscle bed can shuttle oxidizable substrate to the neighboring muscle fibers with higher respiratory rates[48] or to the myocardium which preferentially uses lactate over glucose and FFA.[49] Brooks[48] summarized a number of animal and human studies which support this concept of a lactate shuttle and suggested that lactate may be a quantitatively important oxidizable substrate during exercise.

It is clear that lactate production and oxidation contribute to energy-producing capacity of muscle. However, excessive lactate production can adversely affect muscle fibers by dissociating into lactate and H^+ ions, thereby lowering their pH. Lowering muscle pH may exert a negative effect on the processes involved in excitation–contraction coupling[50] and, thus, appears to be a contributing factor to the development of muscular fatigue.[51]

Decreased lactate production at a given absolute exercise intensity after physical training can be directly attributed to the smaller buildup of pyruvate and NADH to fuel the lactate dehydrogenase reaction. Due to increased FFA oxidation, there is decreased reliance on glycolysis and, thus, less pyruvate formation after training. In addition, a greater percentage of pyruvate formed from glycolysis is transported into the mitochondria because of their increased volume density in trained muscle.[20]

V. REGULATION OF CARBOHYDRATE METABOLISM DURING EXERCISE

Glycogen stores are the most important supplier of glycolytic substrate in muscle during exercise which lasts less than an hour. Glucose tracer studies, which typically underestimate glucose utilization, have demonstrated that blood glucose may provide 20 to 50% of the energy substrate used in muscle during prolonged submaximal exercise. From the previous section it is clear that a number of factors affect carbohydrate utilization during exercise, including state of training, initial muscle glycogen concentration, and intensity and duration of exercise. This section briefly reviews the factors which regulate muscle glycogenolysis, glycogenesis, hepatic glucose production, and glucose utilization by muscle during exercise. For additional information on regulation of carbohydrate metabolism see Murray et al.,[10] Saltin and Gollnick,[20] Stanley and Connett,[22] Coggan,[35] Björkman and Wahren,[36] and Ren and Hultman.[52]

A. Muscle Glycogenolysis and Glycogenesis

The rate of glycogenolysis in exercising skeletal muscle is dependent upon initial muscle glycogen and activation of the enzyme glycogen phosphorylase (PHOS).[20,53] Phosphorylase b, the inactive form, is activated to PHOS a, the active form, in the presence of catecholamines, cyclic AMP, Ca^{2+}, and increased muscle pH. It should also be noted that PHOS b, the "inactive" form, is active in the presence of AMP, while PHOS a does not require AMP to be active. In addition, accumulation of glucose-6-phosphate (G6P) in muscle provides direct feedback inhibition of PHOS. Thus, control of glycogenolysis occurs via neural-muscle activation (Ca^{2+}), endocrine (catecholamine, cyclic AMP), and metabolic (AMP, G6P, and pH) mechanisms.[22]

Skeletal muscle stimulation is accompanied by a release of Ca^{2+} from the sarcoplasmic reticulum and a rise in free cytosolic Ca^{2+}. Free Ca^{2+} in turn activates phosphorylase kinase, which is responsible for the phosphorylation and activation of PHOS.[10] Apparently this initial activation is only transient during exercise and PHOS reverts to the inactive form within minutes.[54] Epinephrine reactivates the enzyme and stimulates glycogen catabolism in contracting muscle via β-adrenergic stimulation and the cyclic AMP–phosphorylase kinase second messenger system. This method of PHOS activation provides for continuous control of glycogenolysis coupled with exercise-induced sympathetic hormone changes, and appears to act synergistically with cellular Ca^{2+} control. During different types of exercise, one mechanism of PHOS activation may predominate. For example, it has been suggested that Ca^{2+} activation predominates during short-term, high-intensity exercise and during heavy-resistance exercise when muscle blood flow is restricted. Prolonged exercise, on the other hand, may require sympathetic stimulation of PHOS.[20]

AMP stimulates both PHOS a and PHOS b activity and Pi has been shown to be a positive allosteric modulator of PHOS. Since both of these metabolites are products of ATP production during exercise, there is potential for excessive glycogenolytic flux following the initial activation during exercise. However, metabolic control of glycogenolysis during exercise is established either directly through G6P negative feedback inhibition of PHOS or indirectly by control of glycolysis. Glucose-6-phosphate may accumulate in muscle with the onset of exercise due to rapid increases in glucose uptake and glycogenolysis.[20,55] In this way, increases in G6P may regulate skeletal muscle glucose utilization and glycogenolysis via inhibition of hexokinase and PHOS, respectively.

Other indirect intracellular regulatory mechanisms affect the rate of glycolysis and, therefore, the rate of glycogenolysis. The most important of these are metabolic controls which influence phosphofructokinase (PFK), the rate-limiting enzyme of glycolysis. PFK is regulated by many allosteric modulators, including activation by ADP, AMP, Pi, fructose-6-phosphate, and NH_3, and inhibition by ATP, H^+, and citrate.[20,22] Thus, glycolytic flux and G6P concentration can be tightly controlled by PFK activity. It has also been shown recently that glycogen synthesis continues under conditions of net glycogen breakdown during skeletal muscle contraction.[56-58] Consequently, the degree of glycogen catabolism may depend upon the interplay between glycogenesis and glycogenolysis.[52]

The activation of glycogen synthase (GS), the rate-limiting enzyme in the formation of glycogen, plays an important regulatory role in glycogen synthesis. Glycogen synthase has two forms. The less active D-form is phosphorylated and is activated by G6P. The more active I-form of GS is dephosphorylated and its activity is independent of G6P. Both exercise and insulin stimulate glycogen synthesis by increasing the proportion of I-form GS. Similarly, when muscle glycogen is depleted a dephosphorylation enzyme catalyzes the conversion of synthase D to the I-form.[59,60] Therefore, there is normally an inverse relationship between muscle glycogen content and glycogen synthase I activity. Although muscle glycogen level itself plays a key role in regulating glycogenesis, other factors, such as G6P formation, insulin sensitivity, and glucose transport, may be equally important.[59]

Friedman et al.[59] make a strong case for glucose transporter activity being the fundamental regulatory mechanism which controls both glucose utilization and glycogen resynthesis. They have suggested that glucose transporter activity increases without an increase in insulin activity. Thus, increases in exercise-induced glucose transport during recovery from exercise may be important for glycogen resynthesis postexercise.[61] The sensitivity of glucose transport to insulin also increases 5- to 10-fold following acute endurance exercise.[62-65] The synergistic effects of exercise and insulin-mediated glucose transport are discussed more fully in the section on glucose transport.

B. Hepatic Glucose Production

The liver provides virtually all of the glucose entry into the circulation during exercise, either by glycogenolysis or gluconeogenesis. During the early phases of exercise of moderate intensity (35 to 50 min), glucose production occurs predominantly by glycogenolysis and this dominance increases with higher exercise intensity.[66] Even with exercise lasting 4 h, the contribution of hepatic gluconeogenesis only rises to 45% of the overall hepatic glucose output.[36] Hepatic glucose production is stimulated by glucagon, catecholamines, and cortisol and is inhibited by insulin. Plasma insulin concentration decreases with exercise of any duration. Plasma glucagon is not altered during mild to moderate exercise and rises during heavy or prolonged exercise. Both insulin and glucagon appear to be regulated by sympathetic activity during exercise rather than by plasma glucose, because blood glucose concentration does not change or may even increase in the first hour of exercise.[35,36] Epinephrine and, more importantly, norepinephrine seem to stimulate pancreatic glucagon output while inhibiting insulin release.[67]

Increases in glucagon do not appear to be necessary for an exercise-induced rise in hepatic glycogenolysis during exercise in humans.[36] Catecholamines seem to play a more important regulatory role in hepatic glucose production than reciprocal stimulation/inhibition by glucagon and insulin, respectively.[68,69] Presumably, either direct sympathetic stimulation of hepatocytes[70] and/or circulating levels of catecholamines play a major role in regulating liver glycogenolysis during exercise. Björkman and Wahren[36] suggested that insulin and glucagon may only play a modulatory role in hepatic glucose production during exercise by regulating that proportion of glucose production needed to supply the brain and other nonworking tissues with glucose. Growth hormone and cortisol are also involved in the regulation of hepatic glucose production, but their role appears to be minor during exercise.

Hepatic gluconeogenesis becomes quantitatively more important as endurance exercise progresses beyond an hour. Splanchnic fractional extraction and uptake of gluconeogenic precursors, such as lactate, pyruvate, and alanine, increases with exercise duration. The fractional extraction of glycerol, another gluconeogenic precursor, is very high at rest and changes little with exercise. Nevertheless, the contribution of glycerol to gluconeogenesis increases during endurance exercise because of the steady rise in arterial glycerol concentration.[35]

Maximal hepatic glucose production is ultimately dependent on liver glycogenolysis because hepatic gluconeogenesis is not able to maintain glucose production as liver glycogen becomes depleted. Therefore, hypoglycemia occurs more readily after hepatic glycogen depletion. Liver gluconeogenesis is regulated in part by glucagon, catecholamines, cortisol, and growth hormone. However, the relative importance of these hormones during exercise is still in question.[71] Much of this endocrine research has been conducted in dogs, a species which appears to differ from humans with respect to the regulation of hepatic glucose production. In summary, both hepatic glycogenolysis and gluconeogenesis appear to be under redundant multiple hormone regulatory control. Even though the catecholamines are of primary importance in the regulation of hepatic glucose production during exercise, other circulating hormones coupled with plasma glucose may still be involved.[35,36]

C. Glucose Transport Into Skeletal Muscle

Both glycogen synthesis and glucose utilization by muscle are primarily controlled by glucose delivery and subsequent transport into muscle cells. As stated previously, skeletal muscle glycogen depletion during exercise coincides with increased glucose uptake into muscle. Blood-borne glucose may then provide between 20 and 50% of the substrate used by skeletal muscle during submaximal aerobic exercise.[35] Blood glucose uptake is also important for glycogen resynthesis following prolonged exercise,[59] as discussed in the last section of this chapter. Insulin plays an important role in regulating glucose transport into skeletal muscle.[71] However, muscle contraction alone appears to increase glucose transport into muscle fibers.[72-74] This section briefly reviews the roles that insulin and contractility play in regulating muscle glucose transport and uptake during exercise. For additional information on skeletal muscle glucose transport, see Friedman et al.[59] and Bonen et al.[74]

Glucose is transported across the muscle membrane down a concentration gradient by carrier-mediated (glucose transporter protein) facilitated diffusion. The glucose uptake capacities of different skeletal muscle fiber types are quite diverse. Slow-oxidative muscle fibers exhibit greater glucose uptake capacity at rest compared to fast-glycolytic fibers.[75-77] This is due to greater insulin sensitivity and responsiveness in oxidative muscle fibers. These differences are also apparent during exercise and are likely due to differential insulin binding, glucose transporter (GT) availability, blood flow to individual fibers, and contraction-induced changes in sarcolemmal permeability.

1. Muscle Contractility and Glucose Transport

Early experiments by Berger et al.[78] and Vranic et al.[79] suggested that glucose uptake into muscle was dependent upon small quantities of insulin. However, more recently, it has been shown that glucose uptake increases during and after exercise in the absence of insulin.[72,73,76,77,80,81] Vranic and Lickley[71] questioned the physiological significance of these findings because insulin is never totally absent in muscle. In addition, Nesher et al.[82] reported that contractile activity exerted an additive effect on glucose uptake in the presence of insulin. Both insulin and contractility appear to stimulate GT recruitment in muscle.[80,82,83] It has been suggested that exercise stimulates translocation of glucose transporters from intracelullar storage sites to the plasma membrane. Exercise also appears to increase the activity of these GTs.[22]

At least two GTs are expressed in muscle. GLUT-1, the insulin-independent form, is minimally present in skeletal muscle. GLUT-4 is the major transporter species found in muscle and is responsible for insulin-dependent glucose transport.[59] Several recent studies have reported that both insulin and exercise increase the concentration and translocation of insulin-dependent transporter GLUT-4 in skeletal muscle.[80,84-86]

2. Insulin-Dependent Glucose Transport

There is still some question whether glucose transport into muscle can be augmented by muscle contractions alone. Vranic and Lickley[71] maintain that insulin plays a pivotal role in the control of glucose uptake by skeletal muscle *in vivo*. This is because of the difficulty in proving that insulin has been completely removed from *in situ* experiments and because insulin-like growth factors could still be present. In addition, Björkman and Wahren[36] noted that while exercise is accompanied by a fall in plasma insulin, the amount of insulin delivered to working muscle may actually increase because of the rise in muscle blood flow during exercise.

Recent research has focused on the characterization and translocation of GTs in skeletal muscle and their regulation by insulin.[74,87] Insulin-dependent glucose uptake into muscle does not seem to be a function of increased insulin binding to skeletal muscle receptors.[76] Similarly, while phosphorylation of the insulin receptor via tyrosine kinase activity was once thought to regulate insulin receptor activity, there is no conclusive evidence that this mediates insulin-dependent glucose transport.[88] Bonen and co-workers[74] indicated that there is at least circumstantial evidence to suggest the following: (1) GTs are activated in both the presence and absence of insulin, (2) GT affinity and activity can be altered by contractile activity, and (3) GT differences between muscle fiber types likely exist. They also suggested the fast-glycolytic muscle fibers which are quite unresponsive to insulin can still exhibit marked increases in glucose uptake during exercise. This may be mediated by a contraction-induced rise in cytosolic Ca^{2+} which increases GT translocation and affinity.[22] However, to date, it has not been established conclusively that contraction alone can increase glucose uptake into skeletal muscle.

VI. DIETARY MANIPULATION OF CARBOHYDRATE INTAKE

A. Preexercise Diet

The importance of high-carbohydrate diets to promote glycogen storage in days preceding an exhaustive endurance event is well established. Individuals who exercise regularly should routinely consume a diet which provides 55 to 70% of the total calories from carbohydrate. Endurance athletes and those who train exhaustively on successive days are likely to require 65 to 75% of calories from carbohydrate to optimize performance.[89] Glycogen depletion during training can be prevented by a high-carbohydrate diet and periodic rest days to allow muscles time to rebuild glycogen stores. Some feelings of tiredness associated with over-training could be partially related to lowered glycogen stores.[90]

Foods rich in complex carbohydrates are preferable to those high in refined sugars because they are more nutrient dense in terms of absolute levels of vitamins, minerals, and fiber and tend to be very low in fat. In addition, complex carbohydrate foods are likely to produce relatively lower blood glucose and insulin levels. However, when consumed as part of mixed meals containing fat and protein, differences between high-carbohydrate foods in glycemic and insulinemic responses are of lesser magnitude and may not be of physiological significance. Numerous selections of grains, legumes, fruits, and vegetables will ensure sufficient glucose absorption for the maintenance of adequate glycogen stores. Specific guidelines regarding the design of diets with appropriate emphasis on carbohydrates can be found in a number of recent publications.[45,91-93]

Liver glycogen is markedly reduced by an overnight fast and muscle glycogen levels will be suboptimal if the daily diet has not been high in carbohydrate.[31] Preexercise meals emphasizing easily digested high-carbohydrate foods can potentially increase liver and muscle glycogen concentrations, thereby delaying the time at which carbohydrate reserves become depleted and improving performance.[94] The meal should be relatively light (approximately 300 kcal), consist primarily of low-fiber carbohydrate-containing foods, and include a moderate amount of protein.[93] Consumption of this meal at least 2 to 3 h before the exercise session will typically allow for complete gastric emptying and minimize the possibility of exercise-induced gastrointestinal upset.[45]

1. Timing of Preexercise Carbohydrate

Some controversy exists regarding optimal timing of the last meal/snack ingested prior to an endurance exercise event. The ingestion of a carbohydrate snack or beverage from 15 min to 1 h before the exercise bout can lead to hypoglycemia[95,96] and in two studies exerted a negative effect on performance.[97,98] Postingestion increases in insulin at the start of exercise could lower blood glucose, due to increased reliance on glucose as an energy substrate and suppression of hepatic glucose output.[95] Increased glucose utilization would be expected to result from the antilipolytic effect of insulin on adipose cells (i.e., an inhibition of triglyceride mobilization) and increased uptake and utilization of glucose by insulin-sensitive tissues.[96] Even when a high-carbohydrate meal was ingested 4 h before exercise, thereby allowing a return of plasma insulin to fasting levels during the 2 h immediately preceding exercise, a decrease in blood glucose during the first hour of exercise and a suppression of the normal exercise-induced increase in plasma FFA and glycerol were observed.[99] These data suggested that a persistent effect of insulin may have been responsible for the observed decreases in blood glucose and in adipocyte lipolysis.

Recent research suggests that in spite of the elevation in blood glucose and insulin at the onset of exercise and fluctuations in blood glucose during exercise, work performance may not be adversely affected and may be actually improved by the preexercise ingestion of carbohydrate.[100] Carbohydrate ingested prior to exercise can be oxidized by active muscle. Improvements in exercise performance, when observed, may result from a delay in the normal decline in blood glucose, since preexercise carbohydrate ingestion has been suggested to aid in maintaining hepatic glycogen reserves[101] but does not appear to affect rate of muscle glycogen utilization.[94]

Three studies have been reported which support the assertion that ingestion of carbohydrate within 1 h of start of exercise can improve cycling performance.[102-104] Gleeson et al.[102] reported that cyclists rode an average of 13 min longer after ingesting 1 g glucose/kg body weight 45 min before cycling to exhaustion. Neufer et al.[103] demonstrated a 10% mean increase in work output during 15 min of cycling preceded by 45 min of cycling at 80% $\dot{V}O_2$ max when subjects consumed either 45 g of a glucose polymer solution or a solid carbohydrate confectionary bar 5 min before exercise.

The third and most recently reported study used trained cyclists and a cycling time-trial performance to simulate athletic competition.[104] Exercise performance was improved by 12.5% when 1.1 g or 2.2 g of liquid carbohydrate/kg body weight was ingested 60 min before 90 min of cycling at 70% $\dot{V}O_2$ max followed by a 45-min cycling-performance trial. Compared to the placebo treatment, carbohydrate ingestion produced markedly higher serum insulin and markedly lower FFA levels at the onset of exercise and was associated with a 12% greater amount of carbohydrate oxidation. The authors suggested that improved performance was related to greater carbohydrate availability, which most likely resulted from continued gastric emptying of preexercise carbohydrate during exercise.

It must be acknowledged that not all studies have reported positive effects of preexercise carbohydrate ingestion on exercise performance.[96-98,105,106] In addition, individual responses to preexercise carbohydrate feedings may vary considerably, which could be partially related to differences in susceptibility and sensitivity to a transient lowering of blood glucose. Thus, individual athletes should experiment to determine whether their performance can be improved.

2. Type of Preexercise Carbohydrate

It has been suggested that fructose might be superior to glucose as a preexercise carbohydrate source due to lower postingestion increases in serum insulin and glucose.[96,107] However, no differences in endurance performance after the ingestion of glucose compared to fructose have been observed.[96,105] Thus, there appears to be little rationale for recommending the use of fructose for preexercise feeding, especially in light of the possibility of incomplete absorption, cramps, and diarrhea resulting from the ingestion of even moderate (50 g) fructose doses.[108]

A recent area of investigation has been to determine whether there are specific advantages to the preexercise ingestion of low-glycemic compared to high-glycemic foods. The relative glycemic potency, or propensity to raise blood glucose, of many carbohydrate-containing foods have been compared, and these data have been published in the form of a glycemic index.[109] Thomas et al.[110] compared biochemical and physiological responses of trained cyclists to equal carbohydrate portions of a low-glycemic-index food (lentils) and two high-glycemic-index foods (glucose and potato) ingested 1 h before cycling to exhaustion. Compared to the consumption of glucose or potato, lentil ingestion produced: lower plasma glucose and insulin for 30 to 60 min postingestion, higher FFA levels and lower total carbohydrate oxidation during exercise, and an endurance time which averaged 9 min and

20 min longer than the corresponding times for glucose and potato, respectively. The investigators suggested the apparent advantage of preexercise ingestion of a low-glycemic-index food may accrue from decreased stimulation of insulin release prior to exercise and maintenance of higher levels of plasma glucose and FFA at critical times during exercise.

Glycemic response can be markedly altered by the levels of protein, fat, and dietary fiber provided by a given food.[111] Jarvis et al.[112] investigated some of these so-called "food matrix" effects on carbohydrate utilization during exercise by comparing ingestion of 70 g liquid glucose, 30 min prior to exercise, to the preexercise ingestion of three test meals (a refined hot cereal with or without a water-soluble fiber and an oat bar). The test meals decreased the initial glycemic and insulinemic responses compared to glucose alone and slowed down the rate of exogenous carbohydrate utilization. The exercise protocol, 4 h of walking at an intensity corresponding to 40% $\dot{V}O_2$ max, did not allow a comparative assessment of endurance performance. However, it appears unlikely that any performance-related advantages would have accrued from ingestion of the test meals compared to glucose alone, since neither the cumulative 4-h utilization of exogenous or endogenous carbohydrate was significantly altered by their ingestion.

Few studies have specifically compared physiological responses to complex carbohydrate-containing foods or meals with widely differing glycemic effects. Whether the glycemic index of different foods used as preexercise carbohydrate sources should be an important consideration in terms of maximizing endurance performance is a question for which few answers are currently available.

In summary, improvements in endurance performance following preexercise carbohydrate ingestion may result from promotion of liver and muscle glycogen synthesis and/or via a direct contribution to the pool of blood glucose which is ultimately oxidized by working muscle. Preexercise carbohydrate feedings can be provided as a solid or liquid, and recommended dosage is between 1 and 5 g/kg body weight, depending on meal timing.[100] The likelihood of gastrointestinal distress is decreased if the carbohydrate content of the meal is reduced as ingestion time before exercise decreases. Liquid meals may be better tolerated than regular meals close to competition before of their shorter gastric emptying time.[45] For additional information regarding preexercise carbohydrate intake and endurance performance, see Sherman and Wimer,[31] Costill and Hargreaves,[90] Sherman,[94] and Sherman and Wright.[100]

B. Carbohydrate Supercompensation

As stated earlier, depletion of muscle glycogen results in a decrease in exercise energy output followed by cessation of exercise.[26] Thus, the use of carbohydrate supercompensation (loading) to maximize muscle glycogen stores at the onset of exercise may be beneficial for athletes engaged in continuous exercise for more than 90 to 120 min. The initially proposed so-called "classical" method of carbohydrate supercompensation included glycogen depletion followed by loading.[28] Glycogen-depleted muscles become supersaturated in a proportional response to high (500 to 600 g) carbohydrate intakes.[89] This method involves the depletion of glycogen by exhaustive exercise and consumption of a low-carbohydrate diet, and then a supercompensation phase in which a very-high-carbohydrate diet (>90% of total kilocalories) is consumed (Figure 5).[113] This is no longer the preferred method for most athletes, because the 3-day low-carbohydrate feeding period may cause hypoglycemia, irritability, and chronic fatigue. In addition, the two bouts of exhaustive exercise only a few days before the event could result in injury, soreness, and fatigue.[60]

A modified version, also depicted in Figure 5, entails the "tapering down" of exercise during the 6 d prior to the event. At the same time, daily carbohydrate intake is progressively

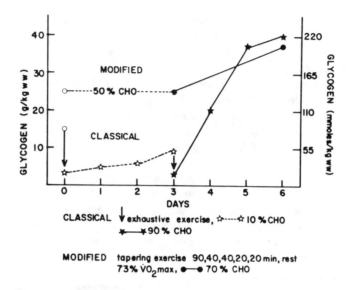

FIGURE 5.   Schematic representation of the "classical" and modified methods of carbohydrate loading. (From Sherman, W. M. and Costill, D. L., *Am. J. Sports Med.*, 12, 44, 1984. With permission.)

increased from an initial level of approximately 350 g to 550 g or 70% of total kilocalories (whichever is larger) during the last 72 h preceding competition.[45,91] Sherman et al.[114] demonstrated that this modified version is as effective as the classical glycogen supercompensation regimen.

The ingestion of at least 550 g of carbohydrates is typically achieved by the consumption of large quantities of pasta, rice, and/or bread, which may cause a minor degree of gastrointestinal fullness and discomfort in some athletes. Lamb and Snyder[115] recently demonstrated that partial substitution of a low-residue, high-calorie, maltodextrin-rich drink for most of the pasta and rice commonly used in glycogen loading diets was at least as effective as a pasta/rice diet in improving glycogen stores and running performance in 14 well-trained males. Ten of the runners reported less gastrointestinal discomfort when consuming the liquid carbohydrate supplement compared to the pasta/rice diet and 90% indicated that they would be more likely to use the supplemented diet for glycogen loading. Thus, a viable option for glycogen loading appears to be a carbohydrate supplement drink which is consumed with normal high-carbohydrate meals and as a snack between meals.

In summary, normal carbohydrate intake and glycogen reserves are adequate for exercise that lasts less than 60 min.[116] Carbohydrate loading can increase high-intensity exercise time (duration) but will not usually affect pace during the first hour of an event.[45] Due to the approximately 3 g of water stored with each extra gram of glycogen, increasing glycogen stores from 15 g/kg to 40 g/kg in 20 kg of muscle would represent an increase in glycogen and water of 1 and 3 lb, respectively. This high degree of glycogen supercompensation and associated weight gain may create a feeling of heaviness or stiffness that could contribute to muscular cramping and premature fatigue.[117] Thus, athletes who use this procedure should experiment to determine the pre-event dietary and exercise modifications which produce an optimal degree of glycogen supercompensation for endurance performance.

C. Supplementation During Exercise

It has been well established that initial muscle glycogen stores directly influence prolonged endurance exercise performance. As previously discussed, daily carbohydrate intake and preexercise carbohydrate feeding clearly affect these skeletal muscle glycogen stores. When muscle glycogen is depleted during exercise, blood glucose utilization becomes increasingly important as a function of both intensity and duration of exercise. In the last decade, numerous studies have evaluated the efficacy of ingesting carbohydrate during prolonged exercise. This section reviews the current literature on carbohydrate ingestion during exercise. It also provides some practical guidelines with regard to the volume, composition, temperature, rate, and timing of carbohydrate supplements taken during exercise. For additional information on this topic, see Coggan and Coyle,[118] Coyle,[119] Maughan and Noakes,[120] Maughan,[121] and Noakes et al.[122]

1. Carbohydrate Ingestion, Glucose Utilization, and Muscle Glycogen

Carbohydrate ingestion during low-intensity exercise (30% $\dot{V}O_2$ max) increases blood glucose and insulin concentrations, which results in a twofold increase in glucose uptake into skeletal muscle. This leads to increased use of blood glucose and decreased use of plasma FFA during exercise.[118] Carbohydrate ingestion during moderate-intensity exercise (50 to 75% $\dot{V}O_2$ max) seems to result in smaller changes in blood glucose and insulin compared to those observed during low-intensity exercise. This is likely due to greater glucose utilization by muscle and increased sympathetic inhibition of pancreatic insulin secretion. The effects of carbohydrate ingestion on blood glucose turnover during moderate exercise have not been extensively studied in humans. However, Coyle et al.[123] estimated that blood glucose utilization accounted for almost all of the carbohydrate oxidized between 3 and 4 h of moderate-intensity exercise. Thus, it is now thought that blood glucose can be oxidized at very high rates during prolonged exercise, and ingested carbohydrates make a significant contribution to the energy substrate used by skeletal muscle.[118,119]

It was initially hypothesized that carbohydrate ingestion during prolonged exercise improved performance by sparing muscle glycogen. This reduction in skeletal muscle glycogenolysis purportedly delayed the onset of fatigue and increased exercise time to exhaustion. However, direct measurements of muscle glycogen before and after exercise, with and without carbohydrate feedings, have disproved this hypothesis.[123-126] Recently, Coyle and co-workers[127] demonstrated that muscle glycogen utilization was unchanged during moderate-intensity exercise, even when hyperglycemia was maintained by continuous glucose infusion. This lent support to the notion that carbohydrate ingestion during continuous moderate-intensity exercise does not reduce muscle glycogen utilization. One caveat to this conclusion still exists for other types of exercise. Several authors have observed that glycogen synthesis is ongoing during low-intensity and intermittent exercise. Carbohydrate feeding, which seems to promote glycogen synthesis and limit muscle glycogenolysis, may, therefore, spare muscle glycogen under these different exercise conditions.[56,128,129]

Both the rate of hepatic glycogenolysis and gluconeogenesis are reduced with carbohydrate ingestion during low-intensity exercise. Variable effects of carbohydrate ingestion on liver glucose production during moderate-intensity exercise have been observed and require further investigation.[118] Nevertheless, it is well established that carbohydrate ingestion helps to maintain blood glucose concentration in the third and fourth hour of prolonged moderate-intensity exercise.[119]

2. Carbohydrate Ingestion, Performance, and Fatigue

In the 1970s, studies yielded conflicting evidence concerning the effects of carbohydrate ingestion on performance during prolonged endurance exercise. Later investigations, published in the 1980s, demonstrated that endurance performance could be improved by carbohydrate ingestion.[118] This was somewhat surprising because no differences in glycogen utilization were found.[123] Fatigue seemed to be associated with the onset of hypoglycemia rather than glycogen depletion. This led to the hypothesis and eventual finding that carbohydrate feeding delayed fatigue and improved endurance performance by helping to maintain euglycemia.[130] During the first 2 h of moderate-intensity exercise, substrate utilization is similar with and without carbohydrate ingestion. Beyond 2 h, if glycogen is depleted and no carbohydrate has been consumed, blood glucose concentration may decline to a critical level (2.5 to 3.0 mmol/l). Low blood glucose promotes fatigue due to inadequate skeletal muscle glucose uptake and oxidation.[118] Coyle[119] further suggested that carbohydrate feedings do not prevent fatigue during moderate-intensity exercise, but only delay it for 30 to 60 min. There also appears to be an upper limit to the intensity of prolonged exercise (75% $\dot{V}O_2$ max) that can be sustained with carbohydrate supplements.[119]

Recently, it has been observed that carbohydrate and electrolyte ingestion during prolonged exercise suppresses activation of the hypothalamic–pituitary–adrenal axis.[131] This could be a potentially beneficial change in light of the known effect of epinephrine on muscle and liver glycogenolysis. While it provides a partial explanation for why fatigue is delayed with carbohydrate feeding, further investigation will be needed to elucidate the overall mechanisms.

Maughan et al.[132] demonstrated that carbohydrate supplementation improved performance in shorter-duration exercise (70 to 90 min). Several studies have evaluated the effects of carbohydrate feeding during running events lasting between 6 and 14 min. While the results were not completely consistent, enhanced performance was generally observed.[133-136] Improvement of shorter-duration exercise performance with carbohydrate ingestion is not well understood, but Maughan and Noakes[120] speculated that it may be linked to a supplementation-induced increase in blood glucose levels.

3. Carbohydrate Ingestion and Gastric Emptying

The most important barrier to the availability of ingested fluid and carbohydrate is the rate of gastric emptying. Gastric emptying controls the rate at which fluids are delivered to, and absorbed from, the small intestine. The rate of gastric emptying is primarily determined by the volume and composition of the fluid ingested.[120,122] In a recent review, Noakes et al.[122] emphasized that volume and, therefore, the pattern of drinking during exercise, is a major factor which regulates the rate of gastric emptying. The volume of ingested water is particularly important in maintaining euhydration during prolonged exercise. Water volume affects carbohydrate availability because carbohydrates are usually ingested in the form of a sports drink. Gastric emptying follows an exponential time course and decreases rapidly as volume remaining in the stomach decreases. Therefore, maintenance of high stomach volume with repeated drinking seems to improve gastric emptying and carbohydrate availability.[137-139]

Glucose concentration, caloric density, and electrolyte content of ingested solutions all seem to influence gastric emptying. Dilute glucose solutions (5% or less) are emptied from the stomach more quickly than concentrated solutions. Therefore, if optimal hydration is the primary goal, dilute glucose–electrolyte solutions should be ingested.[120] In contrast, greater net glucose absorption occurs with increased glucose concentrations in sport drinks. Sodium is also an important constituent of glucose–electrolyte drinks due to its stimulation of rapid absorption of carbohydrate and water in the small intestine.[120]

Osmolality seems to delay the rate of glucose gastric emptying. Therefore, glucose polymers, such as maltodextrin, should theoretically be emptied more rapidly than glucose solutions, because of their lower osmolality.[122] Additional research will be required to determine why this glucose polymer effect on gastric emptying has not been consistently demonstrated.[138,140,141] Palatability has been suggested to be a significant advantage of glucose polymer solutions because they are not nearly as sweet tasting as glucose solutions of the same concentration.[137]

Exercise intensity appears to affect gastric emptying, particularly at higher exercise work loads.[122] The inhibitory effect on gastric emptying is quite small up to an intensity of 70% $\dot{V}O_2$ max and then becomes more important at intensities greater than 80% $\dot{V}O_2$ max.[142] This intensity-linked reduction in gastric emptying may be due to sympathetic inhibition of blood flow and/or gastric motility, and may be partially responsible for the existence of an exercise-intensity threshold (75% $\dot{V}O_2$ max) above which carbohydrate feeding has little effect.

Other factors cited as regulators of gastric emptying include temperature and carbonation. Costill and Saltin[143] originally reported that 5°C solutions were absorbed twice as quickly as 35°C solutions. However, Maughan and Noakes[120] have suggested recently that while cool drinks are more palatable, temperature seems to have little effect on gastric emptying. Similarly, while it was once thought that carbonation would improve gastric emptying of water and carbohydrate, a recent study found little or no effect.[144]

4. Type, Timing, and Rate of Carbohydrate Ingestion

Compared to glucose, sucrose, and glucose polymers, fructose is absorbed less rapidly across the gut, promotes less water uptake, and is metabolized in the liver rather than directly by muscle. Fructose ingestion during exercise results in lower insulin concentrations and lower carbohydrate oxidation than levels reported for other sugars. Since carbohydrate supplements during exercise do not seem to spare glycogen, the lower carbohydrate oxidation may explain why improvements in performance have not been observed with fructose ingestion.[136,145]

Both the timing and rate of carbohydrate ingestion during exercise can influence performance. Carbohydrate supplementation throughout prolonged endurance exercise or provided at least 35 min before the onset of fatigue are both effective in delaying fatigue.[119] Coggan and Coyle[118] suggested that ingesting carbohydrate throughout prolonged exercise may be of greater advantage because of the potential for glycogen resynthesis. Blood glucose concentration is well maintained by supplying supplemental glucose at a rate of 45 g/h during moderate-intensity exercise.[130,146] If the supplementation is provided prior to fatigue during prolonged exercise, the carbohydrate solution should be more concentrated. Recently, Murray and co-workers[147] found no difference in performance after feeding carbohydrate at rates of 26, 52, and 78 g/h during 2 h of moderate-intensity exercise. They concluded that a dose–response relationship does not exist between total carbohydrate ingested and exercise performance. Nevertheless, Coggan and Coyle[118] have recommended that carbohydrate supplementation be sufficient to provide a minimum of 45 to 60 g of total carbohydrate for exercise performance to be improved.

D. Postexercise Diet

Replenishment of liver and muscle glycogen reserves after strenuous physical activity is critical in terms of ability to perform subsequent endurance exercise. This section will discuss the various nutritional factors, including amount, type, and timing of postexercise carbohydrate ingestion, which influence glycogen resynthesis. It should be recalled from Section II of this chapter that only a small fraction of dietary glucose is initially metabolized in the liver. Thus, it appears that muscle glycogen synthesis predominates over liver glycogen synthesis with the ingestion of carbohydrate during recovery.

Blood glucose is the primary precursor for muscle glycogen synthesis and thus must initially be transported across the cell membrane. With the cessation of exercise, the major pathway of glucose disposal in muscle is glycogen synthesis.[59] In 1967, Bergstrom and Hultman[148] reported that the highest rates of glycogen synthesis occur in muscle depleted of its glycogen stores. Work in the early 1970s suggested that following exhaustive exercise, a period greater than 1 d may be required for restoration of glycogen levels to normal.[149,150]

However, more recent work demonstrated that increasing carbohydrate consumption from between 188 to 648 g/d resulted in proportionately greater muscle glycogen resynthesis during the 24-h postexercise period. Muscle glycogen levels could be normalized within 24 h with a carbohydrate intake of 525 to 648 g.[151]

1. Amount and Timing of Postexercise Carbohydrate

Lamb et al.[152] presented data which support the existence of an upper level of carbohydrate intake, ranging from 500 to 600 g/d, above which little additional contribution to glycogen storage or enhancement of athletic performance occurs. Basing carbohydrate intake recommendations on a specific percentage of total energy intake can lead to daily intakes well above this recommended range when overall energy intakes are particularly high. These considerations led to the recommendation that the amount of carbohydrate consumed by athletes is more appropriately based either on total daily consumption (g/d) or, to account for differing body sizes of athletes, total daily consumption per unit body weight (g/kg/d).[31]

A number of recent studies, summarized by Ivy[153] and Friedman et al.,[59] have estimated the upper limit of glycogen synthesis rate for subjects fed varying amounts of carbohydrate immediately following exercise. The overall results suggest that providing 0.7 to 1.0 g glucose/kg body weight every 2 h, for up to 6 h after exhaustive exercise, will maximize glycogen resynthesis rate at between 5 and 8 μmol/g wet weight of muscle tissue/h.[59,153]

This rapid resynthesis of muscle glycogen to near preexercise levels within 24 h has been partially attributed to a glycogen depletion-induced increase in the percentage of the activated I-form of glycogen synthase. Glycogen synthase catalyzes the transfer of glucose from uridine diphosphate–glucose onto the glycogen skeleton which is thought to be the rate-limiting step in glycogen synthesis.[154] As previously discussed, the percentage of synthase in the I form has been shown to be inversely related to the amount of glycogen present in muscle.[155,156] Other critical factors appear to be increases in the permeability of the muscle cell membrane to glucose and in muscle sensitivity to insulin resulting from contractile activity in muscle.[60] For maximal glycogen resynthesis, carbohydrate intake must be high enough to ensure sufficient blood glucose for muscle glucose uptake and sufficient insulin to keep a high percentage of glycogen synthase in the active form.

To determine the effect of relative muscle glycogen depletion on subsequent rate of resynthesis, Zachwieja et al.[156] used one- and two-legged cycling exercise to induce high and low muscle glycogen levels in cyclists. Glycogen resynthesis rate and glycogen synthase activity were higher in the more glycogen-depleted leg. Since both legs were exposed to a similar glucose load, these data suggested glycogenic drive within the muscle, largely dictated by degree of glycogen depletion, was a primary determinant of rate of glycogen resynthesis during postexercise.

The rate of glycogen resynthesis appears to be most rapid in the first 2 h immediately following exercise.[155-157] In addition to the glycogen depletion-induced activation of glycogen synthase, this phenomena may be partially mediated by an increased rate of glucose transport, as there is much evidence which suggests that control of glucose transport across the sarcolemma plays a key role in the overall regulation of glycogen synthesis.[59]

Based on these considerations, maximum glycogen resynthesis should occur when athletes consume carbohydrate soon after exercise, strive to consume the equivalent of 0.7 to 1.5 g glucose/kg body weight ever 2 h during the initial 6 h postexercise,[158,159] and ingest approximately 600 g of carbohydrate during the 24-h postexercise period.[90] High-carbohydrate, low-protein foods or beverages such as fruits, fruit juices, or commercially available carbohydrate drinks are likely to be superior choices for the initial postexercise feedings. Protein ingestion stimulates glucagon secretion,[160] thereby creating a hormonal milieu which may not maximize glycogenesis during recovery from exercise.

2. Type of Postexercise Carbohydrate

The type of carbohydrate consumed following exercise can also affect the rate of muscle glycogen resynthesis. This effect is likely mediated by differential glycemic and insulinemic responses to different carbohydrates. For example, fructose ingestion is associated with markedly lower blood glucose and insulin levels compared to those resulting from glucose or sucrose ingestion.[161] This is consistent with the finding by Blom et al.[158] that glucose and sucrose ingestion were significantly more effective than fructose in promoting postexercise muscle glycogen synthesis. Fructose infusion has led to greater restoration of liver glycogen,[18] which follows from the fact that fructose metabolism is largely confined to the liver.[6]

Potential differences between simple and complex carbohydrates on muscle glycogen resynthesis have also been investigated.[151,162,163] Costill et al.[151] reported that a starch-based diet was more effective than glucose in promoting glycogen synthesis during the second day of recovery from exercise. No differences were observed during the first day nor were any differences observed between simple and complex carbohydrates in the study by Roberts et al.[162] In contrast, simple carbohydrates were demonstrated to promote a greater increase in muscle glycogen content compared to complex carbohydrates during the first 6 h after exercise, but by 20 h postexercise the two diets had produced similar muscle glycogen concentrations.[163]

Unpublished work from Hargreaves' laboratory, recently summarized by Costill and Hargreaves,[90] has bearing on this discussion. Consumption of carbohydrates with a high glycemic index in the 24 h after prolonged exercise resulted in greater glycogen synthesis compared to ingestion of an equivalent amount of low-glycemic-index carbohydrate goods. It is difficult to reconcile this finding with some of the previous work which reported no differential effect of simple vs. complex carbohydrate ingestion on glycogen resynthesis.[151,162] However, the overall data suggest consumption of carbohydrates which maximize glycemic and insulinemic responses (i.e., simple and/or high-glycemic-index carbohydrates) are likely to be most effective for promoting the resynthesis of glycogen immediately following exercise.

3. Muscle Damage and Glycogen Resynthesis

Friedman et al.[59] recently summarized several studies which demonstrated that muscle glycogen resynthesis is impaired following certain types of exercise. Decreased glycogen resynthesis occurs after both eccentric exercise,[164,165] characterized by forced lengthening contraction of muscle, and exhaustive running,[166] which both commonly produce muscle damage and soreness. Decreased availability of glucose for glycogen resynthesis may be attributed to damage to the sarcolemma and subsequent interference with glucose transport.[59] In addition, the inflammatory response to muscle damage results in significantly greater glucose oxidation by white blood cells and promotes release of a factor that stimulates glucose oxidation by the surrounding muscle cells.[165] Thus, Costill et al.[165] suggested that emphasis on high carbohydrate intakes may be of even greater importance after eccentric exercise and exhaustive running because of the potential for this dietary regimen to partially overcome the muscle damage-induced depression of glycogen resynthesis. For additional information regarding the effect of postexercise diet on glycogen resynthesis, see Sherman and Wimer,[31] Friedman et al.,[59] Ivy,[60] Sherman,[94] and Ivy.[153]

VII. SUMMARY

The preferential use of carbohydrate over fat as an energy substrate for exercising muscle is directly related to exercise intensity and initial glycogen levels and inversely related to duration of aerobic exercise and level of physical conditioning. Skeletal muscle glycogen stores and circulating blood glucose originating in liver from glycogenolysis or gluconeo-genesis represent the primary sources of carbohydrate used for energy production by muscle. Glucose derived from muscle glycogen is the most important substrate used during high-intensity anaerobic exercise and during the first 2 h of aerobic exercise. As prolonged exercise continues, the quantitative importance of blood glucose compared to endogenous muscle glycogen as an energy source for muscle oxidation increases. Plasma glucose oxidation can supply 20 to 50% of the total oxidizable substrate during submaximal exercise.

Although plasma glucose is clearly an important energy substrate during prolonged sub-maximal exercise, it should be emphasized that initial skeletal muscle glycogen stores are the primary determinant of one's ability to sustain prolonged moderate to heavy exercise. Glycogen storage in muscle is largely dependent on level of physical conditioning and both the long-term and acute state of carbohydrate nutriture. Trained skeletal muscles have greater glycogen stores which are depleted at a slower rate during exercise.

The dietary manipulation of carbohydrate intake prior to, during, and after exercise can improve exercise performance largely through optimizing muscle and liver glycogen stores or through the maintenance of blood glucose homeostasis. Improved performance is generally associated with maintenance of carbohydrate availability and a high rate of carbohydrate utilization during exercise. Specific recommendations and conclusions related to carbohy-drate intakes are as follows:

1. Individuals who exercise regularly should routinely consume a diet which provides 55 to 70% of the total calories from carbohydrate.
2. The consumption of preexercise meals consisting primarily of low-fiber carbohydrate (solid or liquid) foods, ingested at least 2 to 3 h before the exercise session, can improve performance during endurance-type events.
3. Preexercise carbohydrate ingestion within 1 h of exercise can improve work performance, although some individuals may experience a transient lowering of blood glucose and associated fatigue.
4. Preexercise feedings should contain 1 to 5 g carbohydrate/kg body weight. Liquid carbohydrate intakes at the lower end of this range are better tolerated than solid meals and higher intakes when consumed close to competition, because of shorter gastric emptying time.
5. There appears to be no advantage of preexercise ingestion of fructose over glucose; however, additional research is required to determine whether any advantages accrue from the ingestion of low- compared to high-glycemic-index carbohydrate foods.
6. Carbohydrate supercompensation can improve endurance performance in individuals engaged in continuous exercise for more than 90 min.
7. Carbohydrate ingestion of at least 45 to 60 g during exercise can delay fatigue and improve endurance performance by helping to optimize blood glucose availability.
8. Dilute glucose solutions (5% or less) should be ingested during exercise for optimal hydration because they are emptied from the stomach more quickly than concentrated solutions. However, greater net glucose absorption occurs with increased glucose concentrations in sports drinks.
9. The use of glucose polymer solutions during exercise may be advantageous because of their lower osmolality and potential for more rapid gastric emptying. In contrast, fructose is not the preferred source of carbohydrate because of its relatively slow absorption and its primarily hepatic site of metabolism.
10. Replenishment of liver and muscle glycogen reserves after strenuous physical activity can occur within 24 h and is critical in terms of ability to perform subsequent endurance exercise.
11. Maximum glycogen resynthesis occurs when individuals ingest carbohydrate soon after exercise, strive to consume the equivalent of 0.7 to 1.5 g glucose/kg body weight every 2 h during the initial 6 h postexercise, and ingest approximately 600 g of carbohydrate during the 24-h postex-ercise period.

12. Postexercise ingestion of fructose compared to glucose induces more liver glycogen synthesis but less muscle glycogen synthesis.
13. There is some evidence that the ingestion of carbohydrates which maximize glycemic and insulinemic responses (i.e., simple and/or high-glycemic-index carbohydrates) are most effective for promoting the resynthesis of glycogen immediately following exercise.

REFERENCES

1. National Research Council Subcommittee on the Tenth Edition of the RDAs, *Recommended Dietary Allowances*, 10th ed., National Academy Press, Washington, D.C., 1989, chap. 4.
2. U.S. Department of Agriculture, Nationwide Food Consumption Survey. Continuing Survey of Food Intakes by Individuals: Men 19–50 Years, 1 Day. 1985. Report No. 85-3. Nutrition Monitoring Division, Human Nutrition Information Service, U.S. Department of Agriculture, Hyattsville, MD, 1986.
3. U.S. Department of Agriculture, Nationwide Food Consumption Survey. Continuing Survey of Food Intakes by Individuals: Women 19–50 Years and Their Children 1–5 Years, 4 Days, 1985. Report 85-4. Nutrition Monitoring Division, Human Nutrition Information Service, U.S. Department of Agriculture, Hyattsville, MD, 1987.
4. **Pike, R. L. and Brown, M. L.,** *Nutrition. An Integrated Approach,* 3rd ed., John Wiley & Sons, New York, 1984, chap. 6.
5. **Cori, C. F.,** The fate of sugar in the animal body. I. The rate of absorption of hexoses and pentoses from the intestinal tract. *J. Biol. Chem.,* 66, 691, 1925.
6. **MacDonald, I.,** Carbohydrates, in *Modern Nutrition in Health and Disease,* 7th ed., Shils, M. E. and Young, V. R., Eds., Lea & Febiger, Philadelphia, 1988, chap. 2.
7. **Goodman, M. N.,** Amino acid and protein metabolism, in *Exercise, Nutrition and Energy Metabolism,* Horton, E. S. and Terjung, R. L., Eds., Macmillan, New York, 1988, chap. 6.
8. **Murray, R. K., Granner, D. K., Mayes, P. A., and Rodwell, V. W.,** *Harper's Biochemistry,* 22nd ed., Appleton & Lange, Norwalk, CT, 1990, chap. 20.
9. **Saltin, B. and Gollnick, P. D.,** Skeletal muscle adaptability: significance for metabolism and performance, in *Handbook of Physiology,* Peachy, L. D., Adrian, R. H., and Geiger, S. R., Eds., Williams & Wilkins, Baltimore, 1983, 555.
10. **Murray, R. K., Granner, D. K., Mayes, P. A., and Rodwell, V. W.,** *Harper's Biochemistry,* 22nd ed., Appleton & Lange, Norwalk, CT, 1990, chap. 21.
11. **Nilsson, L. H. and Hultman, E.,** Liver glycogen in man: the effect of total starvation or a carbohydrate-poor diet followed by carbohydrate refeeding, *Scand. J. Clin. Lab. Invest.,* 32, 325, 1973.
12. **Felig, P., Pozefsky, T., Marliss, E., and Cahill, G. F.,** Alanine: key role in gluconeogenesis, *Science,* 167, 1003, 1970.
13. **Felig, P. and Wahren, J.,** Amino acid metabolism in exercising man, *J. Clin. Invest.,* 50, 2703, 1971.
14. **Foster, D. W.,** From glycogen to ketones — and back, *Diabetes,* 33, 1188, 1984.
15. **McGarrey, J. D., Kuwajima, M., Newgard, C. B., and Foster, D. W.,** From dietary glucose to liver glycogen: the full circle round, *Annu. Rev. Nutr.,* 7, 51, 1987.
16. **Radziuk, J.,** Sources of carbon in hepatic glycogen synthesis during absorption of an oral glucose load in humans, *Fed. Proc.,* 41, 110, 1982.
17. **Maehlum, S., Felig, P., and Wahren, J.,** Splanchnic glucose and muscle glycogen metabolism after glucose feeding during post exercise recovery, *Am. J. Physiol.,* 235, E255, 1978.
18. **Nilsson, L. H. and Hultman, E.,** Liver and muscle glycogen in man after glucose and fructose infusion, *Scand. J. Clin. Lab. Invest.,* 33, 5, 1974.
19. **Murray, R. K., Granner, D. K., Mayes, P. A., and Rodwell, V. W.,** *Harper's Biochemistry,* 22nd ed., Appleton & Lange, Norwalk, CT, 1990, chap. 19.
20. **Saltin, B. and Gollnick, P. D.,** Fuel for muscular exercise: role of carbohydrate, in *Exercise, Nutrition and Energy Metabolism,* Horton, E. S. and Terjung, R. L., Eds., Macmillan, New York, 1988, chap. 4.
21. **McArdle, W. D., Katch, F. I., and Katch, V. I.,** *Exercise Physiology: Energy, Nutrition, and Human Performance,* Lea & Febiger, Philadelphia, 1991, 123.
22. **Stanley, W. C. and Connett, R. J.,** Regulation of muscle carbohydrate metabolism during exercise, *FASEB J.,* 5, 2155, 1991.

23. **Katch, F. I. and McArdle, W. D.**, *Nutrition, Weight Control, and Exercise,* Lea & Febiger, Philadelphia, 1988, 53.

24. **Fox, E. L., Bowers, R. W., and Foss, M. L.**, *The Physiological Basis of Physical Education and Athletics,* W. B. Saunders, Philadelphia, 1988, 11.

25. **Phinney, S. D., Bistrian, B. R., Evans, W. J., Gervino, E., and Blackburn, G. L.**, The human metabolic response to chronic ketosis without caloric restriction: preservation of submaximal exercise capacity with reduced carbohydrate oxidation, *Metabolism,* 32, 769, 1983.

26. **Gollnick, P. D. and Saltin, B.**, Fuel for muscular exercise: role of fat, in *Exercise, Nutrition and Energy Metabolism,* Horton, E. S. and Terjung, R. L., Eds., Macmillan, New York, 1988, chap. 5.

27. **Holloszy, J. O.**, Utilization of fatty acids during exercise, in *Biochemistry of Exercise VII,* Taylor, A. W., Gollnick, P. D., Green, H. J., Ianuzzo, C. D., Noble, E. G., Métivier, G., and Sutton, J. R., Eds., Human Kinetics Books, Champaign, IL, 1990, 319.

28. **Bergstrom, J., Hermansen, L., Hultman, E., and Saltin, B.**, Diet, muscle glycogen and physical performance, *Acta Physiol. Scand.,* 71, 140, 1967.

29. **Hermansen, L., Hultman, E., and Saltin, B.**, Muscle glycogen during prolonged severe exercise, *Acta Physiol. Scand.,* 71, 129, 1967.

30. **Saltin, B. and Karlsson, J.**, Muscle glycogen utilization during work of different intensities, in *Muscle Metabolism During Exercise,* Pernow, B. and Saltin, B., Eds., Plenum Press, New York, 1971, 289.

31. **Sherman, W. M. and Wimer, G. S.**, Insufficient dietary carbohydrate during training: does it impair athletic performance?, *Int. J. Sport Nutr.,* 1, 28, 1991.

32. **Wahren, J. P., Felig, P., Ahlborg, G., and Jorfeldt, L.**, Glucose metabolism during leg exercise in man, *J. Clin. Invest.,* 50, 2715, 1971.

33. **Hickson, R. C.**, Carbohydrate metabolism in exercise, in *Ross Symposium on Nutrient Utilization During Exercise,* Fox, E. L., Ed., Ross Laboratories, Columbus, OH, 1983, 1.

34. **Jorfeldt, L. and Wahren, J.**, Leg blood flow during exercise in man, *Clin. Sci.,* 41, 459, 1971.

35. **Coggan, A. R.**, Plasma glucose metabolism during exercise in humans, *Sports Med.,* 11, 102, 1991.

36. **Björkman, O. and Wahren, J.**, Glucose homeostasis during and after exercise, in *Exercise, Nutrition and Energy Metabolism,* Horton, E. S. and Terjung, R. L., Eds., Macmillan, New York, 1988, chap. 7.

37. **Ahlborg, B., Bergstrom, J., Ekelund, L., and Hultman, E.**, Muscle glycogen and muscle electrolytes during prolonged physical exercise, *Acta Physiol. Scand.,* 70, 129, 1967.

38. **Baldwin, K. M., Reitman, J. S., Terjung, R. L., Winder, W. W., and Holloszy, J. O.**, Substrate depletion in differernt types of muscle and in liver during prolonged running, *Am. J. Physiol.,* 225, 1045, 1973.

39. **Ahlborg, G., Felig, P., Hagenfeldt, L., Hendler, R., and Wahren, J.**, Substrate turnover during prolonged exercise in man: splanchnic and leg metabolism of glucose, free fatty acids, and amino acids, *J. Clin. Invest.,* 53, 1080, 1974.

40. **Ahlborg, G. and Felig, P.**, Lactate and glucose exchange across the forearm, legs, and splanchnic bed during and after prolonged leg exercise, *J. Clin. Invest.,* 69, 45, 1982.

41. **Pruett, E. D. R.**, Glucose and insulin during prolonged work stress in men living on different diets, *J. Appl. Physiol.,* 28, 199, 1970.

42. **Coyle, E. F., Hagberg, J. M., Hurley, B. F., Martin, W. H., Ehsani, A. A., and Holloszy, J. O.**, Carbohydrate feeding during prolonged strenuous exercise can delay fatigue, *J. Appl. Physiol.,* 55, 230, 1983.

43. **Holloszy, J. O.**, Metabolic consequences of endurance exercise training, in *Exercise, Nutrition and Energy Metabolism,* Horton, E. S. and Terjung, R. L., Eds., Macmillan, New York, 1988, chap. 8.

44. **Coggan, A. R., Kohrt, W. M., Spina, R. J., Bier, D. M., and Holloszy, J. O.**, Endurance training decreases plasma glucose turnover and oxidation during moderate-intensity exercise in men, *J. Appl. Physiol.,* 68, 990, 1990.

45. **Coleman, E.**, Carbohydrates: the master fuel, in *Sports Nutrition for the 90s,* Berning, J. R. and Steen, S. N., Eds., Aspen Publishers, Gaithersburg, MD, 1991, chap. 3.

46. **Gollnick, P. D., Piehl, K., Saubert, C. W., Armstrong, R. B., and Saltin, B.**, Diet, exercise, and glycogen changes in human muscle fibers, *J. Appl. Physiol.,* 33, 421, 1972.

47. **Hultman, E.**, Regulation of carbohydrate metabolism in the liver during rest and exercise with special reference to diet, in *Biochemistry of Exercise III,* Landry, F. and Orban, W. A. R., Eds., Symposia Specialists, Miami, 1977.

48. **Brooks, G. A.**, The lactate shuttle during exercise and recovery, *Med. Sci. Sports Exercise,* 18, 360, 1986.

49. **Stainsby, W. N. and Brooks, G. A.**, Control of lactic acid metabolism in contracting muscles and during exercise, in *Exercise and Sport Sciences Reviews,* Vol. 18, Pandolf, K. B., Ed., Williams & Wilkins, Baltimore, 1990, 29.

50. **Donaldson, S. K. B. and Hermansen, L.,** Differential, direct effects of H^+ on Ca^{2+}-activated force of skinned fibers from the soleus, cardiac and adductor magnus muscles of rabbits, *Pflügers Arch.,* 376, 55, 1978.

51. **Fitts, R. H. and Metzger, J. M.,** Mechanisms of muscular fatigue, in *Principles of Exercise Biochemistry,* Poortmans, J. R., Ed., S. Karger, Basel, Switzerland, 1988, 212.

52. **Ren, J. M. and Hultman, E.,** Regulation of glycogenolysis in human skeletal muscle, *J. Appl. Physiol.,* 76, 2243, 1989.

53. **Richter, E. A. and Galbo, H.,** High glycogen levels enhance glycogen breakdown in isolated contracting skeletal muscle, *J. Appl. Physiol.,* 61, 827, 1986.

54. **Conlee, R. K., McLane, J. A., Rennie, M. J., Winder, W. W., and Holloszy, J. O.,** Reversal of phosphorylase activation in muscle despite continued contractile activity, *Am. J. Physiol.,* 237, R291, 1979.

55. **Katz, A., Broberg, S., Sahlin, K., and Wahren, J.,** Leg glucose uptake during maximal dynamic exercise in humans, *Am. J. Physiol.,* 251, E65, 1986.

56. **Hutber, C. A. and Bonen, A.,** Glycogenesis in muscle and liver during exercise, *J. Appl. Physiol.,* 66, 2811, 1989.

57. **Kuipers, H., Keizer, H. A., Brouns, F., and Saris, W. H. M.,** Carbohydrate feeding and glycogen synthesis during exercise in man, *Pflügers Arch.,* 410, 652, 1987.

58. **Kuipers, H., Saris, W. H. M., Brouns, F., Keizer, H. A., and ten Bosch, C.,** Glycogen synthesis during exercise and rest with carbohydrate feeding in males and females, *Int. J. Sports Med.,* 10, S63, 1989.

59. **Friedman, J. E., Neufer, P. D., and Dohm, G. L.,** Regulation of glycogen resynthesis following exercise, *Sports Med.,* 11, 232, 1991.

60. **Ivy, J. L.,** Muscle glycogen synthesis before and after exercise, *Sports Med.,* 11, 6, 1991.

61. **Friedman, J. E., Sherman, W. M., Reed, M. J., Elton, C. W., and Dohm, G. L.,** Exercise training increases glucose transporter protein (GLUT 4) in skeletal muscle of obese Zucker (fa/fa) rats, *FEBS Lett.,* 268, 13, 1990.

62. **Cartee, G. D., Young, D. A., Sleeper, M. D., Zierath, J., and Wallberg-Henriksson, H.,** Prolonged increase in insulin stimulated glucose transport in muscle after exercise, *Am. J. Physiol.,* 256, E494, 1989.

63. **Richter, E. A., Garetto, L. P., Goodman, M. N., and Ruderman, N. B.,** Muscle glucose metabolism following exercise in the rat: increased sensitivity to insulin, *J. Clin. Invest.,* 69, 785, 1982.

64. **Richter, E. A., Hanson, S. A., and Hanson, B. F.,** Mechanisms limiting glycogen storage in muscle during prolonged insulin stimulation, *Am. J. Physiol.,* 255, E621, 1988.

65. **Zorzano, A., Balon, T. W., Goodman, M. N., and Ruderman, N. B.,** Additive effects of prior exercise and insulin on glucose and AIB uptake by rat muscle, *Am. J. Physiol.,* 252, E21, 1986.

66. **Stanley, W. C., Wisneski, J. A., Gertz, E. W., Neese, R. A., and Brooks, G. A.,** Glucose and lactate interrelations during moderate-intensity exercise in humans, *Metabolism,* 37, 850, 1988.

67. **Kjaer, M., Engfred, K., Fernandes, A., Secher, N., and Galbo, H.,** Influence of sympathoadrenergic activity on hepatic glucose production during exercise in man, *Med. Sci. Sports Exercise,* 22, S81, 1990.

68. **Hoelzer, D. R., Dalsky, G. P., Clutter, W. E., Shah, S. D., Schwartz, N. S., and Holloszy, J. O.,** Glucoregulation during exercise: hypoglycemia is prevented by redundant glucoregulatory systems, sympathochromaffin activation, and changes in islet hormone secretion, *J. Clin. Invest.,* 77, 212, 1986.

69. **Hoelzer, D. R., Dalsky, G. P., Schwartz, N. S., Clutter, W. E., Shah, S. D., and Holloszy, J. O.,** Epinephrine is not critical to prevention of hypoglycemia during exercise in humans, *Am. J. Physiol.,* 251, E104, 1986.

70. **Freude, K. A., Sandler, L. S., and Zieve, F. J.,** Electrical stimulation of the liver cell: activation of glycogenolysis, *Am. J. Physiol.,* 240, E226, 1981.

71. **Vranic, M. and Lickely, H. L. A.,** Hormonal mechanisms that act to preserve glucose homeostasis during exercise, in *Biochemistry of Exercise VII,* Taylor, A. W., Gollnick, P. D., Green, H. J., Ianuzzo, C. D., Noble, E. G., Métivier, G., and Sutton, J. R., Eds., Human Kinetics Books, Champaign, IL, 1990, 279.

72. **Plough, T., Galbo, H., and Richter, E. A.,** Increased muscle glucose uptake during contraction: no need for insulin, *Am. J. Physiol.,* 247, E276, 1984.

73. **Wallberg-Henriksson, H., and Holloszy, J. D.,** Contractile activity increases glucose uptake by muscle in severely diabetic rats, *J. Appl. Physiol.,* 57, 1045, 1984.

74. **Bonen, A., McDermott, J. C., and Tan, M. H.,** Glucose transport in skeletal muscle, in *Biochemistry of Exercise VII,* Taylor, A. W., Gollnick, P. D., Green, H. J., Ianuzzo, C. D., Noble, E. G., Métivier, G., and Sutton, J. R., Eds., Human Kinetics Books, Champaign, IL, 1990, 295.

75. **Bonen, A., Tan, M. H., and Watson-Wright, W. M.,** Insulin binding and glucose uptake differences in rodent skeletal muscles, *Diabetes,* 30, 702, 1981.

76. **Bonen, A., Tan, M. H., and Watson-Wright, W. M.,** Effects of exercise on insulin binding and glucose metabolism in muscle, *Can. J. Physiol. Pharmacol.,* 62, 1500, 1984.

77. **James, D. E., Kraegen, E. W., and Chisholm, D. J.,** Muscle glucose metabolism in exercising rats: comparison with insulin stimulation, *Am. J. Physiol.,* 248, E575, 1985.

78. **Berger, M., Hagg, S., and Ruderman, N. B.,** Glucose metabolism in perfused skeletal muscle: interaction of insulin and exercise on glucose uptake, *Biochem. J.,* 146, 321, 1975.

79. **Vranic, M., Kawamori, R., Pek, S., Kovacevic, N., and Wrenshall, G. A.,** The essentiality of insulin and the role of glucagon in regulating glucose utilization and production during strenuous exercise in dogs, *J. Clin. Invest.,* 57, 245, 1976.

80. **Goodyear, L. J., King, P. A., Hirshman, M. F., Thompson, C. M., Horton, E. D., and Horton, H. S.,** Contractile activity increases plasma membrane glucose transporters in absence of insulin, *Am. J. Physiol.,* 258, E667, 1990.

81. **Richter, E. A., Plough, T., and Galbo, H.,** Increased muscle glucose uptake after exercise: no need for insulin during exercise, *Diabetes,* 34, 1041, 1985.

82. **Nesher, R., Karl, I. E., and Kipnis, D. M.,** Dissociation of effects of insulin and contraction on glucose transport in rat epitrochlearis muscle, *Am. J. Physiol.,* 249, C226, 1985.

83. **Holloszy, J. O., Constable, S. H., and Young, D. A.,** Activation of glucose transport in muscle by exercise, *Diabetes Metab. Rev.,* 1, 409, 1986.

84. **Douen, A. G., Ramial, T., Klip, A., Young, D. A., Cartee, G. D., and Holloszy, J. O.,** Exercise-induced increase in glucose transporter in plasma membranes of rat skeletal muscle, *Endocrinology,* 124, 449, 1989.

85. **Douen, A. G., Ramial, T., Rastogi, S., Bilan, P. J., Cartee, G. D., Vranic, M., Holloszy, J. O., and Klip, A.,** Exercise induces recruitment of the "insulin-responsive glucose transporter", *J. Biol. Chem.,* 265, 13427, 1990.

86. **Klip, A., Ramial, T., Young, A., and Holloszy, J. O.,** Insulin-induced translocation of glucose transporters in rat hindlimb muscles, *FEBS Lett.,* 224, 224, 1987.

87. **Klip, A. and Paquet, M. R.,** Glucose transport and glucose transporters in muscle and their metabolic regulation, *Diabetes Care,* 13, 228, 1990.

88. **Treadway, J. L., James, D. E., Burcel, E., and Ruderman, N. B.,** Effect of exercise on insulin receptor binding and kinase activity in skeletal muscle, *Am. J. Physiol.,* 256, E138, 1989.

89. **Sherman, W.,** Carbohydrates, muscle glycogen and muscle glycogen supercompensation, in *Ergogenic Aids in Sports,* Williams, M. H., Ed., Human Kinetics Publishers, Champaign, IL, 1983, 3.

90. **Costill, D. L. and Hargreaves, M.,** Carbohydrate nutrition and fatigue, *Sports Med.,* 13, 86, 1992.

91. **Hoffman, C. J. and Coleman, E.,** An eating plan and update on recommended dietary practices for the endurance athlete, *J. Am. Diet. Assoc.,* 91, 325, 1991.

92. **Coleman, E.,** *Eating for Endurance,* Bull Publishing, Palo Alto, CA, 1988, chap. 4.

93. **Clark, N.,** *Nancy Clark's Sports Nutrition Guidebook: Eating to Fuel Your Active Lifestyle,* Leisure Press, Champaign, IL, 1990, 114.

94. **Sherman, W. M.,** Carbohydrate feedings before and after exercise, in *Ergogenics — Enhancement of Performance in Exercise and Sport,* Lamb, D. R. and Williams, M. H., Eds., Benchmark Press, Carmel, IN, 1991, 1.

95. **Costill, D. L., Coyle, E., Dalsky, G., Evans, W., Fink, W., and Hoopes, D.,** Effects of elevated plasma FFA and insulin on muscle glycogen usage during exercise, *J. Appl. Physiol.,* 43, 695, 1977.

96. **Koivisto, V. A., Karvonen, S., and Nikkilä, E. A.,** Carbohydrate ingestion before exercise: comparison of glucose, fructose, and sweet placebo, *J. Appl. Physiol.,* 51, 783, 1981.

97. **Foster, C., Costill, D. L., and Fink, W. J.,** Effects of preexercise feeding on endurance performance, *Med. Sci. Sports,* 11, 1, 1979.

98. **Keller, K. and Schwarzkopf, R.,** Preexercise snacks may decrease exercise performance, *Phys. Sportsmed.,* 12, 89, 1984.

99. **Coyle, E. F., Coggan, A. R., Hemmert, M. K., Lowe, R. C., and Walters, T. J.,** Substrate usage during prolonged exercise following a pre-exercise meal, *J. Appl. Physiol.,* 59, 429, 1985.

100. **Sherman, W. M. and Wright, D. A.,** Preevent nutriton for prolonged exercise, in *The Theory and Practice of Athletic Nutrition: Bridging the Gap,* Grandjean, A. C. and Storlie, J., Eds., Report of the Ross Symposium, Ross Laboratories, Columbus, OH, 1989, 30.

101. **Costill, D. L.,** Carbohydrate for athletic training and performance, *Cont. Nutr.,* 15(9), 1990.

102. **Gleeson, M., Maughan, R. J., and Greenhaff, P. L.,** Comparison of the effects of pre-exercise feeding of glucose, glycerol and placebo on endurance and fuel homeostasis in man, *Eur. J. Appl. Physiol.,* 55, 645, 1986.

103. **Neufer, P. D., Costill, D. L., Flynn, M. G., Kirwan, J. P., Mitchell, J. B., and Houmard, J.,** Improvements in exercise performance: effects of carbohydrate feeding and diet, *J. Appl. Physiol.,* 62, 983, 1987.

104. **Sherman, W. M., Peden, M. C., and Wright, D. A.,** Carbohydrate feeding 1 hr before exercise improves cycling performance, *Am. J. Clin. Nutr.,* 54, 866, 1991.
105. **Hargreaves, M., Costill, D. L., Fink, W. J., King, D. S., and Fielding, R. A.,** Effect of pre-exercise carbohydrate feedings on endurance cycling performance, *Med. Sci. Sports Exercise,* 19, 33, 1987.
106. **Devlin, J. T., Calles-Escandon, J., and Horton, E. S.,** Effects of preexercise snack feeding on endurance cycle exercise, *J. Appl. Physiol.,* 60, 980, 1986.
107. **Decombaz, J., Sartori, D., Arnaud, M. J., Thelin, A. L., Schurch, P., and Howard, H.,** Oxidation and metabolic effects of fructose or glucose ingested before exercise, *Int. J. Sports Med.,* 6, 282, 1985.
108. **Ravich, W. J., Bayless, T. M., and Thomas, M.,** Fructose: incomplete intestinal absorption in humans, *Gastroenterology,* 84, 26, 1983.
109. **Jenkins, D. J. A., Wolever, T. M. S., Taylor, R. H., Barker, H., Fielden, A., Baldwin, J. M., Bowling, J. M., Newman, H. C., Jenkins, A. L., and Goff, D. V.,** Glycemic index of foods: a physiological basis for carbohydrate exchange, *Am. J. Clin. Nutr.,* 34, 184, 1981.
110. **Thomas, D. E., Brotherhood, J. R., and Brand, J. C.,** Carbohydrate feeding before exercise: effect of glycemic index, *Int. J. Sports Med.,* 12, 180, 1991.
111. **Hollenbeck, C. B. and Coulston, A. M.,** The clinical utility of the glycemic index and its application to mixed meals, *Can. J. Physiol. Pharmacol.,* 69, 100, 1991.
112. **Jarvis, J. K., Pearsall, D., Oliner, C. M., and Schoeller, D. A.,** The effect of food matrix on carbohydrate utilization during moderate exercise, *Med. Sci. Sports Exercise,* 24, 320, 1992.
113. **Sherman, W. M. and Costill, D. L.,** The marathon: dietary manipulation to optimize performance, *Am. J. Sports Med.,* 12, 44, 1984.
114. **Sherman, W. M., Costill, D. L., Fink, W. J., and Miller, J. M.,** The effect of exercise and diet manipulation on muscle glycogen and its subsequent utilization during performance, *Int. J. Sports Med.,* 2, 114, 1981.
115. **Lamb, D. R. and Snyder, A. C.,** Muscle glycogen loading with a liquid carbohydrate supplement, *Int. J. Sport Nutr.,* 1, 52, 1991.
116. **McArdle, W. D., Katch, F. I., and Katch, V. I.,** *Exercise Physiology: Energy, Nutrition, and Human Performance,* Lea & Febiger, Philadelphia, 1991, 516.
117. **Fox, E. L., Bowers, R. W., and Foss, M. L.,** *The Physiological Basis of Physical Education and Athletics,* W. B. Saunders, Phiadelphia, 1988, 544.
118. **Coggan, A. R. and Coyle, E. F.,** Carbohydrate ingestion during prolonged exercise: effects on metabolism and performance, *Exercise Sport Sci. Rev.,* 19, 1, 1991.
119. **Coyle, E. F.,** Carbohydrate supplementation during exercise, *J. Nutr.,* 122, 788, 1992.
120. **Maughan, R. J. and Noakes, T. D.,** Fluid replacement and exercise stress, *Sports Med.,* 12, 16, 1991.
121. **Maughan, R. J.,** Carbohydrate-electrolyte solutions during prolonged exercise, in *Ergogenics — Enhancement of Performance in Exercise and Sport,* Lamb, D. R. and Williams, M. H., Eds., Benchmark Press, Carmel, IN, 1991, 35.
122. **Noakes, T, D., Rehrer, N. J., and Maughan, R. J.,** The importance of volume in regulating gastric emptying, *Med. Sci. Sports Exercise,* 23, 307, 1991.
123. **Coyle, E. F., Coggan, A. R., Hemmert, M. K., and Ivy, J. L.,** Muscle glycogen utilization during prolonged strenuous exercise when fed carbohydrates, *J. Appl. Physiol.,* 61, 165, 1986.
124. **Flynn, M. G., Costill, D. L., Hawley, J. A., Fink, W. J., Neufer, P. D., Fielding, R. A., and Sleeper, M. D.,** Influence of selected carbohydrate drinks on cycling performance and glycogen use, *Med. Sci. Sports Exercise,* 19, 37, 1987.
125. **Mitchell, J. B., Costill, D. L., Houmard, J. A., Fink, W. J., Pascoe, D. D., and Pearson, D. R.,** Influence of carbohydrate dosage on exercise performance and glycogen metabolism, *J. Appl. Physiol.,* 67, 1843, 1989.
126. **Noakes, T. F., Lambert, E. V., Lambert, M. I., McArthur, P. S., Myburgh, K. H., and Benade, A. J. S.,** Carbohydrate ingestion and muscle glycogen depletion during marathon and ultramarathon racing, *Eur. J. Appl. Physiol.,* 57, 482, 1988.
127. **Coyle, E. F., Hamilton, M. T., Alonso, J. G., Montain, S. J., and Ivy, J. L.,** Carbohydrate metabolism during intense exercise when hyperglycemic, *J. Appl. Physiol.,* 70, 834, 1991.
128. **Kuipers, H., Keizer, H. A., Brouns, F., and Saris, W. H. M.,** Carbohydrate feeding and glycogen synthesis during exercise in man, *Pflügers Arch.,* 410, 652, 1987.
129. **Kuipers, H., Saris, W. H. M., Brouns, F., Keizer, H. A., and ten Bosch, C.,** Glycogen synthesis during exercise and rest with carbohydrate feeding in males and females, *Int. J. Sports Med.,* 10, S63, 1989.
130. **Coggan, A. R. and Coyle, E. F.,** Reversal of fatigue during prolonged exercise by carbohydrate infusion or ingestion, *J. Appl. Physiol.,* 63, 2388, 1987.
131. **Denster, P. A., Singh, A., Hofmann, A., Moses, F. M., and Chronsos, G. C.,** Hormonal responses to ingesting water or a carbohydrate beverage during a 2 h run, *Med. Sci. Sports Exercise,* 24, 72, 1992.

132. **Maughan, R. J., Leiper, J. B., and McGaw, B. A.,** Effects of exercise intensity on absorption of ingested fluids in man, *Exp. Physiol.,* 75, 419, 1990.

133. **Coggan, A. R. and Coyle, E. F.,** Effect of carbohydrate feedings during high-intensity exercise, *J. Appl. Physiol.,* 63, 2388, 1988.

134. **Mitchell, J. B., Costill, D. L., Houmard, J. A., Flynn, M. G., Fink, W. J., and Beltz, J. D.,** Effects of carbohydrate ingestion on gastric emptying and exercise performance, *Med. Sci. Sports Exercise,* 20, 110, 1988.

135. **Murray, R.,** The effects of consuming carbohydrate-electrolyte beverages on gastric emptying and fluid absorption during and following exercise, *Sports Med.,* 4, 322, 1987.

136. **Murray, R., Paul, G. L., Seifert, J. G., Eddy, D. E., and Halaby, G. A.,** The effect of glucose, fructose and sucrose ingestion during exercise, *Med. Sci. Sports Exercise,* 21, 275, 1989.

137. **Rehrer, N. J., Beckers, E., Brouns, F., Ten Hoor, F., and Saris, W. H. M.,** Exercise and training effects on gastric emptying of carbohydrate beverages, *Med. Sci. Sports Exercise,* 21, 540, 1989.

138. **Rehrer, N. J., Brouns, F., Beckers, E., Ten Hoor, F., and Saris, H. M.,** Gastric emptying with repeated drinking during running and bicycling, *Int. J. Sports Med.,* 11, 238, 1990.

139. **Mitchell, J. B. and Voss, K. W.,** The influence of volume of fluid ingested on gastric emptying and body fluid balance, *Med. Sci. Sports Exercise,* 22, S90, 1990.

140. **Mitchell, J. B., Costill, D. L., Houmard, J. A., Fink, W. J., Robergs, R. A., and Davis, J. A.,** Gastric emptying: influence of prolonged exercise and carbohydrate concentration, *Med. Sci. Sports Exercise,* 21, 269, 1989.

141. **Sole, C. C. and Noakes, T. D.,** Faster gastric emptying for glucose-polymer and fructose solutions than for glucose in humans, *Eur. J. Appl. Physiol.,* 58, 605, 1989.

142. **Foster, C.,** Gastric emptying during exercise. Influence of carbohydrate concentration, carbohydrate source, and exercise intensity, in *Fluid Replacement and Heat Stress,* National Academy of Sciences, Washington, D.C., 1990, chap. 6.

143. **Costill, D. L. and Saltin, B.,** Factors limiting gastric emptying during rest and exercise, *J. Appl. Physiol.,* 37, 679, 1974.

144. **Zachwieja, J. L., Costill, D. L., Widrick, J. J., Anderson, D. E., and McConell, G. K.,** Effects of drink carbonation on the gastric emptying characteristics of water and flavored water, *Int. J. Sports Nutr.,* 1, 45, 1991.

145. **Massicotte, D., Peronnet, F., Brisson, G., Bakkouch, K., and Hilliare-Marcel, C.,** Oxidation of a glucose polymer during exercise: comparison of glucose and fructose, *J. Appl. Physiol.,* 66, 179, 1989.

146. **Murray, R., Seifert, J. G., Eddy, D. E., Paul, G. L., and Halaby, G. A.,** Carbohydrate feeding and exercise: effect of beverage carbohydrate content, *Eur. J. Appl. Physiol.,* 59, 152, 1989.

147. **Murray, R., Paul, G. L., Seifert, J. G., and Eddy, D. E.,** Responses to varying rates of carbohydrate ingestion during exercise, *Med. Sci. Sports Exercise,* 23, 713, 1991.

148. **Bergstrom, J. and Hultman, E.,** Muscle glycogen synthesis after exercise: an enhancing factor localized to the muscle cells in man, *Nature,* 210, 309, 1966.

149. **Piehl, K.,** Time course for refilling of glycogen stores in human muscle fibers following exercise-induced glycogen depletion, *Acta Physiol. Scand.,* 90, 297, 1974.

150. **Costill, D. L., Bowers, R., Branam, G., and Sparks, K.,** Muscle glycogen utilization during prolonged exercise on successive days, *J. Appl. Physiol.,* 31, 834, 1971.

151. **Costill, D. L., Sherman, W. M., Fink, W. J., Maresh, C., Witten, M., and Miller, J. M.,** The role of dietary carbohydrates in muscle glycogen resynthesis after strenuous running, *Am. J. Clin. Nutr.,* 34, 1831, 1981.

152. **Lamb, D. R., Rinehardt, K. F., Bartels, R. L., Sherman, W. M., and Snook, J. T.,** Dietary carbohydrate and intensity of interval swim training, *Am. J. Clin. Nutr.,* 52, 1058, 1990.

153. **Ivy, J. L.,** Carbohydrate supplementation for rapid muscle glycogen storage in the hours immediately after exercise, in *The Theory and Practice of Athletic Nutrition: Bridging the Gap,* Grandjean, A. C. and Storlie, J., Eds., Report of the Ross Symposium, Ross Laboratories, Columbus, OH, 1989, 47.

154. **Soderling, T. R. and Park, C. R.,** Recent advances in glycogen metabolism, in *Advances in Cyclic Nucleotide Research,* Vol. 4, Greengard, P. and Robinson, G. A., Eds., Raven Press, New York, 1974, 283.

155. **Conlee, R. K., Hickson, R. C., Winder, W. W., Hagberg, J. M., and Holloszy, J. O.,** Regulation of glycogen resynthesis in muscles of rats following exercise, *Am. J. Physiol.,* 235, R145, 1978.

156. **Zachwieja, J. J., Costill, D. L., Pascoe, D. D., Robergts, R. A., and Fink, W. J.,** Influence of muscle glycogen depletion on the rate of resynthesis, *Med. Sci. Sports Exercise,* 23, 445, 1991.

157. **Ivy, J. L., Katz, A. L., Cutler, C. L., Sherman, W. M., and Coyle, E. F.,** Muscle glycogen synthesis after exercise: effect of time of carbohydrate ingestion, *J. Appl. Physiol.,* 64, 1480, 1988.

158. **Blom, P. C. S., Hostmark, A. T., Vaage, O., Kardel, K. R., and Maehlum, S.,** Effect of different post-exercise sugar diets on the rate of muscle glycogen synthesis, *Med. Sci. Sports Exercise,* 19, 491, 1987.

159. **Ivy, J. L., Lee, M. C., Brozinick, J. T., and Reed, M. J.,** Muscle glycogen storage after different amounts of carbohydrate ingestion, *J. Appl. Physiol.,* 65, 2018, 1988.

160. **Westphal, S. A., Gannon, M. C., and Nuttall, F. Q.,** Metabolic response to glucose ingested with various amounts of protein, *Am. J. Clin. Nutr.,* 52, 267, 1990.

161. **Vrana, A. and Fabry, P.,** Metabolic effects of high sucrose or fructose intake, *World Rev. Nutr. Diet.,* 42, 56, 1983.

162. **Roberts, K. M., Nobel, E. G., Hayden, D. B., and Taylor, A. W.,** Simple and complex carbohydrate-rich diets and muscle glycogen content of marathon runners, *Eur. J. Appl. Physiol.,* 57, 70, 1988.

163. **Kiens, B., Raben, A. B., Valeur, A. K., and Richter, E. A.,** Benefit of dietary simple carbohydrates on the early postexercise muscle glycogen repletion in male athletes, *Med. Sci. Sports Exercise,* 22, S88, 1990.

164. **O'Reilly, K. P., Warhol, M. J., Fielding, R. A., Frontera, W. R., Meredith, C. N., and Evans, W. J.,** Eccentric exercise-induced muscle damage impairs muscle glycogen repletion, *J. Appl. Physiol.,* 63, 252, 1987.

165. **Costill, D. L., Pascoe, D. D., Fink, W. J., Robergs, R. A., Barr, S. I., and Pearson, D.,** Impaired muscle glycogen resynthesis after eccentric exercise, *J. Appl. Physiol.,* 69, 46, 1990.

166. **Blom, P. C. S., Costill, D. L., and Vollestad, N. K.,** Exhaustive running: inappropriate as a stimulus of muscle glycogen supercompensation, *Med. Sci. Sports Exercise,* 19, 398, 1987.

Chapter 3

CARBOHYDRATE IN ULTRA-ENDURANCE EXERCISE AND ATHLETIC PERFORMANCE

_____ Gregory D. Miller

CONTENTS

0-8493-7911-3/94/$0.00+$.50
© 1994 by CRC Press, Inc.

I. INTRODUCTION

Enhancement of performance through dietary modification has been of interest to athletes since early times. More recently, participation in ultra-endurance sporting events such as ultra-marathon running and cross-country skiing, mountain climbing, and triathlons has increased the attention given to the role that nutrition can play in enhancing performance. Although optimal nutrition is related to endurance and performance, it is only an adjunct to innate ability, training, and honing of skills.

The nutritional requirements of the ultra-endurance athlete will depend on age, sex, body weight and composition, the length, frequency, and duration of the activity, and environmental conditions. Dietary guidelines will vary accordingly, but must contain adequate amounts of carbohydrate, protein, fat, vitamins, minerals, and water. Because carbohydrate intake and subsequent glycogen concentrations are a major determinant of endurance capacity, this review will consider the need for carbohydrates by ultra-endurance athletes. Additional information on carbohydrate metabolism in exercise and sport is given in the companion chapter entitled "Carbohydrate Metabolism and Exercise".

II. ENERGY COST OF ULTRA-ENDURANCE PERFORMANCE

Caloric requirements vary with energy expenditure. Daily energy cost is the result of resting metabolic rate (RMR), the thermic effect of feeding, the thermic effect of activity, and adaptive thermogenesis.[1,2] RMR represents the largest energy cost, accounting for as much as 75% of a person's daily energy requirements[2,3] (Figure 1). RMR is highly variable, due to the influence of many factors such as age, sex, genetics, and body composition.[2,4,5] The results of studies examining the effects of training on RMR have been conflicting. Studies have found that endurance training may potentiate RMR or have no effect.[3,6-8] A failure to observe an enhanced RMR may be the result of inadequate intensity or duration in the training. It has been speculated that there is an intensity–duration threshold that must be met for exercise to produce a prolonged effect on RMR.[9]

The heat produced as a result of the energy expended to digest and absorb food is called the thermic effect of feeding and is only a small portion of daily energy requirements. Similar to thermic effect of food in energy cost is adaptive thermogenesis. Van Zant[2] describes adaptive thermogenesis as the alteration in heat produced with no change in physical activity. For example, nonshivering thermogenesis as a result of cold exposure.[10]

The most critical component of daily energy requirements for the ultra-endurance athlete is that for physical activity. Exercising at 30% of $\dot{V}O_2$ max (maximal oxygen uptake), a 70-kg man burns 350 kcal/h. Increasing the intensity of exercise to 80% of $\dot{V}O_2$ max increases energy consumption to approximately 950 kcal/h.[11] It has been estimated that the highly trained endurance athlete will utilize oxygen at an average of 80% of $\dot{V}O_2$ max over the distance of a marathon (42 km), resulting in an energy cost of 0.95 kcal/kg/km, or a total of 2793 kcal for a 70-kg man.[12,13] Studies examining energy expenditure by athletes during multistage ultra-endurance cycling events have demonstrated energy utilization to be between 7000 and 10,000 kcal/d.[14,15] Kreider[15] estimated the energy expenditure for an ultra-distance triathlon (2-km swim, 90-km bike, and a 21-km run) to be approximately 5000 kcals. Energy consumption during a 24-h ultra-endurance race has been demonstrated to be as high as 18,000 kcal.[12]

Body energy stores will be utilized to meet the large caloric requirement for ultra-endurance athletic performance. The average amount of stored fuels in the nonobese 70-kg man are given in Table 1.[16] Body fat stores provide the largest amount of available energy (approximately 80% of total stores). Although energy stored as protein may be as high as 40,000 kcal, its utilization is limited. Less than 10% of total available energy is in the form of carbohydrate, stored as glycogen in muscle and liver. A small amount of glucose in circulation also is available to meet energy needs.

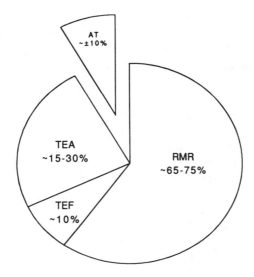

TOTAL ENERGY EXPENDITURE

FIGURE 1.   Components and percentages of total energy expenditure: RMR, resting metabolic rate; TEF, thermic effect of feeding; TEA, thermic effect of activity; AT, adaptive thermogenesis. (From Van Zant, R. S., *Int. J. Sport Nutr.*, 2, 1, 1992. With permission.)

TABLE 1 Average Body Energy Stores of the Nonobese 70-kg Man

Fuel	Amount stored (kg)	Caloric value (kcal)
Triacyglycerols (adipose tissue)	15.56	140,000
Glycogen		
Muscle	0.35	1,400
Liver	0.09	360
Glucose (extracellular fluids)	0.02	80
Protein (muscle)	10	40,000
Total	26.02	181,840

Adapted from Felig, P. and Wahren, J., *N. Engl. J. Med.*, 293, 1078, 1975.

III. UTILIZATION OF ENERGY SOURCES

The quantity of various fuel substrates utilized varies as a function of availability, physical conditioning, exercise intensity, and exercise duration. Substrate utilization is commonly measured in terms of the respiratory exchange ratio (RER), the ratio of the volume of expired CO_2 to the volume of oxygen absorbed by the lungs per unit of time.[17] An RER near 1.0 indicates that carbohydrate is the substrate being consumed. When fat is the major fuel source, an RER near 0.7 is obtained.

Resting muscle derives energy almost exclusively from the oxidation of fatty acids, with a minor amount of energy obtained from glucose.[18,19] During exercise there is a shift from the consumption of fat to carbohydrate to meet energy needs. Early work by Christensen and Hansen[20] demonstrated that RER rises with exercise, indicating a shift to carbohydrate metabolism. Carbohydrate is the principle source of energy during the initial onset (<2 min) of exercise.[21] As exercise continues, depending on intensity, fatty acids will be consumed in conjunction with carbohydrate to meet energy needs. Thus, RER will initially be high and fall toward 0.7 as the contribution of fatty acids increases.[22] During prolonged exercise, protein may contribute a small percentage (<10%) of the fuel substrate utilized for energy.[23] Hermansen et al.[11] observed that RER increases as a function of exercise intensity. Subjects exercising for 80 min at approximately 30, 50, and 80% of their $\dot{V}O_2$ max had average RERs of 0.87, 0.90, and 0.93, respectively. The shift in substrate utilization from fatty acids to carbohydrate during high-intensity (>75% $\dot{V}O_2$ max) exercise, where O_2 availability is reduced, represents a more efficient utilization of O_2 to produce ATP.[17] Thus, it appears that O_2 availability is an important regulator of substrate utilization.[17]

In the first 5 to 10 min of exercise, glycogenolysis in muscle provides carbohydrate for oxidation.[24] However, as exercise continues and glycogen stores decrease, utilization of blood glucose increases. Muscle uptake of glucose depends on intensity of exercise and can reach levels 20 times that found at rest.[25]

Prolonged exercise at a moderate intensity (<60% $\dot{V}O_2$ max) results in increased (by as much as 70%) fatty acid uptake and utilization by muscle.[16,26] Uptake of free fatty acids (FFA) is proportional to blood levels and the rate of fatty acid oxidation is greater in exercised, conditioned vs. unconditioned subjects.[16,17,26] This may be the consequence of a higher proportion of slow twitch fibers with high oxidative capacity and/or an increased ability to release FFA from adipose tissue in conditioned subjects.[27-29] It has been observed that FFA levels are significantly elevated during an ultra-distanced triathlon compared with an olympic-length triathlon.[30] The oxidative capacity of slow twitch fibers can be maximized by conditioning.[31] Utilization of FFA for energy spares muscle glycogen.

During prolonged exercise of moderate intensity, amino acids may be taken up and oxidized by muscle.[19,32,33] However, the contribution to total energy needs is small.[23] Alborg et al.[19] examined the flow of amino acids between visceral tissue and skeletal muscle in men at rest and after 40 min of moderate exercise. They observed the flow of branched-chain amino acids from visceral tissue to skeletal muscle and alanine from skeletal muscle to visceral tissue. The carbon skeleton of alanine returning to the liver can be utilized for gluconeogenesis. Branched-chain amino acids are catabolized to acetoacetate and acetyl coenzyme A (CoA) by skeletal muscle and can be utilized as a source of energy.[34] Amino acids taken up by skeletal muscle are oxidized at a rate of 4 to 6 g/h and provide less than 3% of total oxidative energy.[19,35] After approximately 4 h of exercise, the net output of alanine from skeletal muscle is three times that observed at rest.[35] However, synthesis of glucose in the liver from amino acids is less than 4 g/h, providing little of the energy utilized during prolonged moderate exercise.

As exercise intensity increases to levels greater than 70% of $\dot{V}O_2$ max, dependence on muscle glycogen metabolism for energy increases (Figure 2).[11,36-38] Muscle glycogenolysis is most rapid in the early stages of exercise.[39,40] Hermansen et al.[11] found that reduction in muscle glycogen during exercise was linearly related to $\dot{V}O_2$ max. They investigated the role of muscle glycogen as an energy source during prolonged exercise.[11] Subjects were exercised to complete exhaustion on a bicycle ergometer at workloads averaging 77% of $\dot{V}O_2$ max. Work bouts of 20 min were followed by 15 min of rest. During rest, needle biopsies were taken from working muscle so that glycogen utilization could be measured for comparison with total carbohydrate utilization. It was observed that subjects were unable to continue pedaling when the muscle glycogen content was practically zero. These results suggested that the capacity for prolonged strenuous work is limited by muscle glycogen stores. This is supported by the work of Hultman,[24] who observed that subjects exercised at 75% of $\dot{V}O_2$ max had total work capacities that were related to muscle glycogen levels (Figure 3). There are several factors that can influence the rate of muscle glycogen breakdown. Muscle glycogenolysis will be enhanced as a result of the recruitment of additional

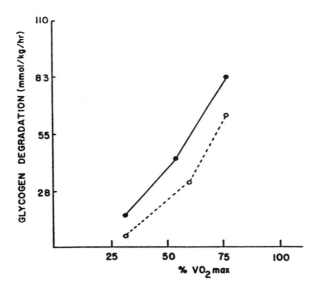

FIGURE 2. Muscle glycogen degradation as a function of exercise intensity in untrained (●) and trained (○) subjects. Note that as exercise intensity increases, there is an "obligate" increase in muscle glycogen degradation and training has a muscle glycogen-sparing effect. (From Sherman, W. M. and Costill, D. L., *Am. J. Sports Med.*, 12, 44, 1984. With permission.)

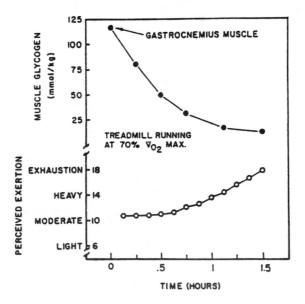

FIGURE 3. Muscle glycogen depletion and ratings of perceived exertion during strenuous running. Note that exhaustion occurs simultaneously with low levels of muscle glycogen. Thereafter, if exercise is to be continued, exercise intensity must be significantly reduced. (From Sherman, W. M. and Costill, D. L., *Am. J. Sports Med.*, 12, 44, 1984. With permission.)

fibers.[41] Increased secretion of adrenaline during high-intensity exercise may stimulate muscle glycogen utilization.[42,43] Enhanced oxidative capacity of muscle as an adaptation to training results in a reduced rate of glycogen utilization.[44] Thus, work capacity can be influenced by training.

Perception ratings of exertion during exercise are inversely related to muscle glycogen levels (Figure 3). However, the perception of exhaustion is less defined during intense

Leg glucose uptake

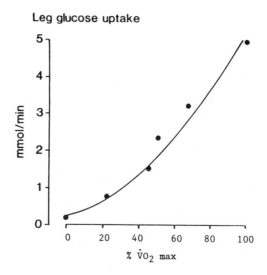

FIGURE 4. Leg glucose uptake during short-term (<15 min) exercise at different intensities. Values of leg glucose uptake are from References 25 and 46 and are mean values of six to ten subjects. (From Sahlin, K., *Ann. Med.*, 22, 185, 1990. With permission.)

running than cycling. Sherman and Costill[38] suggest that the less exact perception of exhaustion during running is due to a reduced rate of muscle glycogen breakdown, the result of a larger muscle mass contributing to the total work output. It is concluded that muscle glycogen stores are an important source of energy during intense, prolonged exercise.

Although depletion of muscle glycogen stores has been associated with exhaustion, it has been suggested that the development of hypoglycemia may also be an important factor. The amount of energy derived from blood glucose increases as a function of intensity/duration of exercise. Blood glucose may supply up to 90% of the carbohydrate consumed by muscle after 40 min, depending on the intensity of exercise.[45] It has been observed that leg muscle uptake of glucose increases with the intensity of the exercise and at maximum intensity (100% $\dot{V}O_2$ max) may be 50 times higher than at rest (Figure 4).[17,25,46]

The mechanisms responsible for the enhanced uptake of glucose by muscle during exercises remains uncertain. There is evidence that muscle contraction induces an increased uptake of glucose and that this is enhanced by insulin.[47,48] Hargraves[40] has observed an inverse relationship between muscle glycogen levels and leg glucose uptake during supine cycling in untrained men. This has been observed by others.[49] These results indicate that muscle glycogen levels (or breakdown) may be involved in the regulation of glucose uptake by muscle.

The available blood glucose is derived from hepatic glycogenolysis and gluconeogenesis. The shift to blood glucose utilization results in an increased rate of glycogen breakdown by the liver, as much as five times basal levels.[17] During prolonged (3- to 4-h) exercise at high intensity, hepatic glycogen stores will be depleted. Under these conditions hepatic glucose production is less than peripheral utilization and hypoglycemia results.[45,50] Hypoglycemia can impair performance by affecting central nervous system functioning. Bergstrom et al.[36] have demonstrated that high levels of dietary carbohydrates prior to exercise will prevent a precipitous fall in blood glucose concentration, delaying the onset of exhaustion (Figure 5). Pruett[51] observed that subjects exercised to exhaustion at 70% $\dot{V}O_2$ max had blood glucose levels 37.5% lower than preexercise levels. Symptoms of dizziness, nausea, and confusion developed with the onset of low blood glucose and disappeared when glucose levels increased.

The pattern of fuel utilization to meet energy needs during exercise depends on the duration and intensity of the exercise. During exercise of low intensity (<40% $\dot{V}O_2$ max), FFA and

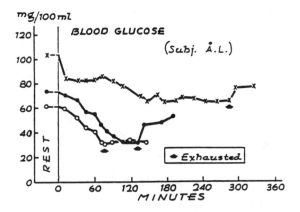

FIGURE 5.   Blood glucose concentration in connection with exercise after different diets. (x) Carbohydrate diet; (●) mixed diet; (○) fat and protein diet. (From Bergstrom, J. et al., *Acta Physiol. Scand.*, 71, 140, 1967. With permission.)

blood glucose are used to meet energy needs. However, as intensity increases, utilization of muscle glycogen increases and depletion of muscle glycogen stores is correlated with exhaustion (Figure 3). Blood glucose may provide energy to muscle with glycogen depletion and delay the onset of exhaustion. Endurance is related to the nature of the fuel source, and factors (such as diet) affecting the composition of fuel stores will affect endurance.

IV. DIETARY MANIPULATIONS OF FUEL STORES AND METABOLISM

There is a long history of investigation on the influence of diet on endurance. Christensen and Hansen[20] examined the effects of a high-carbohydrate/low-fat diet (83%/3%) vs. a high-fat/low-carbohydrate diet (94%/4%) on endurance. They observed that carbohydrate made a significantly higher contribution as a fuel source in subjects consuming the high-carbohydrate diet than in subjects consuming the high-fat diet and increased endurance (210 min to exhaustion vs. 88 min).[52] Similarly, Issekutz et al.[27] observed that the contribution of carbohydrate as a fuel source during work is related to the concentration of carbohydrate in the diet preceding testing.

The observation that endurance during exercise is related to prior carbohydrate intake stimulated research on the contribution of dietary carbohydrate to muscle glycogen stores and their subsequent effect on endurance. Bergstrom and co-workers[36] demonstrated that ingestion of a high-carbohydrate diet increases muscle glycogen stores and improves endurance. It was observed that time to exhaustion of subjects exercised at approximately 75% $\dot{V}O_2$ max was dependent on the level of preexercise muscle glycogen stores. On their usual mixed diet, initial muscle glycogen stores were 1.75 g/100 g muscle (wet weight) and exhaustion occurred at 114 min. The same workload could be tolerated for only 57 min when initial glycogen stores had been lowered to 0.63 g/100 g muscle (wet weight) by consuming a diet high in fat and protein for 3 d. Consumption of a carbohydrate-rich diet for 3 d increased muscle glycogen content to 3.51 g/100 g muscle (wet weight) and time to exhaustion to 167 min. Similarly, Hultman[24] observed that muscle glycogen levels were increased by consumption of a high-carbohydrate diet and that performance time of subjects was significantly correlated with initial muscle glycogen stores (Figure 6).

The demonstration that endurance was proportional to the level of preexercise muscle glycogen stores, and that depletion of muscle glycogen correlated with exhaustion, led to investigation of methods to enhance glycogen stores and minimize breakdown during exercise. Bergstrom and Hultman[53] observed that exercise-depleted muscle glycogen stores could be returned to preexercise levels within 24 h by consumption of a diet which consisted

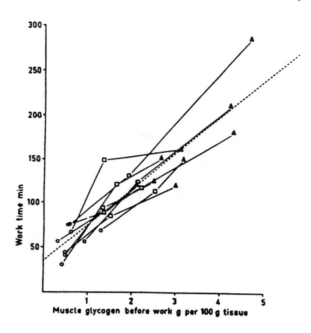

FIGURE 6. Work time vs. muscle glycogen concentration in nine subjects. Each subject was investigated three times with different concentrations of muscle glycogen at start of work. (□) After mixed diet; (○) after carbohydrate-free diet (fat and protein); (▲) after carbohydrate-rich diet; the dashed line is the regression line. (From Hultman, E., *Circ. Res. Suppl.*, 1, 1, 1967. With permission.)

almost exclusively of carbohydrate. Consumption of the high-carbohydrate diet for an additional 2 d increased muscle glycogen stores to twice preexercise levels (Figure 7).[54] Bergstrom and Hultman[53] observed that exercise-induced depletion of muscle glycogen in one leg, using one-legged ergometry, was rapidly replaced in that leg to a level greater than that found in the unexercised leg by a diet consisting almost exclusively of carbohydrate. The high-carbohydrate diet increased the glycogen level in the exercised leg to almost twice that of the unexercised leg (Figure 8).

It is now established that the rate of muscle glycogen repletion is related to the carbohydrate content of the diet.[55] Bergstrom et al.[36] demonstrated that consumption of a high-carbohydrate diet would rapidly replace exercise-depleted muscle stores, while a protein and fat diet only slowly increased glycogen resynthesis (Figure 7). Hultman[24] reported that the repletion of exercise-depleted muscle glycogen stores can take in excess of a week with a diet high in protein and fat. Costill and Miller[56] observed a rapid decline in muscle glycogen as a function of time (days) in hard-training subjects maintained on a diet containing approximately 40% of the calories as carbohydrates. However, when these same subjects were switched to an isocaloric diet, containing about 70% of the calories as carbohydrate, muscle glycogen was only slowly depleted over successive days (Figure 9). More recent work has indicated that rate of muscle glycogen resynthesis will be increased if carbohydrate is consumed immediately following exercise vs. carbohydrate given 2 h later.[57]

In another study, Costill and co-workers[58] examined how types of dietary carbohydrates affect muscle glycogen resynthesis after exercise. Subjects consumed isocaloric diets high (70% of calories) in simple (glucose, sucrose, fructose) or complex (starch) carbohydrates after a 10-mile run at 80% $\dot{V}O_2$ max. Subjects consumed 3700 kcal during the first 24 h and 2383 kcal during the next 24 h. Although gastrocnemius muscle glycogen levels were similar for all groups at 24 h, subjects consuming the complex carbohydrate diet had

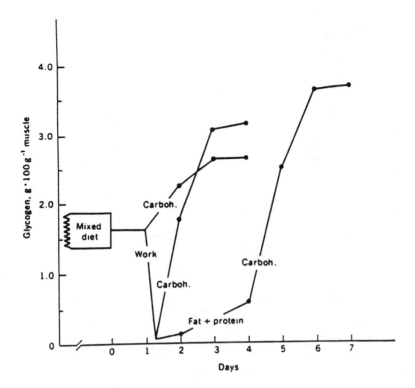

FIGURE 7. Different possibilities of increasing the muscle glycogen content. (From Saltin, B. and Hermansen, L., in *Nutrition and Physical Activity,* Blix, G., Ed., Almquist and Weksells, Uppsala, Sweden, 1967. With permission.)

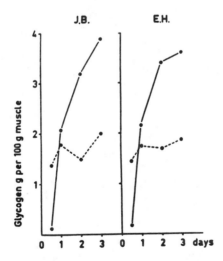

FIGURE 8. Effect of carbohydrate diet on muscle glycogen content after exhaustive work. One-leg exercise during day one. Exercised leg is shown by solid line; nonexercised leg by dashed line. (From Hultman, E., *Circ. Res. Suppl.,* 1, 1, 1967. With permission.)

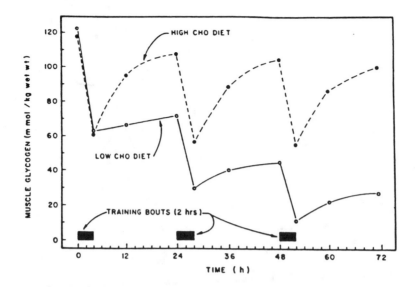

FIGURE 9. Muscle glycogen content during three successive days of heavy training in subjects with diets in which caloric compositions were 40% carbohydrate (low CHO) and 70% carbohydrate (high CHO). (From Costill, D. L. and Miller, J. M., *Int. J. Sports Med.*, 1, 2, 1980. With permission.)

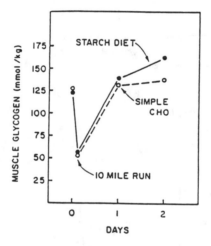

FIGURE 10. Influence of diets rich in starch and simple carbohydrates (glucose and fructose) on muscle glycogen and restoration after exhaustive exercise. (From Costill, D. L. and Miller, J. M., *Int. J. Sports Med.*, 1, 2, 1980. With permission.)

significantly higher muscle glycogen levels at 48 h (Figure 10). Apparently, diets high in complex carbohydrates are more effective than those high in simple carbohydrates for long-term repletion of muscle glycogen stores after exhaustive exercise.

The demonstration that muscle glycogen is influenced by diet and, in turn, influences endurance has led to recommendations for glycogen loading prior to exhaustive exercise. It has been estimated that 500 to 700 g of glycogen can be stored in the body and that carbohydrate loading techniques can increase stores by approximately 500 g, at which time *de novo* lipogenesis occurs.[59] Astrand[60] has suggested that muscle glycogen supercompensation could be achieved by curtailing exhaustive training 1 week prior to competition.

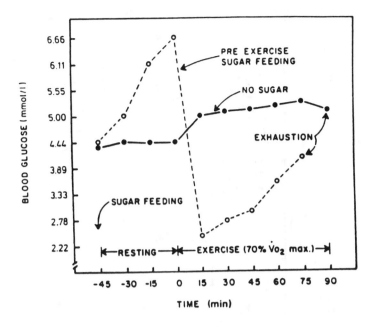

FIGURE 11.   Effects of preexercise carbohydrate feedings on blood glucose, insulin, and work time to exhaustion. (From Costill, D. L. and Miller, J. M., *Int. J. Sports Med.*, 1, 2, 1980. With permission.)

Following the period of exhaustive training, total carbohydrate intake should be restricted for 3 d. This is followed by a carbohydrate-rich diet for the next 4 d. The intensity of training should be sharply reduced during the period of high-carbohydrate intake to maximize glycogen stores (see Figure 7). One problem with this glycogen-loading regimen is that athletes often find it difficult to train during the period of carbohydrate depletion. The severe depletion of glycogen stores results in fatigue, nausea, dizziness, and irritability. Costill and Miller[56] proposed that the glycogen supercompensation regimen include 3 d of mixed diet instead of the carbohydrate-restricted diet. They observed that this loading method can result in muscle glycogen levels that are 2.5 times that found in subjects on a nonloading dietary regimen. Several easy-to-follow dietary plans are available for the general public.[61-63]

The ingestion of carbohydrates before and during an ultra-endurance exercise can have profound effects on performance. Costill et al.[64] demonstrated that ingestion of a 75-g glucose load 45 min prior to exercise results in elevated blood glucose levels and hyperinsulinemia at the onset of exercise (Figure 11). This results in impaired mobilization of FFA and an increase in the utilization of carbohydrate for energy. Subsequently, hypoglycemia and an increased rate of utilization of glycogen develop, which results in an accelerated onset of exhaustion.[60] Costill and Miller[56] suggest that a high-carbohydrate meal be consumed 3 to 4 h before competition so that plasma insulin and glucose have adequate time to return to basal levels. However, it has been demonstrated that consumption of a mixed-macronutrient snack 30 min prior to exercise does increase plasma insulin, but does not increase muscle glycogen depletion and does not impair endurance performance in untrained subjects.[65] These results indicate that the form (liquid vs. solid) or composition may impact the effectiveness of a carbohydrate supplement. This is supported by the data of Neufer et al.,[66] who observed that subjects fed a solid carbohydrate supplement 5 min before the beginning of exercise had a significant improvement in performance in a ride to exhaustion. Recent work by Jarvis et al.[67] indicates that carbohydrate given in a food matrix reduces the initial glycemic and insulinemic response relative to glucose given alone.

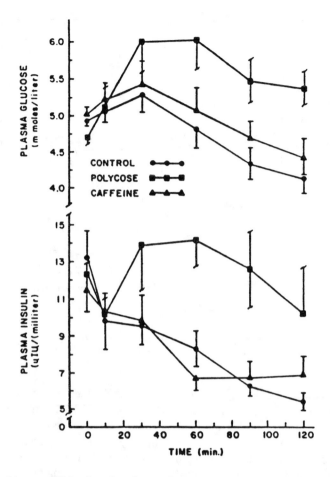

FIGURE 12. Mean ± SEM values for plasma glucose and insulin during exercise in control, glucose polymer, and caffeine trials. (From Ivey, J. L. et al., *Med. Sci. Sports*, 11, 16, 1979. With permission.)

Results of recent studies have demonstrated that the ingestion of carbohydrate during exercise may have a positive effect on endurance. Ivy et al.[68] found that trained subjects exercising at approximately 70% of $\dot{V}O_2$ max had a significant increase in work output during the last 30 min of a 2-h workout when given glucose polymer feedings at 15-min intervals throughout exercise. It is suggested that the reduced rate of fatigue that occurred over the last 30 min of exercise is due to the maintenance of elevated blood glucose levels (Figure 12) and increased utilization and carbohydrates.

Coyle and colleagues[69] observed that trained subjects given a glucose polymer solution at 20, 60, 90, and 120 min of exercise at approximately 75% $\dot{V}O_2$ max had a delayed time to exhaustion compared to subjects receiving a placebo (157 vs. 134 min). Carbohydrate feeding during exercise increased blood glucose concentrations and prevented a decrease in plasma insulin. These results suggest that the maintenance of high blood glucose and insulin levels by feeding carbohydrates during exercise at 70 to 80% $\dot{V}O_2$ max, delays exhaustion by slowing muscle glycogen depletion through an increased utilization of blood glucose. Similarly, Hargraves et al.[70] found that trained subjects given a high-carbohydrate (43 g sucrose) snack at 1-h intervals during 4 h of exercise had a 20% reduction in muscle glycogen loss. It was observed also that during carbohydrate feeding, subjects were able to perform better during a sprint at the end of a 4-h cycling period. Work by Murray et al.[71] indicates that there is no relationship between exercise performance and the rate at which supplemental carbohydrate is ingested. Their data demonstrate that a carbohydrate intake of 25 g/h is sufficient to elicit an ergogenic effect.

Recent data indicate that carbohydrate consumption both taken throughout exercise and 35 min before the point of fatigue can effectively delay the onset of fatigue.[22,69,72,73] Coyle[72] has suggested that carbohydrate feedings prevent the lowering of blood glucose that occurs during the latter stages of prolonged strenuous exercise, which is a major factor in the development of muscular fatigue. Maintaining blood glucose levels allows muscle glucose uptake to offset reduced muscle glycogen availability. Although blood glucose will become the primary energy source during this time, there will be some continued utilization of muscle glycogen. Fatigue can occur with continued carbohydrate consumption and this may occur when the contribution of muscle glycogen to energy utilization is zero.[72]

V. SUMMARY

The results of research into fuel metabolism and its effects on athletic performance demonstrate that nutritional manipulation can be employed to maximize the potential of the ultra-endurance athlete. Thus, it has been demonstrated that glycogen loading techniques can elevate glycogen stores, increasing time to exhaustion, and that consumption of carbohydrates during exercise maintains blood glucose levels as an energy source. In addition to a nutritional strategy, a pacing strategy can improve performance. An initial high rate/intensity of performance may utilize a large portion of muscle glycogen stores while a moderate pace spares muscle glycogen stores by obtaining energy through the metabolism of FFA. Judicious pacing will provide for increased rate/intensity of performance near the end of competition by assuming availability of sufficient muscle glycogen stores. Finally, ultra-endurance athletes competing on successive days should consume a carbohydrate-rich diet to replenish depleted muscle glycogen stores. Simple or complex carbohydrates will replenish muscle glycogen stores at an equal rate over 24 h, while complex carbohydrates are more effective over a 48-h period.

ACKNOWLEDGMENTS

The author thanks Patti Barango and Nancy Warner for reviewing and typing this chapter.

REFERENCES

1. **Horton, E. S.,** Introduction: an overview of the assessment and regulation of energy balance in humans, *Am. J. Clin. Nutr.,* 38, 972, 1983.
2. **Van Zant, R. S.,** Influence of diet and exercise on energy expenditure — a review, *Int. J. Sport Nutr.,* 2, 1, 1992.
3. **Broeder, C. E., Burrhus, K. A., Svanevik, L. S., and Wilmore, J. H.,** The effects of either high-intensity resistance or endurance training on resting metabolic rate, *Am. J. Clin. Nutr.,* 55, 802, 1992.
4. **Bouchard, C., Tremblay, A., Nadeau, A., Despres, J.-P., Theriault, G., Boulay, M. R., Lortie, G., Leldanc, C., and Fournier, G.,** Genetic effect in resting and exercise metabolic rates, *Metabolism,* 38, 364, 1989.
5. **Bogardus, C., Lilliuja, S., Ravussin, E., Abbott, W., Zawadzki, J. K., Young, A., Knowler, W. C., Jacobowitz, R., and Moll, P. P.,** Familial dependance on the resting metabolic rate, *N. Engl. J. Med.,* 315, 96, 1986.
6. **Poehlman, E. T., Melby, C. L., and Badylak, S. F.,** Resting metabolic rate and postprandial thermogenesis in highly trained and untrained males, *Am. J. Clin. Nutr.,* 47, 793, 1988.
7. **Poehlman, E. T., Melby, C. L., Badylak, S. F., and Calles, J.,** Aerobic fitness and resting energy expenditure in young adult males, *Metabolism,* 38, 85, 1989.

8. **Ravussin, E. and Bogardus, C.,** Relationship of genetics, age, and physical fitness to daily energy expenditure and fuel utilization, *Am. J. Clin. Nutr.,* 49, 968, 1989.

9. **Mole, P. A.,** Impact of energy intake and exercise on resting metabolic rate, *Sports Med.,* 10, 72, 1990.

10. **Poehlman, E. T. and Horton, E. S.,** The impact of food intake and exercise on energy expenditure, *Nutr. Rev.,* 47, 129, 1989.

11. **Hermansen, L., Hultman, E., and Saltin, B.,** Muscle glycogen during prolonged severe exercise, *Acta Physiol. Scand.,* 71, 129, 1967.

12. **Davies, C. T. M. and Thompson, M. W.,** Estimated aerobic performance and energy cost of severe exercise of 24-hour duration, *Ergonomics,* 22, 1249, 1979.

13. **Davies, C. T. M. and Thompson, M. N.,** Physiological responses to prolonged exercise in ultra-marathon athletes, *J. Appl. Physiol.,* 61, 611, 1986.

14. **Westerterp, K. R., Saris, W. H. M., Esvan, M., and Ter Hoor, F.,** Use of doubly labeled water technique in humans during heavy sustained exercise, *J. Appl. Physiol.,* 61, 2162, 1986.

15. **Kreider, R. B.,** Physiological considerations in ultra-endurance performance, *Int. J. Sport Nutr.,* 1, 3, 1991.

16. **Felig, P. and Wahren, J.,** Fuel homeostasis in exercise, *N. Engl. J. Med.,* 293, 1078, 1975.

17. **Sahlin, K.,** Muscle glucose metabolism during exercise, *Ann. Med.,* 22, 185, 1990.

18. **Andres, R., Cader, G., and Zierler, K. L.,** The quantitatively minor role of carbohydrate in oxidative metabolism by skeletal muscle in intact man in the basal state. Measurements of oxygen and carbon dioxide and lactate production in the forearm, *J. Clin. Invest.,* 35, 671, 1956.

19. **Alborg, G., Bergstrom, J., Ekelund, L. G., and Hultman, E.,** Muscle glycogen and muscle electrolytes during prolonged physical exercise, *Acta Physiol. Scand.,* 70, 120, 1967.

20. **Christensen, E. H. and Hansen, O. V.,** Respiratorischer Quotient Und O_2-Aufnahme, *Skand. Arch. Physiol.,* 81, 180, 1939.

21. **McCardle, F. I. and Katch, F. L.,** *Energy and Human Performance,* Lea & Febiger, Philadelphia, 1981.

22. **Coggan, A. R. and Coyle, E. F.,** Metabolism and performance following carbohydrate ingestion late in exercise, *Med. Sci. Sports Exercise,* 21, 59, 1989.

23. **Lemon, P. W. R.,** Protein and exercise: update 1987, *Med. Sci. Sports Exercise,* 19, 5179, 1987.

24. **Hultman, E.,** Physiological role of muscle glycogen in man with special reference to exercise, *Circ. Res. Suppl.* 1, Vol. 20/21, 1, 1967.

25. **Wahren, J., Felig, P., and Ahlborg, G.,** Glucose metabolism during exercise in man, *J. Clin. Invest.,* 50, 2715, 1971.

26. **Alborg, G., Felig, P., Hagenfeldt, L., Hendler, R., and Wahren, J.,** Substrate turnover during prolonged exercise in man: splanchnic and leg metabolism of glucose, free fatty acids, and amino acids, *J. Clin. Invest.,* 53, 1080, 1974.

27. **Issekutz, B., Miller, H., Paul, P., and Radah, K.,** Aerobic work capacity and plasma FFA turnover, *J. Appl. Physiol.,* 20, 293, 1965.

28. **Mole, P. and Holloszy, J.,** Exercise-induced increase in the capacity of skeletal muscle to oxidize palmitate, *Proc. Soc. Exp. Biol. Med.,* 134, 789, 1970.

29. **Hultman, E. and Harris, R. C.,** Carbohydrate metabolism, in *Principles of Exercise Biochemistry,* Poortmas, J. R., Ed., S. Karger, Basel, Switzerland, 1988, 78–119.

30. **Jurimae, T., Viru, A., Karelson, K., and Smirnov, T.,** Biochemical changes in blood during the long and short triathlon, *J. Sports Med. Phys. Fitness,* 29, 305, 1989.

31. **Terjung, R. L. and Hood, D. A.,** Biochemical adaptations in skeletal muscle induced by exercise training, in *Nutrition and Aerobic Exercise,* Layman, D. K., Ed., American Chemical Society, Washington, D.C., 1986, 8–26.

32. **Dohm, G. L., Williams, R. T., Jasperek, G. J., and van Rij, A. M.,** Increased excretion of urea and NT-methylhistidine by rats and humans after a bout of exercise, *J. Appl. Physiol.,* 52, 27, 1982.

33. **Layman, D. K. and Hendrix, M. K.,** Protein and amino acid metabolism during exercise, in *Nutrition and Aerobic Exercise,* Layman, D. K., Ed., American Chemical Society, Washington, D.C., 1986, 45–58.

34. **Shinnick, F. L. and Harper, A. E.,** Branched-chain amino acid oxidation by isolated rat tissue preparations, *Biochem. Biophys. Acta,* 437, 477, 1976.

35. **Koivisto, V. A.,** The physiology of marathon running, *Sci. Prog. (Oxford),* 70, 109, 1986.

36. **Bergstrom, J., Hermansen, L., Hultman, E., and Saltin, B.,** Diet-muscle glycogen and physical performance, *Acta Physiol. Scand.,* 71, 140, 1967.

37. **Pernow, B. and Saltin, B.,** Availability of substrates and capacity for prolonged heavy exercise in man, *J. Appl. Physiol.,* 31, 416, 1971.

38. **Sherman, W. M. and Costill, D.,** The marathon: dietary manipulation to optimize performance, *Am. J. Sports Med.,* 12, 44, 1984.

39. **Vollestad, N. K., Vaage, O., and Hermansen, L.,** Muscle glycogen depletion patterns in type 1 and subgroups of type II fibres during prolonged severe exercise in man, *Acta Physiol. Scand.,* 122, 433, 1984.

40. **Hargraves, M.,** Skeletal muscle carbohydrate metabolism during exercise, *Aust. J. Sci. Med. Sport,* 22, 35, 1990.

41. **Vollestad, N. K. and Blom, P. C. S.,** Effect of varying exercise intensity on glycogen depletion in human muscle fibres, *Acta Physiol. Scand.,* 125, 395, 1985.

42. **Galbo, H.,** Endocrinology and metabolism in exercise, *Int. J. Sports Med.,* 2, 203, 1981.

43. **Jansson, E., Hijemdahl, P., and Kaijser, L.,** Epinephrine-induced changes in muscle carbohydrate metabolism during exercise in male subjects, *J. Appl. Physiol.,* 60, 1466, 1986.

44. **Jansson, E. and Kaijser, L.,** Substrate utilization and enzymes in skeletal muscle of extremely endurance-trained men, *J. Appl. Physiol.,* 62, 999, 1987.

45. **Wahren, J.,** Glucose turnover during exercise in man, *Ann. N.Y. Acad. Sci.,* 301, 45, 1977.

46. **Katz, A., Broberg, S., Sahlin, K., and Wahren, J.,** Leg glucose uptake during maximal dynamic exercise in humans, *Am. J. Physiol.,* 251, E65, 1986.

47. **Wallberg-Henriksson, H. and Holloszy, J. O.,** Contractile activity increases glucose uptake by muscle in severely diabetic rats, *J. Appl. Physiol.,* 57, 1045, 1984.

48. **DeFronzo, R. A., Ferrannini, E., Sato, Y., Felig, P., and Wahren, J.,** Synergistic interaction between exercise and insulin on peripheral glucose uptake, *J. Clin. Invest.,* 68, 1468, 1981.

49. **Gollnick, P. D., Perniw, B., Essen, B., Jansson, E., and Saltin, B.,** Availability of glycogen and FFA for substrate utilization in leg muscle of man during exercise, *Clin. Physiol.,* 1, 27, 1981.

50. **Levine, S. A., Gordon, B., and Drick, C. L.,** Some changes in the chemical constituents of the blood following a marathon race, *JAMA,* 82, 1778, 1924.

51. **Pruett, E.,** Glucose and insulin during prolonged work stress in men living on different diets, *J. Appl. Physiol.,* 28, 199, 1970.

52. **Evans, W. J. and Hughes, V. A.,** Dietary carbohydrates and endurance exercise, *Am. J. Clin. Nutr.,* 41, 1146, 1985.

53. **Bergstrom, J. and Hultman, E.,** Muscle glycogen synthesis after exercise: an enhancing factor localized to the muscle cells in man, *Nature,* 210, 309, 1966.

54. **Saltin, B. and Hermansen, L.,** Glycogen stores and prolonged severe exercise, in *Nutrition and Physical Activity,* Blix, G., Ed., Almquist and Weksells, Uppsala, Sweden, 1967.

55. **Piehl, K., Adolfsson, S., and Nazar, K.,** Glycogen storage and glycogen synthetase activity in trained and untrained muscle of man, *Acta Physiol. Scand.,* 90, 779, 1974.

56. **Costill, D. L. and Miller, J. M.,** Nutrition for endurance sport: carbohydrate and fluid balance, *Int. J. Sports Med.,* 1, 2, 1980.

57. **Ivy, J. L., Katz, A. L., Cutler, C. L., Sherman, W. M., and Coyle, E. F.,** Muscle glycogen synthesis after exercise: effect of time of carbohydrate ingestion, *J. Appl. Physiol.,* 64, 1480, 1988.

58. **Costill, D. L., Sherman, W. M., Fink, W. J., Maresh, L. W., Hen, M., and Miller, J. M.,** The role of dietary carbohydrates in muscle glycogen resynthesis after strenuous running, *Am. J. Clin. Nutr.,* 34, 1831, 1981.

59. **Acheson, K. J., Schutz, Y., Bessard, T., Anantharaman, K., Flatt, J.-P., and Jequire, E.,** Glycogen storage capacity and de novo lipogenesis during massive carbohydrate overfeeding in man, *Am. J. Clin. Nutr.,* 48, 240, 1988.

60. **Astrand, P. O.,** Diet and athletic performance, *Fed. Proc.,* 26, 1772, 1967.

61. **Costill, D.,** *Food Power, A Coaches' Guide to Improving Performance,* National Dairy Council, Rosemont, IL, 1984.

62. **Coleman, E.,** *Eating for Endurance,* Bull Publishing, Palo Alto, CA, 1988.

63. **Hoffman, C. J. and Coleman, E.,** An eating plan and update on recommended dietary practices for the endurance athlete, *J. Am. Diet. Assoc.,* 91, 325, 1991.

64. **Costill, D. L., Coyle, E., Dalsky, G., Evans, W., Fink, W. J., and Hoopes, D.,** Effects of elevated plasma FFA and insulin on muscle glycogen usage during exercise, *J. Appl. Physiol.,* 43, 695, 1977.

65. **DeVlin, J. T., Calles-Escandon, J., and Horton, E. S.,** Effects of pre-exercise snack feeding on endurance cycle exercise, *J. Appl. Physiol.,* 60, 980, 1986.

66. **Neufer, D. P., Costill, D. L., Flynn, M. G., Kirwan, J. P., Mitchell, P., and Houmard, J.,** Improvements in exercise performance: effects of carbohydrate feedings and diet, *J. Appl. Physiol.,* 62, 983, 1987.

67. **Jarvis, J., Pearsall, D., Oliner, C. M., and Schoeller, D. A.,** The effect of food matrix on carbohydrate utilization during moderate exercise, *Med. Sci. Sports Exercise,* 24, 320, 1992.

68. **Ivy, J. L., Costill, D. L., Fink, W. J., and Lower, R. W.,** Influence of caffeine and carbohydrate feedings on endurance performance, *Med. Sci. Sports Exercise,* 11, 6, 1979.

69. **Coyle, E. F., Hagberg, J. M., Hurley, B. F., Mardin, W. H., Ehsani, A. A., and Hollszy, J. O.,** Carbohydrate feeding during prolonged strenuous exercise can delay fatigue, *J. Appl. Physiol.,* 55, 230, 1983.

70. **Hargraves, M., Costill, D. L., Coggan, A., Fink, W. J., and Nishibata, I.,** Effect of carbohydrate feedings on muscle glycogen utilization and exercise performance, *Med. Sci. Sports Exercise,* 16, 219, 1984.

71. **Murray, R., Paul, G. L., Seifert, J. G., and Eddy, D. E.,** Responses to varying rates of carbohydrate ingestion during exercise, *Med. Sci. Sports Exercise,* 23, 713, 1991.

72. **Coyle, E. F.,** Carbohydrate supplementation during exercise, *J. Nutr.,* 122, 788, 1992.

73. **Coyle, E. F., Coggan, A. R., Hemmert, M. K., and Ivy, J. L.,** Muscle glycogen utilization during prolonged strenuous exercise when fed carbohydrate, *J. Appl. Physiol.,* 61, 165, 1986.

Chapter **4**

PUTATIVE EFFECTS OF DIET AND EXERCISE ON LIPIDS AND LIPOPROTEINS

Tinker D. Murray
William G. Squires, Jr.
G. Harley Hartung

CONTENTS

0-8493-7911-3/94/$0.00+$.50
© 1994 by CRC Press, Inc.

I. INTRODUCTION

The putative effects of diet and exercise on plasma lipids and lipoproteins have received widespread scientific and media attention for over 35 years. For example, as early as 1961, an ad hoc committee of the American Heart Association (AHA) released an updated report about the possible relation of dietary fat to heart attacks and stroke. The report included the following recommendations:

1. Overweight persons should decrease their caloric intake and attempt to achieve a desirable body weight.
2. The composition of the diet should be altered by reducing intakes of total fats, saturated fats, cholesterol, and by increasing intakes of polyunsaturated fats.
3. Weight reduction should be facilitated by regular moderate exercise.
4. Men at increased risk for coronary heart disease should pay particular attention to dietary alteration.
5. For those at high risk, dietary changes should be carried out with medical supervision.[1]

Follow-up reports by the AHA on dietary guidelines to reduce coronary heart disease (CHD) risk were released in 1965, 1968, 1973, 1978, 1986, 1988, and 1990. The National Heart, Lung, and Blood Institute in 1985 began the National Cholesterol Education Program (NCEP),[2] which reinforced the AHA's position statements (linking cholesterol and CHD) at the national and international levels. Together, these two developments have firmly planted the seed of cholesterol awareness in the public's mind in the 1990s. However, with this increased public awareness, manufacturers have eagerly made nutritional and exercise claims about how their products help reduce or control cholesterol levels. These claims are often reported in various media formats, and may or may not be accurate in regards to cholesterol reduction. The manipulation of lipids and lipoproteins has become the major established treatment modality for atherosclerosis in the 1990s.[3] Yet, numerous unresolved issues remain about how changes in the diet and/or exercise patterns can favorably alter lipid and lipoprotein levels.[4]

Previously, we received studies that emphasized the effects of plasma lipids and lipoproteins and their effects on optimal health and/or athletic performance.[5] We summarized the following findings from the relevant literature:

1. Lipids are a major fuel source for exercise.[6]
2. Plasma lipids and lipoproteins are associated with the etiology of CHD.[7-10]
3. Dietary factors have various effects on plasma lipids and lipoproteins.[11]
4. Lipid metabolism is influenced by physical training.[12]

The purpose of this review is to update what is currently known and unknown about dietary and exercise influences on lipids and lipoproteins. The review will be limited to research findings with implications for the acquisition and maintenance of health and physical fitness in adults.

II. OVERVIEW OF THE CHARACTERISTICS OF PLASMA LIPIDS, LIPOPROTEINS, AND APOLIPOPROTEINS

Lipids are a heterogeneous group of chemicals that include free fatty acids (FFA) and substances found naturally in chemical association with them.[13] The major lipids found in humans are FFA, triglycerides (TG), steroids, phospholipids, prostaglandins, fat-soluble vitamins, provitamins, and lipoproteins. The function of lipids are[13]

1. To provide fuel
2. To serve as insulation
3. To provide protective padding for organs and structures
4. To supply building blocks for other chemicals
5. To provide essential fatty acids
6. To serve as components of cell membranes and other cell structures

A brief description of how plasma lipids and lipoproteins function in the body will provide the basic framework for the remainder of this review. More detailed reviews of lipid metabolism are available elsewhere.[14-17]

Triglycerides are the chief lipid ingested and are stored within the body. They consist of three FFA combined with glycerol. The digestion of TG, cholesterol, and phospholipids originates in the small intestine and concludes with the entry of the chylomicrons into the thoracic duct. Small amounts of FFA are also absorbed directly by the liver via the portal circulation. Triglycerides are stored in the body in adipose tissue, the liver, and skeletal muscle.[18]

The major plasma lipids, including cholesterol (a fatlike pearly substance) and TG, are transported in the form of lipoprotein complexes. The plasma lipoproteins transport both endogenously synthesized products and exogenously ingested dietary lipids. The plasma lipoproteins contain cholesterol, TG, phospholipid, and protein (see Table 1).[19] Lipoproteins are classified into five major classes by their gravitational density, as follows:

1. Chylomicrons (primary exogenous TG)
2. Very-low-density lipoprotein cholesterol (VLDL-C), primarily endogenous triglycerides
3. Intermediate-density lipoprotein cholesterol (IDL-C, LDL-C precursor)
4. Low-density lipoprotein cholesterol (LDL-C, approximately 50% cholesterol transport, 60 to 75% of the total plasma cholesterol)
5. High-density lipoprotein cholesterol (HDL-C, normally transports 20 to 25% of the total plasma cholesterol)

The TG of chylomicrons are hydrolyzed by lipoprotein lipase (LPL) into monoglycerides and FFA in the capillaries of adipose tissue and skeletal muscle. The FFA are re-esterified or oxidized by adipose or muscle cells. The remnants of the chylomicrons are cleared by the liver.[20]

The VLDL-C originates in the liver and small intestine and is increased with excess carbohydrate-rich diets. VLDL-C is hydrolyzed to IDL-C by LPL. The IDL-C remnants are further hydrolyzed to LDL, probably by LPL and hepatic triglyceride lipase (HTGL).[17,21] Some of the IDL-C is cleared from plasma by hepatic LDL receptors that bind apolipoprotein E in the liver. The residual IDL-C forms LDL-C with apolipoprotein B-100 on its surface. Apolipoprotein B-100 is recognized by the hepatic and extrahepatic LDL receptors. The plasma LDL-C levels are influenced by LDL-C receptor number and each cell's need for cholesterol. When the need is low, cells make fewer receptors and LDL-C is removed at lower rates. When this occurs plasma LDL-C rises. Elevated LDL-C levels can accelerate the rate of atherosclerosis, increasing CHD risk.[17]

TABLE 1 Characteristics and Functions of the Plasma Lipoproteins

Characteristics		Chylomicron	VLDL	IDL*	LDL	HDL
				Classes of Lipoproteins		
Density (g/mL)		<0.95	0.95–1.006	1.006–1.019	1.019–1.063	1.063–1.210
Electrophoretic mobility		Origin	Pre-B	Pre-B to B	B	a
Origin		Intestine	Liver and intestine	In circulation secondary to catabolism of other lipoproteins	Liver	Liver & intestine
Physiologic role		Transport of dietary triglyceride	Transport of endogenous triglyceride	Liver LDL precursor	Major cholesterol transport lipoprotein	Reverse cholesterol transport
Relative atherogenicity		0	+	+++	++++	Negatively correlated with atherosclerosis
Composition, %						
	Triglyceride	90	60	40	10	5
	Cholesterol	5	12	30	50	20
	Phospholipid	3	18	20	15	25
	Protein	2	10	10	25	50
Major apolipoproteins		A-I A-IV B-48 CI CII CIII	B-100 CI CII CIII E	B-100 E	B-100	A-I A-II

*IDL, intermediate-density lipoprotein.
a- and B- areas in electrophoretic gradient; a being furthest from origin of gradient, B being nearer, pre-B being even nearer.

Source: Kris Etherton, et al., The effect of diet on plasma lipids, lipoproteins, and coronary heart disease. Copyright the American Dietetic Association. Reprinted by permission from *Journal of the American Dietetic Association*, vol. 88, pp. 1373–1400, 1988.

The LDL-C supplies cholesterol to extrahepatic cells where it is used for cell membrane and steroid hormone synthesis. Some of the LDL-C is degraded by scavenger cells which help control high plasma concentrations. The liver removes the remaining circulating LDL-C. Thus, the LDL-C concentration depends upon the balance between the liver's production of VLDL-C, the partitioning of VLDL-C between hepatic removal and conversion to LDL-C, as well as the activity of LDL-C receptors.[17]

It is thought that HDL-C removes cholesterol from tissues and/or accepts it from VLDL-C metabolism.[22,23] Direct production of HDL-C occurs in both the liver and the intestine. The HDL-C binds unesterified cholesterol and delivers cholesteryl esters to the liver and VLDL-C. Some of the cholesterol is delivered to the liver by HDL-C and is excreted into the gallbladder as bile. HDL-C can be subdivided into 15 subfractions.[24] Two of the major subfractions include HDL_2-C and a more dense HDL_3-C. Mature HDL (HDL_3-C converted to HDL_2-C) is formed by the addition of surface components derived from chylomicron and VLDL-C metabolism.[25]

Low levels of HDL-C (<35 mg/dl) are as predictive for coronary heart disease (CHD) as high blood pressure, cigarette smoking, or diabetes.[2] The major causes of reduced HDL-C include cigarette smoking, obesity, lack of exercise, androgenic and related steroids (androgens, progestional agents, and anabolic steroids), beta-adrenergic blocking agents, hypertriglyceridemia, and genetic factors (i.e., hypoalphalipoproteinemia).[2]

Apolipoproteins are also important to the understanding of plasma lipid and lipoprotein metabolism. The apolipoproteins regulate biochemical reactions by stabilizing lipoprotein particles, providing recognition sites for cell membranes and by acting as cofactors for enzymes. The apolipoproteins determine the structure and regulatory functions of lipoproteins (see Table 2).[26]

Three major enzymes that influence lipid metabolism are lecithin cholesterol acetyltransferase (LCAT), lipoprotein lipase (LPL), and hepatic lipase (HL). The enzyme LCAT can affect the production of HDL. LPL is a lipolytic enzyme that controls TG hydrolysis and is the rate-limiting step in the uptake of lipoprotein, TG, and FFA into adipose tissue and muscle.[27,28] Hepatic lipase interacts with lipoproteins in the liver and may play a role in the reconversion of HDL_2 to HDL_3.[29]

A variety of genetic disorders in lipoprotein metabolism have been identified. These include abnormal functions with all the apolipoproteins and enzymes, as well as certain cell surface receptors that bind apolipoproteins. Genetic abnormalities have been found for gene encoding of LDL-C receptors, defective deregulation of LDL-C receptor synthesis, apo-B 100 structure abnormalities, and defects in VLDL-C metabolism which overproduce LDL-C.[4] Most of these disorders are fairly rare, but they are of clinical significance because they can produce severe hyperlipidemia and predispose individuals to premature CHD.[26]

The aging process itself decreases the activity of LDL-C receptors and causes the TC and LDL-C plasma levels to rise.[4] The mechanism for these increases with age are presently unknown, but may be due to cellular aging or a decrease in the body's overall metabolic rate.[4]

III. PLASMA LIPID/LIPOPROTEIN LEVELS AND CHD RISK

Interest in lipids and lipoproteins greatly intensified in the 1980s and 1990s due to findings that elevated cholesterol levels are causally linked to an increased risk of CHD.[2] Total cholesterol (TC), LDL-C, and HDL-C are all strong predictors of CHD risk.[30] Increased levels of plasma of TC and LDL-C are positively linked to CHD risk, while increased levels of HDL-C are negatively linked to CHD risk. High plasma levels of HDL_2-C are inversely related to the extent of coronary artery disease and HDL_2-C predicts CHD risk better than HDL-C or HDL_3-C.[31] There is also evidence that smaller LDL-C particles are more atherogenic than larger LDL-C particles.[32]

TABLE 2 Major Apolipoproteins of Plasma Lipoproteins

Name	Lipoprotein	Molecular weight	Function
Apo A-I	HDL, chylomicrons	28,000	Structural; activator of LCAT enzyme; reverse cholesterol
Apo A-II	HDL, chylomicrons	16,000	Structural
Apo A-IV	HDL, chylomicrons, VLDL	46,000	Unknown
Apo B-100	LDL, VLDL	550,000	Structural; synthesis and secretion of VLDL; binds to LDL receptor
Apo B-48	Chylomicrons	250,000	Structural; synthesis and secretion from intestine
Apo C-I	HDL, chylomicrons	6,000	Activator of LCAT enzyme
Apo C-II	HDL, chylomicrons, VLDL	7,000	Activator of LPL
Apo C-III	HDL, chylomicrons, VLDL	7,000	Modulates LPL activity
Apo E	Chylomicrons, VLDL, HDL	34,000	Binds to hepatic lipoprotein receptors

HDL = high-density lipoproteins; LCAT = lecithin-cholesterol acyltransferase; VLDL = very-low-density lipoproteins; LDL = low-density lipoproteins; LPL = lipoprotein lipase

From Brown, W. V., Lipoproteins: what, when, and how often to measure, *Heart Disease Stroke*, 1(1), 1992. With permission of the American Heart Association.

The plasma lipid and lipoprotein profile may be more useful for estimating CHD risk than a single value.[9] The combination of a moderately high plasma total cholesterol level, elevated HDL-C, and low LDL-C is not as atherogenic as the same total cholesterol with low HDL-C and high LDL-C values. The HDL-C/TC and HDL-C/LDL-C ratios (or reciprocals) are more powerful predictors of CHD than total cholesterol alone.[30] Although the lipid/lipoprotein ratios are important for predicting CHD risk, the National Cholesterol Education Program's Adult Treatment Panel[2] recommends that plasma TC be measured first (serum cholesterol multiplied by .97 = plasma values). Total cholesterol is more commonly available and less expensive to assess than LDL-C, yet the two are highly correlated. If the TC is higher than 240 mg/dl, then a lipoprotein analysis is recommended. A LDL-C level of 130 to 159 mg/dl places an individual at borderline high risk, while a level of ≥160 mg/dl is indicative of high risk for CHD. When the HDL-C is below 35 mg/dl CHD is significantly increased.[2]

Elevated plasma TG levels are associated with increased risk for CHD. However, the association often disappears when adjustments are made for other risk factors like HDL-C.[3,33] A recent report suggests that TG concentration is a marker of increased CHD risk, especially in subjects with high LDL-C/HDL-C ratios.[34] The measurement of plasma TG is positively related to LDL-C and inversely related to HDL-C, particularly HDL$_2$-C. Although the measurement of TG levels may not be the best current indicator to help monitor CHD risk, they do allow one to estimate LDL-C, if TC and HDL-C are known.[26] Most clinical laboratories can measure TC, HDL-C, and TG, thus, from the Friedwald equation: LDL-C = TC − [HDL + (TG/5)].[35] The equation allows the simple prediction of LDL-C as long as TG are less than 400 mg/dl.[26]

The serum apolipoproteins have been used as specific markers of CHD risk. Apolipoproteins A-I (apo A-I, associated with HDL-C) and B (apo B, associated with LDL-C) have

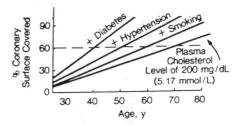

FIGURE 1. The relationship of coronary atherosclerosis (percentage of surface with raised lesions) vs. age as modified by addition of other risk factors. In the absence of other risk factors, patient cholesterol level of 200 mg/dl (5.17 mmol/l) should reach critical stenosis at about age 70 years. Addition of smoking reduces age to 60 years, and addition of more risk factors (i.e., hypertension and diabetes mellitus) reduces age further. (From Grundy, S. M., *JAMA*, 256(20), 2855, 1986. With permission.)

also been used individually and as ratios (A-I:B) to assess CHD risk.[26] Apo B has frequently been found to be elevated, compared to LDL-C, in patients with vascular disease. Apo A-I correlates highly with HDL-C and has been a consistent predictor of coronary artery disease. It has been suggested that HDL-C subfractions containing apo A-I and apo A-II may be better markers of CHD risk than HDL-C alone. However, Stampfer et al.[36] found that neither apolipoprotein levels nor HDL_2-C or HDL_3-C levels add significantly to predicting CHD, compared to the predictive power of measures of LDL-C and HDL-C alone. Currently, the ability to routinely obtain accurate and reliable measures of the apolipoproteins is beyond the capability of most clinical laboratories.[26,37]

IV. RATIONALE FOR INTERVENTION: DIET MODIFICATION AND EXERCISE

Lipid/lipoprotein metabolism is regulated by a variety of physiological variables that can affect the synthesis and catabolism of the various particles. These variables include aging, genetics, hormones, diet composition, calorie intake, alcohol consumption, cigarette smoking, medication, body composition, and exercise.[3,19]

Diet modification and regular exercise are typically recommended by physicians as the first step for adults to lower TC (and thus LDL-C) prior to drug intervention.[2,38] The rationale for this advice is based on epidemiological evidence, which indicates that there is a direct correlation between TC levels and CHD rates.[39-42] The relationship is continuous throughout the range of TC levels based on CHD mortality.[43] When TC exceeds 240 mg/dl, an individual has approximately a twofold increase in CHD risk.[2]

Clinical trials using single or multifactor interventions have shown that lowering LDL-C in men can reduce CHD incidence and actually slows or produces regression of coronary atherosclerosis.[43] This has been found in primary and secondary CHD-prevention trials.[44]

Women are also at high CHD risk when LDL-C levels are elevated, but prior to menopause their LDL-C levels are lower than those found for men. Following menopause, their risk of CHD increases due to loss of estrogen-stimulated LDL receptor activity.[4] Clinical trials on LDL-C lowering in women are not currently available.

When TC levels are lowered by 1%, there is a 2% reduction in CHD rates.[9,44] It does appear that at least an 8 to 9% reduction in TC is needed to reduce CHD mortality significantly. But if an individual could lower their TC by 10 to 15% with diet and exercise, they should reduce their CHD risk by 20 to 30%.[2]

For individuals who have multiple risk factors for CHD, lowering TC (and LDL-C) can have even greater effects.[45,46] For example, Grundy[39] (Figure 1) has shown that there is a hypothetical level (60% of coronary artery with raised plaque) which predicts the severity

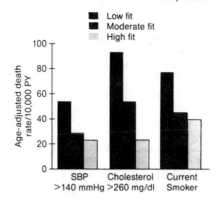

**DEATHS BY FITNESS AND
OTHER RISK FACTORS, MEN**

FIGURE 2. The relationship between fitness and all-cause mortality in men with high levels of other risk factors. Men in the moderate-fitness category have much lower death rates than the lower-fitness men in each of the other risk factor groups. (From Blair, S. N., *Gatorade Sports Science Exchange*, 3(29), 3, 1990. With permission.)

of atherosclerosis by age, at various cholesterol levels in relationship to other established CHD risk factors. If an individual has a TC level of 200 mg/dl, they would most likely become high risk for CHD at age 70, in the absence of other risk factors. If smoking is added, the critical stage is reached at 60. The addition of hypertension and diabetes to the risk profile would drop the ages for significantly increased CHD risk to 50 and 40, respectively. Thus, attention should be focused on managing all CHD risks in concert with controlling one's lipid/lipoprotein levels.

Blair et al.[47] have shown that men who are moderately active (based on treadmill fitness measures) have lower CHD mortality rates than inactive males, even when other risks for CHD are present (Figure 2). Men who had levels of TC >240 mg/dl and who were moderately active had significantly reduced mortality for CHD than men who were less fit. These relationships also appear to apply to women, but the data are based on fewer subjects than that for males.

Dietary modification and regular exercise (which may raise HDL-C) provide the foundation for the initial intervention for hyperlipidemia because they can have significant positive effects on lipid and lipoprotein metabolism.[48] For most Americans, diet modification and regular exercise can help reduce cholesterol-CHD risk, even when they are used as adjunct therapy to medication.[4,17] Diet modification and exercise are also more economical than medication therapy.

V. DIETARY FACTORS
A. Dietary Goals

It has been reported that the most significant factor influencing hypercholesterolemia is diet.[2,4] A variety of dietary strategies can be utilized to lower TC and LDL-C. The cholesterol-lowering response to dietary intervention is variable and depends on several factors, including the following:

1. Composition of the diet
2. The initial TC level (people with the highest levels usually have the greatest decrease per mg/dl, but even those with initially lower levels see a similar percent change)
3. The responsiveness of the individual
4. Acceptance and compliance with diet
5. Changes in body weight (especially body composition changes)[2,19]

The AHA, NCEP, National Research Council, and American Diabetes Association all recommend similar guidelines in regards to dietary composition to control lipid and lipoprotein levels.[2,4] These guidelines include the following:

1.　Consume 50 to 60% of total calories from the intake of carbohydrates with more than half of this amount in the form of complex carbohydrates.
2.　Consume less than 30% of calories from the intake of fats; saturated fats should comprise no more than 10% of the total fat intake, with 10% coming from polyunsaturated fats and the remaining 10 to 15% should come from monounsaturated fats.
3.　Protein should represent 10 to 20% of the dietary intake.
4.　To achieve these dietary composition goals, the diet should contain a variety of nutrients and be palatable.
5.　In addition, the diet should contain less than 300 mg/day intake of cholesterol (<200 mg/day in the Step 2 diet of the NCEP), and the total number of calories should be balanced towards the achievement or maintenance of desirable body weight.

Several detailed reviews of the effects of diet on lipids and lipoproteins can be found in the professional literature.[2,4,11,17,19,48,49] These studies form the basis for our review, which will summarize the following dietary issues related to lipids/lipoproteins: total dietary fat, cholesterol intake, saturated vs. unsaturated fats, carbohydrate intake, fiber intake, vegetarianism, alcohol consumption, coffee consumption, and obesity (weight gain).

B. Total Fat Intake

Americans consume 37 to 40% of their total calories from fat.[49] As mentioned above, many professional organizations like the AHA recommend that there should be no more than 30% total daily calories from fat. The rationale to reduce total fat in the diet is based on the concept that it will decrease saturated fatty acids (SF) intake, decrease the total calories in the diet, and promote weight reduction. However, excessive reduction of fat intake can increase TG levels and lower HDL-C.[3,49,50,51] Reducing the fat intake below 30% of the total dietary calories is not necessary to reduce CHD risk for most individuals, although there can be benefits for high-risk subgroups within the population.[52] It should be noted also that low-fat diets (below 30% of the total calories) are not palatable and may not be accepted well by many individuals.

There are data that demonstrate that fat quality has a more significant effect on plasma lipid/lipoprotein response than fat quantity.[19] Lowering total fat in the diet will reduce SF intake and can be facilitated further when unsaturated fatty acids (UF) are substituted for SF.[19,49]

C. Dietary Cholesterol

In metabolic ward studies, a cholesterol-raising action of dietary cholesterol is a consistent finding.[49] However, individuals vary in their responsiveness from treatment to treatment. In free-living setting studies, increased dietary cholesterol has variable effects on TC, LDL-C, and HDL-C, but generally they are increased. American men consume about 400 mg/d while women consume about 300 mg/d.[19] Raising cholesterol intake from a baseline level of 200 to 400 or 500 mg/d will increase TC 5 to 10 mg/dl.[17,39,53] Mechanisms that cause this increase appear to be related to the suppression of LDL-C receptor synthesis with a secondary increase in hepatic cholesterol content.[17,54] The plasma lipid response to dietary cholesterol will be affected by baseline intake and the type of fat in the diet.

D. Saturated Fatty Acids

The U.S. diet contains about 14% of the total calories as SF, whereas nutritionists recommend that the intake should be 7% or less.[2,17] Saturated fats are those found in animal fats and coconut and palm oils. The hypercholesterolemic effects of SF have been studied for more than 40 years and can be predicted.[19,53,55] The extra 7% of SF in the average person's diet increases TC by about 20 mg/dl, most of which is LDL-C. Generally, for every 1% increase of SF intake, TC increases about 2.7 mg/dl.[19] Increased SF intake decreases LDL-C receptor activity by several possible mechanisms.[17] It has been reported that some of the longer-chain SF (like stearic acid) may be less hypercholesterolemic than medium-chain SF, but more research is needed to determine the relative effects of different SF on lipid/lipoprotein levels.

E. Polyunsaturated Fatty Acids

If SF are reduced in the diet they must be replaced by other sources of fats, including polyunsaturated fats (PF). Americans consume approximately 7% of their total calories in the form of PF.[19] One source of PF includes linoleic acid which is consumed as vegetable oils, like corn oil, soybean oil, sunflower oil, etc. It has been shown that a 1% increase of linoleic acid in the diet decreases TC by 1.4 mg/dl.[19,53] Increasing PF intake is routinely recommended as a substitute to SF intake.[4] The mechanism by which linoleic acid lowers TC and LDL-C may be due to increased LDL-C receptor activity or simply because it replaces SF content in the diet. However, when PF intake in the form of linoleic acid exceeds 10% of the total calories, it has been reported that there is a lowering of HDL-C, suppression of the immune system, increased risk for cholesterol gallstones, promotion of carcinogenesis, and increased LDL-C oxidation (which is associated with rendering LDL-C atherogenic).[4,56-60]

Omega-3 fatty acids (O3FA) are another type of PF and they are found in fish and fish oils. The O3FA have been promoted as an alternative replacement for SF instead of linoleic acid.[19,61] The most consistent finding of O3FA on lipids/lipoproteins is the reduction of TG, which requires high doses.[39,62] They do not appear to lower TC or LDL-C any more than other UF. The O3FA have also been found to be antithrombotic because they reduce platelet aggregation and they are anti-inflammatory.[63] It is prudent to encourage fish consumption as a substitute for meats that are high in SF, which may help reduce CHD risk. However, fish oil supplements (which are commercially available without a prescription) are not recommended for individuals with normal plasma lipid/lipoprotein levels at this time. The clinical benefit of consuming fish oil supplements remains to be fully tested.[19]

F. Monounsaturated Fatty Acids

Monounsaturated fatty acids (MF) have been shown to lower TC and LDL-C without lowering HDL-C.[2] Americans consume approximately 14 to 16% of their total calories from MF. Sources of MF (oleic acid) include animal (the majority of the American diet) and vegetable sources (i.e., olive oil and canola oil). It is recommended by the AHA and NCEP that MF should comprise 10 to 15% of the total dietary intake and vegetable sources should be emphasized.[2,63] None of the side effects found for linoleic acid have been found for oleic acid, and therefore this form of MF may be the preferred replacement for SF.[4] Substituting MF at higher levels than recommended by the AHA or NCEP may promote weight gain, if indeed, the total fat intake exceeds 30% of the total calories. Thus, the diet should be balanced according to the specific fatty acid guidelines for each nutrient.

G. High-Carbohydrate Diets

High-carbohydrate diets have been recommended as one way to reduce TC and LDL-C. By increasing carbos in the diet there will be a reduction of total fat intake and this may promote weight loss. However, high intakes of carbos can stimulate hepatic synthesis of TG and raise VLDL-C levels.[4,64,65] They also lower HDL-C levels and both of these effects do not appear to be as transitional as once believed.[66]

H. Dietary Fiber

The effects of dietary fiber consumption on lipids/lipoproteins have received widespread media attention and have confused consumers due to the release of reports with conflicting conclusions. Much of the confusion is caused by different study designs, different study populations, and the evaluation of different types of fiber. Americans normally consume 10 to 20 g of dietary fiber daily as compared to the recommended levels of 20 to 25 g/d (not to exceed 40 to 50 g/d).[2] Dietary fiber which is water soluble (oats, fruits, beans, rice, and peas, etc.) has been shown in epidemiological studies to lower TC by 5 to 15%, while water-insoluble fiber (cellulose, lignin, and wheat bran, etc.) shows no TC-lowering effect.[2,19] There is evidence that water-soluble fiber can bind bile acids and increase fecal bile acid exertion.[67,68] The use of excessively large fiber intake can cause abdominal discomfort, decreased nutrient absorption, diarrhea, and other negative side effects. These same side effects can occur, when dietary fiber intake is increased, unless it is done gradually over time.[19]

I. Vegetarian Diets

Vegetarian diets are low in total fat, SF, cholesterol, and high in fiber. Vegetarians have been found to have lipid/lipoprotein profiles which are consistent with reduced CHD risk.[19,69,70] Vegetarian diets, which limit red meat consumption and reduce the consumption of animal by-products to control SF intake, are often recommended to patients with hypercholesterolemia to control TC and LDL-C. If one decides to adopt a vegetarian type of diet, they should make sure that they consume a variety of foods to insure proper nutrient balance.

J. Alcohol Consumption

Moderate alcohol consumption has been shown to be associated with reduced CHD risk and increased HDL-C.[5,71] The increases in total HDL-C may be due to increases in HDL$_3$-C vs. HDL$_2$-C, which some investigators have suggested would not be as desirable as the opposite effect.[11] Hartung et al.[72] have found recently that alcohol consumption in habitual male exercisers increased HDL-C, HDL$_2$-C, HDL$_3$-C, and Apo A-I. However, the manipulation of alcohol intake in premenopausal exercising women does not appear to have any significant influence on the same variables.[73] The average intake of alcohol in the U.S. diet is approximately 5% of the total calories, although this value varies greatly. The AHA[74] recommends that alcohol consumption should not exceed 1 to 2 oz/d, because alcohol consumption has been found to increase TG levels, and is associated with hypertension, cirrhosis, certain cancers, fetal alcohol syndrome, psychosocial problems, and accidents.[19] Moderate alcohol consumption (1 to 3 glasses of wine or beer) appears to provide some protection against CHD due to increased plasma HDL-C levels. However, at this time, it is not recommended that individuals increase their alcohol consumption to favorably change lipid/lipoprotein profiles.

K. Coffee Consumption

There is some evidence that increased coffee consumption is correlated and may cause negative lipid/lipoprotein level changes.[19] Although the results of the studies on coffee consumption are quite variable, increases in TC and LDL-C have been found with moderate (1 to 4 cups/d) and high (5 to 9 cups/d) coffee consumption. It is not clear whether caffeine or the other ingredients in coffee affect the lipid/lipoprotein levels. More research is needed before specific recommendations concerning coffee consumption will be formulated.[19]

TABLE 3 Effects of Dietary Modification on Plasma Lipids and Lipoproteins

	Decrease in fat	Decrease in cholesterol	Increase in polyunsaturated/ saturated	Increase in carbohydrates[a]	Increase in alcohol
Total cholesterol	−	−	−	−, n.c.	n.c.
Triglyceride	−, +	−, +	−	+	+
LDL-C	−	−	−	−	−
HDL-C	−, n.c.	−, n.c.	−, n.c.	−	+
HDL-C/total cholesterol	−, n.c.	−, n.c.	n.c.	−	+

Note: + = increase; − = decrease; n.c. = no change.

[a] Carbohydrates, especially simple sugars.

From Hartung, G. H., *Sports Med.*, 1, 413, 1984. With permission.

L. Obesity (Weight Gain)

Obesity (20 to 30 pounds or more over desirable body weight) may be the most underestimated cause of hypercholesterolemia.[4] Diet composition changes are usually recommended prior to weight reduction in those with clinically elevated lipid/lipoprotein levels.[4,75] American adults increase their weight by 20 to 30 pounds on average from age 20 to age 50.[17] It has been reported that the weight gain is associated with increases in TC that average 25 mg/dl. The increase in TC is mainly due to LDL-C increases and partly due to VLDL-C increases. HDL-C levels are usually reduced in obese individuals.[39] Grundy[17] has summarized two metabolic effects that obesity has on lipid/lipoprotein metabolism and they are (1) obesity promotes hepatic output of apo B-lipoproteins, which enhances the conversion of VLDL-C to LDL-C, and (2) whole-body synthesis of cholesterol is increased by obesity, expanding the hepatic cholesterol pool and this suppresses LDL-C receptor synthesis. Thus, obesity may be the number-one nutritional factor responsible for increased CHD risk in the U.S.[4] Controlling obesity is also important in reducing CHD risk for those individuals with elevated lipids/lipoproteins who have related chronic disease processes like hypertension, hyperinsulinemia, and diabetes mellitus. The effects of weight loss on lipid/lipoprotein levels will be discussed in the next section of the review, which highlights exercise as an intervention.

M. Summary

Dietary factors (see Table 3)[11] can have a significant impact on modifying plasma lipids/lipoproteins. Health-care professionals, who provide diet modification advice to individuals for the control of lipid/lipoprotein levels, should consider the following prudent recommendations:

1. Implement diet strategies which parallel those published by organizations like the AHA and the NCEP.
2. Provide flexibility in diet planning, particularly for individuals with multiple CHD risk factors or other hyperlipidemia-related disorders (i.e., hypertension, diabetes mellitus, etc.).
3. Encourage and instruct individuals about how to attain and maintain desirable body weight.

VI. EXERCISE
A. Exercise Goals

Hyperlipidemic individuals are usually encouraged by health-care professionals to increase their physical activity levels, engage in more exercise, or improve their physical fitness

TABLE 4 Effects of Exercise Training on Plasma Lipids and Lipoprotein

	Cross-sectional studies		Longitudinal studies	
	Men	Women	Men	Women
Total cholesterol	−, n.c.	−, n.c.	−, n.c.	−, n.c.
Triglyceride	−	−	−	−, n.c.
LDL-C	−	−	−	−
HDL-C	+	+	+, n.c.	+, n.c.
HDL-C/total cholesterol	+	+	+	+, n.c.

From Hartung, G. H., *Sports Med.*, 1, 413, 1984. With permission.

levels as part of a prudent risk factor modification plan. Although the terms physical activity, exercise, and physical fitness are used synonymously, they are defined by epidemiologists differently, and can confound the interpretations of lipid/lipoprotein-lowering investigations.[3,76] In our review, the term "exercise" will be used as all-encompassing, to include references from the relevant lipid/lipoprotein literature which have evaluated high vs. low physical activity levels, exercise training volumes, or physical fitness levels.

The AHA and the NCEP recommend regular exercise as part of an effective lipid/lipoprotein-lowering strategy.[2,72] Generally, exercise is encouraged by these groups due to the positive associations with weight reduction, fat weight loss, and increased caloric expenditure. Although low levels of exercise (walking 2 miles in 30 min, four to five times per week) have been found to lower all-cause mortality in men and women, higher intensities, durations, and frequencies of exercise training may be required for significant and specific exercise-related lipid/lipoprotein changes.[47,77] The AHA and the American College of Sports Medicine have recommended that adults should be encouraged to exercise three to five times per week, for 30 to 40 min, at an intensity of 60 to 90% of maximal heart rate reserve or 50 to 80% of maximal oxygen consumption, for the maintenance of good cardiovascular health.[77,78] In our previous review,[5] we reported that favorable alterations in lipid/lipoprotein levels may require jogging the equivalent of about 10 miles/week or greater than 1000 kcal/week of caloric expenditure involving endurance exercise over a 3- to 9-month period of time.[79] The specific effects of exercise training on plasma lipids and lipoproteins are illustrated in Table 4[11] and are discussed in the following sections.

The effects of exercise on blood lipids/lipoproteins have been reviewed extensively by several authors prior to 1990.[5,11,29,80-83] Only a few reviews have appeared in the literature since then.[3,83,84] The focus of this review will be to summarize the cross-sectional and longitudinal effects of exercise on blood lipids/lipoproteins by highlighting the following issues: endurance vs. resistance (strength) training influences, influences on men vs. women, influences on lipid metabolism enzymes and particle size, and the influences of the interaction of exercise vs. weight loss effects.

B. Endurance Exercise

Endurance exercise includes sustained aerobic exercise (training) like that required by brisk walking (3.5 to 4.5 miles/h), jogging (4.5 to 6 miles/h), running (>6 miles/h), cross-country skiing, tennis, soccer, or vigorous occupations (e.g., lumberjacks).[5] Cross-sectional studies involving endurance exercise, with few exceptions, have shown that in large epidemiological samples, as well as small study subgroups, exercise increases HDL-C (or its subfractions) and decreases TG, while VLDL-C changes are inversely related to those of HDL-C.[26,72,85-87] The cross-sectional evidence of the effects of exercise training on TC and

LDL-C, is mixed, with usually no effect found on TC, while LDL-C drops due to increases in HDL-C or its subfractions.[3,88]

In longitudinal studies, endurance exercise is generally associated with no significant change in TC, decreases or no change in LDL-C and VLDL-C, increases in HDL-C (or its subfractions), and decreases in TG.[3,85,89,90-92] The effects of exercise in longitudinal studies for women are less than those observed for men (at least for HDL-C) and will be discussed in another section. Acute exercise increases HDL-C and HDL_2-C subfraction in most studies, with HDL-C being influenced the most by high-intensity, long-duration bouts of exercise like marathon runs.[85] The positive longitudinal benefits of exercise on HDL-C levels for men have been reported in numerous studies, and it appears that an exercise dosage of the equivalent of 10 to 15 miles/week of jogging for 6 months is required for significant benefit.[3,85]

C. Resistance (Strength) Exercise

The reports from cross-sectional studies which have evaluated lipid/lipoprotein profiles in strength-trained individuals have produced conflicting results.[83] This may be due to the lack of control of various factors in the study designs, which have been shown to confound the lipid/lipoprotein levels. In longitudinal resistance (strength) training studies prior to 1990, investigators generally found favorable changes in blood lipid/lipoprotein levels. However, the conclusions of these studies are weakened by the following study design flaws: lack of control for day-to-day variation in lipids/lipoproteins, body composition changes, use of anabolic steroids, dietary factors, acute vs. chronic training effects, and plasma volume shifts.[83,93-95] When these methodological concerns were controlled, strength training for 20 weeks did not alter plasma lipid/lipoprotein profiles or regulatory enzymes that influence TG and HDL-C in men who were at risk for CHD.[96]

D. Influences on Men vs. Women

Exercise tends to have the same effects on lipid/lipoprotein levels in men and women (see Table 4), except that HDL-C and TG changes in women are not usually significantly altered, unless there are large increases in exercise intensity and duration.[85] Women, prior to menopause, usually have higher HDL-C levels compared to men and their HDL-C levels may be more difficult to modify by any means.[85] The effects of exercise training on HDL-C in women remains controversial because there have not been any long-term, randomized, controlled studies conducted.[4,85]

E. Influences on Lipid Metabolism Enzymes and Particle Size

Exercise training may influence the following lipid metabolism regulating enzymes: LCAT, LPL, and HL (see Section II). LCAT has been found to be higher in athletes and both LCAT and LPL increase following training.[3,85] HL has been shown to decrease following exercise training. The amount of exercise necessary to create favorable changes in these enzymes is currently unknown.[3]

The particle sizes of various lipoproteins have also been reported to be influenced by exercise.[3] Smaller LDL-C mass particles are considered to be more atherogenic than larger LDL-C particles, and exercise has been reported to lower small mass LDL-C particles.[3,24,97,98] Specific HDL-C particles (HDL_2-C) have been reported to increase in endurance runners compared to nonexercising controls and have been found to be inversely correlated to increased CHD risk.[97,98]

F. The Influence of Exercise vs. Weight Loss

The precise relationship between the influence of exercise on lipids/lipoproteins has been difficult to interpret due to a variety of interacting variables, like age, initial lipid/lipoprotein

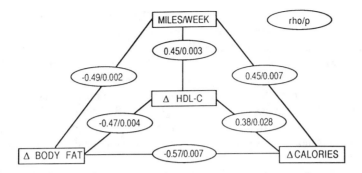

FIGURE 3. Spearman's coefficients among average miles run per week and one-year changes in plasma HDL-C concentration, percent body fat, and caloric intake in nondieting exercisers. Spearman's rho and the significant *p* of the correlation (two-tailed) is shown for each relationship. (From Wood, P. L. et al., *Metabolism*, 32, 31, 1983. With permission.)

levels, length of training, training intensity, level of aerobic fitness, and weight loss (particularly when expressed as percent body fat).[99] It has been reported that plasma lipid/lipoprotein changes are more associated with fat weight reduction than exercise training itself.[3,100,101] These findings suggest that specific thresholds of exercise training and/or fat weight loss must be obtained prior to the observation of favorable changes in HDL-C and TG.[3] The following discussion summarizes what is currently known about the exercise vs. fat weight loss influences on lipids/lipoproteins.

Williams et al.[102] were among the first to find that weight loss was strongly associated with HDL-C and HDL_2-C during exercise training in middle-aged men. In a longitudinal study which compared runners (8 miles/week) and controls, Wood et al.[100] found that significant changes in HDL-C and HDL_2-C were significantly correlated with changes in body fat and caloric intake (see Figure 3).

When overweight men were studied in a 1-year trial, fat loss acquired by either diet or exercise was equally effective in raising HDL-C.[101] Changes in LDL-C and TC were not significantly influenced for the full trial, and an increase in aerobic capacity ($\dot{V}O_2$ max) was associated with decreases in TG for exercisers only. Wood et al.[101] concluded that fat loss was the key to raising HDL-C, whether an individual achieved the results via dieting or exercise.

The issues of exercise vs. weight loss influence on lipids/lipoproteins has been evaluated more recently by Wier et al.[103] These investigators studied over 1500 men, of varying age and fitness levels, cross-sectionally and they also followed up on a subset of 156 men longitudinally (for 3 years), to assess the effects of exercise and weight loss on TC, LDL-C, TG, and HDL-C. In the cross-sectional data, age, fat weight, fat-free weight, and $\dot{V}O_2$ max were independently related to TC and HDL-C. Triglycerides were related to age, fat weight, and $\dot{V}O_2$ max, while LDL-C was related to age and $\dot{V}O_2$ max only. In the longitudinal sample, TC, LDL-C, and TG were only related to changes in weight (LDL-C) or changes in fat weight and changes in fat-free weight (TC and TG), and not $\dot{V}O_2$ max. Changes in both $\dot{V}O_2$ max and fat weight were significantly related with changes in HDL-C.

The authors concluded that their cross-sectional and longitudinal data indicated that:

1. When one assesses changes in lipids/lipoproteins, body composition should be the focus for TC and TG.
2. LDL-C is not influenced much by exercise-related changes in body composition or $\dot{V}O_2$ max.
3. Favorable changes in HDL-C are most responsive to changes in both body composition and $\dot{V}O_2$ max.

It is important to note that a 1 mg/dl increase in HDL-C is associated with a 2% decrease in CHD risk for men, and a 3% decrease in women.[104] In order to raise the HDL-C by 5 mg/dl, Wier et al.[103] predicted that fat weight would have to fall 5 kg and $\dot{V}O_2$ max would have to be increased by 9 ml $\cdot$ kg^{-1} $\cdot$ min^{-1} in their subjects. For a man weighing 79 kg, with 20% body fat and a $\dot{V}O_2$ max of 37 ml $\cdot$ kg^{-1} $\cdot$ min^{-1}, he would have to reduce his body fat to 14.6% and raise his $\dot{V}O_2$ max to 46 ml $\cdot$ kg^{-1} $\cdot$ min^{-1} to achieve the 5 mg/dl HDL-C increase. Although these fitness changes would require significant attention to increasing exercise habits (particularly if one is sedentary), this predictive example is consistent with the threshold of exercise training reported by others[3,5,79,85] to yield beneficial changes in HDL-C.

In contrast to the above findings, other investigators have confirmed that exercise training without weight loss can result in increased HDL-C levels.[85,105,106] In fact Sopko et al.[107] found that the effects of exercise with weight constant and weight loss without exercise on HDL-C were independent and additive in obese men. It has also been reported that young men who participated in exercise training for 20 weeks, and who had significant weight and fat loss with significant gains in $\dot{V}O_2$ max, did not increase their HDL-C levels.[108] The exercise vs. weight loss controversy regarding lipids/lipoproteins remains unresolved, while the specific mechanisms by which exercise increases HDL-C and HDL$_2$-C remains unknown and requires further investigation.

VII. SUMMARY

The NCEP has recommended that every adult over the age of 20 should know what their plasma TC level is, because the measurement of TC is a simple and inexpensive CHD risk screening tool.[2] If the TC level is below 200 mg/dl (LDL-C less than or equal to 129), the person has a desirable TC level and they should be encouraged to follow the AHA prudent diet guidelines and have their TC evaluated in 5-year intervals.[26] If the TC level is 200 to 239 mg/dl (130 to 159 mg/dl), the person should have their TC level measured after 4 to 6 weeks, and if it remains above 200 mg/dl, they should have their lipoprotein profile assessed. Dietary intervention should also be encouraged until the lipid/lipoprotein levels are normalized. In conclusion, based upon our previous review[5] and the current relevant literature, the combined effects of a healthy diet, maintenance of desirable body weight, and appropriate levels of endurance exercise can favorably influence lipid/lipoprotein profiles and reduce CHD risk in adults, as part of a primary prevention benefit.[26] In individuals with diagnosed CHD, the benefit of controlling lipid/lipoprotein levels is much larger than even that found for primary prevention.[98]

ACKNOWLEDGMENT

This paper is dedicated to the memory of Laurette Nichols, who typed our original manuscript for the first edition of this publication, and who was recognized as an outstanding employee at Southwest Texas State University during 1991.

REFERENCES

1. **Gotto, A. M.**, Preface, *Circulation*, 80, 716, 1989.
2. Report of the National Cholesterol Education Program Expert Panel on Detection, Evaluation, and Treatment of High Blood Cholesterol in Adults. The Expert Panel, *Arch. Intern. Med.*, 148, 36, 1988.
3. **Superko, H. R.**, Exercise training, serum lipids, and lipoprotein particles: is there a change threshold?, *Med. Sci. Sports Exercise*, 23, 677, 1991.

4. **Grundy, S. M.,** Cholesterol and coronary disease: future directions, *JAMA,* 264, 3053, 1990.
5. **Murray, T. D., Squires, W. G., and Hartung, G. H.,** Regulation of lipids and lipoproteins by diet and exercise, in *Nutrition in Exercise and Sport,* Hickson, J. F. and Wolinsky, I., Eds., CRC Press, Boca Raton, FL, 1989, 63.
6. **Bowers, R. W. and Fox, E. L., Eds.,** *Sports Physiology,* 3rd ed., Wm. C. Brown, Dubuque, 1988.
7. **Gordon, T., Castelli, W. P., Hjortland, M. C., Kannel, W. B., and Dawber, T. R.,** High density lipoprotein as a protective factor against coronary disease. The Framingham Study, *Am. J. Med.,* 62, 707, 1977.
8. **Castelli, W. P., Doyle, J. T., Gordon, T., Hames, C. G., Hjortland, M. C., Hulley, S. B., Kagan, A., and Zukel, W. J.,** HDL cholesterol and other lipids in coronary disease. The cooperative lipoprotein phenotyping study, *Circulation,* 55, 767, 1977.
9. Lipid Research Clinics Program: The Lipid Research Clinics Coronary Primary Prevention Trial Results. II. The relationship in incidence of coronary heart disease to cholesterol lowering, *JAMA,* 251, 365, 1984.
10. **Miller, G. J. and Miller, N. E.,** Plasma high density lipoprotein concentration and development of ischemic heart-disease, *Lancet,* 1, 16, 1975.
11. **Hartung, G. H.,** Diet and exercise in the regulation of plasma lipids and lipoproteins in patients at risk of coronary disease, *Sports Med.,* 1, 413, 1984.
12. **Dufax, B., Assman, G., and Hollman, W.,** Plasma lipoproteins and physical activity: a review, *Int. J. Sports Med.,* 3, 123, 1982.
13. **Lewis, B., Ed.,** *The Hyperlipidemias: Clinical Laboratory Practice,* Vol. 1–3, Blackwell Scientific, Oxford, 1976.
14. **Goldstein, J. L. and Brown, M. S.,** The low density lipoprotein pathway and its relation to atherosclerosis, *Annu. Rev. Biochem.,* 46, 897, 1977.
15. **Gotto, A. M.,** High-density lipoproteins: biochemical and metabolic factors, *Am. J. Cardiol.,* 52, 2B, 1983.
16. **Brown, M. S. and Goldstein, J. L.,** A receptor-mediated pathway for cholesterol homeostasis, *Science,* 232, 34, 1986.
17. **Grundy, S. M.,** Multifactorial etiology of hypercholesterolemia: implications for prevention of coronary heart disease, *Arteriosclerosis Thrombosis,* 11, 1619, 1991.
18. **Brooks, G. A. and Fahey, T. D.,** *Exercise Physiology: Human Bioenergetics and Its Applications,* Vol. 7, John Wiley & Sons, New York, 1984.
19. **Kris-Etherton, P. M., Krummel, D., Dreon, D., Mackey, S., Borchers, J., and Wood, P. D.,** The effects of diet on plasma lipids, lipoproteins, and coronary heart disease, *J. Am. Diet. Assoc.,* 88, 1374, 1988.
20. **Eisenberg, S. and Levy, R. I.,** Lipoprotein metabolism, *Adv. Lipid Res.,* 13, 1, 1976.
21. **Levy, R. and Rifkind, B. M.,** The structure and metabolism of high density lipoproteins: a status report, *Circulation,* 62, IV-4, 1980.
22. **Glomset, S. A.,** The plasma lecithin cholesterol acyltransferase reaction, *J. Lipid Res.,* 9, 155, 1968.
23. **Carew, T. E., Kroschinsky, T., Hayes, S. B., and Steinberg, D.,** A mechanism by which high-density lipoproteins may slow the atherogenic process, *Lancet,* 1, 1315, 1976.
24. **Williams, P. T., Krauss, R. M., Wood, P. D., Lindgren, F. T., Giotas, C., and Vranizan, K. M.,** Lipoprotein subfractions of runners and sedentary men, *Metabolism,* 35, 45, 1986.
25. **Breslow, J. L.,** Apolipoprotein genetic variation and human disease, *Physiol. Rev.,* 68, 85, 1988.
26. **Brown, W. V.,** Lipoproteins: what, when, and how often to measure?, *Heart Dis. Stroke,* 1, 21, 1992.
27. **Marniemi, J., Dahlstorm, S., Kvist, M., Seppanen, A., and Hietanen, E.,** Dependence of serum lipid and lecithin: cholesterol acyltransferase levels on physical training of young men, *Eur. J. Appl. Physiol.,* 49, 25, 1982.
28. **Kinnunen, P. K., Virtanen, J. A., and Vainio, P.,** Lipoprotein lipase and hepatic endothelial lipase: their roles in plasma lipoprotein metabolism, *Atherosclerosis Rev.,* 11, 65, 1983.
29. **Superko, H. R. and Haskell, W. H.,** The role of exercise training in the therapy of hyperlipoproteinemia, *Clin. Cardiol.,* 5, 285, 1987.
30. **Gordon, T., Kannel, W. B., Castelli, W. B., and Dawber, T. R.,** Lipoproteins, cardiovascular disease and death: the Framingham Study, *Arch. Intern. Med.,* 141, 1128, 1981.
31. **Miller, N. E., Hammett, F., Saltissi, S., Van Zeller, H., Coltart, J., and Lewis, B.,** Relation of angiographically defined coronary artery disease to plasma lipoprotein subfractions and apolipoproteins, *Br. Med. J.,* 282, 1741, 1981.
32. **Williams, P. T., Krauss, R. M., Kindel-Joyce, S., Dreon, D. M., Vranizan, K. M., and Wood, P. D.,** Relationship of dietary fat, protein, cholesterol, and fiber intake to atherogenic lipoproteins in men, *Am. J. Clin. Nutr.,* 44, 788, 1986.
33. **Hartung, G. H., Squires, W. G., and Gotto, A. M.,** Effect of exercise training on plasma high-density lipoprotein cholesterol in coronary disease patients, *Am. Heart J.,* 101, 181, 1981.

82 Nutrition in Exercise and Sport, 2nd Edition

34. **Manninen, V., Tenkanen, L., Koskinen, P., Huttunen, J. K., Manttari, M., Heinonen, O. P., and Frick, M. H.,** Joint effects of serum triglyceride and LDL cholesterol concentrations on coronary heart disease risk in the Helsinki Heart Study: implications for treatment, *Circulation,* 85, 37, 1991.

35. **Friedwald, W., Levy, R., and Fredrikson, D.,** Estimation of the concentration of low-density, lipoprotein cholesterol in plasma, without use of the preparative ultracentrifuge, *Clin. Chem.,* 18, 499, 1972.

36. **Stampfer, M. J., Sacks, F. M., Salvini, S., Willet, W. C., and Hennekens, C. H.,** A prospective study of cholesterol, apolipoproteins, and the risk of myocardial infarction, *N. Engl. J. Med.,* 325, 373, 1991.

37. **Vega, G. L. and Grundy, S. M.,** Does measurement of apolipoprotein B have a place in cholesterol management?, *Arteriosclerosis,* 10, 668, 1990.

38. **McBride, P. E., Plane, M. B., and Underbakke, G.,** Hypercholesterolemia: the current educational needs of physicians, *Am. Heart J.,* 123, 817, 1992.

39. **Grundy, S. M.,** Cholesterol and coronary heart disease: a new era, *JAMA,* 256, 2849, 1986.

40. **Kannel, W. B., Castelli, W. P., and Gordon, T.,** Serum cholesterol lipoproteins and risk of coronary disease: The Framingham Study, *Ann. Intern. Med.,* 74, 1, 1971.

41. Final Report of the Pooling Project Research Group, Relationship of blood pressure, serum cholesterol, smoking habit, relative weight and ECG abnormalities to incidence of major coronary events, *J. Chronic Dis.,* 31, 201, 1978.

42. **Goldbourt, V., Holtzman, E., and Neufeld, H. N.,** Total and high density lipoprotein cholesterol in the serum and risk of mortality: evidence of a threshold effect, *Br. Med. J.,* 290, 1239, 1985.

43. **Stamler, J., Wentworth, D., and Neaton, J.,** Is the relationship between serum cholesterol and risk of death from coronary disease continuous and graded?, *JAMA,* 256, 2823, 1986.

44. **Holme, I.,** An analysis of randomized trials evaluating the effect of cholesterol reduction on total mortality and coronary heart disease incidence, *Circulation,* 82, 1916, 1990.

45. **Stamler, J.,** Major coronary risk factors before and after myocardial infarction, *Postgrad. Med.,* 57, 34, 1975.

46. **Stamler, J.,** Primary prevention of coronary heart disease: the last 20 years, *Am. J. Cardiol.,* 47, 722, 1981.

47. **Blair, S. N., Kohl, H. W., Paffenbarger, R. S., Clark, D. G., Cooper, K. H., and Gibbons, L. W.,** Physical fitness and all-cause mortality: a prospecitve study of healthy men and women, *JAMA,* 262, 2395, 1989.

48. **Conner, W. E. and Conner, S. L.,** The dietary treatment of hyperlipidemia: rationale, technique, and efficacy, *Med. Clin. North Am.,* 66, 485, 1982.

49. **Grundy, S. M., Brown, W. V., Dietschy, J. M., Ginsberg, H., Goodnight, S., Howard, B., La Rosa, J. C., and McGill, H. C.,** Workshop III, Basis for Dietary Treatment, AHA Conference Report on Cholesterol, *Circulation,* 80, 729, 1989.

50. **Grundy, S. M.,** Comparison of monosaturated fatty acids and carbohydrates for lowering plasma cholesterol, *N. Engl. J. Med.,* 314, 745, 1986.

51. **Mensink, R. P. and Katan, M. B.,** Effect of monosaturated fatty acids versus complex carbohydrates in high-density lipoproteins in healthy men and women, *Lancet,* 1, 122, 1987.

52. **Hartung, G. H., Reeves, R. S., Sigurdson, A. S., Traweek, M. S., Foryet, J. P., and Blocker, W. P.,** Effect of a low-fat diet and exercise on plasma lipoproteins and cardiac dysrhythmia in middle-aged men, *Circulation,* 68 (Part 2), III-226, 1983.

53. **Keys, A., Anderson, J. T., and Grande, F.,** Serum cholesterol response to changes in the diet. II. The effect of cholesterol in the diet, *Metabolism,* 14, 759, 1965.

54. **Sorci-Thomas, M., Wilson, M. D., Johnson, F. L., Williams, D. L., and Rudel, L. L.,** Studies on the expression of genes encoding apolipoproteins B100 and B48 and the low density lipoprotein receptor in primates, *J. Biol. Chem.,* 264, 9039, 1989.

55. **Hegsted, D. M., McGandy, R. B., Meyers, M. L., and Stare, F. J.,** Quantitative effects of dietary fat on serum cholesterol in man, *Am. J. Clin. Nutr.,* 17, 281, 1965.

56. **Shepard, J., Packard, C. J., Patsch, J. R., Gotto, A. M., and Taunton, O. D.,** Effects of dietary polyunsaturated and saturated fat on the properties of high-density lipoprotein and the metabolism of apolipoprotein AI, *J. Clin. Invest.,* 61, 1582, 1978.

57. **Weymen, C., Berlin, J., Smith, A. D., and Thompson, R. S. H.,** Linoleic acid as an immunosuppressive agent, *Lancet,* 2, 33, 1975.

58. **Strurdevant, R. A. L., Pearce, M. L., and Dayton, S.,** Increased prevalence of cholelithiasis in men ingesting a serum-cholesterol-lowering diet, *N. Engl. J. Med.,* 288, 24, 1973.

59. **Reddy, B. S.,** Amount and type of dietary fat and colon cancer: animal model studies, *Prog. Clin. Biol. Res.,* 222, 295, 1986.

60. **Parthasarathy, S., Khoo, J. C., Miller, E., Barnett, J., and Witztum, J. L.,** Low-density lipoprotein rich in oleic acid is protected against oxidative modification: implications for dietary prevention of atherosclerosis, *Proc. Natl. Acad. Sci. U.S.A.,* 87, 3894, 1990.

61. **Simons, L. A., Hickie, J. B., and Balasubramanian, S.,** On the effects of dietary omega-3 fatty acids (Max EPA) on plasma lipids and lipoproteins in patients with hyperlipidemia, *Atherosclerosis,* 54, 75, 1985.
62. **Phillipson, B. E., Rothbrock, D. W., Conner, W. E., Harris, W. S., and Illingworth, D. R.,** Reduction of plasma lipids, lipoproteins, and apoproteins by dietary fish oils in patients with hypertriglyceridemia, *N. Engl. J. Med.,* 312, 1210, 1985.
63. **National Dietary Council,** Nutrition and health effects of unsaturated fatty acids, *Dairy Council Dig.,* 59, 1, 1988.
64. **Grundy, S. M.,** Comparison of monounsaturated fatty acids and carbohydrates for lowering plasma cholesterol, *N. Engl. J. Med.,* 314, 745, 1986.
65. **Grundy, S. M., Florentin, L., Nix, D., and Whelan, M. F.,** Comparison of monounsaturated fatty acids and carbohydrates for reducing raised levels of plasma cholesterol in man, *Am. J. Clin. Nutr.,* 47, 965, 1988.
66. **West, C. E., Sullivan, D. R., Katan, M. B., Halferkamps, I. N., and van der Torre, H. W.,** Boys from populations with high-carbohydrate intake have higher fasting triglyceride levels than boys from populations with high fat intake, *Am. J. Epidemiol.,* 131, 271, 1990.
67. **Kay, R. M. and Truswell, A. S.,** Effect of citrus pectin on blood lipids and fecal steroid excretion in man, *Am. J. Clin. Nutr.,* 30, 171, 1977.
68. **Kay, R. M.,** Dietary Fiber, *J. Lipid Res.,* 23, 221, 1982.
69. **Sacks, F. M., Castelli, W. F., Donner, A., and Kass, E. H.,** Plasma lipids and lipoproteins in vegetarians and controls, *N. Engl. J. Med.,* 292, 1148, 1975.
70. **Zetts, R. A., Avent, H. H., Murray, T. D., and Squires, W. G.,** Comparison of high density lipoprotein levels (HDL) between vegetarian and non-vegetarian females, *Med. Sci. Sports Exercise,* 17 (Abstr.), 285, 1985.
71. **Hartung, G. H. and Foreyt, J. P.,** The effect of alcohol intake on high-density lipoprotein cholesterol and coronary heart disease, *Cardiovasc. Rev. Rep.,* 5, 678, 1984.
72. **Hartung, G. H., Foreyt, J. P., Reeves, R. S., Krock, L. P., Patsch, W., Patsch, J. R., and Gotto, A. M.,** Effect of alcohol dose on plasma lipoprotein subfractions and lipolytic enzyme activity in active and inactive men, *Metabolism,* 39, 81, 1990.
73. **Hartung, G. H., Reeves, R. S. Foreyt, J. P., Patsch, W., and Gotto, A. M.,** Effect of alcohol intake and exercise on plasma high-density lipoprotein subfractions and apolipoprotein A-I in women, *Am. J. Cardiol.,* 58, 148, 1986.
74. The Nutrition Committee, American Heart Association, Dietary guidelines for healthy American adults, *Circulation,* 77, 721A, 1988.
75. **Kannel, W. B., Gordon, T., and Castelli, W. P.,** Obesity, lipids and glucose intolerance: The Framingham Study, *Am. J. Nutr.,* 32, 1238, 1979.
76. **Casperson, C. J.,** Physical activity epidemiology: concepts, methods, and applications to exercise science, *Exercise Sci. Rev.,* 17, 423, 1989.
77. American College of Sports Medicine, Position Stand, The recommended quantity and quality of exercise for developing and maintaining cardiorespiratory and muscular fitness in healthy adults, *Med. Sci. Sports Exercise,* 22, 265, 1990.
78. American Heart Association, *1990 Heart and Stroke Facts,* National Center, Dallas, 1990.
79. **Superko, H. R., Haskell, W. L., and Wood, P. D.,** Modification of plasma cholesterol through exercise: rationale and recommendations, *Postgrad. Med.,* 78, 64, 1985.
80. **Wood, P. D., Williams, P. T., and Haskell, W. L.,** Physical activity and high-density lipoproteins, in *Clinical and Metabolic Aspects of High-Density Lipoproteins,* Miller, N. E. and Miller, G. J., Eds., Elsevier, New York, 1984, 133–165.
81. **Haskell, W. L.,** The influence of exercise training on plasma lipids and lipoproteins in health and disease, *Acta Med. Scand. Suppl.,* 711, 23, 1986.
82. **Hurley, B. F.,** Effects of resistive training on lipoprotein-lipid profiles: a comparison to aerobic exercise training, *Med. Sci. Sports Exercise,* 21, 689, 1989.
83. **Kokkinos, P. F. and Hurley, B. F.,** Strength training and lipoprotein-lipid profiles: a critical analysis and recommendations for further study, *Sports Med.,* 9, 266, 1990.
84. **Schieken, R. M.,** Effect of exercise on lipids, *Ann. N.Y. Acad. Sci.,* 623, 269, 1991.
85. **Hartung, G. H.,** High density lipoprotein cholesterol and physical activity: an update: 1983–1991, *Sports Med.,* 1993.
86. **Marti, B., Knobloch, M., Riesen, W. F., and Howald, H.,** Fifteen-year changes in exercise, aerobic power, abdominal fat, and serum lipids in runners and controls, *Med. Sci. Sports Exercise,* 23, 115, 1991.
87. **Stray-Gundersen, J., Denkee, M. A., and Grundy, S. M.,** Influence of lifetime cross-country skiing on plasma lipids and lipoproteins, *Med. Sci. Sports Exercise,* 23, 695, 1991.
88. **Superko, R. M.,** Exercise, lipoproteins, and coronary artery disease, *Circulation,* 79, 1143, 1989.

89. **Baker, T., Allen, D., Lei, K. Y., and Willcox, K. K.,** Alterations in lipid and protein profiles of plasma lipoproteins in middle-aged men consequent to an aerobic exercise program, *Metabolism,* 35, 1037, 1986.
90. **Thompson, P. D., Cullinane, E. M., Sady, S. P., Flynn, M. M., Bernier, D. N., Kanter, M. A., Saritelli, A. L., and Herbert, P. N.,** Modest changes in high-density lipoprotein concentration and metabolism with prolonged exercise training, *Circulation,* 78, 25, 1988.
91. **Ratliff, R., Knehans, A., and McCarthy, M.,** Effects of frequency of exercise training on plasma lipids and lipoproteins, *Med. Sci. Sports Exercise,* 22 (Abstr.), S48, 1990.
92. **Marti, B., Suter, E., Riesen, W. F., Tschopp, A., Wanner, H. U., and Gutzwiller, F.,** Effects of long-term, self-monitored exercise on the serum lipoprotein and apolipoprotein profile in middle-age men, *Atherosclerosis,* 81, 19, 1990.
93. **Hurley, B. F., Hagberg, J. M., Goldberg, A. P., Seals, D. R., Ehsani, A. A., Brennan, R. E., and Holloszy, J. O.,** Resistance training can reduce coronary risk factors without altering VO$_2$ max or percent body fat, *Med. Sci. Sports Exercise,* 20, 150, 1988.
94. **Kokkinos, P. F., Hurley, B. F., Vaccaro, P., Patterson, J. C., Gardner, L. B., Ostrove, S. M., and Goldberg, A. P.,** Effects of low- and high-repetition resistive training on lipoprotein-lipid profiles, *Med. Sci. Sports Exercise,* 20, 50, 1988.
95. **Kokkinos, P. F., Hurley, B. F., Smutok, M. A., Farmer, C., Reece, C., Shulman, R., Charabogos, C., Patterson, J., Will, S., Devane-Bell, J., and Goldberg, A. P.,** Strength training does not improve lipoprotein-lipid profiles in men at risk for CHD, *Med. Sci. Sports Exercise,* 23, 1134, 1991.
96. **Manning, J. M., Dooley-Manning, C. R., White, K., Kampa, I., Silas, S., Kesselhaut, M., and Ruoff, M.,** Effects of a resistance training program on lipoprotein-lipid levels in obese women, *Med. Sci. Sports Exercise,* 23, 1222, 1991.
97. **Wirth, A. C., Diehm, C., Hanel, W., Welte, J., and Vogel, I.,** Training-induced changes in serum lipids, fat tolerance, and adipose tissue metabolism in patients with hypertriglyceridemia, *Atherosclerosis,* 54, 263, 1985.
98. **LaRosa, J. C. and Cleeman, J. I.,** Cholesterol lowering as a treatment for established coronary heart disease, *Circulation,* 85, 1229, 1992.
99. **Tran, Z. V., Weltman, A., Glass, G. V., and Mood, D. P.,** The effects of exercise on blood lipids and lipoproteins: a meta analysis of studies, *Med. Sci. Sports Exercise,* 15, 393, 1983.
100. **Wood, P. D., Haskell, W. L., Blair, S. N., Williams, P. T., Krauss, R. M., Lindgren, F. T., Albers, J. J., Ho, P. H., and Farquhar, J. W.,** Increased exercise level and plasma lipoprotein concentrations: a one-year randomized, controlled study in sedentary, middle-aged men, *Metabolism,* 32, 31, 1983.
101. **Wood, P. D., Stefanick, M. L., Dreon, D. M., Frey-Hewitt, B., Gary, S. C., Williams, P. T., Superko, H. R., Fortmann, S. P., Albers, J. J., Vranizan, K. M., Ellsworth, N. M., Terry, R. B., and Haskell, W. L.,** Changes in plasma lipids and lipoproteins in overweight men during weight loss through dieting as compared to exercise, *N. Engl. J. Med.,* 319, 1173, 1988.
102. **Williams, P. T., Wood, P. D., Haskell, W. L., Krauss, R. M., Vranizan, K. M., Blair, S. N., Terry, R.,and Farquhar, J. W.,** Does weight loss cause the exercise-induced increase in plasma high density lipoproteins?, *Atherosclerosis,* 47, 173, 1983.
103. **Weir, L. T., Jackson, A. S,. and Pinkerton, M. B.,** Effects of body composition and VO$_2$ max on HDL-C: cross-sectional and longitudinal analyses, *Med. Sci. Sports Exercise,* 23, S50, 1991.
104. **Gordon, D. J., Probstfield, J. L., Garrison, R. J., Neaton, J. D., Castelli, W. P., Knoke, J. D., Jacobs, D. R., Bangdiwala, S., and Tyroler, H. A.,** High-density lipoprotein and cardiovascular disease: four prospective American studies, *Circulation,* 79, 8, 1989.
105. **Higuchi, M., Hashimoto, I., Yamakawa, K., Tsuji, E., Nishimuta, M., and Suzuki, S.,** Effect of exercise training on plasma high-density lipoprotein cholesterol at constant weight, *Clin. Physiol.,* 4, 125, 1984.
106. **Kiens, B., Lithell, H., and Vessby, B.,** Further increase in high density lipoprotein in trained males after enhanced training, *Eur. J. App. Physiol.,* 52, 426, 1984.
107. **Sopko, G., Leon, A. S., Jacobs, D. R., Foster, N., Moy, J., Kuba, K., Anderson, J. T., Casal, D., McNally, C., and Frantz, I.,** The effect of exercise and weight loss on plasma lipids in young obese men, *Metabolism,* 34, 227, 1985.
108. **Despres, J.-P., Bouchard, C., Savard, R., Tremblay, A., and Allard, C.,** Lack of relationship between changes in adioposity and plasma lipids following endurance training, *Atherosclerosis,* 54, 135, 1985.

Chapter 5

RESEARCH DIRECTIONS IN PROTEIN NUTRITION FOR ATHLETES

James F. Hickson, Jr.
Ira Wolinsky

CONTENTS

0-8493-7911-3/94/$0.00+$.50
© 1994 by CRC Press, Inc.

I. OVERVIEW

Protein intake has been a primary concern of competitive athletes since ancient times when the Greek Olympic Games were held. The reasons for this enthusiasm over protein nutrition have varied over the years, but one fact stands out: persons engaged in manual labor or athletics have preferred a higher-protein diet when compared with more sedentary persons. However, support for high-protein diets remains a matter of controversy among health care professionals, including dietitians.

Scientists have responded to athletes' claim to the high-protein diet by conducting experiments designed to produce evidence in support of, or to deny, the practice. Over the last two decades, two dominant lines of investigation have emerged. One of these is based on the belief of many athletes that exercise traumatizes or "tears down" skeletal muscle proteins, and to allow for tissue repair and compensatory hypertrophy, a high-protein diet must be consumed. The other one follows the reasoning that exercise enhances the oxidation of amino acids at the skeletal muscle to provide energy for work, and a high-protein diet is necessary to offset the quantity of skeletal muscle protein catabolized for energy.

The purpose of this chapter is to review several studies which fall within each of the two lines of scientific research regarding the validity of athletes' claims for a high-protein diet. In this way, the directions of research in protein nutrition for athletes will be generally defined.

II. PRACTICABLE INTAKES

The study of practicable protein intakes provides information about what has worked relative to common experience. In this regard, it is helpful to consider the practices of modern athletes vs. typical Americans who are likely to be sedentary by comparison. Some athletes believe that they can never consume too much protein, and indeed, there is no human data suggesting that the nutrient is toxic even at extreme levels. However, there is no evidence to indicate that maximum, practicable intakes are advantageous either.

A. Achieving High Protein Intake

Dietary studies of modern athletes generally reveal "high" intakes of protein. Intakes are high for two reasons: (1) high-protein foods are emphasized in the diet, and (2) the total food intake is great in order to meet the energy demands of sport. Each of these effects on protein intake have been documented with teenage and collegiate football players, and adult male and female bodybuilders.[1-5]

1. Emphasis on Protein-Rich Foods

The dietary behaviors of collegiate football athletes in their winter stage of training illustrate the effect of selecting high-protein foods over others.[4] Sixteen men served as subjects over a 3-d period; the mean body weight of subjects was 108 kg. The exercise regimen consisted of 1.0 h of weight training and 1.0 h of distance running and spring training during mid-afternoon on four to five weekdays. Food intake data were collected during Tuesday, Wednesday, and Thursday in February 1985. Subjects took all their meals from a "training table" in a dining facility reserved for athletes. The menu included a complete variety of foods; meats were served at every meal. Food obtained from the tray line was weighed by an investigator on an electronic balance. There were also food and beverage stations located in the dining hall, so two to three investigators watched this area, recording any selections by subjects. Plate waste was visually estimated except for meat refuse (bones and meat), which was weighed.

The results of the study[4] indicate that subjects emphasized meat in their diets. The mean intake of protein was 190 g/d, representing 22% of energy. Considering their mean body weight (108 kg), subjects consumed 1.8 g protein/kg, which is 225% of the recommended dietary allowance (RDA). The major source of dietary protein and energy was meat. For the typical American male, meats make a smaller contribution to energy (28 vs. 33% kcal) and protein (49 vs. 63%) intakes.[4,6] There were two factors at the training table which promoted subjects' meat consumption. First, meat was perceived to be a bodybuilding food. Second, athletes were allowed unlimited access to all foods at the training table. Hence, subjects could return for as many servings of meat as they liked, and they could ask for more than one entree at a time. Furthermore, subjects took advantage of this opportunity to eat meat. Hickson et al.[4] wrote, "We frequently observed subjects receiving 500–600 g of 1–3 meats on their plate."

2. High Energy Intake

Besides emphasizing protein-rich foods, athletes can obtain a high-protein diet simply by eating a lot of food. The intake of many nutrients is known to rise as total food consumption rises.[6,7] This phenomenon is illustrated by a study conducted by Hickson et al.[7] Eighteen members (19.8 ± .3 years, 71.1 ± 1.7 kg) (mean ± SE) of the elite Indiana University soccer team served as subjects in a two-part study. The team won the National Collegiate Athletic Association (NCAA) Division I Championship in soccer before and during the study. Dietary survey data were taken during two stages of training, including preseason conditioning and competition.

During preseason conditioning, subjects participated in two 2.5-h exercise sessions, one focusing on the development of individual athletic skills and the other involving practice scrimmage situations. During the competition season, daily exercise sessions lasted only 2 h, and they focused on strategic elements concerning upcoming matches and short situation scrimmages. During preseason conditioning, all subjects lived on campus and ate three meals per day at a university cafeteria. A wide variety of foods were available at the cafeteria, and subjects could eat as much as they wanted, except that there was a limitation of one entree per person at the dinner meal. Food intakes at the cafeteria were observed and recorded over three weekdays by the investigators.[7] During the competitive season, subjects recorded their own food intakes over three weekdays after receiving instruction in the use of a structured recording form.

Subjects' mean daily energy intake was significantly higher during preseason conditioning than during competition (4492 vs. 3346 kcal).[7] The exclusion of prolonged scrimmages during the competitive season probably accounts for the drop of 1146 kcal from one stage to the next. Mean protein intake was 159 g/d during preseason conditioning, and it was 138 g/d during competition. The fall in protein intake was not statistically significant, but the direction of the change suggests a relationship between energy and protein intakes.

The magnitude of protein intakes is high relative to typical American men aged 19 to 22 years, who consume an average of 99 g at 2395 kcal/d.[6] One explanation for the lower protein intake of typical American males is that the athletic subjects consumed more food, as reflected in their higher energy intake. Importantly, this higher protein intake was not due to a focus on protein-rich foods, since their access to entrees was limited. In conclusion, dietary protein intake may be elevated for the athlete simply because he or she needs to eat a large amount of food in order to satisfy the energy demands of sport participation.

B. Determinants of Food Consumption
1. Mode of Thought

Some athletes think and act regarding diet and nutrition in a way that suggests a "concrete" or physical understanding of nature.[8] In other words, they explain principles of diet and nutrition in terms of what can be physically experienced — seen, touched, heard, smelled, and tasted. Consider the following three examples. First, red meat looks like muscle tissue, so athletes desiring to build a muscular body should eat lots of it.

Second, the relatively low RDA for protein is confusing to athletes because they have learned that "muscles are made of protein". It seems logical that a high-protein diet would be necessary to support a muscular athlete in training to get even bigger in size. For a world-class bodybuilder weighing 105 kg, the RDA would be only 84 g protein. This is less than the protein content of just one of the two to three steaks which Shawn Ray, a professional bodybuilder and contender for the 1992 Mr. Olympia crown, reports eating every day.[9]

Third, the visual experience of a massive bodybuilder is very powerful in presenting a case for the high-protein diet. Curtis[9] writes that one look at Shawn Ray tells the whole story on protein needs and bodybuilding: "You can't argue with a physique like Shawn Ray's. Medical journals are nice, and as a registered dietitian (sic) I depend on them for accurate information about nutrition. But here in the gym in Southern California, the *facts* were standing right in front of me . . . "

By way of contrast, in the "abstract" or intellectual mode of thinking, it is possible to imagine that dietary protein goes through transformations at the gut and is later metabolized at the liver and in the skeletal muscle before being incorporated into tissue proteins.[8] Additionally, the abstract mode of thinking allows for the existence of other factors to influence the process of muscle hypertrophy, particularly energy intake.

2. Sociocultural Determinants

Within the sociocultural environment of the athlete's diet, the specific practice of high-protein feeding is most influenced by group culture. Parraga[10] has identified and described four cultural factors which influence food selection behaviors of athletes, including: (1) values, (2) beliefs, (3) customs, and (4) symbolism. In the short run, the decision to eat a food may be made on the basis of nutritional value. This is an intellectual approach to the problem. However, for long-term decisions all people consider the "emotional, social, and mythical meanings" of food.[10] The decision results in the formation of a symbolic status. Interestingly, nutritional value then becomes a secondary matter. This finding is supported by data from studies of athletes in which nutrition knowledge was compared with food choice behaviors.[10-13]

"Values determine what is desirable and undesirable as food and which foods are held in high esteem. Values, as abstract concepts of worth, are usually not the result of an individual's own valuing. They are social products that have been imposed on and slowly internalized by the individual.''[9] For example, high-protein foods are prized by strength athletes while high-carbohydrate foods are not. The explanation for this phenomenon is that protein is viewed as a direct path to building bigger muscles while carbohydrate does not have the capacity to do so.

Beliefs are interpretations of values, and they help to shape the attitude towards a food.[9] The important point is that they serve to motivate the athlete to eat or to avoid a particular food or selection of foods. Nutritional manipulations, including the use of nutritional ergogenic aids, have become popular with athletes to improve physical performance during competition or the response to training. In this context the athlete is motivated to consume a high-protein diet because he or she believes that it can maximize skeletal muscle gains in the shortest possible time.

Custom is perhaps the most obvious factor directing athletes to a high-protein diet. As members of social subgroups, athletes of all sports are subjected to the norms for diet and nutrition. ''Individuals within a culture respond to approved behavioral pressures by selecting from among the available foods those foods that are acceptable.''[9] For example, bodybuilders are subjected to pressures to consume protein powders, amino acid supplements, and protein-rich foods, to the exclusion of other foods, in order to attain very high protein intakes. These pressures for a high-protein diet are readily apparent in the many advertisements for protein supplements in the popular sports magazines.

Finally, symbolism is a factor relating to the emotional reasons that athletes choose a high-protein diet. All foods are invested with meaning, and these meanings come from the cultural heritage of the group.[9] For example, beef has often been said to be a ''masculine'' food which ''gives strength''.[9] Hence, an athlete may feel more vigorous and stronger after a meal which features broiled steak than one consisting of a non-meat salad. As it regards athletes, protein-rich foods are perceived as superior to others because of the importance of strength to sports performance.

3. Emulation of Winners

Finally, an athlete might decide to emphasize dietary protein because of the observation that winners consume high-protein diets. The fact that high protein intake is consistent with winning has led many athletes and coaches to believe that such diets are essential for maximal sports performance and success. Winners in the sport of bodybuilding are legendary for their focus on dietary protein. Aspiring athletes who read articles in the sports magazines about successful athletes often try to emulate them. An example from the popular bodybuilding literature illustrates how this works.

In an interview for *Bodybuilder* magazine, John DeFendis, an amateur bodybuilder competing on the national level, was asked what his diet consisted of during the time between contests when he was ''bulking up'' or training heavy to make gains in muscle size.[14] ''My year-round diet mainly consists of meat, fish, and eggs and is very low in carbohydrate content. I believe in taking in tremendous amounts of protein instead of carbohydrates . . . in this manner I'm guaranteed maximum muscle gains . . . (if I include) carbohydrates, then my body gets smooth and I don't get maximum muscle growth.''[14]

DeFendis' bulking diet is described in Table 1; it was analyzed for energy and nutrient contents using a computer diet-analysis program.[15] Considering that his body weight could get as high as 105 kg between contests, then his protein intake of 653 g is extraordinarily high at about 6.2 g/kg or 778% of RDA.[16] The distribution of energy is 33% from protein, 65% fat, and 0% carbohydrate. This is consistent with his stated desire for a low-carbohydrate diet. There were no marginal nutrient intakes owing to the large volume of food consumed, but cholesterol intake was high at 12,019 mg. The total energy intake is impressive at about

TABLE 1 Computerized Analyses of Training Diets for Adding Muscle Mass (the Bulking Diet) and for Losing Body Fat Prior to Competition (the Contest Diet)

Diet, Foods eaten	Energy (kcal)	Protein (g)
"Bulking"		
6:30 A.M. — 10-egg cheese omelet	1520	95
11:00 A.M. — 6 eggs + 1 lb steak	2024	153
1:30 P.M. — 6 eggs + 1 lb steak	2024	153
4:00 P.M. — 1 lb turkey breast	691	132
6:30 P.M. — 10-egg omelet	950	60
8:00 P.M. — 10-egg omelet	950	60
Totals	8159	653
"Contest"		
6:30 A.M. — 1/2 cantaloupe	94	2
11:00 A.M. — 1 lb chicken cutlet	754	143
1:30 P.M. — 1 lb chicken cutlet	754	143
3:30 P.M. — 6.5 oz canned, water-packed tuna	268	47
7:00 P.M. — 1 lb chicken cutlet	754	143
Totals	2624	478

Note: Analyses based on diets of amateur bodybuilder John DeFendis.

Data from References 14 and 15.

78 kcal/kg, indicating that bodybuilding can require a high-energy diet; part of this intake would be used to synthesize skeletal muscle proteins for net gains in size.[17,18]

In the 4 to 6 weeks prior to a contest, a bodybuilder's diet changes to produce maximum skeletal muscle definition. DeFendis described his contest diet for the Mr. USA competition as being "rigid and (taking) lots of determination to stick with it."[14] His contest diet is described in Table 1. Because total food intake decreases relative to the off-season diet, energy and total protein fall, too. Considering that his contest body weight is about 91 kg, then his protein intake approximates 5.3 g/kg (6.6 × RDA) at an energy intake of 29 kcal/kg. The distribution of energy is 76% from protein, 20% fat, and 4% carbohydrate. This contest diet is marginal for several nutrients, including calcium, zinc, and vitamins B_1 and B_6. Cholesterol intake is down to 110 mg.

The description and computerized nutritional analyses of the "bulking" and contest diets for DeFendis clearly demonstrate the high level of motivation of some athletes — they will do whatever is necessary to obtain the high-protein diet which they believe is required for successful sports performance. It is noteworthy that DeFendis did not report any ill effects of his high-protein regimen.[14] Subsequent interviews with DeFendis in the bodybuilding magazines over a 12-year period have not detailed any problems resulting from high protein intake.

III. RESEARCH WITH STRENGTH EXERCISE

Research with strength-building modes of exercise, such as weight training or bodybuilding, has centered around its purported effect to "tear down" skeletal muscle tissue. Many athletes express the popular belief that exercise-induced hypertrophy is initially stimulated by trauma. Then, over the course of the next 48 h, the resting muscle tissue is repaired and net growth occurs. Athletes seem to "feel" that exercise is traumatic because of the "good" pain which normally accompanies it. This is the basis for the common expression, "no pain, no gain''. In this section, scientific studies of the torn-tissue hypothesis will be examined.

A. The Torn-Tissue Hypothesis

Some athletes, especially bodybuilders, believe that properly executed strength-building exercise is supposed to traumatize or ''tear down'' skeletal muscle proteins. Ironically, it is this trauma or ''tearing down'' action which is supposed to serve as the stimulus for net growth or hypertrophy of the tissue. From this belief comes the common expression ''no pain, no gain'', implying that one has to work to the point of pain to elicit the trauma which leads to hypertrophy. Protein requirements are said to be enhanced during exercise-induced muscle hypertrophy in order to replace the tissue torn down and to allow for net tissue gains. These popular, common beliefs of athletes have not been scientifically validated.

The modern idea that strenuous exercise tears down skeletal muscle may have originated with Hough[19] around the turn of the 20th century. Hough[19] studied work capacity using an ergograph following exercise-induced skeletal muscle soreness. His findings led him to propose that there are two forms of soreness, one due to the accumulation of waste products during exercise and the other due to exercise which is strenuous enough to ''rupture'' the structure of muscle (acute exertional rhabdomyolysis). Hough[19] was unable to fully investigate his hypothesis because his technology was not specific to the contractile proteins of skeletal muscle tissue (i.e., it was an indirect index of the proposed trauma).

In a follow-up investigation of Hough's[19] torn-tissue hypothesis, Abraham[20] measured urinary myoglobin excretion, because the red pigment is known to be released from skeletal muscle as a result of intense, prolonged physical exertion. Abraham[20] monitored the urine of eight men and seven women for myoglobin after strenuous arm exercise. He attempted to correlate the subjects' perceptions of arm soreness with the appearance of myoglobin in their urine. Eight of the eleven subjects excreted myoglobin after exercise, suggesting that skeletal muscle injury had occurred, and this finding supports the torn-tissue hypothesis. Interestingly, not all of the subjects with myoglobinuria experienced soreness; this suggests that soreness may not be a reliable indicator of skeletal muscle injury. In any event, the measurement of urinary myoglobin is an indirect indicator of protein metabolism at the skeletal muscle since it is not actually a component of the contractile proteins.

B. Acute Bouts of Exercise

1. Novice Bodybuilders

Hickson et al.[21,22] conducted a 15-d controlled feeding period with ten college-age men. Since subjects' urine was to be analyzed for *N*-methylhistidine (3MH) and creatinine, the diet was lacto-ovo-vegetarian to restrict the intake of these metabolites.[23-32] The 3-d cycle menu has been published.[21] The protein intake was set at 0.9 g/kg/d over the last 10 d of the study. Study days 1 to 7 were designated as controls to allow subjects' adaptation to the experimental diet.[23,29-41]

The subjects were not athletes, and they had not participated in a program of chronic exercise over the 12-month period preceding the study. Study days 8 and 12 were designated for bouts of bodybuilding exercise according to the protocol described by Hickson et al.[42]

The workouts were standardized so that the intensity and volume of training among subjects at each exercise bout and for each subject between bouts would be as similar as possible.[42,43] The initial work intensity for each exercise movement was targeted at 75 to 80% 1-RM (one-repetition maximum), which is the maximum amount of weight that can be handled properly one time through a range of motion for any given exercise movement.[44-46]

Work volume refers to the number of repetitions performed in a given exercise bout, all over work sets.[43] In this study, the workload dictated the performance of a range of six to

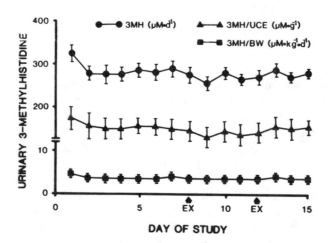

FIGURE 1. Group mean daily urinary excretion (mean ± SE) for 3-methylhistidine (3MH) and excretions expressed by urinary creatinine excretion (UCE) and by body weight (BW); EX, day of strength exercise session. (From Hickson, J. F. et al., *Med. Sci. Sports Exercise*, 18(5), 563, 1986. With permission from the American College of Sports Medicine.)

ten repetitions per work set, and there the number of work sets was fixed in advance at 18 per bout.[42] In summary, when the number of work sets in a bout is fixed, then exercise volume is dependent on the number of repetitions, and that number is dependent on intensity. In this standardized bodybuilding program, the work volume can be described as involving 108 to 180 repetitions.

The bodybuilding program had been tested beforehand in a 28-d study with a different group of young adult men.[47] Strength was assessed weekly using the 1-RM technique. The weekly values for each exercise movement for each subject were totaled.[47] Regression analysis of these totals over time indicated that exercising subjects made significant, linear gains in strength, while there was no change in the strengths of nonexercise subjects.[47] This finding indicates that the program of bodybuilding exercise was correctly designed to produce a desirable training effect over time (i.e., increases in strength).

Subjects made timed urine collections for analysis of protein metabolites including ammonia, creatinine, 3MH, total and urea nitrogen.[23-32,48-52] In order to facilitate study of the data on a 24-h basis and later by shorter time intervals or "partials", subjects were instructed to collect their urine over four time intervals (A, B, C, D) including: 7:00 A.M. to noon (A); noon to 5:00 P.M. (B); 5:00 to 10:00 P.M. (C); and 10:00 P.M. to 7:00 A.M. (D). A 24-h composite was made from the partials to study 24-h effects.[22] Three days of minimal physical activity were allowed following exercise sessions in order to provide time for the complete recovery of urinary 3MH.[23,29] Ammonia and total and urea nitrogen excretions were used as indices of general protein metabolism and trauma.[30,48-52]

There were no statistically significant changes in the urinary excretions of ammonia, creatinine, 3MH, total or urea nitrogen excretions consequent to bodybuilding exercise sessions.[22] The mean group data for each parameter are shown plotted in Figures 1 and 2. The lack of a change in 3MH excretion indicates that skeletal muscle proteins were not "torn down" by weight training exercise (Figure 1). Supporting this conclusion was the lack of any rise in other urinary indices of general protein metabolism, including ammonia, total and urea nitrogen excretions (Figure 2).[22]

If skeletal muscle tissue had been torn down and amino acids released, then total and urea nitrogen excretions would have been expected to rise as excess amino acids were degraded at the liver to maintain homeostasis of the blood pool.[34,35,48-51,53] In addition,

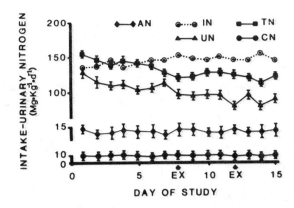

FIGURE 2. Group mean daily urinary excretions (mean ± SE) expressed by body weight of ammonia nitrogen (AN), creatinine nitrogen (CN), total nitrogen (TN), and urea nitrogen (UN), with mean group daily intake nitrogen (IN) expressed by body weight; EX, day of strength exercise session. (From Hickson, J. F. et al., *Med. Sci. Sports Exercise*, 18(5), 563, 1986. With permission from the American College of Sports Medicine.)

subjects were fed just about the RDA for protein.[16] Yet exercise did not increase the urinary excretion of total or urea nitrogen excretions to indicate an enhanced utilization of protein consistent with an exercise-enhanced need for dietary protein. This is in contrast to the belief of some athletes that high-protein diets, in excess of the RDA,[16] are necessary to replace skeletal muscle tissue torn down by strenuous exercise.

While there were no 24-h effects of weight training on urinary excretion of subjects,[22] it is possible that there were shorter-term effects (occurring over time intervals of less than 24 h). Some athletes have proposed that the tearing-down action of strength exercise is followed within hours by the repair of the tissue. Hence, urinary excretion of protein metabolites might be enhanced soon after exercise and then reduced drastically below control levels later in the day. If so, then a 24-h sample might hide or mask an exercise effect. To investigate this possibility, subjects' urine was studied by 5- to 9-h partials. The weight training exercise sessions were conducted during the time when the A partial was collected from 10:00 to 11:00 A.M.

Hourly excretions of 3MH, expressed by body weight, were not affected by bodybuilding exercise on exercise days 8 and 12 or on recovery days.[54] Furthermore, exercise did not change the rate of excretion by partial from one study day to the next. If the torn-tissue hypothesis had been valid, then a raise in 3MH excretions would have been expected in partials A and/or B on exercise days, reflecting subjects' participation in workouts in the morning hours. Additionally, a fall in excretions would have been expected in the C and/or D partials, relative to control days, when repair and net growth are reputed to take place.

The lack of an exercise effect on 3MH excretions was corroborated by the urea excretion data.[21] There was no effect to increase or decrease urea excretions by partials A, B, C, D, when expressed by body weight, on exercise or recovery days relative to control days.[21] Urinary urea content is known to be a reflection of the quantity of amino acids available for catabolism at the liver.[34] If bodybuilding exercise tore down skeletal muscle tissue proteins, then there would be an increase in the size of the cellular amino acid pool. In turn, excess amino acids from the swollen pool would move out into the circulation, where they would be picked up by the liver with subsequent urea formation.[34] Hence, the popular idea that strength exercise tears down skeletal muscle tissue followed by an immediate period of repair over the course of a day was not supported by 3MH or urea excretion data.

There was a diurnal rhythm in the urea excretions when data were analyzed over study days 6 to 15.[34] These fluctuations were not due to exercise but, more likely, they were due to the cyclic input of foodstuffs during the daylight hours.[34,53,55-59] Absorbed amino acids are known to induce the activity of urea cycle enzymes at the liver.[34,53,55] Therefore, short-term fluctuations in protein metabolites can be masked in 24-h sample analyses.

The fact that a diurnal rhythm was not observed with 3MH suggests that the skeletal muscle tissue may not be capable of the same, rapid fluctuations in catabolic activity over the course of a day for which the liver is recognized.[34,53,55-59] Furthermore, it could be that the skeletal muscle is not being traumatized by isolated bouts of "practical" bodybuilding exercise (i.e., consistent with a regular program of exercise resulting in net gains in skeletal muscle size and strength). This might explain the lack of an exercise effect on urinary 3MH excretion from subjects of the present study.[22]

2. Experienced Bodybuilders

It is possible that the findings of the study reported by Hickson et al.[21,22] might have been differernt if experienced bodybuilders had served as subjects instead of novices. Weight-trained athletes would have performed work of greater intensity and volume because they are bigger and stronger. They are also more skilled with weight-training exercise techniques and more motivated to perform because bodybuilding is a part of their "lifestyle". For these reasons, it can be argued that any torn-tissue effect would more likely be observed with experienced than novice bodybuilders.

The objectives of the present study were to investigate the torn-tissue hypothesis with experienced bodybuilders, to compare the findings with prior results for novices, and to test the effect of exercise sessions of varying degrees of perceived difficulty and work volume on urinary indices of protein metabolism.[54] Five experienced male bodybuilders served as subjects in a 12-d study. Inclusion characteristics for subjects were (1) participation in three to six bodybuilding exercise sessions per week over 5 years or longer, and (2) classification as a Level I or II competitor in the National Physique Committee system for amateur, competitive bodybuilders. All of the subjects held titles from national or regional bodybuilding contests in which they had participated. Subjects took all their meals at a metabolic facility; the diet was lacto-ovo-vegetarian in nature to facilitate the analysis of 24-h urine collections for creatinine and 3MH.[23-32]

In setting the dietary protein level for the study, subjects were first assessed by means of dietary surveys to determine typical intakes. The range was wide, from 175 to 350 g/d, and the intake was set at the mean of 2.3 g/kg/d (203 g/d); in so doing, an adaptive response to a new, lower protein intake level was effectively blunted.[23,29-41]

Bodybuilding exercise was performed on study days 4, 7, and 10 according to the program previously described.[42,47,60] By using the same exercise program structure, comparisons between the present study and the previous one by Hickson et al.[21,22] were facilitated. However, certain changes were made in the exercise protocol in order to manipulate the "volume" of training by subjects. The work volume for novice bodybuilders in the study conducted by Hickson et al.[22] was only 108 to 180 repetitions. At the other extreme, nationally competitive bodybuilders report in the popular bodybuilding magazines that they may train for very high work volumes.

For example, in 1979, 21-year-old bodybuilder John DeFendis described his training regimen for the 1980 Mr. USA contest sponsored by the National Physique Committee (NPC) which governs amateur, competitive bodybuilding.[14] He was training at least 6 d per week, three times per day. For each of several body parts that were to be exercised in a session, he performed up to 15 different exercise movements in order to work them from all angles. He alternated his exercise routines daily, so that one day he exercised the chest, back, and biceps (routine "A"), and the next day he exercised the shoulders, legs, and triceps (routine "B"); 300 repetitions of abdominal exercises were performed each day. Each work set was performed to "failure".

In the "A" workout, 195 work sets were performed.[14] Assuming that six to ten repetitions were completed in each work set, then the volume of training was 1470 to 2250 repetitions. In the "B" workout, 220 work sets were performed; assuming that six to ten repetitions were completed in each work set, then the volume of training was 1620 to 2500 repetitions. These intense workouts were dubbed "insanity training" by the bodybuilding media. This account underscores the point that weight training can be successfully practiced with different work volumes depending on the level of the athlete's experience. These volumes of work performed by DeFendis are many times that which was accomplished by novice bodybuilders in the study by Hickson et al.[22]

The choice of an appropriate work volume depends on what is necessary to produce a training effect and that is determined by the experience and motivation of (the) subject(s). When asked about his very strenuous training routine, DeFendis stated, "I feel that I've gotten fantastic results from it . . . when I do such a high number of sets, my body is breaking down muscle tissue and . . . my physique increases in size and maintains a good amount of muscularity while on a tremendously high protein diet" (Section II.B.3).[14]

Since the number of repetitions is constant at six to ten in the standardized program,[22,42,60] then variation in training volume was accomplished for the present study[54] by manipulating the number of work sets per exercise movement and the total number of movements per exercise session. Three workouts were set up to test the effect of volume in eliciting the torn-tissue phenomenon. To establish the volume for each workout, subjects were asked to submit records of their recent workouts, including exercise movements, number of work sets for each movement, and number of repetitions for each work set. Data were compiled for all subjects, and a typical workout was formulated which was labeled "just right". This workout included 44 work sets of 264 to 440 repetitions. A "light" workout was set at the lower volume of 28 work sets per 168 to 280 repetitions for the light workout, and a "heavy" workout has set at 60 work sets per 360 to 600 repetitions.

Subjects' perception of the difficulty of the three workouts was exactly as had been targeted during the design of the research protocol: they differed progressively from easy to challenging to punishing.[54] Despite the punishing nature of the heavy workout, it did not affect the group mean urinary total or urea nitrogen or 3MH excretions. Hence, the volume of strength training performed does not appear to induce skeletal muscle trauma. As with the novice bodybuilders,[22] these findings do not support the torn-tissue hypothesis.

3. Novice and Experienced Weight Lifters

Paul et al.[61] conducted a 5-d study with ten experienced weight lifters and seven who had not lifted before. Subjects consumed a meat-free diet on their own according to instructions from the investigators; the protein intake level was not described. Weight-training exercise was performed on study day 4 in general accordance with that described by Hickson et al.[22,42,60] and others.[43,61] Urine samples were collected at 24-h intervals over study days 1 to 5 for analysis of creatinine[23,24,26,27,30-32] and 3MH as markers for skeletal muscle protein catabolism and trauma.[23-25,28] Blood samples were collected immediately prior to the exercise session (T = 0) and afterwards at T = 12 and 24 h; these samples were assayed also for creatine kinase and myoglobin as indices of skeletal muscle trauma.[62]

The authors did not find any significant change in the urinary excretion of absolute 3MH excretions or as expressed by creatinine excretion from either group, experienced or novice weight lifters.[61] This finding can be interpreted to show that skeletal muscle protein catabolism was not affected by strength exercise, supporting the conclusion of Hickson et al.[22] (Section III.B.2). However, Paul et al.[61] also analyzed the data when it was collapsed into a single pool. When treated this way, there was a significant decrease in group mean 3MH excretion from the baseline value (18.6 μmol 3MH/mmol creatinine) to those at 12 h

(18.6 μmol 3MH/mmol creatinine) and 24 h (18.6 μmol 3MH/mmol creatinine) postexercise. These data treatments suggest that strength exercise has an anabolic effect which is consistent with the common observation that athletes who train with weights become muscular.

Curiously, data for creatinine kinase and myoglobin were elevated following the exercise session, indicating skeletal muscle damage according to traditional interpretations of these blood parameters.[62] This is similar to the conclusion of Abraham,[20] who reported that some of his subjects experienced both soreness and myoglobinuria following exercise. It is difficult to reconcile the fact that Paul et al.[61] did not observe increased 3MH excretions with elevated data for blood parameters. All three parameters are known to be elevated with skeletal muscle trauma.[62-64] Perhaps the measurement of urinary 3MH or the two blood parameters is not valid. Alternatively, these parameters may provide information other than what they are assumed to provide.

4. Experienced Powerlifters

Contrary to the negative findings reported by other investigators[21,22,61] for isolated bouts, Dohm et al.[65] reported that strength exercise led to increased 24-h urea and 3MH excretions from four male subjects. Their subjects were apparently experienced powerlifters who were in various stages of training for the sport of powerlifting. Any dietary restrictions were not described, and subjects could have eaten meat and excess or deficient levels of protein and energy during the study. The exercise session consisted of a "standard power-lift routine . . . of standing press, squats, and curls. The exercise bout lasted about 1 hr." Subjects contributed 24-h urine collections for the time periods before and after the exercise session for analyses of creatinine as an index of skeletal muscle mass and 3MH and urea as indices of trauma.[23-25,48-51,63,64]

There was a nonsignificant trend toward higher absolute urinary urea excretion after exercise (864 ± 124 mmol/24 h) relative to measurements before exercise (654 ± 54 mmol/24 h). When expressed by creatinine excretion, the difference was statistically significant (32 ± 0.05 vs. 0.49 ± 0.07 mmol/mg creatinine). Dohm et al.[65] concluded from these findings that exercise enhances amino acid catabolism. They[65] calculated that the amount of excess protein catabolized due to the exercise session was 37 g for their subjects. This would have contributed about 18% of the energy expended during the exercise bout.

Urinary 3MH excretions were also elevated. Again, there was a nonsignificant trend toward higher absolute excretions after exercise (678 ± 60 μmol/24 h) relative to measurements beforehand (588 ± 52 μmol/24 h). However, excretions expressed by creatinine were significantly higher after exercise (0.28 ± 0.03 vs. 0.38 ± 0.03 μmol/mg creatinine). Dohm et al.[65] interpreted these data to support the common belief of some athletes in the torn-tissue hypothesis. Furthermore, it was suggested that the source of protein for the increased urea excretion was the skeletal muscle. This might mean that the breakdown of muscle proteins during exercise is the result of energy starvation. Consequently, amino acids released during the tearing-down process are oxidized to meet the exercise-enhanced energy requirements of the working muscle cells.

An important difference between the studies conducted by Dohm et al.[65] and by Hickson et al.[22] concerns the nature of workouts performed by subjects and perhaps their level of experience. In the study reported by Hickson et al.,[22] untrained men performed sessions of weight training taken from an introductory-level physical education course offered to university students. In the study reported by Dohm et al.,[65] subjects "performed a standard power-lift routine that consisted of standing press, squats, and curls. The exercise bout lasted approximately 1 hr". This brief description of the exercise session implies that their subjects were familiar with weights, and they may have been weight-trained athletes.

Dohm et al.[65] did not provide information about the number of sets of repetitions of each exercise movement which were performed by their subjects or whether all performed the same number of sets and repetitions. It is not known if the workout was consistent with a regular program of chronic training or if it was intended to be an exhaustive single bout. Hence, it is difficult to compare the volume of exercise performed between the two studies, but the untrained subjects in the study conducted by Hickson et al.[22] may have performed less strenuous bouts.

Hickson et al.[22,47] have suggested that a rise in the urinary total and urea nitrogen excretions might have been observed if subjects had been asked to train harder during exercise sessions. However, more work could have induced trauma by training too hard (i.e., "overtraining"). Increased excretions would be expected with trauma,[23-25,48-51,63,64] but this response should not be taken as healthful.[66] Rather, this conclusion is troublesome, since it suggests that athletes in training will be in negative nitrogen balance on a regular basis.[48-51,66] This is contrary to "morphological evidence" of strength athletes, who are evidently in positive nitrogen balance since they realize net gains in skeletal muscle size with a regular program of weight training.[23,25,66]

With regard to diet, the subjects may have eaten meat immediately before or during the urine collection periods, providing an exogenous source of 3MH.[65] Meat is a rich dietary source of the amino acid, and its consumption increases the urinary excretion.[30,67] Consequently, the actual (endogenous) excretion levels of 3MH would have been camouflaged and the results of Dohm et al.[65] for urinary 3MH excretion would have been confounded.[23,29] In the study reported by Hickson et al.,[21,22] subjects were allowed a 7-d control period to adapt to a meat-free diet. Research with humans has shown that 100% of an orally administered dose of 3MH is recovered within 72 h; a 7-d control period should have been more than adequate to "wash out" 3MH of exogenous origin.[29]

C. Chronic Exercise

1. Novice Bodybuilders without a Control Period

Hickson's laboratory[68] conducted a 28-d study with 13 young adult males distributed among four groups. Five of the subjects were fed the RDA for protein[16] while the others were fed three times this amount (3 × RDA). Since subjects' urine were to be analyzed for creatinine and 3MH, the diet did not contain meat, in order to minimize the intakes of these metabolites.[30] Urinary creatinine excretion was essentially constant for subjects over the last 14 d of the study. The coefficient of variation was only 9.3%, indicating excellent precision of timing, completeness of urine collections, and adherence to the experimental diet.[30]

Two RDA and four 3 × RDA subjects participated in a 6-d/week weight-training program; data for two of the four original RDA group members were omitted from analyses at the end of the study because of suspected cocaine abuse. Exercise subjects began working out on study day 1; therefore, subjects did not serve as their own controls, and comparisons were made between exercise and nonexercise groups at each protein intake level. The weight-training program has been described.[22,42,47,60] Exercising subjects increased in strength over the course of the study, judging from linear increases made in total weight loads lifted at weekly 1-RM sessions.[47] There was no change in the strength of nonexercise subjects.

RDA subjects appear to have decreased their absolute excretion of nitrogen or excretions expressed by intake over nesting periods A to D (Figures 3 and 4).[68] This suggests that the RDA for protein was a lower intake that subjects were used to consuming in their prestudy, free-living diets, and they adapted by improving their efficiency of utilization at the liver.[33-39,41] 3 × RDA subjects do not show this downward ramp in their plotted data, suggesting that their intakes were similar to those of their prestudy, free-living diets. Adaptation to a lower protein-intake level, as with the RDA subjects, provides the necessary flexibility in meeting variations in dietary intakes.[39-41]

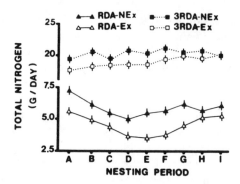

FIGURE 3. Least-squares means (± SE) of absolute urinary total nitrogen excretion vs. time for the four experimental groups with data grouped in 3-d nesting periods (except first period includes study days 1 to 4); RDA, recommended dietary allowance;[16] Ex, exercise subjects; and NEx, nonexercise subjects. (From Hickson, J. F. et al., *Nutr. Res.*, 8, 725, 1988. With permission from Pergamon Press.)

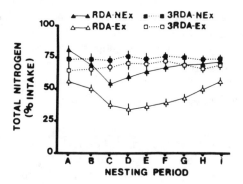

FIGURE 4. Least-squares means (± SE) of urinary total nitrogen excretion expressed as a percentage of intake nitrogen vs. time for the four experimental groups with data grouped in 3-d nesting periods (except first period includes study days 1 to 4); RDA, recommended dietary allowance;[16] Ex, exercise subjects; NEx, nonexercise subjects. (From Hickson, J. F. et al., *Nutr. Res.*, 8, 725, 1988. With permission from Pergamon Press.)

Second, excretions for 3 × RDA subjects are about three times as great as for RDA subjects, indicating that the excess nitrogen they consumed is not stored, but simply excreted (see Figure 3).[68] If excess nitrogen intake could be stored, then skeletal muscle hypertrophy could be accomplished without bodybuilding exercise; common experience has shown this to be false.

Third, excretions for exercising subjects fell below those of nonexercise subjects (see Figure 3).[68] This difference could reflect an adaptive response to exercise if the demand for protein was enhanced, as suggested by Yoshimura.[40] Accordingly, the efficiency of protein metabolism in exercising subjects would be improved by decreasing the activity of catabolic enzymes at the liver to enable positive nitrogen balance consistent with exercise-induced skeletal muscle growth.[33-35,38-41] These findings suggest that it may not be necessary for the bodybuilder or other athlete to consume a high-protein diet to offset any exercise-enhanced demands.[68]

Visual examination of the plotted 3MH excretion data suggests that catabolism was gradually increasing for exercising subjects relative to nonexercise subjects (Figures 5 and 6).[60] In fact, statistical analyses revealed that there was an exercise effect for exercising subjects

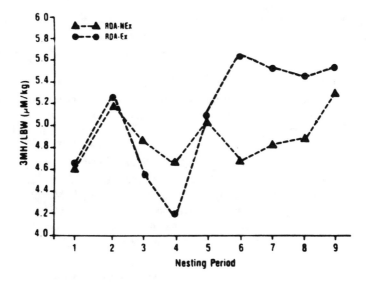

FIGURE 5. Least-squares means of urinary 3-methylhistidine (3MH) excretion, expressed by lean body weight (LBW) to correct for differences in total and lean body weight of subjects, vs. clustering period for exercise (Ex) and nonexercise (NEx) subjects consuming the RDA[16] for protein. (From Hickson, J. F. and Hinkelmann, K., *Am. J. Clin. Nutr.*, 41, 246, 1985. With permission from The American Society of Clinical Nutrition.)

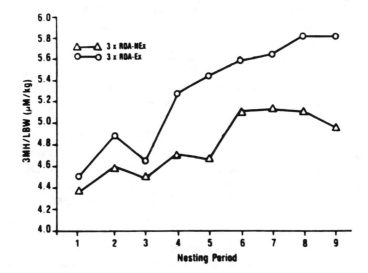

FIGURE 6. Least-squares means of urinary 3-methylhistidine (3MH) excretion, expressed by lean body weight (LBW) to correct for differences in total and lean body weight of subjects, vs. clustering period for exercise (Ex) and nonexercise (NEx) subjects consuming three times the RDA[16] (3 × RDA) for protein. (From Hickson, J. F. and Hinkelmann, K., *Am. J. Clin. Nutr.*, 41, 246, 1985. With permission from The American Society of Clinical Nutrition.)

at both protein intake levels. Apparently, gains in strength, achieved by exercising subjects, were made with increased skeletal muscle protein breakdown.

The findings seem to support those of Dohm et al.,[65] as reported for an isolated bout of powerlifting exercise. These investigators interpreted their data to show that strength exercise enhances skeletal muscle protein catabolism, too.[65] However, Dohm et al.[65] suggested that their findings were specific to an isolated bout of unaccustomed exercise and consistent with negative nitrogen balance. By contrast, subjects training repeatedly would become accustomed to the exercise stress, and there would be no exercise-enhanced skeletal muscle protein catabolism.[65]

In this case, increased urinary 3MH excretions do not necessarily reflect an exercise-induced tissue trauma. If the data did indicate trauma, then urinary total and urea nitrogen excretions should have risen above intake,[48-51] but this did not happen (Figure 3). In fact, just the opposite was observed. Total nitrogen excretions for exercising subjects at both protein intake levels were less than those of nonexercise subjects.[68] The only logical explanation is that increased catabolic rate was offset with an increase in the rate of synthesis.

Hickson and Hinkelmann[60] suggested that the present data reflect the adaptations in the rate of turnover in skeletal muscle proteins. In this case, increased 3MH excretion indicates that the breakdown component of turnover was accelerated. If the rate of synthesis did not also increase, then there would have been a net loss of muscle tissue. Since the urinary nitrogen losses do not suggest a catabolic effect of exercise, it was concluded that the rate of synthesis increased, too.

A possible explanation for an exercise-enhanced rate of turnover is to allow skeletal muscle tissue to be "remodeled" or "reorganized" in order to make gains in size and strength and to attain more highly developed shapes of individual muscles (i.e., morphological adaptation which is visible to the eye) all within a practical period of time.[66,69] New muscle tissue is not simply added on top of existing tissue in the same manner that trees grow. If a tree of good size is sawed across the trunk, the cut surface reveals "annual rings" or layers of growth. Each year a new layer is wrapped around the last one.

Tree-like growth could be accomplished easily in the human simply by increasing the rate of muscle synthesis and turning off the catabolic processes. Existing tissue would be inert and new tissue would be added on top of the old. However, in the human, newly acquired muscle tissue must be integrated with the existing tissue in order to create a single integrated unit that can withstand the stresses of contraction during physical activity. If it were organized like a tree, with layers or rings of tissue, then the stresses induced by contraction might rip away one layer from another.

In order to integrate new proteins into existing tissue, the entire tissue must be reorganized, with existing tissue broken down and resynthesized. During this process, extra proteins are added back into the reorganized muscle to result in net gains in size and strength. This process could not occur in a reasonable period of time without an increase in the rate of muscle tissue turnover.[39,66] If the rate did not rise, then practical adaptation would not occur, and this would be a disadvantage from an evolutionary perspective.

The experience of the subjects in the present study illustrates that a possible increase in skeletal muscle turnover enabled significant gains in strength to be made in a matter of only 4 weeks. That is a practical time period for adaptation as opposed to months or years. Similarly, it is the common experience of bodybuilders that gains in skeletal muscle size can be achieved quickly, too; top national competitors report in the popular sports magazines that they may gain up to 0.5 kg of skeletal muscle in a month. A question which has not been investigated concerns the effect of exercise that does not stimulate morphological adaptation, such as endurance exercise.[70] Perhaps this type of exercise does not give rise to an increase in the rate of skeletal muscle protein turnover with a regular training program.[70-72]

2. Novice Bodybuilders with a Control Period

Hickson et al.[73] conducted a 19-d follow-up study with novice bodybuilders, but this time the 11 young adult males served as their own controls. Subjects were fed by body

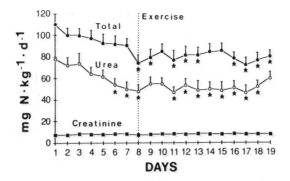

FIGURE 7. Group mean daily urinary total, urea, and creatinine nitrogen (N) excretions expressed by body weight over time. Starred (*) data points indicate significantly lower values ($p < .05$). (From Hickson, J. F. et al., *Nutr. Res.*, 10, 723, 1990. With permission from Pergamon Press.)

weight, taking all their meals in a metabolic kitchen; details of the diet have been published.[73] The protein intake level was set at the RDA of 0.8 g/kg/d.[3] The exercise regimen has been described previously.[42,47,60] Study days 1 to 7 were designated as no-exercise controls; subjects exercised on study days 8 to 19, alternating the upper and lower body to prevent overtraining. Timed, 24-h urine collections were made for analysis of urinary total and urea nitrogen and 3MH excretions.

Visual examination of plotted data for urinary total and urea nitrogen excretions suggests adaptation to a protein intake that was lower than prestudy intakes (Figure 7).[73] Statistical analyses indicate that excretions were significantly lower, beginning study day 6 for urea nitrogen and study day 8 for total nitrogen excretions. These results do not indicate that exercise, beginning on study day 8, decreased excretions, since subjects apparently did not adapt to the experimental diet until the onset of exercise sessions. A previous study with novice bodybuilders did suggest decreased urinary total and urea nitrogen excretions consequent to exercise, but subjects did not serve as their own controls.[68]

An alternative interpretation of the data is that bodybuilding exercise was not catabolic in nature. Excretions did not rise, as would be expected if the torn-tissue hypothesis were valid. Major support among laymen for the proposed catabolic effect of exercise comes from frequent citations in popular sports magazines of two studies by Gontzea and colleagues[74,75] (Sections IV.C.3.e and IV.C.4.a). Subjects in these studies were in zero nitrogen balance until they began strenuous exercise bouts, after which balance became negative.

An important criticism of popular interpretations of the Gontzea et al.[74,75] studies is that they used bicycloergometer exercise, rather than bodybuilding. It is generally recognized that endurance and strength modes of exercise elicit different morphological adaptations.[70,71] Making comparisons of studies not using the same modes of training is akin to comparing apples and oranges; certainly, it is risky to extrapolate the findings of one to another. Attempts to make such comparisons suggest that exercise is a generic activity, when the weight of modern scientific evidence indicates that it is not.[66,70,71]

The data for urinary total and urea nitrogen excretions do not suggest that the RDA for protein was an inadequate intake.[16] A basic premise of the torn-tissue hypothesis is that a high protein intake is necessary to replace tissue damaged by exercise. Again, there was no rise in urinary nitrogen excretions to indicate that tissue was traumatized or protein catabolism was enhanced.[48-51] Of course, urinary nitrogen content should not be taken as an equivalent indicator of the overall relationship between intake and output (i.e., nitrogen balance).

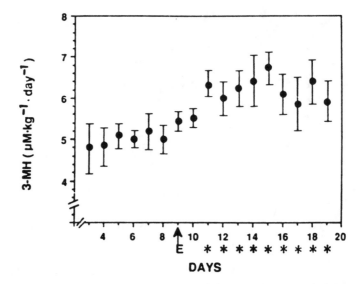

FIGURE 8. Mean (± SE) daily urinary 3MH excretions expressed by body weight; E, first day of weight training exercise; (∗) indicates a significant increase in 3MH excretion ($p < .005$). (From Pivarnik, J. M. et al., *Med. Sci. Sports Exercise*, 21(3), 283, 1989. With permission from the American College of Sports Medicine.)

However, skeletal muscle trauma is well known to be reflected in urinary nitrogen excretions.[48-51] The fact that it was not observed to increase in the present study could be interpreted to mean that the RDA for protein was an adequate intake; high protein intake was not justified.

Just as in the previous reports by Hickson et al.[68] and Hickson and Hinkelmann[60] for a 28-d study of novice bodybuilders, subjects' urinary 3MH excretions rose consequent to exercise,[76] but they did so without an increase in urinary nitrogen excretions.[73] Values for urinary 3MH excretion were significantly increased beginning with study day 11 (Figure 8). The data indicate that there was a short "lag" time between the initiation of the exercise and regimen and the rise in excretions. Furthermore, this rise was not temporary. Therefore, it was concluded that adaptation had occurred, resulting in a "new turnover rate" of skeletal muscle proteins.[76]

In summarizing the data, Pivarnik et al.[76] stated, "An increase in skeletal muscle degradation in the face of (chronic) weight training exercises that are known to result in increases in muscle strength and hypertrophy may appear paradoxical. However, these catabolic events may be initial steps in a muscle tissue rearrangement process . . . " as proposed by Waterlow.[38,39,69] Furthermore, simultaneous rebuilding of catabolized tissue (i.e., increased synthesis at least to balance increased breakdown) would explain why nitrogen excretions did not rise, and hence, why strength exercise does not have a net catabolic effect.

A particularly exciting interpretation of the present findings is that increased 3MH excretions could be a training effect of chronic bodybuilding exercise.[76] If so, then the results of a previous study by Hickson et al.[22] in which subjects performed isolated bouts of bodybuilding exercise can be explained. In that study by Hickson et al.,[22] there was no change in 3MH excretion, suggesting that isolated bouts do not elicit a training effect.[76] This explanation would be consistent with the common observation that athletes must participate in a routine of chronic exercise to achieve increases in skeletal muscle size and strength. Performance of isolated bouts is not sufficient to provide a training effect.

TABLE 2 Characteristics, Mean (± S.D.) Intakes of Selected Nutrients and Overall Nitrogen Balance Data for the Experimental Subgroups

Parameter	Subgroup		
	I	II	III
No. of subjects	3	3	4
Mean body weight (kg)	66 ± 6	75 ± 1	90 ± 11
Protein (g/d)	130 ± 38	143 ± 29	159 ± 28
(g/kg/d)	2.0	1.9	1.8
Energy (kcal/d)	3,577 ± 618	3,800 ± 548	4,321 ± 513
(kcal/kg/d)	54	51	48
Balance (g/d)	−0.47 ± 1.70	+0.38 ± 0.93	+1.30 ± 1.80

Data from Reference 78.

3. Experienced Bodybuilders

Tarnopolsky et al.[77] have reported a nitrogen balance study with several groups of subjects. One of these included experienced bodybuilders. The study has been reported in Section IV.C.4.b because all of the other athletes participated in endurance-type sports.

4. Experienced Weight Lifters

Ten experienced Polish "weight lifters" served as subjects in an 11-d study by Celejowa and Homa;[78] it is not clear if their athletes corresponded to competitive American powerlifters or Olympic lifters. These subjects ranked just below Olympic-caliber athletes as competitors. Subjects were assigned to subgroups according to competitive classification as feather- or lightweights, middle-weights, and heavy-weights (Table 2).

The men took all their meals at a metabolic facility. The diets were fed by the mean body weight of subgroups in an attempt to correct for differences among groups (Table 2). Subjects trained each day with general conditioning exercises and by lifting weights; the mean energy cost of the two components was calculated to be 1458 kcal/d. The investigators designed the study for measurement of true nitrogen balance. Therefore, urine and feces were collected daily, but miscellaneous losses were not measured. Sweat nitrogen was sampled during exercise; for other times of the day, sweat nitrogen was calculated rather than measured. There was no period allowed for adaptation to the new protein- or energy-intake levels or to the exercise regimens.

The group mean nitrogen balance data indicate that subgroup I was in negative balance while subgroups II and III were in positive balance (Table 2). Two factors known to have a strong influence over nitrogen balance include protein and energy intakes.[41,79-85] According to the design of the study, these two nutritional factors were normalized across subgroups, and hence, there is no obvious explanation for the differences in nitrogen balances among subgroups. However, body weight data reveal changes for individual subjects over the course of the study (Table 3). All subjects gained or lost weight, and some changes were large, and this indicates that subjects were not in energy balance.

Kies[31] recommends that experimental protocols be designed for maintenance of initial body weight. It can be expected that subjects who lost weight would have negative nitrogen balance and vice versa.[41,79-85] When balance data ranging between −1.00 and +1.00 are excluded because of their small magnitude,[86] then change in body weight is directly correlated with nitrogen balance in every case (Table 3). This confirms the importance of energy as a factor in nitrogen balance for the subjects of the study. Because energy balance was not attained in all subjects, the data are confounded.

**TABLE 3 Correlation Between Reported
Nitrogen Balance Data and Body Weight
Change**

Subject code	Nitrogen balance	Body weight change (g)	Correlation
J.H.	+1.63	+500	Yes
D.P.	(0)	+200	
H.F.	−2.49	−600	Yes
W.S.	(0)	+200	
J.Kam.	+1.69	+800	Yes
J.K.	(0)	+400	
Z.P.	+1.09	+1100	Yes
K.G.	(0)	−100	
E.M.	+4.20	+400	Yes
J.D.	−1.05	−600	Yes

Note: Nitrogen balance values between −1.00 and +1.00
were set to zero because of their small magni-
tudes.

Data from Reference 78.

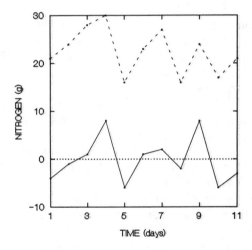

FIGURE 9. Plots of nitrogen intake (dashed line) and nitrogen balance (solid line) in the competitor W.S. (From Celejowa, I. and Homa, M., *Nutr. Metab.*, 12, 259, 1970. With permission from S. Karger AG.)

Nitrogen intake and balance data over the course of the study were presented for one subject (Figure 9).[78] The plot reveals large fluctuations in intake from day to day; energy intake must have varied as well, since the two are directly associated in the diet. Therefore, subjects' consumption of the experimental diets was not controlled despite the stated claim of the investigators.[78]

The failure to achieve adaptation is clearly shown in plotted data of nitrogen intake vs. nitrogen balance; the two mirror one another in a zig-zag fashion (Figure 9). In the adapted state, the plots for both nitrogen balance and intake should be smooth. Hence, the investigators[78] violated a basic premise of the nitrogen balance method calling for adaptation, and again, the data are confounded.

Laymen for the popular sports magazines generally view the plotted nitrogen intake and balance data for one subject with an uncritical eye (Figure 9). They do not recognize that the plot shows that the subject failed to equilibrate either nitrogen intake or excretions. Laymen generally conclude that the days of positive balance correlate with high protein intakes, and this indicates that a high-protein diet is required for athletes, but these particular data cannot be used in this manner. Additionally, laymen make frequent reference to another group of data presented in this report by Celejowa and Homa.[78] These are the mean balance data for the ten individual subjects over all study days. Five of the subjects are shown to be in positive balance, and five are shown to be in negative balance with the inclusion of calculated sweat nitrogen data. This is interpreted to reveal that the mean protein intake of about 2 g/kg/d does not provide a reasonable safety margin to allow for interindividual differences in protein requirements.

Laymen often express the belief that interindividual differences in nutrient requirements are great relative to actual requirements. Colgan[87] writes, "Most medical assessments of nutritional requirements are inadequate (because) they fail to allow for genetic individuality . . . Claiming that two people need the same amount of protein is as stupid as saying that dark-skinned and light-skinned people can take the same amount of sunlight. Yet some health professionals still uphold the sacred number of RDA for protein as if the Almighty had designed it straight in the human system." At a later time, Colgan[87] wrote, "Certainly the RDA was designed for Mr. and Ms. Average America. As the handbook states on the first page, 'RDA should not be confused with requirements for a specific individual.' The 'average' fallacy reminds me of the statistician who drowned in a hole in a lake he knew was of three feet average depth." Yet, the accumulated body of science indicates that interindividual differences in nutrient requirements are small relative to actual requirements. This fact is an underlying assumption used in the formulation of the RDA.[16]

The individual data for subjects in the present study must be viewed carefully.[78] Laymen often take nitrogen balance data to be exact values in which they can place great confidence. With assumptions, calculations, and methodological errors in the present study, especially the inconstancy of the diet and body weights, it is not realistic to assign importance to small numbers. For example, a cautious interpretation of the mean balances for subgroups I and II (Table 2) would take them to be no different from zero.[86]

In summary, the study reported by Celejowa and Homa[78] is well known and widely cited in the sports magazines as strong evidence supporting the need for high protein intakes among athletes. The importance of subjects' sweat nitrogen losses on nitrogen balance determinations is generally considered to be an important finding by laymen. However, it does not seem to be appreciated that at least some of these data were calculated rather than measured. Careful analysis of the methods and data indicate the need for caution, since the data are confounded by lack of adaptation to the diet, fluctuating protein and energy intakes, and inconstant body weight.[30,31]

IV. RESEARCH WITH ENDURANCE EXERCISE

Recently, scientists' thinking about dietary protein requirements for endurance athletes has been influenced by reports of data indicating exercise-enhanced catabolism of amino acids at the skeletal muscle despite abundant carbohydrate and fat stores elsewhere in the body.[88-92] These observations have been interpreted to mean that endurance exercise induces "local energy starvation" which depresses skeletal muscle protein synthesis.

With the rate of protein synthesis depressed, the turnover of proteins is imbalanced with net degradation, and the cellular amino acid pool swells. Coupled with possibly inadequate supplies of other fuel sources, excess amino acids are oxidized.[41] It is argued that this means the dietary need for protein is enhanced by endurance exercise.[88-92] Importantly, the proposed catabolic nature of endurance exercise is not a variant of the torn-tissue hypothesis, which is hypothesized to be a response to trauma.

Ironically, it seems that scientists have come full circle in their thinking. About 150 years ago, protein was thought to be the exclusive source of energy for muscular activity.[93,94] Twenty-seven years later, the first of a series of experiments revealed that protein could not account for all of the energy utilized during exercise. In fact, protein only accounted for a small fraction; it could not be the preferred energy substrate during work.

It was this perspective on protein, that it was not the preferred energy source for exercise,[93,94] which predominated in nutrition science up until recently, when new findings suggested that protein utilization actually was increased during endurance exercise.[90,91] The challenge for nutritionists today is to reconcile this recently collected data with that of the more distant past. Additionally, it is necessary to consider the need for making recommendations for protein intakes which might be higher than the RDAs which have been set for "typical Americans", but not specifically athletes.[16]

A. Liebig's Dogma

With the dawn of organic chemistry in the mid-19th century, an influential force in nutrition science was the European chemist named Liebig. He proposed in 1845 that protein provided the energy for muscle contraction through its breakdown within muscle tissue.[93-96] He believed that dietary protein was first incorporated into tissue before being catabolized on demand to provide energy for work: "There can be no greater contradiction, with regard to the nutritive process, than to suppose that the nitrogen of the food can pass into the urine as urea, without having previously become part of an organized tissue . . . the amount of tissue metamorphosed in a given time may be measured by the quantity of nitrogen in the urine."[94]

The role of dietary fat and carbohydrate in energy production for exercise was not recognized by Liebig. Instead, he thought that the role of carbohydrate and fats was to react with oxygen at the lungs to produce heat, thus preventing "oxygen poisoning". Hence, he termed these substances "respiratory" foods.[93-96] Therefore, only protein was truly nutritive since it served as the structural component of skeletal muscle tissue as well as its sole energy source.[93,95]

Liebig strongly influenced the thinking of his students and of other investigators at the time because his views were accepted as dogma within the European scientific community. This was not an unusual problem; it was not considered appropriate to challenge the views of a master even if they could not be supported by data. Consequently, there was an emphasis on protein in the diet which eventually reached the layman. According to Chittenden,[93] " . . . ever since Liebig advanced his theory . . . there has been a deep rooted belief that meat is the most efficient kind of food, keeping up the strength of the body, and hence, [it was] especially demanded by all whose work is mainly physical [including the athlete]."

B. The Traditional View

If Liebig's views had been correct, then it would be expected that a linear relationship would exist between the extent of exercise and the breakdown of muscle proteins as reflected in the content of nitrogen in the urine. Furthermore, Liebig's views would have made it possible for the urinary excretion of nitrogen to be unrelated to protein intake. For example, excess protein consumed would be stored as skeletal muscle tissue until the stimulus of work initiated its catabolism. On the other hand, there might be a large amount of nitrogen in the urine following exercise despite a lack of protein intake over many days.

It is now recognized that protein intake in excess of need is not stored as skeletal muscle tissue, but most likely catabolized for energy.[35,38,97] Chittenden[93] stated in 1907, "It is one of the cardinal laws of proteid metabolism that the store of nitrogenous substances in the body is not increased by, or not in proportion to, an increase in the nitrogen intake." When protein and energy intake are greater than necessary to meet immediate demands, as in overfeeding, the excesses can only be stored as glycogen and/or adipose (fat cannot be stored as glycogen). "Flesh" (skeletal muscle tissue) cannot be increased by overfeeding.[93] If it could, then athletes could make gains in muscle size and strength simply by eating a high-protein diet. Common experience, with athletes consuming great amounts of protein, has shown that this does not occur.

1. Mountain Climbing

Carpenter[95] writes that it was Fick and Wislicenus who reported in 1869 the results of a study which dealt a "death blow" to Liebig's views. In the experiment, the urinary nitrogen excretions of the two scientists were measured during and after they climbed Swiss Mount Faulhorn, which was 6500 ft. high. A diet free of protein was consumed during the experimental period. Analysis of Fick and Wislicenus' urine revealed that the quantity of nitrogen excreted during and immediately after the climb could not have accounted for more than half of the energy expended. Hence, energy sources other than protein must have contributed to meet the demands imposed by exercise. In contrast to Liebig's view, this finding clearly demonstrated that the energy for muscular work does not come exclusively from the catabolism of tissue proteins.[93] Additionally, the experiment demonstrated that the energy for muscular work does not come from dietary protein, since none was eaten during the experiment.

2. Cross-Country Skiing

The report by Fick and Wislicenus (see Reference 95) laid the groundwork for others to demonstrate that non-nitrogenous, energy-yielding macronutrients, carbohydrate, and fat, were the primary sources of fuel for man during exercise. The relatively recent experiment by Hedman,[98] reported in 1957, is a good example. The experiment involved three young, adult, well-trained cross-country skiers, but urinary nitrogen excretion data was obtained for only one. Each subject was sedentary the day before a bout of skiing; subjects slept in the laboratory during the night.

Food was available and subjects were encouraged to eat up to 10:00 P.M. on the preexercise day, then subjects fasted. No food was given immediately before or during the exercise bout, and subjects had been fasting at least 12 h when the skiing bout began. The exercise took place on a level, circular track 750 m in length. Lap time was set at approximately 180 to 200 s, giving rise to an average workload of 82% $\dot{V}O_2$ max.

The subject for whom urinary nitrogen determinations were made performed 47 laps over 2 h 42 min. The nitrogen content of this subject's urine on the preexercise day was 19.2 g (8.9 g from the day and 10.2 g during the night). On the day of exercise, his total urinary nitrogen excretion was 12.0 g (5.4 g from the day and 6.6 g from the night). Hedman[98] measured the energy cost of exercise for this subject to be 2899 kcal. The nitrogen content of the urine on the exercise day reflects no more than 300 kcal protein catabolized, just 10% of the total energy cost of the exercise bout.

Clearly, protein was not the sole fuel for exercise. Furthermore, measurement of expired gases indicated that glycogen stores provided about 60% of energy expended, with fat contributing most of the rest. This demonstrates further that protein is not the preferred source of fuel for muscular work, even in a fasting subject. In other words, these findings show that skeletal muscle tissues are not excessively catabolized to provide energy during exercise. Finally, this report is widely cited as the most recent to provide strong evidence against the views of Liebig and to confirm the findings of investigators from the 19th century.

3. Exceptions to the Rule

While it is firmly established that protein is not the usual or preferred source of energy for exercise, there are noteworthy exceptions. Chittenden[93] reports that two 19th-century scientists, Pfluger and Argutinsky, showed that protein could be the primary source of fuel for dogs or humans during exercise if carbohydrate and fat intakes were minimized or if protein intake was very high. "While proteid is plainly not the material from which the energy of muscular contraction is ordinarily derived, it is equally evident that in emergency, as when the usual store of carbohydrate and fat is wanting, proteid can be drawn upon, and in such cases vigorous work may be attended with increased nitrogen output."[93]

In 1972, Krebs[35] also proposed that protein could be the preferred source of energy if the diet contained an excess amount of protein in relation to the body's needs. In support of his assertion, Krebs[35] argued that surfeit protein consumption enhanced the activity of inducible enzymes at the liver. Interestingly, the switch to protein as an energy source would occur despite a ready supply of carbohydrate and fat. Therefore, high-protein diets can apparently shift energy metabolism to protein and away from carbohydrate and fat. One explanation for this effect of protein is that it cannot be stored in the short run, as can both carbohydrate and fat. Hence, the body is obliged to metabolize excess protein in preference to other fuel sources.

C. Departure from the Traditional Value

During the 1970s, scientists were quietly gathering and reporting various kinds of data showing exercise-enhanced changes in nitrogen metabolism. In these reports, endurance exercise was associated with increased levels of serum, sweat, and urinary urea. The study of radioactive isotope and amino acid metabolism also indicated changes suggesting a catabolic effect of exercise. Then Lemon and Nagle published a review and summary of these reports in 1981.[91] This paper became a watershed in modern thinking about exercise and protein requirements. Lemon and Nagle[91] concluded, "Although clearly not as important as either [carbohydrate or fat], recent investigations employing both humans and laboratory animals suggest that protein/amino acids, under some conditions, may contribute significantly to total exercise calories."

A key term in their conclusion was the use of the word "significant" to describe the potential contribution of protein to the energy cost of exercise.[91] The issue is how to interpret the use of this word. Not too long ago, scientists and health professionals, particularly nutritionists and physiologists, were of a mind that the contribution of protein to the total daily energy requirement could be safely ignored. As an essential nutrient, protein was considered to be too important to be oxidized for energy — it would be wasteful to use it for energy production. Instead, energy production was thought best left to the nonessential nutrients, carbohydrate and fat.

Scientists turned a blind eye to the energy potential of protein many years ago. For example, as far back as 1924, Lusk[57] published his calculations of the respiratory quotient, and he assumed that protein made no contribution at all to the energy requirement. These calculations were widely accepted both then and now in measurements of indirect calorimetry. Therefore, Lemon and Nagle's[91] discussion of protein as a significant energy source may have been a surprise for some. It was no longer safe to assume that protein builds proteins exclusively while fat and carbohydrate provide for energy needs.

Still there is the question of what constitutes a significant contribution to total energy needs. Nutritionists have long been aware that protein contributes to the total daily energy needs of the American population. For example, in 1984, U.S. Department of Agriculture[6] nutrient intake data indicated that the distribution of dietary energy over all ages and both sexes was approximately 17% of kilocalories from protein, 41% from fat, and 43% from carbohydrate.

TABLE 4 Effect of 3-h, 45-min Mild Treadmill Exercise on the Catabolism of Protein in Young Adult Men

Time of measurement	Protein catabolism	
	Overall (mg protein/h/kg)	Change relative to control day (%)
Control day, $n = 5$		
Rest	26	—
Exercise day, $n = 6$		
Rest	27	+4
During	98–146	+277–462
After	27–57	+4–119

Data from Reference 99.

Rennie et al.[99] assessed how much extra protein is catabolized as a result of athletes' participation in a bout of endurance exercise (Table 4). Their subjects ran on a treadmill for 3 h 45 min, and urinary urea was elevated relative to a control day, which they[99] took to indicate an exercise-enhanced oxidation of 28 to 44 g amino acids. At 4 kcal/g, this amount of protein represents 112 to 176 kcal or 4 to 8% of the total energy cost of exercise, which was estimated to range from 2032 to 3728 kcal.

While the contribution of protein to exercise calories does not seem to be large judging from the data of Rennie et al.,[99] Lemon and Nagle[91] may be correct in asserting that the metabolism of amino acids is greatly enhanced as the magnitude of amino acid oxidation can rise almost 500% above resting values (Table 4). Therefore, it is necessary to keep in mind the larger picture; the report by Rennie et al.[99] suggests that the increased contribution of protein is relatively unimportant in regards to the total energy metabolism of the body. For example, if subjects' maintenance requirements for energy are arbitrarily estimated to be 2000 kcal/d, and the cost of exercise is added to this, then the contribution of exercise-enhanced protein catabolism would only have been in the neighborhood of 3% of kilocalories overall.

As a caveat, it is important to remember that the utilization of protein as a source of energy at skeletal muscle tissue is dependent on the protein and energy intake levels, as well as the availability of carbohydrate and fat sources of fuel.[84,86] Specifically, high protein intake and/or limiting energy intake will enhance the catabolism of protein at rest and during exercise.[33,34,36-41,84,94,97,100-104] On the other hand, when coupled with adequate energy to maintain balance, manifest in stable body weight, the use of protein as a source of fuel will be minimized.[105] Furthermore, research with carbohydrate and fat has revealed desirable levels/patterns of macronutrient intake to optimize endurance sports performance.[100,106-109]

1. Leucine Catabolism

The studies of leucine metabolism conducted by Wolfe[92] have yielded data to suggest that exercise may be catabolic in nature. The work was based on a series of measurements and one or more major assumptions since it was not known how to take all of the needed measurements. Basically, the following describes the general experimental approach. Leucine is an essential amino acid which is incorporated into skeletal muscle proteins. Additionally, as a branched-chain amino acid, it is preferentially catabolized at the skeletal muscle rather than the liver.[91] Hence, the study of leucine metabolism should give more relevant information about the effect of exercise on protein metabolism at the working tissues.

Well after feeding, in the postabsorptive state, blood samples were taken and assayed for a radioisotope of the amino acid, $[1\text{-}^{13}C]$leucine. It was assumed that any of the labeled

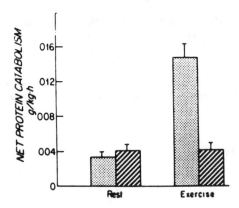

FIGURE 10. Estimation of net balance between protein synthesis and catabolism agree in resting period when urea (striped area) and leucine data (stippled area) are used. During exercise, leucine data indicate a significant increase in net protein catabolism, whereas estimation based on urea production indicates no change in catabolism. (From Wolfe, R. R., *Med. Sci. Sports Exercise,* 19, S172, 1987. With permission from the American College of Sports Medicine.)

amino acid present in the blood had come from the breakdown of skeletal muscle proteins; this logic reflects scientists' understanding that leucine catabolism would not be dominated by the liver during exercise. Measurements made over time allowed for determination of the rate at which labeled leucine was being released. Then the rates during rest and exercise were compared.

The comparisons indicated that leucine release was relatively greater during exercise, suggesting a catabolic effect. However, this finding was contradicted by measurements of urea labeled with the ^{15}N-isotope. As shown in Figure 10, the height of the urea bar was unchanged with exercise, while that for leucine rose substantially.[92] Contradictory data are disappointing, but not unexpected in the study of nutrient metabolism when radioisotopes are employed. There can be no question that the assumptions made when using radioisotopes are critical. For example, with the tagged leucine, it was not known how much was reutilized within the skeletal muscle cell for new tissue proteins after catabolism. Wolfe[92] had to make an assumption in this regard. However, this was not the only problem; others have been carefully discussed by Wolfe[92] in his review on the subject.

In summary, no modern investigator is free of the problems which come with the use of radioisotopes in the study of nutrient metabolism. The resultant data should be viewed cautiously — a piece of the puzzle is always missing, opening the door for assumptions and error. It is not appropriate to give the radioisotope technology credibility simply because it represents an advancement in the sophistication of research methods available in nutrition science. The studies of past scientists over many years, which are based on very old technologies, are still valid and reliable, having stood the test of time. They should not be dismissed in favor of blind progress.

2. The Glucose–Alanine Cycle

The output of alanine from the skeletal muscle tissue into the blood has been found to rise with exercise, in proportion to its intensity. This observation has led to the hypothesis that exercise enhances protein catabolism at the skeletal muscle.[88,89] Hence, this is another reason to suggest that the protein needs of athletes are greater than nonathletes.[91]

Explaining the rise in alanine output with exercise was a problem at first, since there is no alanine-rich protein in the skeletal muscle tissue to serve as a source. After all, the

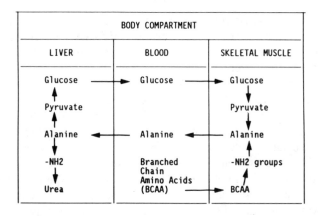

FIGURE 11. Glucose–alanine cycle showing input of branched-chain amino acids leucine, isoleucine, and valine.

precursor could not be a typical protein with a balanced variety of amino acids because this variety would be observed in the output. The solution to the problem came when scientists hit upon the idea that exercise increased the *de novo* synthesis of alanine. The carbon skeleton was derived from glucose, and the amino groups came from the deamination of other amino acids at the skeletal muscle, particularly the branched-chain amino acids: leucine, isoleucine, and valine.[91]

The exercise-induced synthesis of alanine is hypothesized to serve as a nontoxic, water-soluble carrier of amino groups produced through protein catabolism.[91] The carrier, alanine, moves these groups out of the tissue and prevents the build up of toxic ammonia molecules. Once in the blood, the carrier is picked up by the liver. At this organ, the "cargo" of amino groups is lost to the urea cycle with formation of urea. What remains is the carbon skeleton of the carrier; it is converted to glucose via gluconeogenesis. This glucose is released into the blood stream from the liver, and the skeletal muscle picks it up during circulation. To complete the cycle, the "fresh" glucose in the skeletal muscle, just having been taken up from the blood, is converted to pyruvate and is then transaminated to form alanine all over again. This cycle is depicted in Figure 11.

It should be recognized that the glucose–alanine cycle may not result in the formation of a net increase in blood glucose for uptake at the skeletal muscle. Again, the purpose of the cycle is hypothesized to be the outward movement of toxic ammonia groups. However, there is another, indirect benefit: it permits the catabolism of amino acids in the skeletal muscle tissue that can yield energy for work.[91] The question is whether or not this catabolism is meaningful in terms of the dietary protein requirement. It has been argued by scientists and laymen that any loss of amino acids is detrimental to the organism if these nutrients could have been used to maintain or increase skeletal muscle mass.[91]

3. Studies of Acute Bouts
a. 16- to 19-km Run
Dohm et al.[65] studied 10 young adult male runners who participated in a run of 10 or 12 miles with an average time of 1.4 ± 0.1 h. The subjects selected their own diets, but were instructed to maintain protein intake constant during the 3 days prior to, and 1 day after, the run. In addition, five did not eat meat during this time in order to facilitate the analysis of urines for 3MH; those who ate meat were asked to keep intake constant. The dietary protein level was not described. All subjects contributed 24-h urine collections before and after the run.

Urinary urea excretions rose from 406 ± 106 mmol/24 h (mean ± SE) before exercise to 730 ± 202 mmol/24 h after exercise.[65] This result indicates an exercise-enhanced protein catabolism. However, urinary excretion of creatinine also rose from one collection to the other. Urinary creatinine excretion is generally accepted as an indicator of the precision of timing and of the completeness of urine collections.[23,30-32] Hence, subjects' urine collections should be viewed with caution. When urea excretion is expressed by creatinine, there is no significant difference to indicate an exercise-enhanced protein catabolism. Dohm et al.[65] discount the rise in urinary creatinine excretion by suggesting that it can be attributed to an exercise-enhanced creatine metabolism. The rate of creatinine formation is affected by body temperature, which is elevated during work; it is possible that increased creatinine excretion was a function of exercise and not due to deviation from the experimental protocol.

Running also increased the urinary excretion of 3MH in the study conducted by Dohm et al.[65] There was an increase for subjects who ate meat and for those who did not, and thus, the data were combined. Urinary 3MH excretion was 286 ± 51 μmol/24 h before exercise and 514 ± 73/24 h after exercise. These data suggest that the source of protein for the proposed exercise-enhanced catabolism was the skeletal muscle, providing that urinary 3MH excretion is a reliable marker for catabolism of this tissue.[23,25,110] When expressed by creatinine excretion, urinary 3MH was still significantly elevated following exercise.

Dohm et al.[65] calculate that the quantity of excess protein catabolized by their subjects because of their participation in the run amounted to 57 g or 18% of the energy expended during work. At this level of input, protein is a significant, but not major, source of energy for exercise. This observation led Dohm et al.[65] to suggest that the purpose of protein degradation during exercise, possibly from the skeletal muscle, was to provide precursors for glucose production at the liver. This suggestion is consistent with that of Lemon and Nagle,[91] as discussed above.

b. 100-km Run

In a report consistent with those of other investigators,[74,91] Decombaz et al.[111] reported elevated urinary urea excretions from participants in a 100-km marathon. Eleven trained male marathon runners served as subjects in the study. Food intake was not controlled. Urine was collected for the 24-h preexercise period, over the last 40 km of the race, and postexercise to 8:00 A.M. the following morning (18- to 25-h period). The ratio of urea to creatinine was higher in the postexercise period than in the preexercise period (approximately 15–16:1 vs. 11:1), indicating an exercise-enhanced catabolism of protein.

In contrast to Dohm et al.,[65] mean urinary 3MH excretions for the subjects of the study reported by Decombaz et al.[111] were not different between pre- and postexercise periods when expressed by time (μmol/min). This was interpreted to mean that the catabolism of skeletal muscle was not enhanced consequent to exercise. Caution should be used in evaluating this interpretation, since subjects' diets were not controlled. This finding of no exercise effect on the excretion of 3MH is just the opposite of that reported by Dohm et al.[65] However, Decombaz et al.[111] suggest that the skeletal muscle may still have been the source of excess protein catabolized due to exercise. If the synthesis of tissue proteins was depressed during the marathon, then an excess of amino acids would have been available for catabolism at the liver to form urea.

c. Mild Treadmill Exercise

Rennie et al.[99] have reported a 6-d study of four 32- to 45-year-old males. It was not specified whether or not the subjects were athletes. Subjects ate their usual diet except they refrained from eating meat. Then on study days 5 and 6, a milk-based liquid formula diet was fed, providing 40 g protein/m² along with 5 MJ energy/m² of body surface area. On study day 5, subjects rested; on study day 6 subjects exercised at 50% $\dot{V}O_2$ max on a treadmill for 3.75 h. The treadmill was located in an air-conditioned room in order to keep ventilation and air temperature at a level to inhibit sweating and consequent loss of urea nitrogen across the skin.

Plasma urea concentrations were measured every 45 min, and levels rose over time; postexercise plasma urea levels were elevated for at least 5 h.[99] This rise may be explained in part by decreased urine formation, since plasma creatinine rose during the exercise period, too. However, urinary excretion of urea was elevated over the 22- to 25-h period following exercise when compared with no-exercise, control day 5.[99]

In contrast to urea, there was a statistically significant fall in the 24-h urinary excretion of 3MH from 252 ± 32 μmol (mean ± SE) on preexercise study day 5 down to 220 ± 41 μmol on postexercise study day 6.[99] The fall in excretion of this amino acid suggests that skeletal muscle protein catabolism decreased due to exercise. Therefore, the rise in plasma urea during exercise and in urinary urea excretion after exercise would have been due to the catabolism of proteins from sources other than the skeletal muscle tissue.

Rennie et al.[99] speculated that the source of amino acids for an exercise-enhanced catabolism may have been the liver. If the controlling factor on protein catabolism at the liver is the influx of amino acids from the portal blood, then a fall in portal blood flow consequent to exercise may result in an increase in catabolism of liver proteins.[99] Since the energy contribution of the protein catabolized is small relative to the energy cost of exercise, it seems likely that the catabolism was not intended to meet energy needs. Rather, the protein catabolized may have been used to provide precursors for gluconeogenesis, as suggested by Dohm et al.[65] and Lemon and Nagle,[91] and/or it may reflect an increase in the obligatory loss of protein during exercise.[74,75,90,91,112,113]

d. Intense Treadmill Exercise

Radha and Bessman[114] reported a study that is different in results from either Decombaz et al.[111] or Dohm et al.[65] The subjects of the study were five trained male runners. The men ate no meat over the 3-week study period, but the protein intake level was not specified. Exercise sessions were conducted during weeks 2 and 3, and they consisted of running on a treadmill for 1 h per day at an intensity of 70% $\dot{V}O_2$ max. Urine samples were collected each day of the study. The urinary excretion of 3MH was significantly lower on exercise days than on control days (2.4 vs. 2.9 nmol/min/kg). Although the excretion of creatinine fell significantly, too, the decrease was smaller than that for 3MH. The ratio of 3MH to creatinine was 0.243 vs. 0.218; the differences in these ratios was not statistically significant. Urinary urea excretion data were not reported. Hence, it is not known if there was an exercise-enhanced protein catabolism.

Radha and Bessman[114] interpreted their results to indicate that " . . . diminishing methylhistidine excretion is possibly explicable on the diversion of energy from protein breakdown to muscle activity for it has been shown that protein breakdown is dependent upon available energy." Furthermore, the authors[114] speculated that other investigators showing increased urinary excretions of 3MH may have exercised their subjects to exhaustion, leading to trauma and destruction of skeletal muscle tissue. Hence, there is a question of making fair comparisons between studies when exercise protocols are not standardized.[66] In other words, it is important to be able to distinguish between studies designed to produce an effect by overtraining vs. those that are intended to reflect "real life" bouts from practical exercise programs.

e. Bicycloergometer Exercise

Gontzea et al.[74] have suggested that the catabolic effect of endurance exercise is a reflection of increased "obligatory" losses of amino acids. Accordingly, the prolonged elevation in

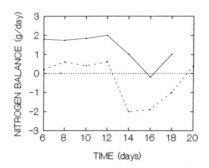

FIGURE 12. Effect of exercise over study days 13 to 16 on nitrogen balance at protein intake levels of 1.0 g/kg/d (dashed line) and 1.5 g/kg/d (solid line). (From Gontzea, I. et al., *Nutr. Rep. Int.*, 10, 35, 1974. With permission from Butterworths Publishers.)

skeletal muscle cell metabolism due to exercise results in the "unfortunate" and unavoidable loss of more than usual numbers of amino acids from the skeletal muscle cell pool into oxidative pathways. By contrast, Lemon and Nagle[91] explain the catabolic effect of endurance exercise as being the result of inadequate carbohydrate and fat molecules to serve as energy sources. In this state of "starvation", the skeletal muscle turns to its own protein reserves to meet the energy demands of work.

Gontzea et al.[74] conducted a controlled-feeding nitrogen balance study with 30 adult men to test the effect of bicycloergometer exercise on nitrogen balance. The subjects were hospitalized and sedentary for 12 d during phase I. The diet supplied 1.0 g protein/kg/d and 110% of energy needs as determined by energy expenditure measurements. The excess energy intake was fed to promote efficient protein metabolism.[80,115,116] Over study days 13 to 16, they exercised for six or seven 20-min periods, which were separated by 30-min rest breaks. This was followed by a no-exercise recovery period over study days 17 to 20. Six subjects continued their participation in the study during phase II, but they consumed a higher protein intake level of 1.5 g protein/kg/d. After allowing 8 d for adaptation to the new diet, the exercise protocol was repeated. During most of the study, subjects contributed urine, fecal, and sweat samples to enable a good approximation of "true" nitrogen balance.[31]

The investigators[74] hypothesized "that muscular activity increases consumption of proteins and consequently there must be an increased excretion of nitrogen, resulting in negative nitrogen balance." The results of the study are shown in Figure 12. During the sedentary period, zero nitrogen balance was achieved for subjects consuming 1.0 g protein/kg/d; this is normal in adults. However, balance became negative during the exercise period, indicating an abnormal condition. Because total energy intake was more than adequate to meet the demands of exercise, increased utilization of proteins cannot be attributed to a lack of fuel. Therefore, the investigators attributed the finding of negative balance to an "augmentation of the energy expense during exertion [which] increases protein metabolism." In other words, the unavoidable or obligatory losses of proteins were enhanced significantly during prolonged exercise.

The results for the six subjects who continued on to the second phase of the study are also shown in Figure 12. Visual inspection of the plotted data suggests that nitrogen balance did not become negative during the exercise period for these subjects. This finding was interpreted by Gontzea et al.[74] to indicate that a high-protein diet is beneficial to the athlete in maintaining a healthy balance between nitrogen intake and output. It may give "protection" against obligatory catabolism by flooding skeletal muscle cells with excess amino acids which can be sacrificed instead of those derived from skeletal muscle proteins.

An important problem with the findings of the second phase of the study is that adult subjects were in positive nitrogen balance during the sedentary period.[79,86,94,97,102-104] This

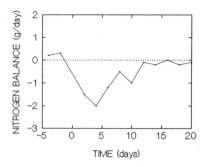

FIGURE 13. The effect of a 20-d program of endurance exercise on nitrogen balance when subjects consumed 1.0 g protein/kg;[75] exercise began after a 2-week control period on study day +1 on the plot. (From Gontzea, I. et al., *Nutr. Rep. Int.*, 11, 231, 1975. With permission from Butterworths Publishers.)

is unexpected because positive balance is ordinarily associated with growth; for example, growing children would be expected to be in positive balance. A partial explanation for the finding is that sweat nitrogen losses were apparently not measured during the sedentary period of phase II, and this could have resulted in a substantial error in calculations of balance.[91,116-123] Hence, nitrogen balance during this time interval may actually be more negative than plotted. If the plot for phase II were corrected to reflect zero balance during the sedentary, control period, then it would overlay that for phase I. Then there would be no difference in the response to endurance exercise between phases I and II, indicating there is no advantage to a high protein intake.

4. Studies of Chronic Exercise
a. Bicycloergometer Exercise
Gontzea et al.[75] have also conducted the only long-term nitrogen balance study to date of men engaged in a program of chronic endurance exercise. Twelve young adult men participated in the 32-d study. The diet provided 1.0 g protein/kg/d. Energy intake was set at 10% higher than necessary to maintain body weight during both the control and experimental phases in order to promote efficient protein metabolism.[80,115,116] Zero nitrogen balance was obtained during the no-exercise, control period (study days 1 to 12). However, Gontzea et al.[75] observed increased urine, fecal, and sweat nitrogen excretions and negative nitrogen balance immediately with the onset of the exercise regimen (Figure 13). This initial response to the exercise regimen, indicating increased protein catabolism, is like that reported by some other investigators of isolated exercise bouts.[65,74,91]

An exciting and often-overlooked result of the long-term study by Gontzea et al.[75] was the occurrence of an adaptation in protein utilization to the chronic exercise stress over the 20-d exercise period. This adaptation resulted in subjects return to zero nitrogen balance by study day 32. This finding suggests that more efficient protein metabolism is a training effect, occurring over time, to a regular regimen of endurance exercise. This effect not only prevents the loss of body reserves of protein in the long run, particularly skeletal muscle, but it also enables the athlete's body to adapt to the stress without having to increase dietary protein intake. This adaptation phenomenon to endurance exercise has also been observed by Yoshimura.[40] However, the time course of adaptations in protein metabolism for his subjects[40] was relatively brief (days) relative to those of Gontzea et al.[75] (between 2 and 3 weeks).

TABLE 5 Characteristics, Mean (±SD) Intakes of Selected Nutrients, and Overall Nitrogen Balance Data for the Experimental Subgroups

Parameter	Group		
	Sedentary	Bodybuilders	Endurance
No. of subjects	6	6	6
Age (years)	22 ± 1	24 ± 1	22 ± 1
Mean body weight (kg)	76 ± 2	80 ± 2	73 ± 1
Body fat (%)	15 ± 1	10 ± 2	7 ± 1
Low-protein diet			
Protein (g/kg/d)	1.1 ± 0.04	1.0 ± 0.02	1.7 ± 0.03
Energy (kcal/d)	3,222 ± 39	4,807 ± 21	4,539 ± 18
Balance (g/d)	+1.73 ± .72	+1.06 ± .56	+1.75 ± 0.62
High-protein diet			
Protein (g/kg/d)	1.9 ± 0.04	2.7 ± 0.02	2.7 ± 0.02
Energy (kcal/d)	3,141 ± 41	4,802 ± 22	4,562 ± 26
Balance (g/d)	+6.15 ± 1.05	+13.35 ± 1.54	+7.09 ± 0.76

Data from Reference 77.

	EXPERIMENT A <------NORMAL DIET------>	EXPERIMENT B <------ALTERED DIET------>
10 days <-----------> Food History and Diet Analysis	10 days <-----------> Adaptation . 3 days <---------> N Balance	10 days <-----------> Adaptation . 3 days <----------> N Balance
Group:		
Sedentary	3220 kcal/d .--> 1.1 g pro/kg.	3141 kcal/d .--> 1.9 g pro/kg.
Bodybuilders	4802 kcal/d .--> 2.8 g pro/kg.	4807 kcal/d .--> 1.1 g pro/kg.
Endurance	4590 kcal/d .--> 1.7 g pro/kg.	4562 kcal/d .--> 2.7 g pro/kg.

FIGURE 14. Experimental design for subject groups, endurance athletes, bodybuilders, and sedentary individuals. (From Tarnopolsky, M. A. et al., *J. Appl. Physiol.*, 64, 187, 1988. With permission from the American Physiological Society.)

b. Elite Runners, Skiers, and Bodybuilders

Tarnopolsky et al.[77] conducted two nitrogen balance experiments with the same three groups of six subjects each (Table 5). Group 1 included sedentary persons (nonathletes). Group 2 included elite endurance athletes in the sports of running or nordic skiing. Group 3 was comprised of bodybuilders. The experimental design is depicted in Figure 14. The purpose of having two experiments with the same subjects was to compare their response to two different levels of protein intake (Table 5). During the adaptation phase of each experiment, subjects self-prepared food distributed by the investigators. During balance periods, the investigators prepared the food for the subjects. The diets were designed to maintain body weight. Both groups of exercising subjects were in "maintenance" phases of training. Urine and fecal collections were made for actual measurement of nitrogen losses; sweat nitrogen losses were estimated on the basis of sweat samples taken at rest and during exercise.

Mean nitrogen balance data for groups indicate that subjects were in zero or slight positive balance during periods of "low protein intake" (Table 5).[77] Balance became strongly positive

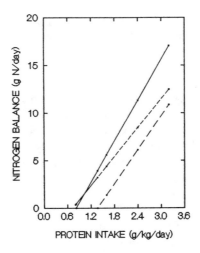

FIGURE 15. Predicted protein intakes to achieve zero nitrogen balance based on extrapolated data for endurance athletes (— —), bodybuilders (—), and sedentary individuals (– – – –). (From Tarnopolsky, M. A. et al., *J. Appl. Physiol.*, 64, 187, 1988. With permission from the American Physiological Society.)

for all groups with "high protein intake". High protein intake is known to induce strong positive balance even when energy intake is generous.[94,97,102-104] The fact that the sedentary group went into strong positive balance on the high-protein diet demonstrates that the balances for the other groups were not the result of an exercise effect. Additionally, body composition assessments revealed that there were no changes over the course of the study for any of the groups. Therefore, high protein intake did not facilitate gains in lean body mass.[77] Therefore, it cannot be concluded from these data that there is any advantage in the feeding of high-protein diets to athletes.

Tarnopolsky et al.[77] found that a plot of nitrogen balance vs. protein intake shows that the balance becomes more positive as the dietary protein content rises for each experimental group (Figure 15). This phenomenon is known to occur in persons who are not athletes.[94,97,102-104]

Interestingly, the plots for the groups of sedentary subjects and bodybuilders overlay one another while that for endurance athletes is offset to the right (Figure 15). These data could mean that endurance athletes need more protein than bodybuilders per unit of body weight. Perhaps the obligatory nitrogen losses induced by exercise are important for endurance athletes, but not for bodybuilders, whose training sessions are relatively short.[65,74,75,88-92] Minimum acceptable intakes for bodybuilders and endurance athletes were determined from extrapolated data to be approximately 0.8 and 1.4 g protein/kg/d, respectively. This is contrary to the common wisdom that muscular athletes like bodybuilders need more protein than others because "muscle is made of protein".

c. Summary

The results of acute effects studies clearly indicate that endurance exercise is catabolic in nature.[65,88-92] Because the phenomenon of adaptation has not been explored, except by Tarnopolsky et al.,[77] most of these studies have been interpreted to mean that a high-protein diet is necessary for endurance athletes.[65,74,75,90-92] Additionally, it may be appropriate to re-interpret acute effects studies in light of the fact that athletes train in regimens of chronic exercise rather than isolated, disconnected bouts. Over the long run, participation in an exercise regimen promotes good health, but without adaptation, athletes would slowly waste away.[66] The work of Gontzea et al.[75] demonstrates that there can be an adaptation in protein metabolism in response to chronic endurance exercise, and this effect can mitigate the need for a high-protein diet.

V. SUMMARY AND CONCLUSIONS

Exercise is not a generic activity. It can be classified according to training effects, including modes that build strength and endurance. Research with novice and experienced subjects in studies of acute and chronic bouts of strength and endurance exercise have produced some data to show that the two modes influence protein metabolism in different ways. Strength exercise does not appear to increase protein catabolism, according to most reports. On the other hand, endurance exercise does increase breakdown measurably (i.e., it could be "catabolic in nature"). However, the magnitude of the increase may not be important from a nutritional standpoint.

Recommended intakes — The RDA[16] is a good place to begin formulating recommendations for generous and safe protein intakes for athletes. To that ground level of intake, additional allowances can be made. For strength athletes, an allowance for making gains in skeletal muscle tissue with training is appropriate. For endurance athletes, an allowance for covering a potentially important rise in obligatory nitrogen losses due to exercise is appropriate. The size of additional allowances made to the RDA has generally been left up to the athlete's discretion. There is no particular set of guidelines on which to make such decisions. Furthermore, very high intakes have not proved to be toxic, which has encouraged the practice of overconsumption. Many athletes take the attitude that "it is better to be safe than sorry". Commonly recommended levels of protein intake for strength and endurance athletes run about $3 \times$ RDA and $2 \times$ RDA, respectively.

Future research — Studies of isolated bouts of exercise, eliciting short-term adaptation responses, probably do not yield information which can be directly applied to athletes. Future research might focus on investigations of standardized programs of chronic exercise, to elicit long-term adaptation, and strict dietary protocols with the potential to be interpreted in an applied manner directly to athletes. No-exercise, control periods should be incorporated for all subjects before beginning the experimental phase of studies. Subjects were must be allowed to adapt to the dietary protein and energy intake levels, which may require a control period of 7 to 14 d. Research with high protein intakes would be both interesting and beneficial to athletes seeking a competitive edge.

REFERENCES

1. **Faber, M. and Benade, A. J. S.,** Nutrient intake and dietary supplementation in body-builders, *S. Afr. Med. J.*, 72, 831, 1987.
2. **Heyward, V. H., Sandoval, W. M., and Colville, B. C.,** Anthropometric, body composition and nutritional profiles of bodybuilders during training, *J. Appl. Sports Sci. Res.*, 3(2), 22, 1989.
3. **Hickson, J. F., Duke, M. A., Risser, W. L., Johnson, C. W., Palmer, R., and Stockton, J. E.,** Nutritional intake from food sources of high school football athletes, *J. Am. Diet Assoc.*, 87, 1656, 1987.
4. **Hickson, J. F., Wolinsky, I., Pivarnik, J. M., Neuman, E. A., Itak, J. F., and Stockton, J. E.,** Nutritional profile of football athletes eating from a training table, *Nutr. Res.*, 7, 27, 1987.
5. **Kleiner, S. M.,** Performance-enhancing aids in sport: health consequences and nutritional alternatives, *J. Am. Coll. Nutr.*, 10, 336, 1991.
6. **Human Nutrition Information Service,** *Nutrient Intakes: Individuals in 48 States, Year 1977–78,* U.S. Department of Agriculture, Washington, D.C., 1984.
7. **Hickson, J. F., Schrader, J. W., Pivarnik, J. M., and Stockton, J. E.,** Nutritional intake from food sources of soccer athletes during two stages of training, *Nutr. Rep. Int.*, 34, 85, 1986.

8. **Ginsburg, H. and Opper, S.,** *Piaget's Theory of Intellectual Development,* 2nd ed., Prentice-Hall, Englewood Cliffs, NJ, 1979, 75.
9. **Curtis, D.,** Pump up your protein powder?, *Muscle & Fitness,* 52(10), 75, 1991.
10. **Parraga, I. M.,** Determinants of food consumption, *J. Am. Diet. Assoc.,* 90, 661, 1990.
11. **Douglas, P. D. and Douglas, J. G.,** Nutrition knowledge and food practices of high school athletes, *J. Am. Diet. Assoc.,* 84, 1198, 1984.
12. **Perron, M. and Endres, J.,** Knowledge, attitudes, and dietary practices of female athletes, *J. Am. Diet. Assoc.,* 85, 573, 1985.
13. **Werblow, J. A., Fox, H. M., and Henneman, A.,** Nutritional knowledge, attitudes, and food patterns of women athletes, *J. Am. Diet. Assoc.,* 73, 242, 1978.
14. **Gruskin, R.,** John DeFendis: update on a champion, *Bodybuilder,* 2(3), 8, 1980.
15. **Hickson, J. F. and Stockton, J. E.,** RECALL: computerized dietary recall program, in *Proceedings of the Ninth Annual Indiana University Computing Network Conference on Academic Computing Applications,* Glenn, P., Huls, S., and Michael, R., Eds., Indiana University Southeast, New Albany, IN, 1982, 34.
16. **Food and Nutrition Board,** *Recommended Dietary Allowances,* 10th ed., National Academy of Sciences, Washington, D.C., 1989.
17. **Kielenowski, J.,** in *Pig Production,* Cole, D. J. A., Ed., Butterworths, London, 1972.
18. **Payne, P. R. and Waterlow, J. C.,** *Lancet,* 2, 210, 1971.
19. **Hough, T.,** Ergographic studies in muscle soreness, *Am. J. Physiol.,* 7, 76, 1902.
20. **Abraham, W. M.,** Factors in delayed muscle soreness, *Med. Sci. Sports,* 9, 11, 1977.
21. **Hickson, J. F., Pivarnik, J. M., and Wolinsky, I.,** Diurnal urinary urea excretion and bodybuilding exercise, *Nutr. Rep. Int.,* 39(4), 845, 1989.
22. **Hickson, J. F., Wolinsky, I., Rodriguez, G. P., Pivarnik, J. M., Kent, M. C., and Shier, N. W.,** Failure of weight training to affect urinary indices of protein metabolism in men, *Med. Sci. Sports Exercise,* 18, 563, 1986.
23. **Buskirk, E. R. and Mendez, J.,** Sports science and body composition analysis: emphasis on cell and muscle mass, *Med. Sci. Sports Exercise,* 16, 584, 1984.
24. **Lukaski, H. C.,** Methods for the assessment of human body composition: traditional and new, *Am. J. Clin. Nutr.,* 46, 537, 1987.
25. **Young, V. R. and Munro, H. N.,** N-Methylhistidine (3-methylhistidine) and muscle protein turnover: an overview, *Fed. Proc.,* 37, 2291, 1978.
26. **Boileau, R. A., Hornstman, D. H., Buskirk, E. R., and Mendez, J.,** The usefulness of urinary creatinine excretion in estimating body composition, *Med. Sci. Sport,* 4, 85, 1972.
27. **Forbes, G. B. and Bruining, G. J.,** Urinary creatinine excretion and lean body mass, *Am. J. Clin. Nutr.,* 29, 1359, 1976.
28. **Lukaski, H. and Mendez, J.,** Relationship between fat-free weight and urinary 3-methylhistidine excretion in man, *Metabolism,* 29, 758, 1980.
29. **Long, C. L., Haverberg, L. N., Young, V. R., Kinney, J. M., Munro, H. N., and Geiger, J. W.,** Metabolism of 3-methylhistidine in man, *Metabolism,* 24, 929, 1975.
30. **Bodwell, C. E.,** Biochemical indices in humans, in *Evaluation of Proteins for Humans,* Bodwell, C. E., Ed., Avi, Westport, CT, 1977, chap. 6.
31. **Kies, C. V.,** Techniques in human nitrogen balance studies, in *Evaluation of Proteins for Humans,* Bodwell, C. E., Ed., Avi, Westport, CT, 1977, chap. 8.
32. **Heymsfield, S. B., Ateaga, C., McManus, C., Smith, J., and Moffitt, S.,** Measurement of muscle mass in humans: validity of the 24-hr urinary creatinine method, *Am. J. Clin. Nutr.,* 37, 478, 1983.
33. **Das, T. K. and Waterlow, J. C.,** The rate of adaptation of urea cycle enzymes, amino transferases and glutamic dehydrogenase to changes in dietary protein intake, *Br. J. Nutr.,* 32, 353, 1974.
34. **Elwyn, D. H.,** The role of the liver in regulation of amino acid and protein metabolism, in *Mammalian Protein Metabolism,* Vol. 4, Munro, H. N., Ed., Academic Press, New York, 1970, 523.
35. **Krebs, H. A.,** Some aspects of the regulation of fuel supply in omnivorous animals, in *Advances in Enzyme Regulation,* Vol. 10, Weber, G., Ed., Pergamon Press, New York, 1972, 397.
36. **Schimke, R. T.,** Adaptive characteristics of urea cycle enzymes in the rat, *J. Biol. Chem.,* 237, 459, 1962.
37. **Schimke, R. T.,** The importance of both synthesis and degradation in the control of arginase levels in rat liver, *J. Biol. Chem.,* 239, 3808, 1964.
38. **Waterlow, J. C.,** Observations on the mechanism of adaptation to low protein intakes, *Lancet,* 2, 1091, 1968.
39. **Waterlow, J. C.,** Nutritional adaptation in man: general introduction and concepts, *Am. J. Clin. Nutr.,* 51, 259, 1990.
40. **Yoshimura, H.,** Adult protein requirements, *Fed. Proc.,* 20 (Part III, Suppl. 7), 103, 1961.

41. **Young, V. R. and Marchini, J. S.**, Mechanisms and nutritional significance of metabolic responses to altered intakes of protein and amino acids, with reference to nutritional adaptation in humans, *Am. J. Clin. Nutr.*, 51, 270, 1990.
42. **Hickson, J. F., Wilmore, J. H., Buono, M. J., and Constable, S. H.**, Energy cost of weight training exercise, *Natl. Strength Conditioning Assoc. J.*, 6, 22, 1984.
43. **Fleck, S. J. and Kraemer, W. J.**, *Designing Resistance Training Programs*, Human Kinetics, Champaign, IL, 1987.
44. **DeLorme, T. L. and Watkins, A. L.**, Techniques of progressive resistance exercise, *Arch. Phys. Med.*, 3, 25, 1948.
45. **Berger, R. A.**, Effect of varied weight training programs on strength, *Res. Q. Am. Assoc. Health Phys. Educ. Recreat.*, 33, 168, 1962a.
46. **Berger, R. A.**, Optimum repetitions for the development of strength, *Res. Q. Am. Assoc. Health Phys. Educ. Recreat.*, 33, 334, 1962b.
47. **Hickson, J. F. and Wolinsky, I.**, Protein intake level and introductory weight training exercise on selected blood measurements in untrained men, *Nutr. Rep. Int.*, 37(3), 575, 1988.
48. **Cuthbertson, D. P.**, The disturbance of metabolism produced by bony and non-bony injury with notes on certain abnormal conditions of bone, *Biochem. J.*, 24, 1244, 1930.
49. **Cuthbertson, D. P.**, Physical injury and its effects on protein metabolism, in *Mammalian Protein Metabolism*, Vol. 2, Munro, H. N. and Allison, J. B., Eds., Academic Press, New York, 1964, chap. 19.
50. **Cuthbertson, D. P. and Tilston, W. J.**, Metabolism during the postinjury period, in *Advances in Clinical Chemistry*, Vol. 12, Bodansky, O. and Steward, C. P., Eds., Academic Press, New York, 1969, 1.
51. **Cuthbertson, D. P., Fell, G. S., Smith, C. M., and Tilston, W. J.**, Metabolism after injury. I. Effects of severity, nutrition, and environmental temperature on protein, potassium, zinc, and creatine, *Br. J. Surg.*, 59, 925, 1972.
52. **Mutch, B. J. C. and Banister, E. W.**, Ammonia metabolism in exercise and fatigue: a review, *Med. Sci. Sports Exercise*, 15, 41, 1983.
53. **Wurtman, R. J.**, Diurnal rhythms in mammalian protein metabolism, in *Mammalian Protein Metabolism*, Vol. 4, Munro, H. N., Ed., Academic Press, New York, 1970, chap. 36.
54. **Hickson, J. F.**, unpublished data, 1991.
55. **Garlick, P. J., Clugston, G. A., Swick, R. W., and Waterlow, J. C.**, Diurnal pattern of protein and energy metabolism in man, *Am. J. Clin. Nutr.*, 33, 1983, 1980.
56. **Kato, H., Mizutani-Funahashi, M., Shiosaka, S., and Nakagawa, H.**, Circadian rhythms of urea formation and arginosuccinate synthetase activity in rat liver, *J. Nutr.*, 108, 1071, 1978.
57. **Lusk, G.**, *The Elements of the Science of Nutrition*, 2nd ed., W. B. Saunders, Philadelphia, 1909.
58. **Parsons, H. G., Wood, M. M., and Pencharz, P. B.**, Diurnal variation in urine 15N-urea content, estimates of whole body protein turnover, and isotope recycling healthy meal-fed children with cystic fibrosis, *Can. J. Physiol. Pharmacol.*, 61, 72, 1983.
59. **Sitren, H. S. and Stevenson, N. R.**, Circadian fluctuations in liver and blood parameters in rats adapted to a nutrient solution by oral, intravenous and discontinuous intravenous feeding, *J. Nutr.*, 110, 558, 1980.
60. **Hickson, J. F. and Hinkelmann, K.**, Exercise and protein intake effects on urinary 3-methylhistidine excretion, *Am. J. Clin. Nutr.*, 41, 246, 1985.
61. **Paul, G. L., DeLany, J. P., Snook, J. T., Seifert, J. G., and Kirby, T. E.**, Serum and urinary markers of skeletal muscle tissue damage after weight lifting exercise, *Eur. J. Appl. Physiol.*, 58, 786, 1989.
62. **McCully, K. K.**, Exercise-induced injury to skeletal muscle, *Fed. Proc.*, 45, 2933, 1986.
63. **Long, C. L., Birkhahn, R. H., Geiger, J. W., and Blakemore, W. S.**, Contribution of skeletal muscle protein in elevated rates of whole body protein catabolism in trauma patients, *Am. J. Clin. Nutr.*, 34, 1087, 1981.
64. **Williamson, D. H., Farrell, R., Kerr, A., and Smith, R.**, Muscle-protein catabolism after injury in man, as measured by urinary excretion of 3-methylhistidine, *Clin. Sci. Mol. Med.*, 52, 527, 1977.
65. **Dohm, G. L., Williams, R. T., Kasperek, G. J., and Van Rij, A. M.**, Increased excretion of urea and N-methylhistidine by rats and humans after a bout of exercise, *J. Appl. Physiol.*, 52, 27, 1982.
66. **Booth, F. W. and Watson, P. A.**, Control of adaptations in protein levels in response to exercise, *Fed. Proc.*, 44, 2293, 1985.
67. **Huszar, G., Golenwsky, G., Maiocco, J., and Davis, E.**, Urinary 3-methylhistidine excretion in man: the role of protein-bound and soluble 3-methylhistidine, *Br. J. Nutr.*, 49, 287, 1983.
68. **Hickson, J. F., Hinkelmann, K., and Bredle, D. L.**, Protein intake level and introductory weight training exercise on urinary total nitrogen excretions from untrained men, *Nutr. Res.*, 8, 725, 1988.
69. **Waterlow, J. C.**, Protein turnover in the whole body, *Nature*, 253, 157, 1975.
70. **Keul, J.**, The relationship between circulation and metabolism during exercise, *Med. Sci. Sports*, 5, 209, 1973.

71. **Keul, J., Doll, E., and Keppler, D.,** *Energy Metabolism of Human Muscle,* University Park, Baltimore, 1972, 111.
72. **Pollock, M. L., Wilmore, J. H., and Fox, S. M.,** *Exercise in Health and Disease,* W. B. Saunders, Philadelphia, 1984, 119.
73. **Hickson, J. F., Wolinsky, I., and Pivarnik, J. M.,** Repeated days of bodybuilding exercise do not enhance urinary nitrogen excretions from untrained young adult males, *Nutr. Res.,* 10, 723, 1990.
74. **Gontzea, I., Sutzescu, P., and Dumitrache, S.,** The influence of muscular activity on nitrogen balance and on the need of man for proteins, *Nutr. Rep. Int.,* 10, 35, 1974.
75. **Gontzea, I., Sutzescu, P., and Dumitrache, S.,** The influence of adaptation to physical effort on nitrogen balance in man, *Nutr. Rep. Int.,* 11, 231, 1975.
76. **Pivarnik, J. M., Hickson, J. F., and Wolinsky, I.,** Urinary 3-methylhistidine excretion increases with repeated weight training exercise, *Med. Sci. Sports Exercise,* 21(3), 283, 1989.
77. **Tarnopolsky, M. A., MacDougall, J. D., and Atkinson, S. A.,** Influence of protein intake and training status on nitrogen balance and lean body mass, *J. Appl. Physiol.,* 64, 187, 1988.
78. **Celejowa, I. and Homa, M.,** Food intake, nitrogen and energy balance in Polish weight lifters, during a training camp, *Nutr. Metab.,* 12, 259, 1970.
79. **Chiang, A.-N. and Huang, P.-C.,** Excess energy and nitrogen balance at protein intakes above the requirement level in young men, *Am. J. Clin. Nutr.,* 48, 1015, 1988.
80. **Garza, C., Scrimshaw, N. S., and Young, V. R.,** Human protein requirements: the effect of variations in energy intake within the maintenance range, *Am. J. Clin. Nutr.,* 29, 280, 1976.
81. **Kishi, K., Miyatani, S., and Inoue, G.,** Requirement and utilization of egg protein by Japanese young men with marginal intakes of energy, *J. Nutr.,* 108, 658, 1978.
82. **Munro, H. N.,** General aspects of the regulation of protein metabolism by diet and by hormones, in *Mammalian Protein Metabolism,* Vol. 1, Munro, H. N. and Allison, J. B., Eds., Academic Press, New York, 1964, chap. 10.
83. **Rao, C. N., Naidu, A. N., and Rao, B. S. N.,** Influence of varying energy intake on nitrogen balance in men on two levels of protein intake, *Am. J. Clin. Nutr.,* 28, 1116, 1975.
84. **Young, V. R.,** Metabolic and nutritional aspects of physical exercise, *Fed. Proc.,* 44, 341, 1985.
85. **Young, V. R., Munro, H. N., Matthews, D. E., and Bier, D. M.,** Relationship of energy metabolism to protein metabolism, in *New Aspects of Clinical Nutrition,* S. Karger, Basel, 1983, 43.
86. **Allison, J. B. and Bird, J. C.,** Elimination of nitrogen from the body, in *Mammalian Protein Metabolism,* Vol. 1, Munro, H. N. and Allison, J. B., Eds., Academic Press, New York, 1964, chap. 11.
87. **Colgan, M.,** The bottom line on your bodybuilding protein needs, *Muscle & Fitness,* 49(12), 121, 1988.
88. **Felig, P., Pozefsky, I., Marliss, E., and Cahill, G. F.,** Alanine: key role in gluconeogenesis, *Science,* 167, 1003, 1970.
89. **Felig, P. and Wahren, J.,** Amino acid metabolism in exercising man, *J. Clin. Invest.,* 50, 2703, 1971.
90. **Lemon, P. W. R.,** Protein and exercise: update 1987, *Med. Sci. Sports Exercise,* 19(Suppl.), 179, 1978.
91. **Lemon, P. W. R. and Nagle, F. J.,** Effects of exercise on protein and amino acid metabolism, *Med. Sci. Sports Exercise,* 13, 141, 1981.
92. **Wolfe, R. R.,** Does exercise stimulate protein breakdown in humans: isotopic approaches to the problem, *Med. Sci. Sports Exercise,* 19, S172, 1987.
93. **Chittenden, R. H.,** *The Nutrition of Man,* Stokes, New York, 1907.
94. **Munro, H. N.,** Historical introduction: the origin and growth of our present concepts of protein metabolism, in *Mammalian Protein Metabolism,* Vol. 1, Munro, H. N. and Allison, J. B., Eds., Academic Press, New York, 1964, chap. 1.
95. **Carpenter, K. J.,** The history of enthusiasm for protein, *J. Nutr.,* 116, 1364, 1986.
96. **Guggenheim, K. Y. and Wolinsky, I.,** *Nutrition and Nutritional Diseases: The Evolution of Concepts,* Collamore, Lexington, MA, 1981.
97. **Steffee, W. P., Goldsmith, R. S., Pencharz, P. B., Scrimshaw, N. S., and Young, V. R.,** Dietary protein intake and dynamic aspects of whole body nitrogen metabolism in adult humans, *Metabolism,* 25, 281, 1976.
98. **Hedman, R.,** The available glycogen in man and the connection between rate of oxygen intake and carbohydrate usage, *Acta Physiol. Scand.,* 40, 305, 1957.
99. **Rennie, M. J., Edwards, R. H. T., Krywawych, S., Davies, C. T. M., Halliday, D., Waterlow, J. C., and Millward, D. J.,** Effect of exercise on protein turnover in man, *Clin. Sci.,* 61, 627, 1981.
100. **American Dietetic Association,** Position of the American Dietetic Association: Nutrition for physical fitness and athletic performance for adults, *J. Am. Diet. Assoc.,* 87, 933, 1987.
101. **Waterlow, J. C., Garlick, P. J., and Millward, D. J.,** *Protein Turnover in Mammalian Tissues and in the Whole Body,* North-Holland, New York, 1978, 179.
102. **Kurzer, M. S. and Calloway, D. H.,** Nitrate and nitrogen balances in men, *Am. J. Clin. Nutr.,* 34, 1305, 1981.

103. **Oddoye, E. A. and Margen, S.,** Nitrogen balance studies in humans: long-term effect of high nitrogen intake on nitrogen accretion, *J. Nutr.,* 109, 363, 1979.

104. **Young, V. R.,** Nutritional balance studies: indicators of human requirements or of adaptive mechanisms, *J. Nutr.,* 116, 700, 1986.

105. **Poortmans, J. R.,** Protein metabolism, in *Principles of Exercise Biochemistry,* Vol. 27, Poortmans, J. R., Ed., S. Karger, Basel, 1988, 164.

106. **Murray, R., Paul, G. L., Seifert, J. G., and Eddy, D. E.,** Responses to varying rates of carbohydrate ingestion during exercise, *Med. Sci. Sports Exercise,* 23, 713, 1991.

107. **Sherman, W. M.,** Carbohydrate, muscle glycogen, and improved performance, *Physician Sportsmed.,* 15, 157, 1987.

108. **Fielding R. A., Costill, D. L., Fink, W. J., King, D. S., Hargreaves, M., and Kovaleski, J. E.,** Effect of carbohydrate feeding frequencies and dosage on muscle glycogen use during exercise, *Med. Sci. Sports Exercise,* 17, 472, 1985.

109. **Sherman, W. M. and Costill, D. L.,** The marathon: dietary manipulation to optimize performance, *Am. J. Sports Med.,* 12, 44, 1984.

110. **Harris, C. I.,** Reappraisal of the quantitative importance of non-skeletal-muscle source of N-methylhistidine in urine, *Biochem. J.,* 194, 1011, 1981.

111. **Decombaz, J., Reinhardt, P., Anantharaman, K., Von Glutz, G., and Poortmans, J. R.,** Biochemical changes in a 100 km run: free amino acids, urea, and creatinine, *Eur. J. Appl. Physiol.,* 41, 61, 1979.

112. **Felig, P.,** The glucose-alanine cycle, *Metabolism,* 22, 179, 1973.

113. **Viru, A.,** Hormones in plastic attainment of function in exercise, *Hormones in Muscular Activity, Vol. 2, Adaptive Effect of Hormones in Exercise,* CRC Press, Boca Raton, FL, 1985, 35.

114. **Radha, E. and Bessman, S. P.,** Effect of exercise on protein degradation: 3-methylhistidine and creatinine excretion, *Biochem. Med.,* 29, 96, 1983.

115. **Goranzon, H. and Forsum, E.,** Effect of reduced energy intake versus increased physical activity on the outcome of nitrogen balance experiments in man, *Am. J. Clin. Nutr.,* 41, 919, 1985.

116. **Todd, K. S., Butterfield, G. E., and Calloway, D. H.,** Nitrogen balance in men with adequate and deficient energy intake at three levels of work, *J. Nutr.,* 114, 2107, 1984.

117. **Ashworth, A. and Harrower, A. D. B.,** Protein requirements in tropical countries: nitrogen losses in sweat and their relation to nitrogen balance, *Br. J. Nutr.,* 21, 833, 1967.

118. **Calloway, D. H., Odell, A. C. F., and Margen, S.,** Sweat and miscellaneous nitrogen losses in human balance studies, *J. Nutr.,* 101, 775, 1971.

119. **Consolazio, C. F., Johnson, H. L., Nelson, R. A., Dramise, J. G., and Skala, J. H.,** Protein metabolism during intensive physical training in the young adult, *Am. J. Clin. Nutr.,* 28, 29, 1975.

120. **Consolazio, C. F., Nelson, R. A., Matoush, L. O., Harding, R. S., and Canham, J. E.,** Nitrogen excretion in sweat and its relation to nitrogen balance requirements, *J. Nutr.,* 79, 399, 1963.

121. **Mitchell, H. H. and Hamilton, T. S.,** The dermal excretion under controlled environmental conditions of nitrogen and minerals in human subjects, with particular reference to calcium and iron, *J. Biol. Chem.,* 178, 345, 1945.

122. **Pellett, P. L.,** Protein requirements in humans, *Am. J. Clin. Nutr.,* 51, 723, 1990.

123. **World Health Organization,** *Energy and Protein Requirements,* Report of a Joint FAO/WHO/UN Expert Consultation, Technical Report Ser. 724, World Health Organization, Geneva, 1985.

Chapter 6

AMINO ACID METABOLISM DURING EXERCISE

Donald K. Layman
Gregory L. Paul
Melissa H. Olken

CONTENTS

0-8493-7911-3/94/$0.00+$.50
© 1994 by CRC Press, Inc.

I. METABOLIC CONSEQUENCES OF EXERCISE

Exercise produces significant changes in whole body metabolism. The forces determining these changes are the factors which define exercise: intensity, duration, and resistance. At a molecular level, these changes are driven by energy needs, availability of substrates, and hormone regulations. During exercise, these metabolic responses appear designed to assure adequate energy to sustain myofibrillar contractions, while long-term responses result in modification of protein structures and body composition to maximize performance. This chapter will focus on short-term metabolic responses with emphasis on regulation of protein synthesis and use of amino acids as energy substrates.

Energy to maintain the body is derived from oxidation of carbon chains contained in carbohydrates, fatty acids, and amino acids. Each of these molecules can be oxidized to carbon dioxide and water through respiration, with the body trapping energy from the carbon–carbon bonds. The selective use of carbohydrates, fatty acids, and amino acids for energy is dependent on their relative concentrations in the blood and within tissues. Conditions of food intake and physical activity plus previous nutrition and exercise status ultimately determine the mixture of fuels at a given moment.

Fatty acids and carbohydrates serve as primary fuels for the body.[1,2] These macronutrients provide 80 to 100% of the metabolic fuel at any particular point in time. On the surface, these numbers suggest that the roles of amino acids as metabolic fuels are relatively insignificant. However, use of amino acids as fuel is more important than usually thought. During nongrowing maintenance conditions, as found in adults, dietary intake provides an indication of the composition of the fuels. For most Americans, intakes range from 40 to 60% for carbohydrates, 25 to 42% for lipids, and 12 to 20% for protein.[3] If the composition of the body is not changing, these intakes reflect the fuels available to the body and suggest constant degradation of amino acids for energy.

The roles and fates of amino acids in the body are diverse, ranging from a primary role in synthesis of protein to the ultimate fate of catabolism to energy and nitrogen waste products. The role of amino acids for protein synthesis is obvious and extensively studied.[4,5] While much is known about the mechanism for incorporation of amino acids into protein, questions remain about the physiological regulations of this process, differences among tissues, and controls exerted by factors such as diet and exercise. Catabolism of amino acids has also been studied extensively, with the degradative pathways for most amino acids well defined,[6] but, again, the physiological regulations and the relationships among individual tissues within the body remain to be elucidated.

Evaluation of amino acid metabolism requires understanding of the roles of multiple tissues in nitrogen metabolism and the movement of amino acids through "pools" or compartments in the body. The principal tissues involved with amino acid and nitrogen metabolism are the liver, kidney, gut, and skeletal muscle. Skeletal muscle accounts for 40 to 45% of total body amino acids and contains approximately half of the free amino acids. Based on its mass alone, skeletal muscle is a significant component of whole body amino acid metabolism; however, somewhat surprisingly, the role of skeletal muscle in amino acid metabolism has been largely ignored. These tissues and their roles in amino acid metabolism during exercise will be examined in this review.

II. FATES OF AMINO ACIDS: FREE POOLS AND FLUX

The vast majority of the amino acids in the body are in protein structures. Only 0.5 to 1.0% of the total amino acids in the body are present as free amino acids in plasma or intracellular and extracellular space.[6] However, the relatively small amounts of amino acids present in the "free pools" are responsible for the metabolic or substrate influences of all amino acids.

TABLE 1 Amino Acid Concentrations in Serum and Muscle (μmol/dl)

Amino acid	Serum	Muscle
Dispensable		
Alanine	32.6	110
Glutamate	12.0	826
Glutamine	65.2	1038
Glycine	33.6	62
Indispensable		
Lysine	38.0	93.0
Threonine	20.3	33.0
Phenylalanine	6.9	5.9
Leucine	16.6	11.2
Valine	18.8	14.7
Isoleucine	10.8	6.8

Adapted from Morgan et al.[7]

TABLE 2 Amino Acid Pool Size and Flux

	Rat	Man
Free amino acids[a] (mmol/kg)	4.0	2.4
Amino acid flux (mmol/kg/d)	200	12
Half-life of free pool (minutes)	20	200

[a] Represents total concentration of dispensable amino acids in the free pool.

Adapted from Waterlow et al.[4]

Plasma and tissue amino acid concentrations for selected amino acids are presented in Table 1. The amino acids in highest concentration in the plasma and tissues are the dispensable amino acids glutamine, glycine, and alanine. Among the indispensable amino acids, the ones present in the highest concentrations are lysine, threonine, and the branched-chain amino acids (BCAA), valine, leucine, and isoleucine.[7] In most cases, amino acids are transported into tissues by active transports, which assures that even relatively small changes in plasma concentrations will be reflected in tissue levels.[8]

While the free amino acid pool is small and relatively stable in size, amino acid concentrations change associated with conditions such as food intake or exercise, but they change within relatively narrow limits. However, the free pool is highly active. Changes in plasma concentrations are not reflective of the movement or flux of amino acids through the free pool. To appreciate the "real size" of the amino acid pool, one must consider both the amino acid concentration and the movement of amino acids into or out of the pool over time.[4,9] Estimates of free pool size and flux are presented in Table 2. Note that the amounts of amino acids moving through the free pool each day are many times the actual free pool size. In the rat, amino acids in the free pool are replaced on the order of 50 times per day, while in the human the total free pool is replaced approximately 6 times each day.

Flux rates presented in Table 2 represent averages for all amino acids. Significant differences exist among individual amino acids. For example lysine, which has a relatively large and stable free pool, has a half-life within the free pool of approximately 10 h in the human, while leucine, which is much more metabolically active, has a half-life of 45 min.

These differences are important to consider when selecting an amino acid to represent the total free pool or as a metabolic tracer.[9]

III. PROTEIN TURNOVER DURING EXERCISE

Muscle protein mass is determined by the relationship between the processes of protein synthesis and degradation. During periods of growth or protein accretion, synthesis exceeds degradation, resulting in a net accumulation of protein or positive balance of protein turnover. If synthesis is equal to degradation, then the period is defined as maintenance or net balance. Most of the research addressing changes in amino acid metabolism during exercise have examined effects of endurance exercise and have focused on use of amino acids as fuels. Few studies have examined changes in protein turnover during resistance exercise designed to produce muscle hypertrophy.

Studies examining the molecular basis for muscle hypertrophy have relied on animal models and used surgical procedures, weights, or chronic electrically stimulated contractions to produce chronic resistance or stretch on specific muscles.[11-15] Muscle hypertrophy appears to require full extension of the muscle and resistance, while high levels of intensity and duration of the activity are not useful. These procedures produce rapid increases in muscle weight and protein content and corresponding increases in muscle RNA content and the rate of protein synthesis. At the molecular level, these experimental models suggest that hypertrophy of skeletal muscle is dependent on stimulation of transcription to increase muscle protein synthesis. The regulatory controls and limits of this response remain unknown.

Physical activity and exercise training are generally assumed to result in maintenance or enlargement of skeletal muscles; however, there is also general consensus that during endurance exercise protein synthesis is suppressed.[10,16-19] The magnitude of the depression in protein synthesis appears to be proportional to the duration and intensity of the activity.

While protein synthesis is suppressed during exercise, the effects of exercise on protein degradation are less clear. Reports indicate that protein degradation is increased,[10,20] decreased,[21] or unchanged.[18,19] Changes in protein degradation appear to be highly dependent on conditions and methodologies used.

One of the first reports of the influence of exercise on protein synthesis was by Dohm et al.,[17] examining protein synthesis in perfused rat muscles after exercise. These investigators found that exercise decreased the rate of protein synthesis and that the magnitude of the effect was proportional to the level of exertion. Mild exercise produced by swimming rats for 1 h decreased protein synthesis by 17%. More intense treadmill running reduced synthesis by 30% and an exhaustive run of 3 h inhibited synthesis by 70%. These data suggest that exercise produces catabolic conditions in skeletal muscles and that these effects are dependent on the intensity and duration of the exercise.

Dohm et al.[20] also examined the effects of exhaustive running on protein degradation. They ran rats at 28 m per minute for 4 h and measured the urinary excretion of urea and 3-methylhistidine. Urea excretion increased by 31% during the first 12 h after the exhaustive bout of exercise. Urinary 3-methylhistidine, which is an indicator of muscle protein breakdown, also increased after exercise. However, the increase in 3-methylhistidine did not occur until 12 to 36 h after exercise. These studies by Dohm et al.[17,20] indicate that exhaustive exercise suppresses protein synthesis and stimulates protein degradation in skeletal muscle.

The finding that exercise produces a catabolic condition was further supported by Rennie et al.,[10] studying aerobic exercise in humans. They exercised six male subjects on a treadmill for 3.75 h at 50% $\dot{V}O_2$ max and measured the rates of protein synthesis and degradation (Table 3). During the exercise, the rate of synthesis decreased by 14% while the rate of degradation increased by 54%. This study is also important, because it is one of the few studies to make measurements during recovery after exercise. These investigators found that

TABLE 3 Protein Turnover at Rest, and During and After Exercise

Condition	Synthesis	Degradation
Rest	33.0 ± 2.0	26.5 ± 2.1
Exercised	28.4 ± 1.6	40.9 ± 2.6
Postexercise	40.3 ± 1.9	35.4 ± 1.2

Note: Six male subjects were exercised on a treadmill for 3.75 h at 50% $\dot{V}O_2$ max. Synthesis and degradation values are measured in milligrams of nitrogen per kilogram per hour.

Data from Rennie et al.[10]

after exercise the rate of synthesis increased above the initial resting levels while protein degradation returned to preexercise levels. These changes in protein turnover suggest that recovery is driven by increases in protein synthesis.

Wolfe et al.,[18,19] using multiple amino acid tracers, further elucidated the changes in protein synthesis and degradation which occur during prolonged, aerobic exercise. These investigators exercised male subjects on a bicycle ergometer at 30% of $\dot{V}O_2$ max for 105 min. Using constant infusion of labeled leucine and lysine, they found decreases in protein synthesis of 48% using leucine and 17% using lysine. While both amino acids demonstrated that exercise inhibited protein synthesis, the magnitude of the response was significantly different depending on the amino acid tracer selected. Using sophisticated isotope methodology, these investigators did not find any changes in protein degradation or any net increase in urea production associated with this relatively light workload. These studies indicate that the intensity of the exercise and the metabolic tracers used are important to the findings about amino acid metabolism and protein turnover.

While the acute effect of exercise on protein turnover is catabolic, the long-term effects of exercise do not lead to muscle atrophy. Routine exercise produces maintenance or hypertrophy of muscle mass. There are few studies which have looked at the postexercise recovery of protein turnover. The report by Rennie et al.[10] and a later report by Devlin et al.[22] suggest that recovery occurs through stimulation of protein synthesis. Preliminary studies in our laboratory provide additional support for this recovery pattern (Figure 1). We have found that after a 2-h bout of running on a motor-driven treadmill at 26 m per minute, protein synthesis in the gastrocnemius muscle was suppressed by 26 to 30% in fasted male rats. Recovery of protein synthesis occurred during the next 4 to 8 h even if the animals are withheld from eating. These data suggest that muscles have a very high capacity for recovery even during conditions of food restriction. Exercise training and food intakes before and after exercise are likely to be important to the effects of exercise on muscle protein synthesis and on subsequent recovery.

Controls of muscle protein synthesis during exercise remain unknown. High-intensity, exhaustive bouts of exercise produce a transient catabolic effect on protein synthesis. This effect is controlled presumably at the translation level of protein synthesis. Transcription is depressed but RNA concentrations are unchanged during the relatively brief period of the exercise bout. At the level of translation, potential regulatory controls include (1) availability of substrates, (2) hormones, (3) energy states, and (4) initiation factors (Figure 2).

During exercise, there are changes in amino acid concentrations in the plasma and tissues. These changes suggest that individual amino acids may be limiting as substrates for protein

Recovery of Protein Synthesis after Exercise

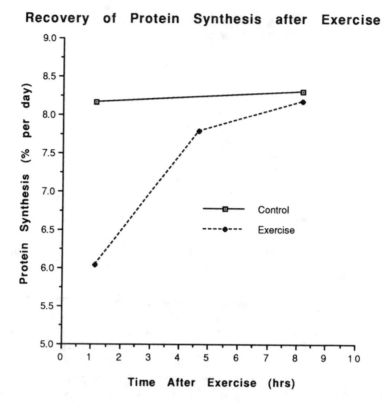

FIGURE 1. *In vivo* protein synthesis was determined in rats by constant infusion of 1-^{14}C-leucine after a 2-h exhaustive run on a motor-driven treadmill at 26 m/min. Control animals receive no exercise. All animals were restricted from food for 20 h prior to the experiment. Animals were killed at three time points during recovery and the fractional synthesis rate was determined for the gastrocnemius muscle. Pooled SEM was ±0.2%/d, $n = 4$. (Paul and Layman, unpublished data.)

Regulation of Protein Synthesis

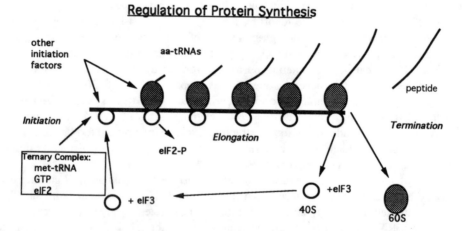

FIGURE 2. The ribosome cycle as pictured begins with initiation (left side of picture), proceeds through elongation to termination (right side of picture). elF2, Eukaryotic initiation factor 2, which represents one of a group of protein factors which serve to regulate/catalyze the initiation of protein synthesis; 40S and 60S, the ribosomal subunits which combine on the mRNA into an 80S ribosome.

synthesis. Primary changes in amino acids during exercise include increases in plasma levels of the three BCAA and alanine and decreases in glutamine and glutamate. While plasma levels of amino acids change during exercise, availability of amino acid substrates for muscle protein synthesis appears to be an unlikely level of control, for a number of reasons. First, muscle contraction has been shown to stimulate amino acid transport and uptake into muscle cells.[23] Second, decreases in protein synthesis and increase in protein degradation produce net release of amino acids into the intracellular free pool, which assures a constant supply of precursors. Finally, Tischler et al.[24] have shown that the rate constant (Km) for the tRNA synthetase for charging of the tRNAs is likely to be far below the amino acid concentration within skeletal muscle. Thus, availability of amino acids is unlikely to limit protein synthesis in skeletal muscles.

Exercise produces changes in hormone levels, with the most dramatic changes occurring after prolonged endurance exercise. Hormones important to protein synthesis include insulin, glucagon, and glucocorticoids. Decreases in the insulin–glucagon ratio and increases in glucocorticoids seen during exercise are consistent with reduced muscle protein synthesis. The molecular mechanism for the action of these hormones on translation remains equivocal, but most evidence points to changes in the initiation phase of translation.[25-27] Additional research is needed to define the role of these hormones in changes in protein turnover which occur during and after exercise.

The energy status of the cell may also be a limiting factor for muscle protein synthesis. Morgan et al.[7] reported that decreases in protein synthesis that occur in proportion to the number of contractions induced by electrical stimulation were in proportion to the decline in the level of ATP in muscle cells. Findings from other laboratories suggest that dephosphorylation of the initiation factor elF2 and subsequent formation of the ternary complex (comprised of the methionine initiator tRNA [met-tRNAf], the initiation factor elF2, and energy in the form of GTP) are energy-requiring steps and appear to be likely control sites for translational regulation of protein synthesis (Figure 2).[28,29]

Formation of the ternary complex (met-tRNA + elF2 + GTP) is viewed by many as a rate-limiting step in translational control of protein synthesis. Efforts have focused on the phosphorylation/dephosphorylation regulation of the initiation factor elF2.[28,29] Protein kinase phosphorylates elF2 to an inactive form which must be regenerated prior to initiation. This protein kinase is known to be stimulated by increased levels of glucagon, cAMP, and calcium and inhibited by insulin. These conditions are all likely to exist within skeletal muscle during exhaustive exercise. Morgan and colleagues reported that insulin may exert its stimulatory effect on translation via the elF2 initiation factor.[7] Further evaluation of these mechanisms is essential for our understanding of the controls and potential to modify protein synthesis during exercise and subsequent recovery.

IV. AMINO ACID METABOLISM DURING EXERCISE

During endurance exercise, changes in protein turnover produce net breakdown of protein with release of amino acids into the free pools. The metabolic roles and importance of these amino acids released during exercise remain uncertain, but our understanding of the pathways is expanding rapidly. It is clear that the principal amino acids involved are the BCAA, alanine, and glutamine and that there is an elaborate interorgan exchange.[30-33]

The dominate features of this interorgan exchange are movement of the branched-chain amino acids (leucine, valine, and isoleucine) from the splanchnic bed (liver and gut) to skeletal muscles, with the return of alanine to the liver and glutamine to the gut (Figure 3). Movement of these amino acids among tissues serves to maintain amino acid precursors for protein synthesis, assists in the elimination of nitrogen wastes, provides substrates for gluconeogenesis, maintains glutamine levels, and maintains the purine nucleotide cycle.

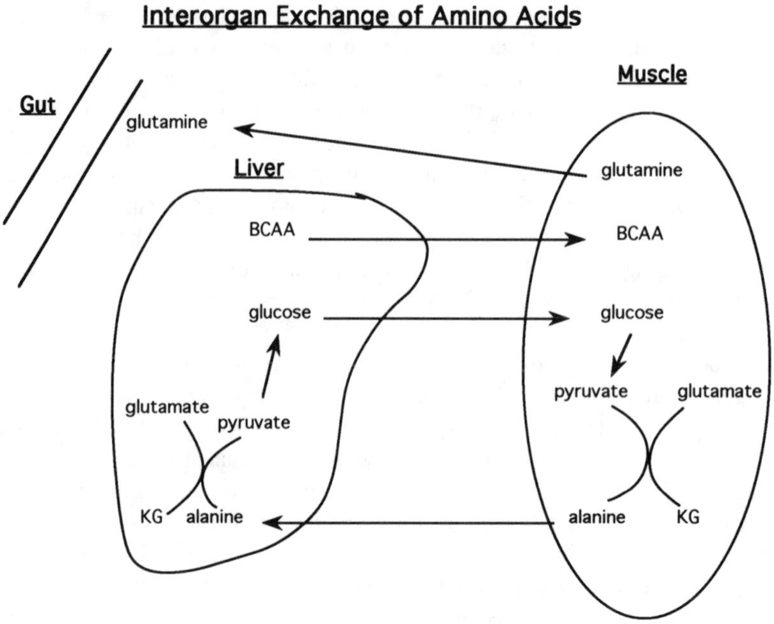

Interorgan Exchange of Amino Acids

FIGURE 3. Diagram indicates movement of substrates through the blood to specific organs. Abbreviations: BCAA, branched-chain amino acids; KG, alpha-ketoglutarate.

Felig et al.[30] provided early evidence about amino acid movement among tissues. By examining arterial–venous differences in substrate concentrations across tissues, they observed that skeletal muscle had net uptake of BCAA with release of alanine in amounts in excess of its content in muscle proteins. The alanine released by skeletal muscle was removed by the splanchnic bed. On the basis of these observations, these investigators proposed the existence of a glucose–alanine cycle for maintenance of blood glucose and the shuttling of nitrogen and gluconeogenic substrate from muscle to liver.

Ahlborg et al.[34] extended these findings to exercise conditions using six untrained adult males exercised at 30% of $\dot{V}O_2$ max on a bicycle ergometer. They examined arterial–venous differences across the splanchnic bed and across the leg during 4 h of cycling. They observed decreases in plasma glucose and insulin, and increases in glucagon and free fatty acids. Plasma glucose declined from a preexercise level of 90 mg/dl but stabilized at 60 mg/dl as release of glucose by the liver continued throughout the exercise period. Glucose remained an important fuel throughout exercise, but there was a significant increase in use of free fatty acids. There was also a significant increase in amino acid flux, including a fourfold increase in the release of branched-chain amino acids from the splanchnic area and a corresponding increase in the uptake by exercising muscles. In return, muscles released alanine, which was removed by the liver for gluconeogenesis. These data demonstrate a change in amino acid flux during exercise with movement of branched-chain amino acids from visceral tissues to skeletal muscles and the return of alanine as a precursor for hepatic synthesis of glucose.

Lemon and Mullin further established the relationship of amino acid metabolism to glucose homeostasis.[35] These investigators demonstrated a dramatic increase in sweat urea nitrogen in men previously depleted of glycogen stores and exercised for 1 h at 61% $\dot{V}O_2$ max. They did not find any change in urinary urea nitrogen. These investigators calculated that in carbohydrate-depleted individuals amino acid catabolism provided 10.4% of total energy for the exercise while in the carbohydrate-loaded group protein provided 4.4% of the energy needs. These results suggest that production of nitrogen wastes during exercise is related to carbohydrate status and that sweating may be an important mechanism for elimination of nitrogen wastes. Subsequent studies by Lemon and Nagle[36] and White and Brooks[37] also support the relationship of increased amino acid degradation with maintenance of hepatic glucose production.

Amino acid metabolism during exercise is similar to conditions observed during periods of food restriction or fasting. There is net release of amino acids from protein due to suppression of protein synthesis, with protein breakdown remaining approximately constant.[4,5,38] This change in protein turnover results in an increase in tissue levels of free amino acids and net release of amino acids from most tissues.[31] Tissues with high rates of protein turnover are most affected, with the liver and gastrointestinal tract incurring the largest losses during short-term fasts.[4,39] Skeletal muscle, which has lower rates of protein turnover, responds somewhat less dramatically, but because of its total mass, muscle is the predominate source of free amino acids during prolonged periods of food restriction.[4,5,31]

The primary site for degradation of most amino acids is the liver. The liver is unique because of its capacity to degrade amino acids and to synthesis urea for elimination of the amino nitrogen. Hepatic tissue contains high concentrations of the degradative enzymes, including the aminotransferases which remove the alpha-amino groups during the first step in amino acid degradation. The exceptions are the branched-chain amino acids (BCAA). The liver is very low in content of the branched-chain aminotransferase which results in the release of BCAA into circulation.[31,32]

Extrahepatic tissues, including kidney and skeletal muscle, contain branched-chain aminotransferase and are responsible for initiation of the degradative pathway. Among these tissues, skeletal muscle appears to be the predominate tissue for degradation of the BCAA.[32,40,41]

Degradation of the BCAA is initiated by the reversible transamination of the BCAA to the alpha-keto acid with transfer of the alpha-amino group to alpha-ketoglutarate, forming glutamate. This step appears to be nearly at equilibrium with little physiological control. The second and rate-limiting step is decarboxylation of the branched-chain keto acids by branched-chain keto acid dehydrogenase (BCKAD). BCKAD activity is highly regulated by phosphorylation and dephosphorylation to the inactive and active forms, respectively. This step is stimulated by increases in the concentration of the leucine keto acid, alpha-ketoiso-caproate (KIC). During periods of increased energy needs, such as starvation, trauma, and exercise, increased levels of BCAA stimulate BCKAD and the BCAA are degraded to energy within skeletal muscle. During absorptive periods when muscles are using glucose as a primary fuel, muscle transaminates the BCAA and releases the keto acids into circulation for complete oxidation by the liver or kidney.[32,40]

Within skeletal muscle, BCAA degradation involves transfer of the alpha-amino group to glutamate via transamination. Glutamate serves as an important intermediate in nitrogen metabolism.[31,33] While glutamate is formed *de novo* in skeletal muscle, there is no net release. Once the amino group is transferred to glutamate, there are two primary fates. The amino group can be transferred either to pyruvate in synthesis of alanine or onto oxaloacetate for the synthesis of aspartate. Alanine is released from muscle into circulation and is ultimately removed by the liver for gluconeogenesis. Aspartate is an important component of the purine nucleotide cycle which is central to maintaining the pool of ATP in muscle.[33] The purine nucleotide cycle serves to regenerate IMP and also produces fumarate and free ammonia (NH_3). The ammonia can be combined with glutamate in the epsilon position via glutamine synthetase to form glutamine. Glutamine is ultimately released from muscle, with the majority of glutamine being used by the gut as a primary energy source. Together, alanine and glutamine represent 60 to 80% of the amino acids released from skeletal muscle while they account for only 18% of the amino acids in muscle protein.[31,32] During exercise glutamine synthesis and glutamine levels in muscle decline due to inhibition of glutamine synthetase.

Amino acids have been shown to play important roles in energy homeostasis during periods of high energy need or low energy intake. While the qualitative role is becoming clear, the quantitative level of this role remains uncertain. Most of these studies have been designed using leucine and alanine as metabolic tracers. These studies establish changes in protein turnover, increases in amino acid flux, and increases in leucine oxidation. However, questions remain about the potential to generalize from these findings to other amino acids or to dietary protein requirements. Endurance exercise causes a reduction in muscle protein synthesis and net protein breakdown, but is there a real loss of amino acids; are there increases in urea production during exercise; are the effects unique to leucine or do they relate to other amino acids? These questions remain to be fully answered.

Using multiple isotopic tracers, Wolfe et al.[18,19] examined amino acid metabolism during aerobic exercise. They found inhibition of protein synthesis, increased leucine oxidation, and increased flux of alanine. These findings are consistent with most earlier reports. However, using direct isotopic measures, they failed to find any increase in urea synthesis. Further, using lysine, a second indispensable amino acid, they demonstrated that the inhibition of protein synthesis was less than half that estimated by leucine (17 vs. 48%) and that there was no increase in lysine oxidation. These data indicate that the exercise effect on leucine is not uniform for all amino acids and the failure to find any increase in urea synthesis suggests that the effect is unique to leucine. In a subsequent study, these investigators found that production of some acute-phase proteins occurs in the liver during endurance exercise.[42] Synthesis of these proteins, which are relatively low in leucine content, may provide a transient pool for other amino acids released by protein breakdown during exercise. The roles and fates of other indispensable amino acids, including valine and isoleucine, need to be investigated.

Leucine appears to be unique among amino acids in its role in protein synthesis[43,44] and its contributions to gluconeogenesis.[19] The effects of diet and exercise training on amino acid metabolism remain to be defined. We recently completed a series of studies designed to define dietary and exercise conditions which influence leucine oxidation. Previous studies have indicated that leucine oxidation is increased by high leucine intakes[45] and exhaustive exercise.[46,47] We examined the interrelationships of dietary protein and exercise training.

In Study 1, we examined the impact of dietary protein on leucine oxidation during aerobic exercise. Female rats were fed diets containing 8 or 23% protein by weight for 2 weeks. Animals were assigned to either sedentary or exercise groups. The exercise group received a single bout of exercise on a motor-driven treadmill at 24 m/min on a 10% incline for 40 min. Animals were used for *in vivo* measurements of leucine oxidation and *in vitro* measurements of branched-chain ketoacid dehydrogenase activity. Animals fed the high-protein diet oxidized 2.2 times more leucine than the animals fed the low-protein diet (Figure 4, groups LC vs. HC). This increase in leucine oxidation was also evident in an increase in the total amount of BCKAD in the liver but not in skeletal muscle (Figure 5).

Exercise increased leucine oxidation in animals fed either low- or high-protein diets (Figure 4). This increase in leucine oxidation was associated with increased levels of BCKAD in the active form in muscle and liver. The amount of BCKAD in the active form in muscle increased by more than 100% (Figure 6) while the liver activity increased approximately 40% (data not shown). As expected, the single bout of exercise had no effect on the total amount of the enzyme present in muscle or liver. In the combined treatment, the effects of protein and exercise were not found to be additive and exercise had minimal effect on the BCKAD enzyme or leucine oxidation in animals fed the high-protein diet. Thus, if the capacity for leucine oxidation is already high, then exercise appears to have a much smaller

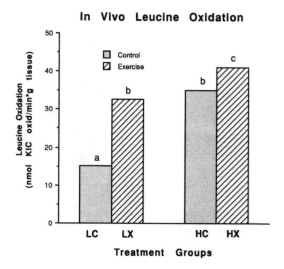

FIGURE 4. Effects of exercise and dietary protein on *in vivo* leucine oxidation determined as $^{14}CO_2$ expired from an intraperitoneal injection of 1-^{14}C-leucine. All animals were studied in a fasted condition and exercise groups were studied after 40 min of running on a motor-driven treadmill. Abbreviations: LC, low-protein control; LX, low-protein exercised; HC, high-protein control; HX, high-protein exercised; KIC, alpha-keto isocaproate. Letters above bars indicate statistical significance at $p < 0.05$. (Olken and Layman, unpublished data.)

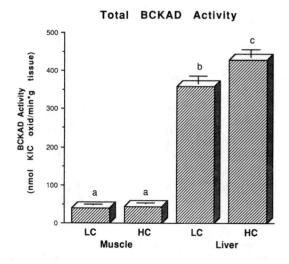

FIGURE 5. Dietary protein effects on total branched-chain keto acid dehydrogenase (BCKAD) activity in muscle and liver. BCKAD activity was determined from *in vitro* oxidation of 2-keto-[1-^{14}C]-isocaproate with collection of $^{14}CO_2$ after full activation of the enzyme complex with MgSO$_4$ and dichloroacetic acetic acid. Abbreviations: LC and HC, low- and high-protein diets, respectively. Letters above bars indicate statistical significance at $p < 0.05$. (Olken and Layman, unpublished data.)

effect on this catabolic pathway. These data suggest that the response of leucine oxidation to exercise is highly dependent on the dietary conditions and specifically the protein intake.

Study 2 was designed to determine the effects of prolonged training on leucine oxidation. We examined leucine metabolism after a bout of exercise in animals that were trained or not trained. Animals were trained for 20 weeks with exercise 5 d/week at 21 m/min for

Muscle BCKAD Activity

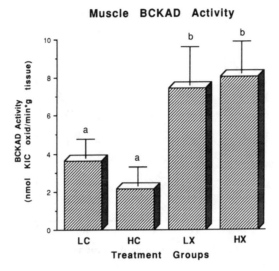

FIGURE 6. Exercise and dietary protein effects on BCKAD activity in skeletal muscle. Activities represent the amount of the BCKAD enzyme that is in the active form within the muscle. Activity was determined from *in vitro* oxidation of 2-keto-[1-^{14}C]-isocaproate with collection of $^{14}CO_2$. Abbreviations: LC, low-protein control; LX, low-protein exercised; HC, high-protein control; HX, high-protein exercised; KIC, alpha-keto isocaproate. Letters above bars indicate statistical significance at $p < 0.05$. (Olken and Layman, unpublished data.)

Effects of Training on Total BCKAD Activity

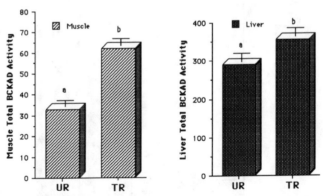

FIGURE 7. Effects of training on total branched-chain keto acid dehydrogenase (BCKAD) activity in the gastrocnemius muscle and liver. Values are expressed as nanomoles of alpha-ketoisocaproate oxidized per minute per gram tissue $\pm$ SEM. UR, not trained; TR, trained. Bars with different letters indicate groups are different at $p < 0.05$, $n = 12$. (Olken and Layman, unpublished data.)

60 min/d on a 10% incline. All animals were fed an adequate diet containing 15% protein. After 20 weeks of training, trained and nontrained control animals were examined either in a sedentary condition or after an exercise bout. Training increased the total amount of BCKAD in both the liver and skeletal muscle (Figure 7). While the capacity for oxidation of the BCAA increased, there was no increase in the rate of leucine oxidation in the trained animals at rest (Figure 8).

Leucine oxidation and the BCKAD responded similarly to results seen in Study 1 for nontrained animals. Specifically, the exercise bout stimulated leucine oxidation (53%) and increased the amount of BCKAD in the active form in the muscle (330%) and liver (211%).

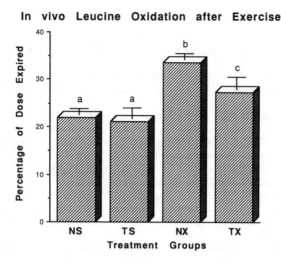

In vivo Leucine Oxidation after Exercise

FIGURE 8. Effects of exercise training on *in vivo* oxidation of 1-^{14}C-leucine at rest and immediately following an exercise bout. Values represent percentage of injected dose expired as $^{14}CO_2$. N, not trained; T, trained; S, not exercised; X, exercised. Bars with different letters indicate groups are different at $p < 0.05$. (Olken and Layman, unpublished data.)

However, in the trained animals the response to the exercise bout was much less. Leucine oxidation increased by 25% and there was no change in the activity of the muscle or liver BCKAD expressed per unit of tissue weight. These data indicate that training increases the enzymatic capacity for leucine oxidation but reduces the actual rate of oxidation at a specific exercise level. It will be important for future investigations to also compare trained and nontrained animals at the same relative workloads.

In total, these studies serve to define conditions for amino acid oxidation during exercise. The highest rates of leucine oxidation occurred in nontrained animals exposed to prolonged aerobic exercise and the response was further elevated if animals were consuming a low-protein diet.

V. SUMMARY

Exhaustive aerobic exercise produces a transient catabolic condition. There is net breakdown of protein due to inhibition of protein synthesis, with protein breakdown remaining constant or possibly increasing. The magnitude of this catabolic condition is dependent on the intensity and duration of exercise and results in release of amino acids from visceral tissues and skeletal muscle. This condition is transient, with recovery occurring from 4 to 8 h postexercise and driven by increases in protein synthesis.

Breakdown of proteins during exercise increases amino acid flux and oxidation of the BCAA, leucine. During exercise, leucine oxidation occurs predominantly in skeletal muscle. Catabolism of the BCAA in skeletal muscle requires elimination of an amino group which results in stimulation of alanine production. There is extensive release of alanine from exercising muscles, with the alanine being ultimately removed from circulation by the liver for gluconeogenesis and maintenance of blood glucose during endurance exercise.

Leucine appears to be unique as the only indispensable amino acids serving as an energy substrate for exercise. Evaluation of conditions for amino acid degradation suggests that leucine oxidation is highest during exhaustive exercise in subjects who are not trained. Training serves to reduce leucine oxidation at a specific workload. The effect of exercise on leucine oxidation is also higher under conditions of low dietary protein intake. Future investigations are needed to define the effects of exercise on other indispensable amino acids and define the diet and exercise conditions that enhance postexercise recovery.

REFERENCES

1. **Hood, D. A. and Terjung, R. L.,** Amino acid metabolism during exercise and following endurance training, *Sports Med.,* 9, 23, 1990.
2. **Goodman, M. N.,** Influence of aerobic exercise on fuel utilization by skeletal muscle, in *Nutrition and Aerobic Exercise,* Layman, D. K., Ed., ACS Symp. Ser. 294, American Chemical Society, Washington, D.C., 1986, 27.
3. **Committee on Diet and Health, Food and Nutrition Board,** *Diet and Health. Implications for Reducing Chronic Disease Risk,* National Academy of Science, National Academy Press, 1989.
4. **Waterlow, J. C., Garlick, P. J., and Millward, D. J.,** *Protein Turnover in Mammalian Tissues and in the Whole Body,* Elsevier/North Holland, New York, 1978.
5. **Young, V.,** The role of skeletal and cardiac muscle in the regulation of protein metabolism, in *Mammalian Protein Metabolism,* Munro, H. N., Ed., Academic Press, New York, 1970, 585.
6. **Meister, A.,** *Biochemistry of the Amino Acids,* Academic Press, New York, 1965.
7. **Morgan, H. E., Earl, D. C. N., Broadus, A., Wolpert, E. B., Giger, K. E., and Jefferson, L. S.,** Regulation of protein synthesis in heart muscle. I. Effect of amino acid levels on protein synthesis, *J. Biol. Chem.,* 246, 2152, 1971.
8. **Christensen, H. N.,** Role of amino acid transport and counter transport in nutrition and metabolism, *Physiol. Rev.,* 70, 43, 1990.
9. **Wolfe, R. R.,** in *Tracers in Metabolic Research,* Alan R. Liss, New York, 1984, 151.
10. **Rennie, M. J., Edwards, R. N. T., Krywawych, S., Davies, C. T. M., Halliday, D., Waterlow, J. C., and Millward, D. J.,** Effect of exercise on protein turnover in man, *Clin. Sci.,* 61, 627, 1981.
11. **Goldberg, A. L.,** Work-induced growth of skeletal muscle in normal and hypophysectomized rats, *Am. J. Physiol.,* 213, 1193, 1967.
12. **Goldberg, A. L.,** Biochemical events during hypertrophy of skeletal muscle, in *Cardiac Hypertrophy,* Alpert, N. R., Ed., Academic Press, New York, 1971, 301.
13. **Goldspink, D. F.,** The influence of passive stretch on the growth and protein turnover of the denervated extensor digitorium longus muscle, *Biochem. J.,* 174, 595, 1978.
14. **Laurent, G. J., Sparrow, M. P., and Millward, D. J.,** Muscle protein turnover in the adult fowl. II. Changes in rates of protein synthesis and breakdown during hypertrophy of the anterior and posterior latissimus dorsi muscle, *Biochem. J.,* 176, 407, 1978.
15. **Wong, T. S. and Booth, F. W.,** Protein metabolism in rat tibialis anterior muscle after stimulated chronic eccentric exercise, *J. Appl. Physiol.,* 69, 1718, 1990.
16. **Dohm, G. L., Hecker, A. L., Brown, W. E., Klain, G. J., Puente, F. R., Askew, E. W., and Beecher, G. R.,** Adaptation of protein metabolism to endurance training, *Biochem. J.,* 164, 705, 1977.
17. **Dohm, G. L., Tapscott, E. B., Barakat, H. A., and Kasperek, G. J.,** Measurement of in vivo protein synthesis in rats during an exercise bout, *Biochem. Med.,* 27, 367, 1982.
18. **Wolfe, R. R., Goodenough, R. D., Wolfe, M. H., Royle, G. T., and Nadel, E. R.,** Isotopic analysis of leucine and urea metabolism in exercising humans, *J. Appl. Physiol.,* 52, 458, 1982.
19. **Wolfe, R. R., Wolfe, M. H., Nadel, E. R., and Shaw, J. H. F.,** Isotopic determination of amino acid-urea interactions in exercise in humans, *J. Appl. Physiol.,* 56, 221, 1984.
20. **Dohm, G. L., Williams, R. T., Kasperek, G. J., and van Rij, A. M.,** Increased excretion of urea and N^T-methylhistidine by rats and humans after a bout of exercise, *J. Appl. Physiol.,* 52, 27, 1982.
21. **Bylund-Fellenius, A., Ojamaa, K. M., Flaim, K. E., Li, J. B., Wassner, S. J., and Jefferson, L. S.,** Protein synthesis versus energy state in contracting muscles of perfused rat hindlimb, *Am. J. Physiol.,* 246, E297, 1984.
22. **Devlin, J. T., Brodsky, I., Scrimgeour, A., Fuller, S., and Bier, D. M.,** Amino acid metabolism after intense exercise, *Am. J. Physiol.,* 258, E249, 1990.
23. **Goldberg, A. L., Jablecki, C., and Li, J. B.,** Effects of use and disuse on amino acid transport and protein turnover in muscle, *Ann. N.Y. Acad. Sci.,* 228, 190, 1974.
24. **Tischler, M. E., Desautels, M., and Goldberg, A. L.,** Does leucine, leucyl-tRNA, or some metabolite of leucine regulate protein synthesis and degradation in skeletal and cardiac muscle, *J. Biol. Chem.,* 257, 1613, 1982.
25. **Hirsch, C. A., Cox, M. A., van Vemrooij, W. J. W., and Henshaw, E. C.,** The ribosome cycle in mammalian protein synthesis. I. Association of the native smaller ribosomal subunit with protein factors, *J. Biol. Chem.,* 248, 4377, 1973.
26. **Rannels, D. E., Pegg, A. E., Rannels, S. R., and Jefferson, L. S.,** Effect of starvation on initiation of protein synthesis in skeletal muscle and heart, *Am. J. Physiol.,* 235, E126, 1978.
27. **Kelly, F. J. and Jefferson, L. S.,** Control of peptide-chain initiation in rat skeletal muscle. Development of methods for preparation of native ribosomal subunits and analysis of the effect of insulin on formation of 40 S initiation complexes, *J. Biol. Chem.,* 260, 6677, 1985.

28. **Scorsone, K. A., Panniers, R., Rowlands, A. G., and Henshaw, E. C.**, Phosphorylation of eukaryotic initiation factor 2 during physiological stresses which affect protein synthesis, *J. Biol. Chem.*, 262, 14538, 1987.

29. **Sarre, T. F.**, The phosphorylation of eukaryotic initiation factor 2: a principle of translational control in mammalian cells, *Biosystems*, 22, 311, 1989.

30. **Felig, Pozefsky, T., Marliss, E., and Cahill, G. F., Jr.**, Alanine: key role in gluconeogenesis, *Science*, 167, 1003, 1970.

31. **Ruderman, N. M.**, Muscle amino acid metabolism and gluconeogenesis, *Annu. Rev. Med.*, 26, 245, 1975.

32. **Harper, A. E., Miller, R. H., and Block, K. P.**, Branched-chain amino acid metabolism, *Annu. Rev. Nutr.*, 4, 409, 1984.

33. **Hood, D. A. and Terjung, R. L.**, Amino acid metabolism during exercise and following endurance training, *Sports Med.*, 9, 23, 1990.

34. **Ahlborg, G., Felig, P., Hagenfeldt, L., Hendler, R., and Wahren, J.**, Substrate turnover during prolonged exercise in man, *J. Clin. Invest.*, 53, 1080, 1974.

35. **Lemon, P. W. R. and Mullin, J. P.**, Effect of initial muscle glycogen levels on protein catabolism during exercise, *J. Appl. Physiol.*, 48, 624, 1980.

36. **Lemon, P. W. R. and Nagle, F. J.**, Effects of exercise on protein and amino acid metabolism, *Med. Sci. Sports Exercise*, 13, 141, 1981.

37. **White, T. P. and Brooks, G. A.**, U^{14}-C glucose, -alanine, and -leucine oxidation in rats at rest and two intensities of running, *Am. J. Physiol.*, 240, E155, 1981.

38. **Hong, S.-O. and Layman, D. K.**, Effects of leucine on in vitro protein synthesis and degradation in rat skeletal muscles, *J. Nutr.*, 114, 1204, 1984.

39. **Addis, T., Poo, L. J., and Lew, W.**, The quantities of protein lost by the various organs and tissues of the body during a fast, *J. Biol. Chem.*, 115, 111, 1936.

40. **Adibi, S. A.**, Metabolism of branched-chained amino acids in altered nutrition, *Metabolism*, 25, 1287, 1976.

41. **Hutson, S. M., Cree, T. C., and Harper, A. E.**, Regulation of leucine and alpha-ketoisocaproate metabolism in skeletal muscle, *J. Biol. Chem.*, 253, 8126, 1978.

42. **Carraro, F., Hartt, W. H., Stuart, C. A., Layman, D. K., Jahoor, F., and Wolfe, R. R.**, Whole body and plasma protein synthesis in exercise and recovery in human subjects, *Am. J. Physiol.*, 258, E821, 1990.

43. **Garlick, P. J. and Grant, J.**, Amino acid infusion increased the sensitivity of muscle protein synthesis in vivo to insulin, *Biochem. J.*, 254, 579, 1988.

44. **Wibert, G. J., Layman, D. K., and Hong, S.-O.**, An in vivo examination of the effects of leucine on skeletal muscle protein synthesis in the fasting rat, *Nutr. Res.*, 11, 1155, 1991.

45. **Harper, A. E. and Benjamin, E.**, Relationship between intake and rate of oxidation of leucine and α-ketoisocaproate in vivo in the rat, *J. Nutr.*, 114, 431, 1984.

46. **Henderson, S. A., Black, A. L., and Brooks, G. A.**, Leucine turnover and oxidation in trained rats during exercise, *Am. J. Physiol.*, 249, E137, 1985.

47. **Hood, D. A. and Terjung, R. L.**, Effect of endurance training on leucine metabolism in perfused rat skeletal muscle, *Am. J. Physiol.*, 253, E648, 1987.

Chapter 7

ENERGY METABOLISM IN EXERCISE AND TRAINING

David R. Bassett, Jr.
Francis J. Nagle

CONTENTS

0-8493-7911-3/94/$0.00+$.50
© 1994 by CRC Press, Inc.

I. INTRODUCTION

Over 200 years ago, Lavoisier demonstrated the similarity of combustion outside the body to the process of metabolism occurring within the body. Von Mayer's contribution to our knowledge, formulated in 1845, became known as the "law of conservation of energy", which was finally validated in 1893 with Rubner's classical experiments. In the past 50 years, the oxidative processes by which energy is transferred from foodstuffs to high-energy phosphate compounds have been elucidated. These are but a few highlights of the remarkable history of energy metabolism. The reader is referred to Asmussen's historical survey[1] for further details.

In this chapter, we propose to review some basic tenets of energy metabolism to provide the reader with baseline information for the subsequent discussion of energy metabolism in exercise. Under exercise metabolism, the range of man's adaptation will be treated, including the topic of economy in meeting the demands of physical effort. We will go on to address some of the more subtle influences of chronic exercise training relating to its effects on substrate use, resting metabolic rate, and body composition.

II. REST STATE AND DAILY ENERGY BALANCE
A. Measuring Metabolism

Energy expenditure may be assessed by direct calorimetry, a measurement of heat dissipated from the body over time, or by indirect calorimetry, which requires the measurement of the physiological gases, oxygen and carbon dioxide, over a fixed time period. In the latter method, energy expended is estimated from the quantity of oxygen used to metabolize substrate and form high-energy phosphate (adenosine triphosphate and creatine phosphate). The energy equivalent of 1.0 liter of oxygen is 20.2 kJ (4.8 kcal). While this does not represent a precise determination of the energy equivalent for humans deriving energy from a mixed diet of foodstuffs, the error of measurement does not exceed 5%. More precision can be attained with the additional assessment of protein utilization. Since direct calorimetry continues to require expensive and sophisticated equipment, indirect calorimetry remains the popular choice for metabolic measurements.

B. Basal Metabolism

This is defined as a minimal rate of energy expenditure compatible with life.[2] It is measured under standardized rest conditions, i.e., after at least 8 h of complete rest, 12 to 18 h in a postabsorptive state and in quiet, comfortable surroundings. While a basal metabolism assessment may have clinical or other special applications, a measurement of rest metabolism, 3 to 4 h postabsorptive, serves most purposes as well, and often does not differ significantly from a basal assessment.[2]

C. Units Expressing Energy Metabolism

Using either direct or indirect calorimetry for assessing human metabolism, energy is measured over time and thus is an expression of human power (energy/time). Table 1, adapted from Durnin and Passmore,[2] shows rest metabolism data for groups of men and women expressed with a variety of units.

It is well known that heat is continually lost from the skin surface and that smaller bodies have a larger surface relative to weight. For this reason, it is conventional to express rest metabolic rate per unit of surface area. Durnin and Passmore[2] make the point that the surface area "law" is a useful generalization, but it does not explain differences in metabolism among members of the same species. For example, Table 1 shows that women have a lower rest metabolic rate than men per unit of surface area (115 vs. 141 ml $\times$ min^{-1} $\times$ m^{-2}).

This might suggest, among other things, inherent differences in the energetics of the tissues. However, when differences in fat weight for men and women are accounted for,

TABLE 1 Physical and Metabolic Data Relative to the Metabolic State in Man

	Women	Men
No. of subjects	25	24
Weight (kg)	58.2	68.5
	(42.4–70.5)	(53.1–8.3)
Height (cm)	165	176
	(156–179)	(168–190)
Body fat (%)	25.6	10.7
	(18.4–34.8)	(4.5–26.)
LBM	43.1	61.1
	(37.8–55.3)	(44.8–74.6)
Resting O_2 consumption		
(ml/min)	186	258
	(148–225)	(188–326)
(ml/min/m²)	115	141
(ml/min/kg LBM)	4.31	4.22
(ml/min/kg body weight)	3.20	3.77
(J/min/kg body weight)	67.2	79.2

Note: Observe that when resting O_2 consumption is expressed per square meter (m²) of surface area, the difference between men and women is large, 141 vs. 115 ml $\times$ kg^{-1} $\times$ m^{-1}, respectively. However, expressed in ml $\times$ kg^{-1} lean body mass (LBM), this difference is minimal, 4.22 vs. 4.31 ml $\times$ min^{-1} $\times$ kg^{-1} LBM, respectively. Note also expression of resting metabolism in ml $\times$ min^{-1} $\times$ kg^{-1} body weight is generally assumed to be 3.5 ml $\times$ min^{-1} $\times$ kg^{-1} irrespective of sex.

Adapted from Durnin and Passmore.[2]

with metabolism expressed per kilogram of lean body mass (LBM), the metabolic costs are nearly equal, 4.22 and 4.31 ml O_2 $\times$ min^{-1} $\times$ kg LBM^{-1}, respectively (Table 1). This is attributed to the fact that fat is less active metabolically than muscle and other tissues.

In Table 1, rest metabolism is also expressed per kilogram body weight and is reported as 3.77 and 3.20 ml O_2 $\times$ kg^{-1} $\times$ min^{-1} for men and women, respectively. The expression of metabolism per kilogram body weight has common use in the exercise literature. In non-weight-supported activities such as level walking and running, body weight constitutes the exercise load. As a general approximation for males and females, the American College of Sports Medicine[3] recommends the use of 3.5 ml O_2 $\times$ kg^{-1} body weight $\times$ min^{-1} as the rate of O_2 consumption of a resting individual. This value is defined as 1.0 MET. Exercise energy demands are then expressed as multiples of this baseline value. For example, an exercise energy demand of 35.0 ml O_2 $\times$ kg^{-1} $\times$ min^{-1} is equivalent to 10.0 METS.

D. Energy Input

It is apparent from Table 2 that energy input is closely related to body size, sex, and age.[4] Climate could be a factor, although this is largely controlled in modern societies.[5] After attaining peaks in the teenage years, energy intake declines at a rate of 2% per decade.[5] These estimates of energy intake are, of course, consistent with those of energy utilized per day.[6] From an analysis of the U.S. National Health Survey statistics, Bray[7] has reported that carbohydrate contributes 40 to 45%, fat 37 to 40%, protein 15%, and alcohol 3 to 5% of the total energy consumed per day. While numerous body tissues may utilize carbohydrate, fat, and protein, alcohol metabolism appears to be limited to the liver.[5]

TABLE 2 Median Energy Intake per Day (kJ) by Age, Sex, and Race

Age (years)	Male		Female	
	Whites	Blacks	Whites	Blacks
1.0	5,384	4,814	4,880	4,964
2–3	6,317	5,792	5,628	5,712
4–5	7,228	6,917	6,502	6,695
6–7	8,497	7,430	7,493	7,106
8–9	8,807	7,993	7,699	6,909
10–11	9,156	7,883	7,917	7,753
12–14	10,252	8,887	7,804	7,270
15–17	12,138	9,706	6,867	6,724
18–19	12,226	10,424	6,724	6,292
20–24	11,726	9,190	6,636	6,800
25–34	10,882	11,164	6,548	5,678
35–44	10,261	9,005	6,350	5,561
45–54	9,425	8,102	6,153	4,948
55–64	8,350	6,859	5,590	4,855
>65	7,216	6,044	5,267	4,637

Adapted from Bray.[5]

III. EXERCISE ENERGY EXPENDITURE
A. Requirements of Common Activities

Walking on level ground at 54.0 m $\times$ min^{-1} (2.0 mph) doubles the metabolic rate (2.0 METS), and walking at 80 m $\times$ min^{-1} (3.0 mph) increases the rest metabolic rate by three times (3.0 METS). Figure 1 shows energy requirements for level grade walking and running. Energy requirements are shown only to the approximate limit of man's aerobic power, i.e., 80.0 ml O_2 $\times$ kg^{-1} $\times$ min^{-1} (1.68 kJ $\times$ kg^{-1} $\times$ min^{-1}) attained in running. These data are readily predicted from formulae established through empirical measurements of oxygen uptake ($\dot{V}O_2$) during physical activity.[3]

For level walking — $\dot{V}O_2$ (ml $\times$ kg^{-1} $\times$ min^{-1}) = speed (m $\times$ min^{-1}) $\times$ 0.1 ml $\times$ kg m^{-1} + (3.5 ml $\times$ kg^{-1} $\times$ min^{-1}), where 0.1 ml $\times$ kg m^{-1} = increase in cost/kg body weight/m distance traversed, and 3.5 ml $\times$ kg^{-1} $\times$ min^{-1} = assumed resting metabolic rate (1.0 MET).

For gradient walking add — $\dot{V}O_2$ (ml $\times$ kg^{-1} $\times$ min^{-1}) = speed (m $\times$ min^{-1}) $\times$ % gradient $\times$ 1.8 ml $\times$ kg m^{-1}, where 1.8 ml $\times$ kg m^{-1} = the increase in energy required to move 1.0 kg 1.0 m vertically.

For level running — $\dot{V}O_2$ (ml $\times$ kg^{-1} $\times$ min^{-1}) = speed (m $\times$ min^{-1}) $\times$ 0.2 ml $\times$ kg m^{-1} + (3.5 ml $\times$ kg^{-1} $\times$ min^{-1}), where 0.2 m $\times$ kg m^{-1} = increase in cost/kg body weight/m distance traversed.

For gradient running add — $\dot{V}O_2$ (ml $\times$ kg^{-1} $\times$ min^{-1}) = Speed (m $\times$ min^{-1}) $\times$ % gradient $\times$ 1.0 ml $\times$ kg m^{-1}, where 1.0 ml $\times$ kg m^{-1} = increase in energy required to move 1.0 kg body weight 1.0 m vertically.

The constant 1.8 ml O_2 $\times$ kg m^{-1} is applicable to gradient walking and doing vertical work in stepping.[3] Why this constant does not apply in running on a gradient has not been determined. A number of investigators have shown that there are no differences in energy requirements between overground and treadmill level or grade walking and running.[8-10] Overground, wind resistance must be considered, however, as an additional energy cost.[11]

For cycle ergometry — $\dot{V}O_2$ (ml $\times$ min^{-1}) = power output (kg m $\times$ min^{-1}) $\times$ 2.0 ml $\times$ kg m^{-1} + (3.5 ml $\times$ kg^{-1} $\times$ min^{-1} $\times$ kg body weight).

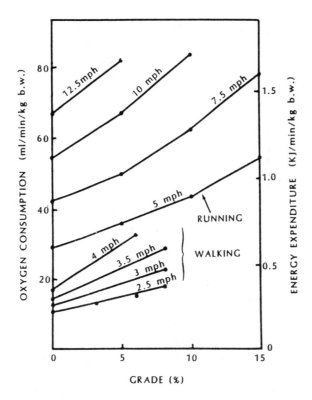

FIGURE 1. Energy costs for walking and running on a treadmill at various speeds and grades. (Adapted from Fletcher, J. B., in *Bioastronautics Data Book*, NASA-SP-3006, Webb, P., Ed., Webb Associates, Yellow Springs, OH, 1964. With permission.)

The above formula can be used to predict the energy cost of pedaling a cycle ergometer for power outputs between 300 and 1200 kg m/min. Since cycling is not a weight-bearing activity, the energy cost is practically independent of body weight. At the same power requirement, two individuals of different body weight would have almost the same absolute $\dot{V}O_2$ (ml $\times$ min^{-1}). However, in proportion to body weight the lighter individual would have a greater relative $\dot{V}O_2$ (ml $\times$ kg^{-1} $\times$ min^{-1}).

B. Walking and Running Economy

Montoye et al.[12] have shown that the treadmill formula for estimating energy requirements in walking underestimates energy costs for teenagers under 17 to 18 years of age. The widest differences were observed for the youngest group (age 10 to 11 years). The same phenomenon has been observed in running.[13,14] Daniels and Oldridge[14] and Daniels et al.[13] observed a difference of 22% in the energy cost of running at 200 m/min for males between 10 and 18 years of age. They also reported that both growth and training contributed to the reduction in the $\dot{V}O_2$ requirement as the 18th year of age was approached. Davies[15] found that when weight was added to child runners their efficiency improved. He concluded that due to their light weight they were unable to transfer energy in the horizontal plane.

Conley and Krahenbuhl[16] showed that greater economy in run energy expenditure occurs in trained runners. Data from the study shown in Figure 2 show that trained runners performed with a 20% greater economy than other nontrained adults. Daniels et al.[17] observed that the greater economy demonstrated in trained runners did not carry over to other activities, e.g., cycling, stepping, walking, and arm cranking. There is evidence that the greater economy

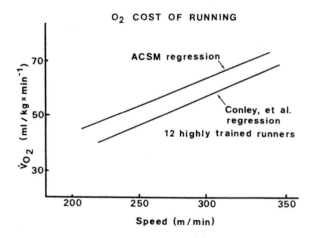

FIGURE 2. A comparison of O_2 cost in running, ACSM, regression represents predicted O_2 cost for normal adult humans. Conley and Krahenbuhl regression represents measured O_2 costs for highly trained runners at various running speeds. Figure demonstrates greater economy of trained runners. (From Conley, D. L. and Krahenbuhl, G. S., *Med. Sci. Sports Exercise,* 12, 357, 1980. With permission.)

in running is attributable, in part, to the proportions of energy used in vertical and horizontal displacement of the body.[18] The greater economy with training has been observed in both men and women.[17]

In sum, energy prediction formulae have broad application in populations of male and female adults. However, the walk and run formulae underestimate energy requirements of young people up to 18 years of age. Furthermore, the run formulae overestimates the energy requirements for many trained runners.

C. Human Limits for Energy Expenditure

Figure 3 shows that healthy men are capable of a maximal power output of 210 kJ $\times$ min^{-1} for a period of 6 s.[19] This is energy equivalent to more than 10.0 liters of oxygen per minute. The figure shows that power output decreases exponentially with time to a point where power can be maintained with small decrements at 50.0 to 75.0 kJ/min (2.5 to 3.5 liters of oxygen per minute). Runs for 24 h—covering 160 miles at an average energy expenditure of 50.0 kJ $\times$ min^{-1}—have been documented.[20] The longest endurance run reported was one of 141 h, during which 623 miles were covered at an average energy expenditure of 42 kJ $\times$ min^{-1}. The range of man's adaptive capacity is extensive.

The way in which total energy needs are met for maximal efforts of varying durations is depicted in Table 3.[21] With maximal efforts of 10 s to 10 min, anaerobic metabolism plays a very important role in meeting the energy need. The anaerobic contribution includes the use of stored adenosine triphosphate (ATP) and creatine phosphate (CrP), which together generate approximately 40.0 kJ;[21] only ATP is used directly for energy by muscle. Glycolysis, the chemical process by which carbohydrate (CHO) is degraded without a need for oxygen, yields a relatively small amount of ATP (3 vs. 39 mol from aerobic CHO metabolism) and produces lactic acid. Beyond these sources of high-energy phosphate (ATP, CrP), active muscles must turn to aerobic metabolism for their energy. The time dependence in generating ATP through anaerobic glycolysis and aerobic oxidation highlights the importance of stored high-energy phosphates in meeting energy needs in short-term maximal efforts (<2.0 min). It is at least 1 min into exercise before maximal activity of glycolysis occurs and it is 2 to 3 min before maximal aerobic metabolism is attained.[22]

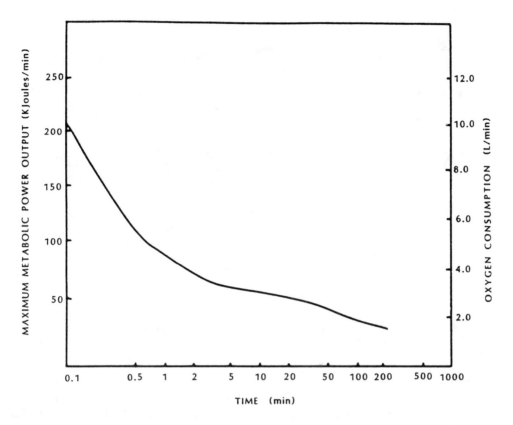

FIGURE 3. Semilog plot of maximum metabolic power output vs. time. (Adapted from Fletcher, J. B., in *Bioastronautics Data Book,* NASA-SP-3006, Webb, P., Ed., Webb Associates, Yellow Springs, OH, 1964. With permission.)

TABLE 3 The Anaerobic and Aerobic Contribution to Total Energy Needs in Maximal Performances of Various Durations

Process	10 s	1 min	2 min	4 min	10 min	30 min	60 min	120 min
Anaerobic								
kJ	100	170	200	200	150	125	80	65
kcal	25	40	45	45	35	30	20	15
%	85	65–70	50	30	10–15	5	2	1
Aerobic								
kJ	20	80	200	420	1,000	3,000	5,500	10,000
kcal	5	20	45	100	250	700	1,300	2,400
%	15	30–35	50	70	85–90	95	98	99
Total								
kJ	120	250	400	620	1,150	3,125	5,580	10,065
kcal	30	60	90	145	285	730	1,320	2,415

Note: Energy needs are expressed in kilojoules and kilocalories for the performance duration indicated. Percent contribution of anaerobic energy sources are also shown.

From Åstrand, P.-O. and Rodahl, K., Eds., *Textbook of Work Physiology,* 3rd ed., McGraw-Hill, New York, 1986, 325. With permission.

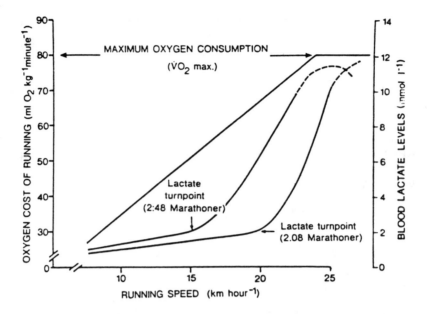

FIGURE 4. The relationship of speed in running to O_2 cost and blood lactate levels for two marathon runners with widely different performance times, i.e., states of training. Figure shows running speeds at which lactate in blood begins to accumulate for the two performers. (From Noakes, T., Ed., *Lore of Running*, Oxford University Press, Capetown, 1986. With permission.)

Given maximal aerobic power ($\dot{V}O_2$ max) of 3.0 to 4.0 $l \times min^{-1}$, a 10-s maximal effort (Figure 3) requires energy equivalent to 2.5 to 3.0 times $\dot{V}O_2$ max. Karlson and Saltin[23] reported that trained individuals who performed a cycling effort at 130% $\dot{V}O_2$ max could continue for 2 min (50% anaerobic), an effort at 100% $\dot{V}O_2$ max could be continued for 7 min (15 to 30% anaerobic), and effort at 90% $\dot{V}O_2$ max for 16 min (5 to 15% anaerobic) before exhaustion ensued. That the exact duration of maximal effort will vary with the state of training and the mode of exercise is indicated by the observation that elite 10,000-m runners perform at 90% $\dot{V}O_2$ max for a 28- to 30-min period.[24]

The wide differences in the ability of humans to sustain maximal exercise efforts in the time frame of 4.0 to 60 and even 120 min are related to two factors. These are (1) the magnitude of an individual's $\dot{V}O_2$ max and (2) the percent $\dot{V}O_2$ max at which lactic acid accumulates in muscle (onset of blood lactate accumulation [OBLA]).[25-27] Better aerobic performers have higher $\dot{V}O_2$ max values and a higher threshold at which lactic acid begins to accumulate. Pollock[28] found $\dot{V}O_2$ max values as high as 84.4 ml $\times$ kg^{-1} $\times$ min^{-1} in elite middle-long distance runners, consistent with values reported by Robinson et al.[29] and Saltin and Astrand.[30] Figure 4 shows $\dot{V}O_2$ and lactate values vs. speed in running.[31] Typical lactate curves highlighting OBLA differences for marathon runners capable of widely differing performances are indicated.

Lactic acid is known to induce an acidotic state with undesirable effects on the homeostasis.[32] Lactic acid production increases with physical effort and accumulates in active muscle and blood at exercise intensities demanding 60 to 75% $\dot{V}O_2$ max. Given an aerobically trained and an untrained individual of the same size, exercising at the same percent $\dot{V}O_2$ max, the untrained would accumulate more lactic acid in muscles and blood. A greater difference would be observed if they exercise at the same absolute O_2 requirement. There is controversy as to whether this training effect is due to decreased lactate production or increased removal. In support of decreased production, researchers have found a lesser lactate accumulation in isolated muscles of trained vs. control animals,[33] and a smaller

TABLE 4 Sources of Substrate Stores in Humans (70 kg body weight)

Fuel	Weight	Energy (kJ)
Circulating fuels		
Glucose (extracellular H_2O)	0.020	336
Free fatty acids (plasma)	0.0004	17
Triglycerides (plasma)	0.004	168
Total		521
Tissue stores		
Fat		
Adipose tissue triglycerides	15.0	588,000
Intramuscular	0.3	11,760
Protein (mainly muscle)	10.0	172,000
Glycogen		
Liver	0.085	1,470
Muscle	0.350	6,090
Total		779,320

Note: Weight of carbohydrate, fat, and protein stores are indicated, as well as the energy in the kilojoules represented by these substrate stores.

From Wahren, J., *Endocrinology*, DeGroot, L. J., Ed., Grune & Stratton, New York, 1979. With permission.

arteriovenous lactate difference after training in humans.[34] However, other investigators suggest that training may result in an increased ability to clear lactate via the liver and other metabolically active tissues.[35-37]

IV. SUBSTRATE UTILIZATION IN EXERCISE

A. Energy Storage

The healthy human in a normal nutritional state derives rest energy needs from carbohydrate, lipids, and protein.[6] The respiratory quotient (ratio of CO_2 produced to O_2 consumed) of 0.82 to 0.85 reflects the mixed diet sources of energy. Table 4 shows the available substrate from which these energy needs are drawn while in the postabsorptive state.[38] Observe that carbohydrate sources stored in muscle, liver, and in extracellular space, total approximately 7900 kJ. Lipids are stored in adipose tissue and muscle, with a negligible amount in extracellular water. Stored energy as lipids (adipose tissue and muscle) amounts to nearly 600,000 kJ. Assuming all body protein as an energy source, some 172,000 kJ could be derived. It is estimated that only 3% of body protein is normally available for energy turnover at any time.[39] This would reduce the readily available protein source to 5000 kJ.

B. Factors Influencing Substrate Use

Four factors have been identified which influence substrate use in exercise. The first of these is the health state. It is well known that a variety of metabolic diseases, e.g., diabetes mellitus, McArdle's syndrome, and Cushing's disease result in a derangement in substrate used for energy. The second factor is the diet, the third, exercise intensity and duration, and the fourth is the training state.

1. Diet

The profound effect of diet on substrate use has been known since the classical experiments of Christensen and Hanson in 1939.[40] Using the respiratory quotient (RQ) during cycling

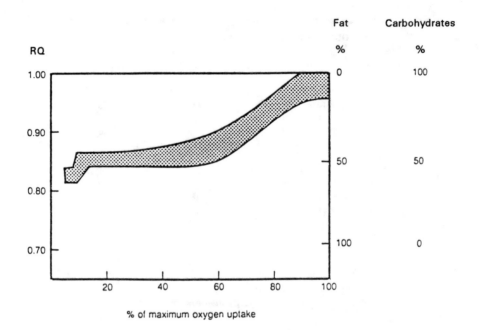

FIGURE 5. The relationship of the respiratory quotient (RQ) to relative intensity of effort in cycling, expressed as percent of maximal O_2 uptake ($\dot{V}O_2$ max). Duration of effort is assumed to be the same for all intensities. As intensity of effort increases, the RQ approaching 1.0 indicates greater use of carbohydrate as metabolic substrate. (From Astrand, P. O. and Rohdahl, K., Eds., *Textbook of Work Physiology,* McGraw-Hill, New York, 1986, 325. With permission.)

exercise as the measure of substrate use, they showed that, when available, carbohydrate was the preferred substrate. Furthermore, the duration of effort was dependent on available carbohydrate. Radioisotope studies have confirmed these findings,[41] as have muscle biopsy assessments of energy stores before and after exercise.[42,43]

2. Exercise Intensity and Duration

Figure 5 shows the nonprotein RQ response to dynamic exercise, such as cycling or running, as exercise intensity is increased.[44] Exercise intensity is expressed as the percentage of $\dot{V}O_2$ max. An RQ of 0.7 indicates lipids as the sole source of energy, and an RQ of 1.0 indicates carbohydrate as the sole source. Since exercise at 100% $\dot{V}O_2$ max can be tolerated for approximately 7 to 15 min,[23] depending on training state, this duration must be assumed at all exercise intensities indicated in Figure 5. It is evident that RQ increases with increasing intensity and approximates 1.0 at 100% $\dot{V}O_2$ max. At intensities exceeding 60 to 70% $\dot{V}O_2$ max, there is a progressively greater dependence on carbohydrate for substrate; glycolysis is accelerated and greater use is made of muscle stores of glycogen. The carbohydrate dependence is also indicated by increased lactate levels in muscle and blood as an exercise effort exceeds 60 to 70% $\dot{V}O_2$ max.[31]

While the rate with which muscle glycogen is used increases progressively with exercise intensity, only in exercise at 70 to 80% $\dot{V}O_2$ max, continued to exhaustion over 90 min (requiring trained performers), it is approaching total depletion (Figure 6).[45] Only under these circumstances can glycogen depletion be invoked as the cause for limiting exercise duration. At higher exercise intensities the absolute level of glycogen depletion is less, so that exhaustion must be attributed to another cause (Figure 6).

Long-duration exercise (>90 to 240 min) is marked by an apparent sparing of the smaller carbohydrate stores and greater dependence on lipids. In the first hour of exercise, mobil-

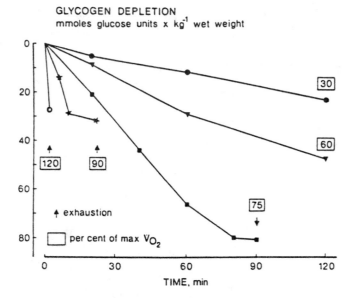

GLYCOGEN DEPLETION
mmoles glucose units x kg^{-1} wet weight

FIGURE 6. The relationship of muscle glycogen to the duration of effort in two-leg cycling to exhaustion at 30, 60, 75, 90, and 120% of $\dot{V}O_2$ max. Quadriceps muscle biopsy samples were taken for glycogen assays at points in time indicated on graph. Only with effort at 75% $\dot{V}O_2$ max is glycogen severely depleted. (From Saltin, B. and Karlsson, J., in *Muscle Metabolism During Exercise*, Pernow, B. and Saltin, B., Eds., Plenum Press, New York, 1971, 289. With permission.)

ization of lipid stores from adipose tissue occurs and this is accompanied by increasing release of glucose from the liver.[38] This occurs as circulating lipolytic hormones, i.e., glucagon, catecholamines, and growth hormone are increased. The adaptations are such that even after 3 h of marathon running circulating glucose levels may remain close to normal.[46]

When glycogen stores are limited, protein may contribute a significant amount to the total energy calories during exercise. Lemon and Mullin[47] reported that protein degradation accounted for 13.7 g/h (10.4%) of the total caloric cost in a cycling effort at 61% $\dot{V}O_2$ max over 1 h, when subjects were in a glycogen-depleted state. In the glycogen-loaded state the contribution was 5.8 g/h (4.4%) of the total cost. In these experiments sweat urea nitrogen and urinary nitrogen, products of protein degradation, were measured. When only urinary nitrogen was measured as the protein marker, Refsum et al.[48] estimated protein breakdown at 2.5 g/h during a 70- to 90-km cross-country ski race. Decombaz et al.[49] found a 44% increase in urinary urea production, equivalent to a degradation of 3.8 g/h of protein during a 100-km run. Lemon and Nagle[50] pointed out that, had sweat urea nitrogen been accounted for in these same experiments, the protein contribution determined would have been much larger. Furthermore, Lemon et al.[51] suggest that urea nitrogen at best provides only a conservative estimate of protein breakdown for energy calories in exercise.

Wahren[38] characterized fuel utilization in longer-duration mild to moderate exercise as a triphasic sequence in which the intramuscular substrate glycogen, then blood glucose and fatty acids, successively, predominate as the major energy-yielding substrate. A clear role for protein use in this sequence remains to be delineated. What is clear relative to protein in the exercise state is (1) protein synthesis is depressed,[51,52] (2) circulating alanine increases and is a precursor for gluconeogenesis, and (3) leucine oxidation is increased.[53]

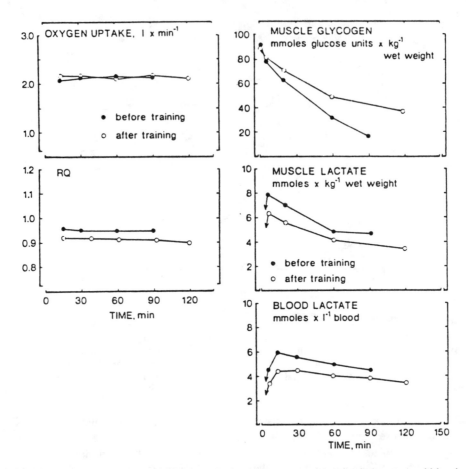

FIGURE 7. Changes in RQ, muscle glycogen (quadriceps muscle), muscle lactate, and blood lactate for five subjects before and after 6 to 8 weeks of endurance training. Mean $\dot{V}O_2$ 2.1 l/min before and after training. (From Saltin, B. and Karlsson, J., in *Muscle Metabolism During Exercise*, Pernow, B. and Saltin, B., Eds., Plenum Press, New York, 1971, 289. With permission.)

3. Training

Figure 7 shows that aerobic training results in alterations in substrate utilization in exercise.[45] Cycling at the same intensity ($\dot{V}O_2 = 2.1$ l $\times$ min^{-1}), trained subjects metabolized less carbohydrate than untrained subjects. This is indicated in Figure 7 by the lower RQ, lower muscle and blood lactate levels, and higher muscle glycogen levels in the trained subjects. Had the exercise been completed even at the same relative intensity (percent $\dot{V}O_2$ max), the differences in substrate use would still be observed.[54]

Such changes occur with aerobic training as mitochondria size and number increase. In addition, induction of critical enzymes of the Krebs cycle and oxidative phosphorylation chain occurs.[55] Figure 8 illustrates the changes in $\dot{V}O_2$ max, and succinic dehydrogenase and cytochrome oxidase with 8 weeks of aerobic training.[55] The result is a greater capacity to utilize lipids and an increase in the threshold at which lactic acid accumulates. In untrained individuals this threshold is reached at 60 to 70% $\dot{V}O_2$ max, whereas in the aerobically trained the threshold is reached near 80% $\dot{V}O_2$ max.[56] Gollnick[57] suggests that the increase in mitochondrial volume and number provides a greater surface area for transport of fatty acids and pyruvate into mitochondria. This reduces cytosol pyruvate that is converted to lactate. Additionally, the greater oxidative capacity of the cell maintains a higher ATP–ADP ratio, which has an inhibiting influence on glycolysis.[57]

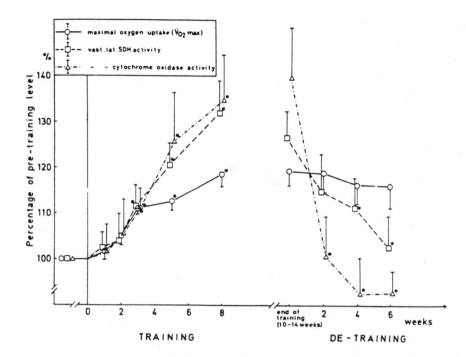

FIGURE 8. Time course of changes in mitochondrial enzymes, succinic dehydrogenase (SDH), cytochrome oxidase, and $\dot{V}O_2$ max over 8 weeks of aerobic training and 6 weeks of detraining. (From Henriksson, J. and Reitman, J. S., *Acta Physiol. Scand.*, 99, 91, 1977. With permission.)

C. Glycogen Storage

Since 1966, with the investigations of Bergstrom and Hultman,[58] we have known that a combined exercise–diet regimen is effective in depositing higher-than-normal levels of glycogen in muscle. Normal stores are 60 to 100 mmol glycosyl units/kg wet muscle. An exercise glycogen-depleting bout followed by a high-carbohydrate diet results in muscle glycogen stores exceeding 200 mmol glycosyl units/kg wet muscle.[59] Earlier reports indicated glycogen deposition was most effectively accomplished by a glycogen-depletion exercise bout, followed by 2 to 3 d on a low-carbohydrate diet and then an additional 3 d on a high-carbohydrate diet.[58,59] More recently, Sherman et al.[60] showed that it was unnecessary to introduce a low-carbohydrate diet to attain high levels of glycogen storage. Following a glycogen-depleting exercise bout, 3 d of a mixed diet containing carbohydrate, followed by 3 d on a high-carbohydrate diet (542 g CHO/d), was equally effective in inducing glycogen deposition.

Repeated days of endurance training have been observed to decrease glycogen stores in muscle when carbohydrate intake is reduced to 250 g/d. However, a diet rich in carbohydrate, 500 to 600 g CHO/d, effectively restores glycogen in 22 h.[61] The same investigators found a trend for greater glycogen storage over 2 d when a diet of complex carbohydrates rather than one of simple sugars was consumed.[62]

V. ACUTE EXERCISE AND REST METABOLISM

Earlier review on this topic[63,64] suggested that acute bouts of exercise had no significant effect on metabolism postexercise. More recently, Freedman-Akabas et al.[65] have reported data supporting this view. They exercised 23 subjects, categorized at levels of low, medium, and high fitness, at approximately 60% $\dot{V}O_2$ max. They measured rest metabolism of the subjects at the same time of day, 4 h postprandial. On one occasion they measured metabolism without preceding exercise and on a second occasion after exercise. Metabolic measurements were made up to 3 h in recovery from exercise. The authors state that the exercise was consistent with that used in weight-control exercise programs (60% $\dot{V}O_2$ max) and conclude that claims for sustained effects of exercise on resting metabolic rate seem unwarranted. Other studies support the view that short bouts of moderate exercise (30 to 70% $\dot{V}O_2$ max) do not significantly alter long-term resting metabolic rate.[66,67]

On the other hand, Gaesser and Brooks,[68] basing their view on several reported studies, state that $\dot{V}O_2$ remains elevated for several hours following prolonged exercise. This is attributed, for the most part, to body temperature and/or circulating catecholamine effects. However, the results of some of these studies are suspect because food intake was not controlled and the thermic effect of food could have contributed to an increased metabolic rate.[69]

Hagberg et al.[70] found that when cycling exercise was sustained at >65% $\dot{V}O_2$ max for 20 min, a marked effect was observed on recovery metabolism due to elevated core temperatures. The persistence of elevated temperatures after exercise may be due partially to "futile cycling" of substrate.[71]

Bielinski et al.[72] studied the residual effect of exercise on metabolism with subjects on a mixed diet. The exercise required 3 h of walking on a treadmill at 50% $\dot{V}O_2$ max, and metabolic measurements were made over 18 h on a nonexercise and an exercise day. The investigators found that the postabsorptive resting metabolism was still elevated 9 h after exercise. Body temperature elevation ($\dot{Q}_{10}$ effect) was cited as a possible cause, and they noted that urinary catecholamines were still elevated 4.5 h postexercise. The resting metabolic rate the morning after exercise was elevated significantly (4.7%) over that measured when no exercise preceded the metabolic rate determination.

Two recent studies[73,74] in which acute exercise was performed at 70% $\dot{V}O_2$ max showed that metabolism was elevated by as much as 12 to 14% for 12 h postexercise. In one of these studies,[73] the excess postexercise oxygen consumption was proportional to the duration of the cycling effort at 70% $\dot{V}O_2$ max.

Training studies in which restricted dieting was combined with exercise strongly suggested an effect of the exercise regimen on metabolic rate. Pavlov et al.[75] conducted a study of Boston policemen judged to be 21% over ideal body weight. After 8 weeks on a diet–exercise regimen the authors accounted for 32% of the total energy expenditure that had to be attributed to an elevated metabolic rate in recovery from exercise. The exercise performed was walk–jog and the average time–distance was 46 min for 5 miles during the 8th week.

A study of Donahue et al.,[76] combining diet and exercise in overweight females, observed the characteristic decrease in resting metabolic rate with weight loss in their control group. However, in their exercising group this trend was reversed. Lennon et al.,[77] in a similar study with both men and women 15 to 35% overweight, showed a 10% increase in resting metabolic rate after 12 weeks of a diet–exercise regimen. This group followed a prescribed exercise regimen expending at least 1240 kJ, 3 d/week. In another daily exercise group where the average exercise energy expenditure was 630 kJ/d, the increase in resting metabolic rate was 5%. While both groups expended about the same energy on a weekly basis, the greater daily caloric expenditure for the prescribed group appeared to contribute to the difference in metabolic rate. Residual effects of acute exercise on resting metabolic rate may well depend on the intensity and/or the duration of the physical activity.

VI. EXERCISE TRAINING AND BODY COMPOSITION

A variety of techniques, including determinations of total body water, total body potassium, and body density (densitometry) are used to assess body composition. These procedures assume the body to be a two-component system consisting of fat and lean body mass (LBM). While this assumption is an oversimplification, the fat–LBM concept remains a useful one.[78]

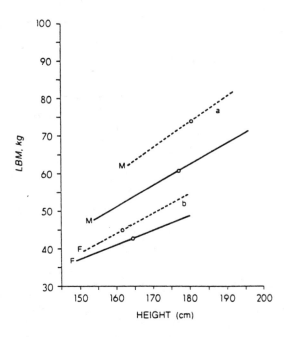

FIGURE 9. Relationship of stature to lean body mass (LBM) for 20- to 30-year-old males and 18- to 30-year-old females. Heavy lines: normal males (*N* = 161) and females (*N* = 135). Line a: male athletes (*N* = 36) and line b: female athletes (*N* = 8). (Adapted from Forbes, G. B., *Fed. Proc.*, 44, 343, 1985. With permission.)

Forbes[78] points out that isolation of exercise-training effects on body composition is a complex issue since other factors such as sex, age, stature, race, and especially nutrition influence fat–LBM proportions. From puberty through the adult years, males have significantly more LBM than females. LBM peaks at 17 to 18 years in females and 20 to 21 years in males, with a subsequent decline with age in both sexes.

In Figure 9, LBM values are plotted vs. stature in normal and athletic, male and female adults.[79] Athletes are shown to possess greater LBM than their less active counterparts. Cross-sectional and longitudinal studies on trained and untrained children and adults of both sexes[80-82] support the contention that athletes do indeed have a larger LBM than nonathletes of the same age, sex, and stature.

Wilmore[83] has summarized the results of 55 studies in which body composition was assessed with controlled physical training. The duration of training varied from 6 to 104 weeks and training frequency was 2 to 3 d/week. Average weight loss was 0.96 kg, the mean LBM increased 0.4 kg, and the mean fat decreased 1.6%. These data are consistent with those reported by Forbes[78] (Figure 10) in similar types of training studies (duration 40 d to 2 years). It will be observed in Figure 10 that exercise training only modestly altered weight and fat-LBM proportions. Increases in LBM amount to approximately 3%. Only with training and administration of nonpharmacological doses of anabolic steroids (190 to 900 mg/d) was LBM increased by 5 to 19% with training (line b, Figure 10).

According to Forbes,[79] the effect of training per se on body composition is obscured by the lack of data on the nutritional status of subjects used in such experiments. Based on our present knowledge, Forbes,[79] in Figure 11, identified exercise training as at least a minor influence among a number of perturbations that affect metabolism and ultimately body composition. A need exists for controlled, longitudinal exercise-training studies.

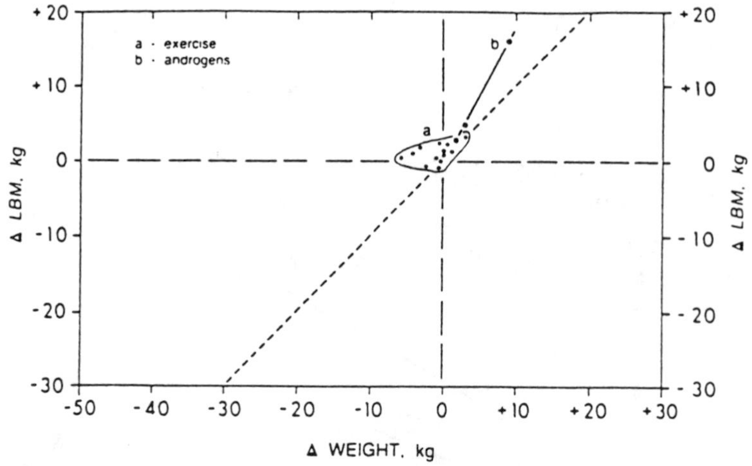
a · exercise
b · androgens
a
b
+20
+10
0
-10
-20
-30
Δ LBM, kg
-50
-40
-30
-20
-10
0
+10
+20
+30
Δ WEIGHT, kg

FIGURE 10. Relationship of change in LBM to change in body weight for various groups of subjects. Diagonal dashed line defines LBM with weight. Values to left of dashed line denote decrease in body fat, to the right an increase in body fat. Area a: effect of exercise training (from a compilation of studies[84-88]). Line b: effect of exercise plus anabolic steroids.[89-90] (Adapted from Forbes, G. B., *Fed. Proc.*, 44, 343, 1985. With permission.)

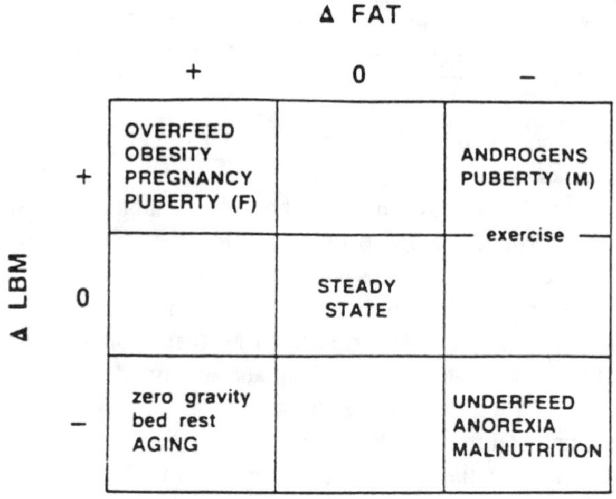
Δ FAT
+
0
–
Δ LBM
+
0
–
OVERFEED
OBESITY
PREGNANCY
PUBERTY (F)
ANDROGENS
PUBERTY (M)
exercise
STEADY
STATE
zero gravity
bed rest
AGING
UNDERFEED
ANOREXIA
MALNUTRITION

FIGURE 11. Changes in LBM and fat effected by a variety of metabolic perturbations of steady state. Exercise training is shown to effect a modest increase in LBM and a modest decrease in body fat. (From Forbes, G. B., *Fed. Proc.*, 44, 343, 1985. With permission.)

VII. SUMMARY

A. Measuring Metabolism

Indirect calorimetry with measurement of O_2 consumption ($\dot{V}O_2$) is the most widely used method for assessing energy expenditure. For purposes of comparison, resting energy expenditure is most often expressed per unit of body surface area. Lower values for women than men are attributable to differences in fat content, which is higher in females and relatively less active metabolically. Expressing metabolism per kilogram LBM minimizes sex differences.

Exercising $\dot{V}O_2$ is commonly expressed per kilogram of body weight for comparative purposes. As a general approximation, resting metabolism is assumed to be 3.5 ml × kg body weight^{-1} × min^{-1} and exercise metabolism may be expressed in multiples of this value.

B. Exercise Energy Expenditure

Exercise energy expenditure in walking, running, and cycling for the adult population is readily predicted from empirical formulae. However, measured values in walking for young males and females (<18 years) exceed prediction estimates. Additionally, well-trained runners, running at fixed speeds, do so more economically than prediction formulae estimate.

Man has a wide range in adaptive capacity for exercise. Anaerobic reserves sustain efforts of 5 to 6 s at power outputs of 210 kJ × min^{-1}, and aerobic sources of energy may sustain efforts of 50 kJ × min^{-1} for as long as 24 h. The principal factors governing maximal exercise efforts are (1) the magnitude of $\dot{V}O_2$ max and (2) the percentage of $\dot{V}O_2$ max marking the onset of lactic acid accumulation.

C. Substrate in Exercise

Lipids provide an abundance of stored energy, whereas calories from carbohydrate and accessible protein are far more limited. Use of substrate stores for energy in exercise depends on (1) health state, (2) diet, (3) exercise intensity and duration, and (4) the state of training. In a normal nutritional state, carbohydrate and fat provide the majority of energy calories in exercise. Long-term exercise and glycogen deficiency have been shown to increase the contribution of protein to exercise energy calories.

D. Acute Exercise and Resting Metabolism

There is considerable controversy regarding the effects of acute exercise on resting metabolism. The literature would suggest that the acute exercise must exceed some threshold in intensity and/or duration to elicit an effect on metabolism.

E. Exercise Training and Body Composition

There are insufficient controlled, longitudinal studies dealing with the effects of exercise training on body composition. The available evidence suggests that regimens of exercise training may increase LBM by 3%. Only in cases where training is accompanied by administration of nonpharmacological doses of anabolic steroids was a highly significant increase in LBM observed.

REFERENCES

1. **Asmussen, E.**, Muscle metabolism during exercise in man: a historical survey, in *Muscle Metabolism During Exercise*, Pernow, B. and Saltin, B., Eds., Plenum Press, New York, 1971, 1.
2. **Durnin, J. V. G. A. and Passmore, R., Eds.**, *Energy, Work and Leisure*, Heinemann, London, 1967.
3. **American College of Sports Medicine**, *Guidelines for Exercise Testing Training*, 3rd ed., Lea & Febiger, Baltimore, 1991.
4. **National Center for Health Statistics**, Dietary intake findings of the United States, 1971–74. Vital and health statistics: Series 11; No. 202, DHEW Publication (HRA) 77-1647, U.S. Department of Health, Education and Welfare, Washington, D.C., 1977.
5. **Bray, G. A.**, Obesity: a human energy problem, in *Human Nutrition Research*, Beacher, G. R., Ed., Beltsville Symposium in Agricultural Research, Allanheld, Ormun Publishers, London, 1979.
6. **McArdle, W. D., Katch, F. I., and Katch, V. L., Eds.**, *Exercise Physiology: Energy, Nutrition and Human Performance*, 2nd ed., Lea & Febiger, Baltimore, 1986.
7. **Bray, G. A.**, The energetics of obesity, *Med. Sci. Sports Exercise*, 15, 32, 1983.
8. **Daniels, J. T.**, A physiologist's view of running economy, *Med. Sci. Sports Exercise*, 17, 332, 1985.

9. **Bassett, D. R., Giese, M. D., Nagle, F. J., Ward, A., Raab, D. M., and Balke, B.,** Aerobic requirements of overground vs. treadmill running, *Med. Sci. Sports Exercise,* 17, 477, 1985.

10. **McMiken, D. F. and Daniels, J. T.,** Aerobic requirements and maximum aerobic power in treadmill and track running, *Med. Sci. Sports Exercise,* 8, 14, 1976.

11. **Pugh, L. G. C. E.,** Oxygen intake in track and treadmill running with observations on the effect of air resistance, *J. Physiol. (London),* 207, 823, 1970.

12. **Montoye, H. J., Ayen, T., Nagle, F. J., and Howley, E.,** The oxygen requirement for horizontal and grade walking on a motor driven treadmill, *Med. Sci. Sports Exercise,* 17, 640, 1985.

13. **Daniels, J., Oldridge, N., Nagle, F. J., and White, R.,** Differences and changes in $\dot{V}O_2$ among young runners 10–18 years of age, *Med. Sci. Sports Exercise,* 10, 200, 1978.

14. **Daniels, J. and Oldridge, N.,** Changes in oxygen consumption of young boys during growth and running training, *Med. Sci. Sports Exercise,* 3, 161, 1971.

15. **Davies, C. T. M.,** Metabolic cost of exercise and physical performance in children with some observations on external loading, *Eur. J. Appl. Physiol.,* 45, 95, 1980.

16. **Conley, D. L. and Krahenbuhl, G. S.,** Running economy and distance running performance of highly trained athletes, *Med. Sci. Sports Exercise,* 12, 357, 1980.

17. **Daniels, J., Scardina, N. J., and Foley, P.,** $\dot{V}O_2$ submax during five modes of exercise, in *Current Topics in Sports Medicine,* Bachl, N., Prokop, L., and Suckert, R., Eds., Urben and Schwarzenberg, Baltimore, 1984.

18. **Miyashita, M., Miura, M., Murase, Y., and Yamanji, K.,** Running performance from the viewpoint of aerobic power, in *Environment Stress, Individual Human Adaptations,* Folinsbee, L. J., Ed., Academic Press, New York, 1978.

19. **Fletcher, J. B.,** in *Bioastronautics Data Book,* NASA-SP-3006, Webb, P., Ed., Webb Associates, Yellow Springs, OH, 1964.

20. **Lloyd, B. B.,** World running records as maximal performance, in *Physiology of Muscular Exercise,* Chapman, C., Ed., Monograph No. 15, American Heart Association, New York, 1967, 218.

21. **Astrand, P. O. and Rohdahl, K., Eds.,** *Textbook of Work Physiology,* McGraw-Hill, New York, 1986, 325.

22. **Keul, J., Doll, E., and Keppler, D., Eds.,** *Energy Metabolism of Human Muscle,* University Park Press, Baltimore, 1972.

23. **Karlsson, J. and Saltin, B.,** Lactate, ATP and CP in working muscles during exhaustive exercise in man, *J. Appl. Physiol.,* 29, 598, 1970.

24. **Daniels, J. T. and Oldridge, N.,** The effects of alternate exposure to altitude and sea level on world class middle distance runners, *Med. Sci. Sports Exercise,* 2, 107, 1970.

25. **Farrell, P. A., Wilmore, J. H., Coyle, E. F., Billings, J. C., and Costill, D. L.,** Plasma lactate accumulation and distance running performance, *Med. Sci. Sports Exercise,* 11, 338, 1979.

26. **Komi, P. V., Ito, A., Sjodin, B., Wallenstein, R., and Karlsson, J.,** Muscle metabolism, lactate breaking point, and biomechanical features of endurance running, *Int. J. Sports Med.,* 2, 148, 1981.

27. **Wasserman, K.,** Anaerobiosis, lactate and gas exchange during exercise, *Fed. Proc.,* 45, 2904, 1986.

28. **Pollock, M. L.,** Submaximal and maximal working capacity of elite distance runners. I. Cardiorespiratory aspects, *Ann. N.Y. Acad. Sci.,* 301, 310, 1977.

29. **Robinson, S., Edwards, H. T., and Dill, D. B.,** New records in human power, *Science,* 85, 409, 1937.

30. **Saltin, B. and Astrand, P. O.,** Maximal oxygen uptake in athletes, *J. Appl. Physiol.,* 23, 353, 1967.

31. **Noakes, T., Ed.,** *Lore of Running,* Oxford University Press, Capetown, 1986.

32. **Costill, D. L., Thomason, H., and Roberts, E.,** Fractional utilization of the aerobic capacity during distance running, *Med. Sci. Sports Exercise,* 5, 248, 1973.

33. **Favier, R. J., Constable, S. H., Chen, M., and Holloszy, J. O.,** Endurance exercise training reduces lactate production, *J. Appl. Physiol.,* 61, 885, 1986.

34. **Henrickson, J.,** Training induced adaptations of skeletal muscle and metabolism during submaximal exercise, *J. Physiol. (London),* 270, 661, 1977.

35. **Brooks, G.,** Lactate production under fully aerobic conditions: the lactate shuttle during rest and exercise, *Fed. Proc.,* 45, 2924, 1986.

36. **Donovan, C. M. and Brooks, G. A.,** Endurance training affects lactate clearance, not lactate production, *Am. J. Physiol.,* 244, E83, 1983.

37. **Donovan, C. M. and Pagliassotti, M. J.,** Enhanced efficiency of lactate removal after endurance training, *J. Appl. Physiol.,* 68, 1053, 1990.

38. **Wahren, J.,** Metabolic adaptation to physical exercise in man, in *Endocrinology,* DeGroot, L. J., Ed., Grune & Stratton, New York, 1979, 1911–1926.

39. **Cahill, G. F.,** Metabolic role of muscle, in *Muscle Metabolism During Exercise,* Proceedings of a Karolinska Institute Symposium, Stockholm, Sweden, Pernow, B. and Saltin, B., Eds., Plenum Press, New York, 1971, 103–110.

40. **Christensen, E. H. and Hanson, O.**, Arbeitsfähigkeit und Ehrnahrung, *Skand. Arch. Physiol.*, 81, 160, 1939.
41. **Issekutz, B., Jr., Shaw, W. A. S., and Issekutz, T. B.**, Effect of lactate on FFA and glycerol turnover in resting and exercising dogs, *J. Appl. Physiol.*, 39, 345, 1975.
42. **Karlsson, J. and Saltin, B.**, Diet, muscle glycogen and endurance performance, *J. Appl. Physiol.*, 31, 203, 1971.
43. **Coyle, E. F., Coggan, A. R., Hemmert, M. K., and Ivy, J.**, Muscle glycogen utilization during prolonged strenuous exercise when fed carbohydrate, *J. Applied Physiol.*, 61, 165, 1986.
44. **Astrand, P. O. and Rodahl, K., Eds.**, *Textbook of Work Physiology*, 3rd ed., McGraw-Hill, New York, 1986, 544.
45. **Saltin, B. and Karlsson, J.**, Muscle glycogen utilization during work of different intensities, in *Muscle Metabolism During Exercise*, Pernow, B. and Saltin, B., Eds., Plenum Press, New York, 1971, 289.
46. **Hartung, G. H., Myrhe, L. G., Nunneley, S. A., and Tucker, D. M.**, Plasma substrate response in men and women during marathon running, *Aviat. Space Environ. Med.*, 455, 128, 1984.
47. **Lemon, P. W. R. and Mullin, J. P.**, Effect of initial glycogen levels on protein catabolism during exercise, *J. Appl. Physiol.*, 48, 624, 1980.
48. **Refsum, H. E., Jessing, R., and Stromme, S. B.**, Changes in plasma amino acid distribution and urine amino acid excretion during prolonged heavy exercise, *Scand. J. Clin. Lab. Invest.*, 29, 407, 1979.
49. **Decombaz, J., Reinhardt, P., Anantharaman, K., Von Glutz, G., and Poortmans, J. R.**, Biochemical changes in 100 km run: free amino acids, urea and creatinine, *Eur. J. Appl. Physiol.*, 41, 61, 1979.
50. **Lemon, P. W. R. and Nagle, F. J.**, Effects of exercise on protein and amino acid metabolism, *Med. Sci. Sports Exercise*, 13, 141, 1981.
51. **Lemon, P. W. R., Yarasheski, K., and Dolny, D. G.**, The importance of protein for athletes, *Sports Med.*, 1, 474, 1984.
52. **Dohm, G. L., Kasparek, G. J., Tapscott, E. B., and Barakat, H. A.**, Protein metabolism during endurance exercise, *Fed. Proc.*, 44, 348, 1985.
53. **Wolfe, R. R., Goodonough, R. D., Wolfe, M. H., Royle, G. T., and Nadel, E. R.**, Isotopic analysis of leucine and urea metabolism in exercising humans, *J. Appl. Physiol.*, 52, 458, 1982.
54. **Karlsson, J., Nordesjo, L. O., Jorfeldt, L., and Saltin, B.**, Muscle lactate, ATP and CP levels after physical training in man, *J. Appl. Physiol.*, 33, 199, 1972.
55. **Henriksson, J. and Reitman, J. S.**, Time course of activity changes in human skeletal muscle succinate dehydrogenase and cytochrome oxidase activities and maximal O_2 uptake with physical activity and inactivity, *Acta Physiol. Scand.*, 99, 91, 1977.
56. **Costill, D. L., Thomason, H., and Robetts, E.**, Fractional utilization of aerobic capacity during distance running, *Med. Sci. Sports Exercise*, 5, 248, 1973.
57. **Gollnick, P. D.**, Metabolism of substrates: energy substrate metabolism during exercise and as modified by training, *Fed. Proc.*, 44, 353, 1985.
58. **Bergstrom, J. and Hultman, E.**, Muscle glycogen synthesis after exercise: an enhancing factor localized to the muscle cells in man, *Nature*, 210, 309, 1966.
59. **Bergstrom, J., Hermansen, L., Hultman, F., and Saltin, B.**, Diet, muscle glycogen and physical performance, *Acta Physiol. Scand.*, 71, 140, 1963.
60. **Sherman, W. M., Costill, D. L., Fine, W. J., and Miller, J. M.**, Effects of exercise-diet manipulation on muscle glycogen and its consequent utilization during performance, *Int. J. Sports Med.*, 2, 1, 1981.
61. **Costill, D. L. and Miller, J. M.**, Nutrition for endurance sports: carbohydrate and fluid balance, *Int. J. Sports Med.*, 1, 2, 1980.
62. **Costill, D. L., Sherman, W. M., Fink, W. J., Maresch, C., Witten, M., and Miller, J. M.**, The role of dietary carbohydrate in muscle glycogen resynthesis after strenuous running, *Am. J. Clin. Nutr.*, 34, 1831, 1981.
63. **Steinhaus, A.**, Studies in the physiology of exercise. Exercise and basal metabolism in dogs, *Am. J. Physiol.*, 83, 658, 1927.
64. **Karpovich, P. V.**, Metabolism and energy used in exercise, *Res. Q. Am. Assoc. Health Phys. Educ. Recreat.*, 12, 423, 1941.
65. **Freedman-Akabas, S., Colt, E., Kissoloft, H. R., and Pi-Sunyer, F. X.**, Lack of sustained increase in $\dot{V}O_2$ following exercise in fit and unfit subjects, *Am. J. Clin. Nutr.*, 41, 545, 1985.
66. **Brehm, B. A. and Gutin, B.**, Recovery energy expenditure for steady state exercise in runners and nonexercisers, *Med. Sci. Sports Exercise*, 18, 205, 1986.
67. **Pacy, P. J., Barton, N., Webster, J., and Garrow, J. S.**, The energy cost of aerobic exercise in fed and fasted normal subjects, *Am. J. Clin. Nutr.*, 42, 764, 1985.
68. **Gaesser, G. A. and Brooks, G. A.**, Metabolic bases of excess post-exercise oxygen consumption: a review, *Med. Sci. Sports Exercise*, 16, 29, 1984.

69. **Horton, E. S.**, Metabolic aspects of exercise and weight reduction, *Med. Sci. Sports Exercise*, 18, 10, 1985.
70. **Hagberg, J. M., Mullin, J. P., and Nagle, F. J.**, Effect of work intensity and duration on recovery O_2, *J. Appl. Physiol.*, 48, 540, 1980.
71. **Newsholme, E.**, Substrate cycles: their metabolic, energetic and thermic consequences in man, *Biochem. Soc. Symp.*, 43, 183, 1978.
72. **Bielinski, R., Schutz, Y., and Jequier, E.**, Energy metabolism during post-exercise recovery in man, *Am. J. Clin. Nutr.*, 42, 69, 1985.
73. **Bahr, R., Ingnes, I., Vaage, O., Sejersted, O. M., and Newsholme, E. A.**, Effect of duration of exercise on excess post exercise O_2 consumption, *J. Appl. Physiol.*, 62, 485, 1987.
74. **Maehlum, S., Grandmontagne, M., Newsholme, E. A., and Sjersted, M.**, Magnitude and duration of excess post exercise oxygen consumption in healthy young subjects, *Metabolism*, 35, 425, 1986.
75. **Pavlov, K. N., Steffe, W. P., Lorman, R. H., and Burrows, B. A.**, Effects of dieting and exercise on lean body mass, oxygen uptake and strength, *Med. Sci. Sports Exercise*, 17, 466, 1985.
76. **Donahue, C. P., Lin, D. H., Kirschenbaum, D. J., and Keesey, R. E.**, Metabolic consequences of dieting and exercise in the treatment of obesity, *J. Consult. Clin. Psychol.*, 52, 827, 1984.
77. **Lennon, D. F., Nagle, F. J., Stratman, F., Shrago, E., and Dennis, S.**, Diet and exercise training effects on resting metabolic rate, *Int. J. Obesity*, 9, 39, 1984.
78. **Forbes, G. B., Ed.**, *Human Body Composition*, Springer-Verlag, New York, 1987, chap. 11.
79. **Forbes, G. B.**, Body composition as affected by physical activity and nutrition, *Fed. Proc.*, 44, 343, 1985.
80. **Brozek, J.**, Physical activity and body composition, *Arch. Ind. Hyg.*, 5, 193, 1954.
81. **Novak, L. P., Hyatt, R. E., and Alexander, J. F.**, Body composition and physiologic function of athletes, *JAMA*, 205, 764, 1968.
82. **Parizicova, J., Ed.**, *Body Fat and Physical Fitness*, Martinus Nijhoff, The Hague, 1977.
83. **Wilmore, J. H.**, Body composition in sport and exercise: directions for future research, *Med. Sci. Sports Exercise*, 15, 21, 1983.
84. **Boyden, T. W., Pamenter, R. S., Grosso, D., Stanforth, P., Rotkis, T., and Wilmore, J. H.**, Prolactin responses, menstrual cycles, and body composition in women runners, *J. Clin. Endocrinol. Metab.*, 54, 711, 1982.
85. **Brown, C. H. and Wilmore, J. H.**, The effects of maximal resistance training on the strength and body composition of women athletes, *Med. Sci. Sports Exercise*, 6, 174, 1974.
86. **Franklin, B., Buskirk, E., Hodgson, J., Gahagan, H., Kollias, J., and Mendez, J.**, Effects of physical conditioning on cardiorespiratory function, body composition, and serum lipids in relatively normal weight and obese middle-aged women, *Int. J. Obesity*, 3, 97, 1979.
87. **Lewis, S., Haskell, W. L., Wood, P. D., Mahoogian, N., Bailey, J. E., and Pereira, M. B.**, Effects of physical activity on weight reduction in obese middle-aged women, *Am. J. Clin. Nutr.*, 29, 151, 1976.
88. **Skinner, J. S., Holloszy, J. O., and Cureton, T. K.**, Effects of a program of endurance exercise on physical work, *Am. J. Cardiol.*, 14, 747, 1964.
89. **Forbes, G. B.**, Some influences on lean body mass: exercise androgens, pregnancy and food, in *Diet and Exercise Synergism in Health Maintenance*, White, P. L. and Mondeika, T., Eds., American Medical Association, Chicago, 1982, 75.
90. **Harvey, G. R., Knibbs, A. V., Burkinshaw, L., Morgan, D. B., Jones, P. R. M., Chettle, D. R., and Vertsky, D.**, Effects of methandienone on the performance and body composition of men undergoing athletic training, *Clin. Sci.*, 60, 457, 1981.

Chapter 8

VITAMINS AND PHYSICAL ACTIVITY

_____ Robert E. Keith

CONTENTS

0-8493-7911-3/94/$0.00+$.50
© 1994 by CRC Press, Inc.

I. INTRODUCTION

Vitamins are generally thought of as a group of organic compounds needed in minute amounts by the body and necessary for normal cellular metabolism, growth, and maintenance of tissue. Vitamins are usually divided into two broad classifications, water soluble and fat soluble. A listing and classification of the vitamins can be found in Table 1. The solubility of the vitamin does affect the way it functions within cells. Water-soluble vitamins include the B-complex group and ascorbic acid (vitamin C). These vitamins all have the common trait that most of their functions relate to their ability to act as coenzymes or cofactors in metabolic reactions. These reactions regulate energy, protein and amino acid metabolism, as well as cell division. An overview of where these water-soluble vitamins function in metabolism can be seen in Table 2. Another common trait of water-soluble vitamins is that body storage is relatively small, thus regular ingestion is required.

Fat-soluble vitamins do not function as coenzymes. Several of the fat-soluble vitamins may actually function more in the manner of hormones. Fat-soluble vitamins can be stored in appreciable amounts within body tissue, thus daily or regular ingestion is not necessarily required. Based upon function and storage, water-soluble vitamin metabolism is more apt to be influenced by physical activity as compared to the fat-soluble group. The exception to this, as noted in Table 2, may be vitamin E.

Whether proper or improper, vitamin use and abuse by athletes is evidently quite common. In one study, Grandjean et al.[1] reported that 75% of college athletes surveyed believed they needed more vitamins than nonathletes. Percy,[2] in discussing ergogenic acids, has also stated that vitamins are one of the most common supplements used by athletes. A report has also been presented to the U.S. Senate concerning vitamin use in Olympic athletes.[3] Olympic athletes were reported to be consuming multivitamins, vitamin B_{12} (injections of 1000 mg), and vitamin C (10,000 mg/d), among others. Bentivegna has reported that a majority of coaches surveyed had at one time recommended vitamin supplements to athletes.[4] Stensland and Sobal have also reported that 60% of a group of dancers took vitamin and mineral supplements on a regular basis.[5] Vitamin supplementation has also been reported in college athletes,[6] nonelite marathon runners,[7] female bodybuilders,[8] and various other professional and amateur athletes.[9,10] Thus, it does appear that a significant number of athletes are probably taking some form of vitamin supplementation in the belief that it will aid in their performance.

Because vitamins are essential nutrients it is virtually certain that a deficiency or suboptimal status of any vitamin will, at some point, impair physical performance. This has been shown by Archdeacon and Murlin[11] and, more recently, by van der Beek et al.,[12] who reported a significant decrease in aerobic power ($\dot{V}O_2$ max decreased 9.8%) and onset of blood lactate accumulation in male subjects receiving a diet low in vitamins B_1, B_2, B_6, and C over an 8-week period. Many studies report improvements in function with vitamin supplementation. This would be expected if the vitamin addition were correcting a deficiency state. The literature is replete with reports of decreased physical function during vitamin-deficient states. It is not the purpose of this chapter to review this literature. However, a list of deficiency symptoms of the various vitamins as they pertain to physical performance is presented in Table 3.

The literature also contains papers reporting low intakes of certain vitamins in some athletic groups. Generally, female athletes have lower intakes than male athletes. In addition, diet-restricted athletes such as gymnasts, dancers, wrestlers, and bodybuilders are more apt to have low intakes of vitamins. Vitamin B_6 may be the vitamin most often found to be low in the diets of athletes, although intakes of vitamins A, C, and B_{12} have been found to be suboptimal in some athletes. The reader is referred to Clarkson[10] for a more extensive review of suboptimal vitamin intakes in athletes. This chapter will address scientific publications that try to answer two questions:

TABLE 1 A Listing and Classification of the Vitamins Known to be Essential to Humans

Water-soluble	Fat-soluble
Thiamin (B_1)	Vitamin A (retinoids)
Riboflavin (B_2)	Vitamin D (calciferols)
Niacin (B_3)	Vitamin E (tocopherols)
Pantothenic acid	Vitamin K (quinones)
Biotin	
Pyridoxine (B_6)	
Folic Acid	
Cobalamin (B_{12})	
Ascorbic acid (Vitamin C)	

TABLE 2 An Overview of Vitamins Involved in Various Metabolic and Physiologic Systems Related to Optimal Physical Performance

Metabolic/physiologic system	Vitamins needed for optimal functioning
Glycolysis (processing of glucose)	Niacin
Gluconeogenesis (conversion of lactate, alanine, glycerol to glucose)	Niacin
Glycogen degradation/synthesis	Pyridoxine[a]
Oxidation of fatty acids	Niacin, riboflavin, pantothenic acid[b]
Krebs (TCA) cycle	Thiamin, riboflavin, niacin, pantothenic acid
Electron transport chain	Riboflavin, niacin
Amino acid degradation/synthesis	Pyridoxine[c]
DNA, RNA synthesis/cell division (synthesis of red blood cells)	Folic acid, cobalamin
Neurological function	Thiamin, pyridoxine, cobalamin, ascorbic acid
Antioxidant functions (protects cells against oxidative damage)	Ascorbic acid, vitamin E

[a] Associated with glycogen storage; does not act as a coenzyme.
[b] Ascorbic acid, biotin, and cobalamin may also have functions related to fatty acid oxidation.
[c] Several other B-complex vitamins may also have functions in the processing of certain amino acids.

1. Does vitamin supplementation above current recommended levels enhance physical performance in individuals already adequately nourished with respect to that vitamin?
2. Does strenuous physical activity increase vitamin requirements in otherwise healthy subjects?

II. WATER-SOLUBLE VITAMINS
A. Vitamin B Complex
1. Thiamin

Thiamin, vitamin B_1, functions in mammalian tissues predominantly as the coenzyme, thiamin pyrophosphate (TPP). TPP is required for the oxidative decarboxylation of

TABLE 3 Vitamin Deficiency Symptoms that Would Adversely Affect Physical Performance

Vitamin	Deficiency symptom
Thiamin	Muscular weakness, fatigue, altered heart function, depression
Riboflavin	Anemia, peripheral neuropathy of the hands and feet
Niacin	Weight loss, strength loss, vertigo, mental confusion, decreased ability to concentrate
Pantothenic acid	Depression, fatigue, muscular weakness
Biotin	Extreme lassitude, muscle pain, anemia
Pyridoxine	Depression, peripheral neuritis, ataxia, anemia
Folic acid	Anemia
Cobalamin	Anemia, weakness, fatigue, loss of weight, neurological damage
Ascorbic acid	Muscular weakness, decreased use of fatty acids, anemia, poor healing of injuries
Vitamin A	Blindness, anorexia, increased infections, depressed growth
Vitamin D	Weak bones, increased fractures, depressed growth
Vitamin E	Increased hemolysis of red blood cells, creatinuria, neurological dysfunction, muscle lesions
Vitamin K	Prolonged blood clotting time

alpha–keto acids. These reactions include the conversion of pyruvate to acetyl coenzyme A (CoA) and α-ketoglutarate to succinyl CoA, as well as the decarboxylation of the branched-chain amino acids valine, leucine, and isoleucine. TPP is necessary for the transketolase reaction of the pentose shunt. Thiamin also plays a role in neurophysiology seemingly separate from its coenzyme function. Thiamin is widely distributed within the various food groups. However, the best sources tend to be whole grain or enriched cereals and breads. Lean pork and wheat germ are also excellent sources of the vitamin. The Recommended Dietary Allowance (RDA) for thiamin is 0.5 mg/1000 kcal consumed, but not less than 1.0 mg/d. Thus, athletes with increased energy expenditures may have increased total thiamin needs. Thiamin requirements appear to increase as the carbohydrate content of the diet increases. Thiamin deficiency has been shown to increase blood lactic acid levels at set carbohydrate intakes compared to well-nourished subjects. This may have important implications for athletes consuming high-carbohydrate diets.[13-16]

Animal studies have addressed the issue of thiamin and exercise. Bialecki and Nijakowski studied the effects of swimming on thiamin content on various tissues and blood in rats.[17] Three groups of rats, including a resting control, were used. Training (4 h of swimming per day for 10 d) significantly decreased the thiamin content in liver, kidney, and blood, but not skeletal and cardiac muscle. A single acute bout of swimming to exhaustion had no effect on the thiamin content of the tissues assayed. All rats were fed a "normal standard diet". Stewart measured the speed of racehorses before and after supplementation of the horses' diets with thiamin.[18] Improvements in speed were noted with vitamin supplementation. McNeil and Mooney studied the relationship among carbohydrate loading, thiamin supplementation, and cardiovascular endurance in mice after a 4-week conditioning program.[19] Mice were trained by swimming with tailweights for 30 min/d. At the end of the conditioning program animals were randomly divided into four groups: (1) high-fat/protein diet, minimum daily requirement (MDR) for thiamin; (2) high-fat/protein diet, 100 × MDR; (3) high-carbohydrate diet, MDR; (4) high-carbohydrate diet, 100 × MDR. Mice in the 100 × MDR groups received their supplemental thiamin by a single ip injection 30 min prior to final exercise data collection. The test measure in the final study was a final timed swim to exhaustion. Results were as follows: low carbohydrate, MDR — 45.6 min; low carbohydrate, 100 × MDR — 41.5 min; high carbohydrate, MDR — 63.1 min; high carbohydrate, 100 × MDR — 88.7 min. Thus, mice receiving high-carbohydrate, 100 × MDR diets swam longer than all other groups. However, this was significantly different from only the low-carbohydrate, 100 × MDR group. It is difficult to interpret the results of this paper because supplemental thiamin was given as a single, large injected dose rather than through diet over a longer period of time.

Human studies involving supplemental thiamin and physical performance are few in number. McCormick studied the effects of giving 5.0 mg of thiamin daily for 1 week on the arm-holding and breath-holding times of young swimmers.[20] The arm-holding test consisted of holding the arms in a horizontal plane for as long as possible. All subjects improved their test results following vitamin supplementation. However, no statistical tests were used and no placebo control groups were utilized. Karpovich and Millman[21] repeated McCormick's work, but included a placebo control group as well as psychological "pep talks". Under these controlled conditions no significant effect was seen on arm-holding or breath-holding times due to thiamin supplementation at 5.0 mg/d for 1 week.

Keys et al.[22] performed a series of four controlled experiments (10 to 12 weeks each) involving thiamin intake and physical performance in young men. Thiamin intakes ranged from 0.23 to 0.96 mg/1000 kcal with subjects consuming approximately 3000 kcal/d (48% carbohydrate, 16% protein, 36% fat). Subjects were given various psychomotor tests as well as exercise on a treadmill for periods of 60 to 90 min. Heart rates were monitored and blood glucose, lactate, pyruvate, and hemoglobin values were measured at various times. Strength tests with leg, grip, and back dynamometers were also performed. Increasing thiamin intakes from 0.23 to 0.96 mg/1000 kcal had no significant effects on any of the variables measured.

Nijakowski reported that blood levels of thiamin decreased in a group of 12 trained skiers after 3 weeks of ski training and also after a single 4-h bout of skiing.[23] A group of nonathletic controls were used in a 4-h ski test. Blood levels of thiamin in the controls did not decrease. Early and Carlson reported decreased fatigue in a group of young male subjects running repeat 50-yard dashes and taking vitamin supplements, as compared to a placebo control group performing the same exercises.[24] These investigators attributed the decreased fatigue to the fact that the experimental subjects were taking thiamin (100 mg) and pantothenic acid (30 mg) supplements each day for a week before the exercise trials. However, no initial assessment of the vitamin status of the subjects was made. Haralambie has reported that erythrocyte transketolase was activated by more than 25% with added thiamin in 12 of 18 athletes studied.[25] Thiamin stimulation of >25% is indicative of severe thiamin deficiency. Read and McGuffin, in a study using male college students, reported a significant positive correlation between thiamin intake and treadmill running times to exhaustion in some, but not all, of their exercise trials.[26] Bonke has reported that supplemental thiamin (90 or 300 mg/d) given for 8 weeks (along with supplemental B_6 and B_{12}) significantly improved firing accuracy in experienced marksmen.[27] Finally, Caster and Mickelsen[28] reported initial significantly decreased urinary thiamin excretion in subjects exercising at 1500 kcal per day on a treadmill as compared to controls. However, a repeated test produced no decrease. The authors suggested that the subjects adapted to the stress of the exercise.

In summary, the data on thiamin and exercise are equivocal. Further well-controlled and designed studies involving thiamin and physical performance are needed. Animal and human studies looking at the effects of training/exercise on tissue and blood thiamin content as well as other markers of biochemical changes (increased blood pyruvate and lactate) are needed. Human studies measuring erythrocyte transketolase activity with training/exercise at different levels of thiamin intake would be valuable. Studies evaluating the effects of high-carbohydrate diets and exercise on thiamin status, as well as thiamin's effect on neurological functioning, would be beneficial.

2. Riboflavin

Riboflavin, vitamin B_2, functions in mammalian tissues in two active coenzyme forms, flavin mononucleotide (FMN) and flavin adenine dinucleotide (FAD). The coenzymes aid in oxidation–reduction reactions within the cell and function as hydrogen carriers in the mitochondrial electron transport system. Riboflavin coenzymes are involved in fatty acid metabolism, the Kreb's cycle, and oxidative deamination of certain amino acids. Thyroid hormone production and riboflavin coenzyme activity seem to be related. The major dietary sources of riboflavin include milk and other dairy products, as well as meat. Liver contains appreciable amounts of riboflavin. The current RDA for riboflavin is 0.6 mg/1000 kcal consumed. In the past riboflavin needs have also been related to lean body mass and body size.[13-16]

In an animal study, Hunter and Turkki studied the effects of exercise on riboflavin status of rats.[29] Exercised animals ran on a treadmill for 6 to 8 weeks and received diets containing 2.0 to 2.5 mg riboflavin/kg of diet (marginally adequate). Tissue riboflavin concentrations and erythrocyte glutathione reductase activity coefficients (EGRAC) were evaluated. A sedentary control group was included. Exercise did not affect EGRAC values and did not increase total riboflavin requirements; however, total riboflavin retention and enzyme activity per gram muscle in gastrocnemius and soleus muscles were increased. The authors suggested decreased B_2 turnover and decreased nonfunctional metabolism of riboflavin may have been the reasons for the normal EGRAC in light of the increased muscle retention.

In early work with humans, urinary excretion of riboflavin was reported to decrease during several hours of mountain climbing and during physical activity.[30,31] Potenza has reported that resistance to fatigue increased in subjects following riboflavin supplementation.[32] However, statistical analysis of the data were inadequate. Tucker et al.[33] maintained nine young males on a constant intake of 2.0 mg of riboflavin per day for a number of months. During this control period the subjects walked on a treadmill such that 3300 kcal/d were required to maintain their body weight. Urinary excretion of riboflavin averaged 285 μg/d. When the walking schedule was increased such that 5500 to 6000 kcal/d were required for weight maintenance, urinary riboflavin decreased to a low value of 137 μg/d. No explanation for the reduced riboflavin was given. However, Tucker et al.[33] did suggest that riboflavin may have been incorporated into new muscle tissue. Tucker's findings agreed with the earlier reports of Delachaux and Ott[30] and Friedemann et al.[31]

More recently, Haralambie has reported EGRAC of greater than 1.25 in 8 of 18 athletes studied.[25] This value is indicative of inadequate riboflavin status. Belko et al.[34-36] have published several studies concerned with the riboflavin status of exercising and nonexercising young women. In one study,[34] the riboflavin requirement of 12 young women was estimated by incrementally increasing their riboflavin intake while measuring the EGRAC. This was done initially for 6 weeks with no exercise followed by a 6-week exercise protocol which consisted of running on a track 20 to 50 min/d. Using this protocol, individual riboflavin requirements ranged from 0.62 to 1.21 mg/1000 kcal before exercise to 0.63 to 1.40/1000 kcal during exercise. The authors concluded that healthy young women have riboflavin requirements greater than the current RDA (0.6 mg/1000 kcal) and that exercise increased riboflavin requirements. In another study,[36] a group of young, weight-reducing women were fed 0.96 mg riboflavin/1000 kcal or 1.16 mg/1000 kcal. Women in each group consumed these levels of B_2 during both nonexercise and exercise periods. EGRAC values increased significantly with exercise at both levels of riboflavin intake. The authors concluded that 0.96 mg B_2/1000 kcal was inadequate for both nonexercise or exercise groups. Yoon et al.[37] have also reported that exercise increased EGRAC values in older women.

Using a different approach, Tremblay et al.[38] evaluated physical performance and the EGRAC in a group of elite swimmers (male and female) before and after supplementation. Subjects were found to be adequately nourished with respect to riboflavin at the beginning of the study. One group of swimmers received 60 mg of riboflavin per day for 16 to 20 d, while a second group received a placebo. No differences were seen in swimming performance, $\dot{V}O_2$ max, ventilatory anaerobic threshold, or glutathione reductase activity between the supplemented and placebo groups. The authors concluded that athletes performing large amounts of training can maintain normal riboflavin status without supplementation and that riboflavin supplementation does not affect physical performance in nondeficient subjects. Keith and Alt[39] measured riboflavin status of trained female (tennis, track, and triathlon) athletes consuming normal diets with riboflavin intakes at approximately the RDA. These athletes were compared to untrained controls. The authors found that EGRAC values of the athletes were normal and not different from controls. The authors concluded that well-trained female athletes with dietary riboflavin intakes near the RDA level could maintain adequate riboflavin stores. Lewis et al.[40] also showed that a vigorous walking program did not affect riboflavin status in pregnant women consuming ample quantities of the vitamin.

Several studies reported to date would suggest an increased riboflavin requirement and/ or altered riboflavin metabolism with increased levels of physical activity. However, not all studies find suboptimal B_2 status with increased exercise training. It is not clear as to why the studies by Belko et al.[34-36] and Yoon et al.[37] report increased EGRAC values with increased exercise while studies by Tremblay et al.[38] and Keith and Alt[39] report normal EGRAC values in their trained subjects. The most obvious difference between the two sets of studies is that the former studies used untrained subjects and initiated a training program. In the latter studies subjects were already highly trained. Perhaps B_2 needs are increased at the beginning of a training program while adaptation may occur in trained subjects, thus allowing them to maintain B_2 status on intakes approximating the RDA.

3. Niacin

Niacin, or vitamin B_3, can exist in foods and supplements in two forms, as nicotinic acid and as nicotinamide. In the body niacin functions as a component of the coenzymes nicotinamide adenine dinucleotide (NAD) and as NAD phosphate (NADP). These coenzymes function as hydrogen acceptors and donors and are essential in numerous oxidation–reduction reactions within the body. Niacin in its coenzyme form plays an essential role in glycolysis, fatty acid oxidation and biosynthesis, the tricarboxcyclic acid cycle, the electron transport chain, and protein metabolism. Niacin can be obtained in foods in the preformed state. Niacin can also be synthesized in the body from the amino acid tryptophan. Thus, foods that are high in niacin and/or tryptophan would be considered good sources of the vitamin. The best food sources would include liver, meat, fish, poultry, beans, seeds, and nuts. The requirement for niacin is closely tied to energy turnover. The RDA for niacin is 6.6 mg/ 1000 kcal or 13 to 19 mg/d for the average healthy adult.[13-16]

Several studies have investigated the effects of nicotinic acid administration on substrate availability in skeletal and cardiac muscle during exercise.[41-45] Findings were virtually unanimous; nicotinic acid was found to block the release of fatty acids from adipose tissue, thus making this source of energy less available during work. As a result, blood glucose and muscle glycogen were relied upon to a greater extent to supply energy. Glycogen depletion during exercise was more rapid following nicotinic acid administration, respiratory (R) values were higher and blood glucose tended to fall more rapidly. These findings would indicate that nicotinic acid should not be used as a supplement for endurance athletes.

Other studies have reported findings on relationships between niacin (nicotinamide) and work performance. Frankau conducted a series of experiments using air-crew cadets as subjects.[46] The exercise protocol was basically of an anaerobic nature but involving some coordination skills. Subjects received either a placebo or 50 mg of nicotinamide daily for 3 to 6 d or 200 mg as a single dose 1.5 to 3 h prior to exercise. In all trials subjects performed the test significantly faster after receiving the B_3 supplement as compared to the control. No mention was made of the initial vitamin status of the subjects. However, Hilsendager and Karpovich gave 75 mg of niacin to subjects 2 h prior to exercise and found no effect of the supplement on endurance performance or changes in blood pressure.[47] Borisov measured N-methyl-nicotinamide excretion, a major urinary niacin metabolite, in 277 physical culture students.[48] Mean excretion was below acceptable levels, despite the fact that the students were consuming what would have appeared to be adequate quantities of the vitamin (7.0 to 9.5 mg/1000 kcal). Jett'e et al.[49] also reported a decrease in N-methyl-nicotinamide excretion in subjects following training and a high-carbohydrate diet. In this particular study the authors did not see increased endurance performance following a high-carbohydrate diet. They hypothesized that reduced niacin intake during the high-carbohydrate diet may have impaired the aerobic oxidative pathways. In an animal study, Yefremov and Faburken reported that nicotinic acid excretion in the urine decreased in rats that were forced to swim (3 h/d, 14 d) as compared to control rats on similar dietary intakes.[50]

In summary, data is strong to support the fact that nicotinic acid supplementation impairs adipose tissue fatty acid mobilization. This, in all likelihood, would impair endurance performance. It also appears that strenuous physical activity results in a decrease in niacin metabolite excretion. Whether or not this represents an increased requirement for niacin, however, is not clear. Currently there are not enough data to determine whether or not nicotinamide supplementation would improve physical performance.

4. Pyridoxine

Vitamin B_6 (pyridoxine, pyridoxal, pyridoxamine) requirements in man are closely associated with protein and amino acid needs. Vitamin B_6 requirements appear to increase when high-protein diets are consumed. The pyridoxine coenzymes (mostly pyridoxal phosphate) function in virtually all aspects of amino acid metabolism; transamination, decarboxylation, desulfhydration, and nonoxidative deamination. Via these reactions, B_6 is involved in catecholamine, hemoglobin, and general protein synthesis. In addition, the enzyme, glycogen phosphorylase, necessary for the breakdown of muscle glycogen, contains pyridoxal phosphate. In this case, pyridoxine seems to be necessary for proper enzyme conformation. Thus, there are metabolic reasons why vitamin B_6 could affect muscular activity. The best food sources include liver, wheat germ, meat, fish, poultry, legumes, bananas, and brown rice. The RDA for vitamin B_6 is 1.6 mg/d for adult females, 2.0 mg/d for adult males, or approximately 0.016 mg B_6/g protein consumed per day.[13-16]

Several animal studies have been conducted involving vitamin B_6 and exercise. Shock and Sebrell determined the work output of perfused frog gastrocnemius muscle following addition of pyridoxine hydrochloride at concentrations of 0.00001 to 1.0 mM per liter of perfusate.[51] A significant improvement in total work output and extent of muscle contraction was observed with concentrations up to 0.05 mM/l. Yefremov and Faburken reported a decrease in excretion of vitamin B_6 and its metabolites in a group of rats forced to swim

3 h/d for 14 d as compared to controls.[50] The authors suggested that prolonged swimming increased the vitamin B_6 requirement. Richardson and Chenman reported increased muscular endurance in the gastrocnemius muscle of rats receiving a dietary vitamin B_6 supplement for 30 d as compared to control animals.[52] However, it is unclear whether the control animals were in fact vitamin B_6 deficient. McMillan et al.[53] looked at the effects of supplemental vitamin B_6 and exercise (climbing with body weights) on the contractile properties of rat muscle. Vitamin B_6 given at 100 times the minimum daily requirement had no positive effects on muscle contractile properties, as compared to a minimum daily requirement group. The authors actually suggested that the additional B_6 may have had adverse effects on the different values measured.

Human studies involving vitamin B_6 and exercise can also be found in the literature. Lawrence et al.[54] investigated the effects of giving supplemental pyridoxine hydrochloride (51 mg) daily for 6 months on endurance performance of trained competitive swimmers. A matched placebo control group was included. No effect of vitamin B_6 on repeat 100-yard swim times was noted. Borisov measured 4-pyridoxic acid excretion in 297 students in a physical culture institute over a 1-year time period.[55] A majority of the students (83%) had excretion values that were considered low to deficient. No mention of dietary intake was made. The authors suggested that physically active students had vitamin B_6 requirements 1.5 to 2.0 times as high as the requirement for the normal population. Moretti et al.[56] exercised six subjects on a cycle ergometer at 80% of maximum heart rate for 60 min. Subjects were infused with either 600 mg of pyridoxine or saline (placebo). The subjects did not know which infusion was given. Pyridoxine infusion produced significant increases in plasma growth hormone levels and significant decreases in prolactin levels as compared to saline values. The authors suggested that the results were probably due to the increase of dopaminergic activity by pyridoxine.

Researchers have investigated the relationships among carbohydrate intake, vitamin B_6 supplementation, and exercise.[57,58] Hatcher et al.[57] reported that postexercise plasma values for B_6 and pyridoxal phosphate were significantly decreased when subjects were on a low-carbohydrate diet as compared to moderate- and high-carbohydrate diets. Furthermore, urinary 4-pyridoxic acid excretion was elevated postexercise for the high- and moderate-carbohydrate diets, but not for the low-carbohydrate diet. The authors suggested an increased vitamin B_6 need with exercise and a low-carbohydrate diet. In contrast, deVos et al.[58] concluded that free fatty acid use as a fuel source on low-carbohydrate diets is decreased with B_6 supplementation. The authors concluded that B_6 supplementation accentuates glycogen depletion. Due to the role of vitamin B_6 in glycogen phosphorylase activity, supplementation of the vitamin may cause a more rapid emptying of muscle glycogen stores. Manore and Leklem[59] also reported that vitamin B_6 supplementation (8.0 mg/d) tended to reduce plasma free fatty acid levels following a bout of exercise.

Leklem and Shultz found increased circulating plasma pyridoxal phosphate levels in trained adolescent boys following a 4500-m run.[60] The authors concluded that exercise in the form of long-distance running dramatically alters plasma pyridoxal phosphate levels. Hofman et al.[61] found that plasma pyridoxal phosphate values were significantly elevated following a 2-h run in subjects receiving either water or a glucose polymer drink. Vitamin B_6 utilization has also been studied in a group of trained male runners.[62] Values were compared to an inactive control group of comparable age and sex. Each group received 4.2 mg of B_6 per day. Basal 4-pyridoxic acid excretion in a 24-h urine sample was significantly lower in the trained group as compared to the inactive controls. However, the authors stated that the reduced 4-pyridoxic acid excretion provided no conclusive evidence for increased need for vitamin B_6 in athletes. They suggested that athletes may have increased storage of pyridoxine. In contrast, Manore et al.[63] reported that 4-pyridoxic acid excretion increased significantly postexercise in a group of untrained subjects. Finally, Yates et al.[64] reported that a walking program did not alter vitamin B_6 status in a group of pregnant women.

In summary, exercise does appear to alter B_6 metabolism in the body. Alterations in plasma levels and metabolite excretion with exercise have been reported in several studies with the level of muscle glycogen and the amount of carbohydrate in the diet affecting these changes. This may represent an increased requirement; however, Dreon and Butterfield[62] suggest that exercise may promote storage of B_6 that is then available for redistribution at needed times. No firm conclusions can be drawn at the present time. The effects of vitamin B_6 supplementation on physical performance have produced equivocal, but mostly negative, results.

5. Pantothenic Acid

Pantothenic acid functions in tissues predominately as part of the structure of coenzyme A (CoA). In this capacity pantothenic acid is involved in carbohydrate, fat, and amino acid metabolism. CoA is also a necessary cofactor in the Krebs cycle and is involved in steroid biosynthesis and acetylcholine formation. Thus, pantothenate as part of CoA occupies a key place in energy metabolism and has a theoretical basis for being related to work output and energy utilization. Pantothenic acid is widely distributed in various food groups and it is highly improbable that anyone eating sufficient kilocalories would become deficient in pantothenic acid. Pantothenic acid is found in higher concentrations in animal tissue, whole grain products, beans, and peas. Pantothenic acid deficiency in humans is rare. There is no RDA for pantothenic acid, although intakes of 4 to 7 mg/d are considered sufficient. Typical American diets provide 5 to 20 mg of pantothenic acid each day for adults.[13-16]

Pantothenic acid, exercise studies are few in number. However, most of the studies to date have reported positive effects of pantothenic acid supplementation on work performance. Three animal studies involving pantothenic acid and work were uncovered. Shock and Sebrell studied the effects of pantothenic acid on the work output of perfused frog gastrocnemius muscle.[65] The investigators reported increased work output as pantothenate concentrations in the buffered glucose–Ringers solution increased from 0.001 to 0.5 milliequivalents/liter. A pantothenate concentration of 1.0 mEq/l did not cause a further increase in work output. Ralli and Dumm fed rats pantothenic acid-deficient, -adequate, or -excessive diets for 40 to 50 d.[66] Animals then swam to exhaustion. Swimming times were 16, 29, and 62 min for the deficient, adequate, and excessive diets, respectively. Bialecki and Nijakowski fed rats a diet containing 35 mEq/d of pantothenic acid.[67] Animals were then subjected to swimming 4 to 5 h/d for periods of 1 to 30 d. A resting control group was used for comparisons. Statistically significant decreases in kidney concentration of pantothenic acid were found at all time periods measured. Significant decreases in pantothenic levels in skeletal muscle, heart muscle, and blood were found in animals swimming 10 to 30 d.

Only a few studies involving pantothenic acid and exercise have been performed with human subjects. As addressed in the section on thiamin, Early and Carlson reported decreased fatigue in young male subjects performing repeat 50-yard dashes.[24] These investigators attributed the decrease in fatigue to the thiamin and pantothenic acid (30 mg) supplements the subjects were consuming. Nijakowski reported higher resting blood pantothenic acid levels in 12 sportsmen as compared to sedentary controls.[23] Pantothenic acid levels in the blood decreased in the sportsmen after short-lasting work on a cycle ergometer. Nice et al.[68] fed 1.0 g of pantothenic acid or a matched placebo to 18 highly conditioned runners (20 to 35 years old) for a period of 2 weeks. Procedures were performed in a double-blind manner. Each subject completed a pre-supplement and post-supplement run to exhaustion. No significant differences between supplement and placebo groups were found for run time, heart rate, and blood levels of cortisol, glucose, creatine phosphokinase, urea nitrogen, albumin,

Na^+, K^+, Cl^-, or HCO_3^-. Litoff et al.[69] gave 2.0 g of pantothenic acid or a placebo to seven highly trained distance runners for a period of 2 weeks. Double-blind procedures were used and all subjects received the supplement and the placebo. Subjects rode the cycle ergometer at 75% $\dot{V}O_2$ max in a series of trials lasting 40 min to exhaustion. Results indicated that pantothenic acid supplementation decreased mean lactate levels 16.7% and O_2 consumption at steady state by 8.4% as compared to placebo values.

Several studies reviewed in this section reported or suggested a positive effect of pantothenic acid on performance. Exercise also decreased pantothenate status in an animal study. Only the well-controlled study by Nice et al.[68] found no effects of supplementation. These papers would suggest a possible relationship between exercise and pantothenic acid metabolism. However, so little well-controlled work has been performed that firm conclusions cannot be reached. Further research involving pantothenic acid is warranted.

6. Cobalamin

Cobalamin, vitamin B_{12}, is essential for the function of all cells, but particularly those with rapid turnover, such as found in the gastrointestinal tract and bone marrow. Cobalamin coenzymes are necessary for normal folic acid metabolism and are involved in neural tissue development. Through its relationship with folic acid, B_{12} is necessary for normal DNA synthesis. Cobalamin is found almost exclusively in foods of animal origin. Liver is very rich in B_{12}. Whole milk, eggs, fish, meat, and cheese are all good sources. The RDA for adults for vitamin B_{12} is 2.0 $\mu g/d$, while the typical American diet contains 5.0 to 15.0 $\mu g/d$.[13-16] Vitamin B_{12} is perhaps one of the more abused vitamins among athletes. Several reports have stated that B_{12} megadosing is common in athletics, with some athletes receiving injections of 1000 mg shortly before competition.[3,70]

Despite the abuse of vitamin B_{12} by athletes, very few studies have actually reported on the effects of supplemental B_{12} and physical performance. Four have been uncovered by this author and three reported no effect of B_{12} on various performance indices, while results of the fourth study are unclear with respect to B_{12}.

Wetzel et al.[71] measured the back, leg, and grip strength of children receiving 10 μg of supplemental B_{12} per day. Addition of the vitamin seemed to have no effect on the parameters measured. Montoye et al.[72] gave healthy adolescent males either 50 μg of B_{12} or a placebo daily for 7 weeks. A third group served as controls. The protocol was performed in a double-blind manner. Supplement and placebo groups were performance matched from preliminary tests. Variables included pre- and post-measurements for half-mile run time, Harvard Step-Test performance, height, and weight. No effects of vitamin supplementation were observed. In a third study, Tin-May-Than et al.[73] measured physical performance capacity in 31 young, healthy male subjects. Anemic subjects were excluded. Males were "weight–age" paired and randomly assigned to a B_{12} or placebo group. B_{12} subjects received injections (1 mg) of the vitamin three times per week for 6 weeks. The placebo group received injections in a similar manner. Injections were given on a double-blind basis. Pre- and post-tests were administered. Results indicated that B_{12} and placebo groups were not different for height, weight, resting heart rate, $\dot{V}O_2$ max, recovery heart rates, pull-ups, leg-lifts, hand-grip strength, standing broad jump, or plate-tapping (a coordination test).

Read and McGuffin reported a significant negative correlation between vitamin B_{12} intake and treadmill running time to exhaustion in a group of male college students.[26] However, the authors suggested that differences in the carbohydrate and fat content of the subjects' diets were the reason for the differences in run times, rather than B_{12} intake. Because vitamin B_{12} is found in animal products, high B_{12} intakes would be associated with higher protein and fat intakes and lower carbohydrate intakes.

The majority of the above-mentioned studies indicated no positive effect of megadoses of the vitamin on any of the values measured. However, the number of studies is small and the subjects young and largely untrained. Future well-controlled studies dealing with vitamin B_{12} status and supplementation in highly trained adult athletes (strength/power athletes in particular) would be worthwhile. Studies utilizing doses (1000 mg by injection) similar to those reportedly being used by athletes would also be interesting.

7. Folic Acid and Biotin

Folic acid functions in tissues in various coenzyme forms. The metabolic function of the vitamin is to act as a donor or acceptor of one-carbon units in several reactions involved in nucleotide and amino acid metabolism. Through these reactions folic acid coenzymes play a strong role in cell division. Tissue with rapid turnover, such as red and white blood cells, and tissue of the gastrointestinal tract and uterus, are most susceptible to deficiencies of folic acid. The best food sources of folic acid include liver, dark green leafy vegetables, various beans, wheat germ, and egg yolk. The adult RDA for folacin is 180 μg for females and 200 μg for males.[13-16]

Biotin functions as a coenzyme for a number of carboxylase enzymes. Thus, biotin functions in CO_2 transfer. In its coenzyme form biotin is necessary for the conversion of pyruvate to oxaloacetate, acetyl CoA to malonyl CoA, and the catabolism of leucine. Biotin, therefore, does have a metabolic role in energy and amino acid metabolism, as well as fat biosynthesis. Not only can biotin be obtained through dietary means, but intestinal bacterial synthesis and subsequent absorption also provides significant amounts of the vitamin in humans. Thus, simple deficiency, which is rare, must occur at two levels, lack of dietary intake, with either concomitant destruction of intestinal microflora or blocking of biotin absorption from bacterial synthesis. These conditions can be met in some individuals on long-term drug therapy or in persons consuming large quantities of raw egg whites on a daily basis. Raw egg whites contain a protein, avidin, which binds to biotin, making the vitamin unavailable for absorption. The consumption of raw eggs (white and yolk) is not uncommon in some athletic groups. This practice could have adverse effects on biotin status. Good food sources of biotin include liver, sardines, walnuts, peanuts, pecans, egg yolks, oats, chicken, and legumes. There is no RDA for biotin. Intakes of 30 to 100 μg/d would be considered adequate.[13-16]

Folic acid and physical performance studies have not been performed. Thus, no conclusions can be drawn as to how, or whether, this vitamin might interact with physical activity. Only two studies were found that involved biotin. Nijakowski reported no changes in blood biotin values after 3 weeks of ski training.[23] Poston and McCartney reported that brook trout displayed decreased swimming stamina when diets were deficient in biotin.[74] Current data are insufficient to make any statements on the relationships between biotin and physical performance.

B. Ascorbic Acid

Ascorbic acid, or vitamin C, has multiple functions in the body, although a coenzyme for the vitamin has never been identified. Vitamin C functions as a water-soluble antioxidant. The study of antioxidants and exercise is of increasing interest and it is possible that ascorbic acid may have some role in this area. Ascorbic acid is involved in various hydroxylation reactions necessary for the synthesis of collagen, carnitine, epinephrine, norepinephrine, and serotonin. Vitamin C also seems to be involved in normal steroid hormone synthesis and/or release from the adrenals. Finally, vitamin C is needed for proper nonheme iron absorption, transport, and storage. Only certain fruits and vegetables contain vitamin C. Good food sources include citrus fruits, strawberries, cantaloupe, broccoli, green peppers, brussel sprouts, dark green leafy vegetables, and cauliflower. While there is debate as to the optimal level of intake, the RDA is 60 mg/d for adults. Doses of 10 to 20 mg/d will prevent outward signs of scurvy while doses of 100 to 200 mg/d will saturate body pools of the vitamin.[13-16]

Over the course of the last 50 years, numerous investigators have reported a positive effect of vitamin C on various biochemical and physiological parameters of physical performance. Sieburg reported that the physical condition of athletes undergoing training was improved with the addition of vitamin C.[75] Lemmel studied 110 institutionalized children receiving a diet low in ascorbic acid.[76] The addition of 100 mg daily of ascorbic acid over a 4-month period improved the work capacity and liveliness (as assessed by teachers unaware of the study) of 48% of the children as compared with 12% of the children in a control group. Wiebel reported that students receiving vitamin C showed an improved capacity for sports, sleep, and appetite, as compared to students receiving a placebo.[77]

Basu and Ray[78] gave four subjects 600 mg of vitamin C and noted that the onset of fatigue in the finger muscles was definitely delayed as compared to that of controls. Brunner reported improved training in men receiving 200 mg vitamin C per day.[79] Dupain and Loutfi reported that vitamin C delayed fatigue and increased work efficiency in their subjects.[80] Harper et al.[81] studied 69 cadets over a period of 21 weeks. One of two groups received 50 mg ascorbic acid daily, the other a placebo. Treatments were reversed at the end of 10 weeks. Subjects receiving vitamin C had a greater resting vital capacity, greater endurance in breath holding, and a faster resting pulse rate. Hoitink worked subjects on a bicycle ergometer before, during, and after being given 300 mg of vitamin C per day for 1 or 2 weeks.[82] He concluded that ascorbic acid (1) increased the amount of work done; (2) reduced glucose levels, red cell count, hemoglobin values, pulse rate, respiration rate, and systolic blood pressure; and (3) had no effect on blood glycogen, inorganic P, blood Ca, blood lactic acid, urinary creatinine, number of leukocytes, diastolic blood pressure, or pulse pressure.

Another investigator reported that performance of bodily work had a considerable effect on ascorbic acid metabolism in the blood, musculature, and organs, as compared to values of resting controls.[83] These results indicated that for heavy work, vitamin C must be in abundant supply. Namyslowski and Desperak-Secomska[84] determined the whole-blood ascorbic acid levels of 100 students attending a physical culture school and concluded that the students' diet was low in vitamin C and that strenuous exercise had helped produce a state of vitamin C deficiency. Namyslowski also reported that urinary and blood serum ascorbate values decreased in long-distance skiers performing endurance exercise while receiving 100 mg of vitamin C per day;[85] doses of 300 mg daily tended to increase ascorbate values. Comparisons of 30 untrained medical students to 33 physical culture students who performed daily exercise revealed that the physical culture students excreted only half as much ascorbic acid as the sedentary medical students. It was concluded that persons taking physical exercise need extra vitamin C.[86] Nitzescu et al.[87] reported that 500 mg of ascorbic acid given intravenously reduced blood lactic acid levels in cardiac patients at rest and after mild exercise.

Babadzanjan et al.[88] studied 40 train engineers, 20 to 50 years of age, over a 2-month period. Half received a vitamin C supplement (200 mg daily) and the other half received a placebo. Blood ascorbate levels of the supplemented group rose from 0.1 to 0.5 mg per 100 ml before treatment to 0.5 to 1.25 mg per 100 ml after treatment. Tests of nervous system function and visual and auditory acuity were made. Performance of engine drivers given the supplement improved and fatigue of the nervous system during work was reduced. Several other studies have also reported that vitamin C supplementation improved performance in human subjects.[89-93] Hoogerwerf and Hoitink worked 33 male, untrained students on a bicycle ergometer at a rate of 120 W for 10 min.[90] The study was double-blind with 15 students receiving 1000 mg vitamin C daily for 5 days while another group of 15 received a placebo. Blood ascorbate values of the vitamin group rose from 0.81 to 1.58 mg per 100 ml. Excess metabolism due to work decreased and mechanical efficiency rose significantly as compared to that of the placebo group. Three men with initially high blood ascorbic acid levels showed decreased work metabolism and increased mechanical efficiency from the outset. Margolis gave one group of 20 adult male workers 100 mg daily of vitamin C while 20 other workers served as controls.[91] The vitamin C supplement was helpful in reducing fatigue and in increasing or preventing a decrease in muscular endurance. Spioch et al.[92] gave 30 healthy men 500 mg of vitamin C intravenously and reported that O_2 consumption was reduced by 12%, pulmonary ventilation by 18%, O_2 debt by 40%, total energy output by 18%, and pulse by 11%. The coefficient of mechanical efficiency increased by 25%.

Another report has demonstrated increased ascorbic acid utilization and requirements in men subjected to hypoxia and physiological stress.[93] Boddy et al.[94] reported a decrease in leukocyte ascorbic acid content in soccer players following 2 h of physical activity.

Meyer et al.[95] investigated the effect of a predominately fruit diet (500 to 1000 mg vitamin C daily) on the athletic performance of six male and three female university and high school students. Performance included 1 h of exercise per day in addition to running 20 km each day. Measurements were taken before, during, and after the diet. After 14 d on the diet, running times, serum lipids, and serum cholesterol levels of the subjects were reduced. No changes were seen in body mass, hematocrit, hemoglobin concentration, or resting heart rates.

Howald et al.[96] studied 13 athletes on a continuous training program of moderate intensity. Subjects were given a placebo initially for 14 d and then received 1000 mg vitamin C daily for the last 14 d of the study. Tests were performed on a bicycle ergometer. A significant increase in physical working capacity at a heart rate of 170 beats per minute was seen with the administration of vitamin C. Blood glucose levels fell and plasma free fatty acid levels of the subjects rose with the vitamin C intake as compared with values of the placebo. In a study on the acute effects of ascorbic acid, van Huss[97] gave 10 well-trained male subjects a drink containing 3 mg ascorbic acid/kg body weight and at another time, a drink containing 15 mg vitamin C or no vitamin C. Drinks were administered 1, 2, or 3 h before work. The author found no difference between treatments for treadmill performance. However, recovery (heart rate, blood pressure, oxygen consumption) was faster in the supplemented group. Keith and Lawson[98] evaluated the postexercise response to vitamin C supplementation in a group of well-trained cyclists. Subjects performed a 1-h workout at a steady-state workload of 150 W, once after 2 weeks at 86 mg vitamin C per day and once after 2 weeks at 687 mg per day. Plasma cortisol was significantly lower postexercise following the 687-mg treatment. In addition, working heart rates were significantly decreased following the 687-mg supplement. No differences were seen in plasma lactate dehydrogenase (LDH) or creatine phosphokinase (CPK).

Garry and Appenzeller reported that plasma concentrations of vitamin C were significantly greater than baseline levels in subjects finishing a 46-km, high-altitude marathon.[99] Similar results were also reported by Duthie et al.[100] and Gleeson et al.[101] Fishbaine and Butterfield have also reported that serum ascorbic acid levels were higher in a group of men running 5 miles/d for 4 weeks as compared to the sedentary control group.[102] Both groups consumed the same amount of vitamin C (315 mg/d) and plasma values for both groups were within the well-nourished range. Thus, it would seem clear that exercise causes at least a temporary increase in plasma ascorbic acid content. Gleeson et al.[101] suggest that the adrenal gland may be the predominant source of ascorbic acid efflux into plasma during physical activity.

Several studies have examined the effects of ascorbic acid supplementation and work under heat stress conditions. While one study[103] found no effect of 500 mg of vitamin C on recovery heart rate, sweat rate, rectal temperature, or strength in subjects required to work in a hot environment, several other studies[104-107] have demonstrated some interrelationship between vitamin C and the ability of humans to adapt to heat stress. Karnaugh found that vitamin C excretion was increased with exercise in the heat.[105] Strydom et al.[106] and Kotze et al.[107] studied the effects of vitamin C intake upon heat acclimatization. They reported that ascorbic acid at 250 or 500 mg per day reduced total sweat output and rectal temperature in working men undergoing heat acclimatization. Their results indicated that ascorbic acid may be effective in reducing heat strain in unacclimatized individuals. Akamatsu et al.[108] have also reported that adrenal gland ascorbic acid levels are reduced in rats subjected to swimming and heat stress.

Other studies involving animals have also shown relationships between ascorbic acid and physical activity. Early investigations with guinea pigs reported that the addition of vitamin C to the diet raised the basal metabolic rate and respiratory quotient of healthy animals.[109-110] Altenburger demonstrated that the simultaneous administration of glucose and ascorbic acid led to increased liver glycogen stores in normal healthy guinea pigs as compared to animals receiving glucose alone.[111] Stojan and co-workers reported that swimming rats until exhaustion reduced the ascorbic acid content of the adrenal glands to 50 to 65% of baseline values.[112] The same swimming stress, but at simulated high altitude, reduced adrenal ascorbic acid content to even lower levels. Hughes et al.[113] also reported that guinea pigs that swam 1 h daily had lower ascorbic acid content in the adrenal glands, brain, and spleen as compared to control animals on similar vitamin C intakes. Keith and Hicks[114] reported results similar to Hughes et al.[113] for guinea pigs that had been exercised on a treadmill for 1 h/d, 5 d/week for 8 weeks.

Three other animal studies have looked at the effects of supplemental vitamin C on muscular performance. Bushnell and Lehmann have reported that high doses of vitamin C (125 and 500 mg/kg) prevented swimming impairment in mice exposed to ethanol.[115] Richardson and Allen have shown that dietary supplementation of rat diet with vitamin C delayed the onset of fatigue in isolated striated muscle.[116] In a similar fashion, Basu and Biswas[117] also noted that contractions of the gastrocnemius muscle of frog's leg were larger in amplitude, and the development of fatigue delayed, when vitamin C was present in the Ringers solution bathing the muscle.

Not all investigative findings in the half-century of research involving ascorbic acid and physically related parameters have found changes. Many researchers and scientists have found no relationship between vitamin C intake and exercise.

Jetzler and Haffler could not find any difference in endurance capabilities in a 50-km ski race between subjects who had been supplemented with 300 mg of vitamin C and those who had not received the supplement.[118] Fox et al.[119] and Jokl and Suzman[120] gave 40 mg of vitamin C daily to a test group of mine workers and no supplements to a control group (572 total subjects). No differences were seen in strength, skill, or endurance (putting the shot, sprinting 100 yards, and running 1 mile) between the groups. Keys and Henshell studied the effect of the addition of 100 to 220 mg daily of ascorbic acid plus other vitamins upon the ability of 26 young soldiers to perform severe exercise on a motor-driven treadmill.[121] The soldiers were divided into two groups, one receiving a placebo during the first half of the experimental period, the other in the second half. Vitamin C had no effect on pulse rate, urinary excretion of nitrogen, or blood content of lactate, glucose, or ketone bodies. Jenkins and Yudkin found no differences in the resting pulse rate, vital capacity, breath holding time, and endurance abilities of 87 children (11 to 12 years of age) who had received an extra 25 mg of vitamin C daily and a control group of 91 children who had received no extra vitamins.[122] Staton found no differences in delayed muscle soreness as measured by a sit-up test between subjects receiving 100 mg of vitamin C and those receiving a placebo.[123]

Yet another researcher found no difference in the running and training records (over 7 months) of two identical twins when one received a daily tablet containing 300 mg vitamin

C and the other received a placebo containing citric acid.[124] Likewise, Rasch also found no differences in performance in a group of cross-country runners receiving 500 mg vitamin C per day as compared to a matched control group receiving a placebo.[125] The experiment lasted one cross-country season. Diets of the two groups were not controlled. Margaria et al. gave 240 mg of ascorbic acid to subjects 90 min prior to exercise and found no effects on treadmill run time to exhaustion or $\dot{V}O_2$ max as compared to control conditions.[126]

Snigur[127] studied 65 school children for 2 years. Half the children were given a supplement of 100 mg of vitamin C daily. The other half were given no supplement. The diet was calculated as providing 40 mg of ascorbic acid per day. No differences were found in fatigability as estimated by strength of the wrist muscles or vital capacity of the lungs. Krichhoff found no difference in O_2 consumption, CO_2 production, respiratory quotient, respiration rate, respiratory volume, pulse rate, or blood pressure between subjects receiving a placebo and those receiving a vitamin C supplement.[128] The experiment was double-blind and work was performed on a motor-driven treadmill.

Gey et al.[129] studied 286 soldiers for 12 weeks. Subjects were given either 1000 mg of ascorbic acid daily or a placebo in a double-blind manner. No differences were seen between placebo or vitamin C groups in endurance performance or overall improvement as measured by the average distance on a 12-min, walk/run test. Bailey et al.[130,131] worked young male subjects on a level motor-driven treadmill at various speeds. The studies were conducted in a double-blind manner, with volunteers receiving either a placebo or 2000 mg of vitamin C daily for 5 d. No differences were seen between treatment groups, as well as smoking and nonsmoking subjects, for minute ventilation, O_2 uptake, oxygen pulse, or the ratio of tidal volume to vital capacity. Bender and Nash studied the effects of giving 250 to 1000 mg of vitamin C per day, either as orange juice or in tablet form, to normal athletic subjects.[132] A placebo and untreated group were included. Tests involved competitive athletic performance in short and long events (sprints and long-distance running), as well as work efficiency as measured by the Harvard Step Test. There were no differences found between any of the groups and no significant change took place within any group.

Horak and Zenisek gave two groups of well-trained athletes either 200 mg vitamin C daily or a diet high in vitamin C foods.[133] These investigators found no significant relationship between resting ascorbic acid levels and work efficiency. Keren and Epstein studied the effects of vitamin C supplementation on both aerobic and anaerobic performance.[134] Ascorbic acid (1000 mg/d) or a placebo were given in a double-blind manner to 33 males. No differences in $\dot{V}O_2$ max or anaerobic capacity were noted between groups following 21 d of training. Keith and Merrill also reported no differences in maximum grip strength or muscular endurance in 15 subjects receiving 600 mg vitamin C or a placebo.[135] The procedures were performed in a double-blind manner with crossover. Keith and Driskell found no differences in forced expiratory volume, forced vital capacity, resting heart rate, blood pressure, treadmill workload, or postexercise lactic acid in a group of 12 smokers and 10 nonsmokers receiving 300 mg of vitamin C or a placebo for 21 d.[136] Once again the study was performed in a double-blind manner with crossover. In a follow-up study,[137] 1.0 g of vitamin C was given daily for 6 weeks and no significant differences were noted between smokers and nonsmokers, except for reduced postexercise blood lactate values in nonsmokers at 3 weeks. Subjects in the last three studies[135-137] had adequate vitamin C status at the beginning of the study, as measured by plasma and diet evaluations.

Summarizing the vitamin C data is difficult. If the question is "Does extra vitamin C improve physical performance?" then the data are equivocal. Of the studies cited in this review, approximately 50% report increased performance and 50% report no effect. These differences may be related to the initial vitamin C status of the subjects, which is often not reported. Subjects with low initial status might be more apt to improve than subjects with adequate status. Most of the later, well-controlled studies, which did monitor initial vitamin status, found no effect of supplementation on performance. However, several instances of reduced working heart rates have been reported. In addition, in only a couple of studies were vitamin C doses above 1 g per day given (and no effect was seen). Most studies gave between 100 and 1000 mg/d of the vitamin. Thus, even if extra vitamin C has an effect on performance, doses greater than 1.0 g do not seem to be warranted.

The second question one could ask is "Does physical performance affect vitamin C metabolism?" Of the studies addressing this question all reported that physical activity did, in some manner, affect vitamin metabolism (increases or decreases in blood, decreases in urine, decreases in tissues such as adrenals, spleen, and brain, decreased postexercise cortisol). While more work is warranted in this area, the present data do indicate that strenuous physical activity alters vitamin C metabolism. The changes in tissue levels of the vitamin and the reduction in cortisol seen in one study would seem to indicate an increased use of vitamin C with exercise. The studies showing relationships between vitamin C and heat stress also tend to support an increased need for the vitamin. This may mean a higher requirement for the vitamin in persons performing strenuous work. While firm levels of recommendation cannot be made at the present time, persons involved in strenuous physical activity on a regular basis may be advised to consume vitamin C at a level approximating those reported to produce tissue saturation (100 to 200 mg/d).

III. FAT-SOLUBLE VITAMINS
A. Vitamins A, D, and K

The fat-soluble vitamins do not function as coenzymes in metabolism, as do the B complex vitamins. In several instances, the fat-soluble vitamins act more as hormone-like compounds. Because vitamins A, D, and K can be stored in appreciable quantities in the body, exercise or physical activity would be less apt to affect requirements. In addition, because the fat-soluble vitamins are not closely involved, from a metabolic standpoint, in energy metabolism or muscle hypertrophy, the addition of these vitamins to an already adequate diet would be less likely to affect performance.

Vitamin A (retinol) is necessary for normal vision, bone growth, and epithelial tissue integrity and reproduction. The leading food sources of vitamin A include liver, fortified milk and milk products, and fish liver oils. Vitamin A activity can also be obtained by consuming the provitamin beta-carotene from various dark green and bright orange fruits and vegetables: sweet potatoes, spinach, cantaloupe, carrots, broccoli, and others. The 1989 RDA for vitamin A is 1000 retinol equivalents (5000 IU) for adult males and 800 retinol equivalents (4000 IU) for adult females. Vitamin A toxicity or hypervitaminosis A has been observed in adults and young athletes consuming more than 50,000 IU per day of retinol (not beta-carotene).[13-16,138]

Vitamin D (calciferol) is necessary in its active forms for normal formation and mineralization of bones and teeth. The mode of action of vitamin D is similar to that of other steroid hormones. Vitamin D is not found in plentiful supply in foods. Some is present in liver, butter, and egg yolks. The best supply of vitamin D would come from fish liver oils and fortified milk and milk products. However, vitamin D can be produced in the body by exposure of the skin to ultraviolet radiation from the sun. This exposure converts a sterol compound, 7-dehydrocholesterol, into cholecalciferol, which can then be used by the body. Thus, with adequate exposure to sunlight an adult may not have a dietary requirement for calciferol. The RDA for adults for vitamin D is 5 μg (200 IU) each day. As is the case with vitamin A, excessive dietary consumption of vitamin D can lead to toxicity. Adults consuming daily doses of more than 2000 IU over a long period of time should be monitored for toxicity.[13-16]

Vitamin K (quinone) compounds are necessary for normal blood clotting. In the liver, vitamin K is necessary as a cofactor for the enzymatic posttranslational conversion of glutamic acid into alpha-carboxyglutamic acid. This amino acid is an important part of the structure of various blood clotting proteins. Vitamin K-dependent proteins may also play a role in bone metabolism. Vitamin K is found in appreciable quantities in green leafy vegetables such as spinach, turnip greens, cabbage, lettuce, and broccoli. Cheese, egg yolks, and liver also contain some vitamin K. Vitamin K is also produced by the microflora of the gastrointestinal tract in humans. Some of the vitamin produced in this manner is available for absorption. Thus, part of the vitamin K requirement of man is met by nondietary means. Deficiencies of vitamin K in adults are unlikely. Dietary sources must be removed while a concomitant destruction of GI microflora occurs. In addition, some storage of the vitamin does occur in body tissues, thus decreasing chances of a deficiency. The RDA for vitamin K is 65 μg/d for adult females and 80 μg/d for adult males.[13-16]

Very few studies have been performed involving vitamins A and D and physical performance. No studies were uncovered involving vitamin K and performance.

Wald et al.[139] placed five young, adequately nourished men on a low-vitamin A diet (100 IU/day) for a period of 6 months, followed by a vitamin A/beta-carotene supplement (25,000 to 75,000 IU/day) for a period of 6 weeks. There were no significant differences in plasma vitamin A throughout the 6-month deficient period. Performance as measured by a walk/run treadmill test was not different for the subjects at any time measured during the low or supplemented periods. Abrams supplemented a group of four racehorses that had low or marginal vitamin A status with retinol (110 to 125 IU/kg/d) for a 1-year period.[140] Another group of unsupplemented racehorses served as controls. All horses had a history of leg problems. Retinol supplements significantly increased the number of races run by the horses, basically due to a decrease in ligament and tendon problems in the supplemented group. The authors suggested the retinol supplements had improved tendon integrity in the supplemented horses. Garry and Appenzeller measured plasma vitamin A in runners before and after a marathon at high altitude.[99] No significant differences were found.

Very few studies with vitamin D and performance are available. Seidl and Hettinger had six subjects perform cycle ergometer tests intermittently over a 2-year period.[141] The authors reported that subjects exposed to UV radiation improved performance but that vitamin D supplements had no effect. Berven gave children a series of PWC170 tests on a cycle ergometer over a 2-year time period.[142] Some children received UV radiation while others received vitamin D (1500 IU/d) for 2 months followed by a single large dose of vitamin D (400,000 IU) at a later date. One group of children received no treatments and served as controls. No significant effects of UV radiation or vitamin D supplementation on work performance were seen. Bikle et al.[143] tried to determine if vitamin D deficiency in rate would retard the ability of muscle to hypertrophy in response to mechanical stress. No differences in muscle size were noted between deficient and sufficient animals in response to the stress. However, Bell et al.[144] found that blood levels of vitamin D were higher in subjects involved in muscle-increasing exercises as compared to controls. The authors suggested that the exercise may have stimulated the production of active vitamin D, possibly to provide calcium to new muscle tissue.

In conclusion, there appears to be little evidence for vitamin A and D to be extensively involved in physical performance. This seems to be substantiated by the few studies that have been performed using these vitamins in an exercise protocol.

B. Vitamin E

Vitamin E is a common term for a group of compounds identified as tocopherols. Vitamin E function(s) in the body have not been completely elucidated; however, it is known to function *in vitro* as a lipid-soluble antioxidant. Vitamin E apparently protects membranes, both cellular and subcellular, from lipid peroxidation by acting as a free radical scavenger. Other functions for vitamin E have not been clearly defined, although possible relationships to prostanoid biosynthesis have been reported. Good food sources include wheat germ, vegetable oils, nuts, liver, spinach, and fresh corn. The RDA for vitamin E in adults is 8 mg tocopherol equivalents/day (12 IUs) for adult females and 10 mg tocopherol equivalents (15 IUs) for males. However, requirements do vary depending on the type of dietary fat consumed and the presence or absence of other antioxidants and/or pro-oxidants. For example, polyunsaturated fats, iron, aspirin, and ozone exposure would increase vitamin E requirements, while saturated fats, ascorbic acid, selenium, and zinc may decrease requirements.[13-16]

Numerous investigators have reported findings relating vitamin E and physical performance. These reports are described in detail elsewhere in this text. Several studies have reported on the effects of supplemental vitamin E on physical performance.[54,145-153] With a couple of exceptions,[151,152] no improvements were noted. One paper has addressed enzyme changes in relation to vitamin E supplementation and physical stress, finding no effects of the vitamin.[154] Other studies have reported on oxidative damage in tissues with exercise, with and without extra vitamin E.[155-161] Findings generally indicate or suggest that peroxidative damage associated with exercise was reduced with supplemental vitamin E. One paper found no effect of vitamin E on delayed muscle soreness.[162]

IV. SUMMARY

Summarizing the data concerning physical performance and vitamin metabolism is difficult. This is due, in part, to the large number of different vitamins but also to the different types of studies performed (humans vs. different animal species, different dose levels, different forms of physical activity, different performance variables, etc.). In addition, the initial vitamin status of human subjects was not ascertained in many cases.

Physical activity does seem to alter the metabolism of a number of the B-complex vitamins (riboflavin, niacin, pyridoxine, pantothenic acid) as well as ascorbic acid. Whether these alterations represent actual increases in requirement values or just a redistribution of the vitamin in body tissues is often not clear. Some of the data concerning ascorbic acid do, however, give some indication that requirements for this vitamin are increased with physical activity. There are also some data concerning thiamin and riboflavin which may suggest that vitamin needs are increased at the initiation of training programs but that adaptations to reduce those needs may occur as training progresses. Overall, data are generally insufficient at the present time to allow actual requirement values to be established for physically active persons. There is little or no indication that physical activity alters fat-soluble vitamin metabolism to the point where requirements would change. The possible exception may be vitamin E, which is discussed elsewhere.

Does vitamin supplementation in large amounts to adequately nourished subjects increase performance? This is a difficult question to answer. Several studies do suggest an ergogenic effect of vitamin megadoses. However, in most well-controlled studies in which subjects' initial vitamin status was adequate, no effect of vitamin megadoses on performance were seen. Pantothenic acid supplementation and thiamin supplementation with high-carbohydrate diets seem to warrant further research in this area. With the exception of perhaps vitamin C and vitamin E, most vitamins have not been adequately studied.

Many of the studies in the vitamin/physical activity area have been poorly controlled and designed. Future studies should determine the initial vitamin status of their subjects. Subjects whose initial status for a vitamin is low or persons taking large quantities of a vitamin prior to entry into a study should be eliminated from the study. Only when this point is addressed will valid results be obtained to the questions addressed in this chapter.

REFERENCES

1. **Grandjean, F., Hursh, L. M., Majure, W. C., and Hanley, D. F.,** Nutrition knowledge and practices of college athletes, *Med. Sci. Sports Exercise,* 13, 82, 1981.
2. **Percy, E.,** Ergogenic aids in athletics, *Med. Sci. Sports,* 10, 298, 1978.
3. **United States Senate,** Proper and improper use of drugs by athletes, June 18, and July 12–13, 1973. U.S. Government Printing Office, Washington, D.C., 1973.
4. **Bentivegna, A.,** Diet, fitness and athletic performance, *Phys. Sports Med.,* 7, 99, 1979.
5. **Stensland, S. H. and Sobal, J.,** Dietary practices of ballet, jazz and modern dancers, *J. Am. Diet. Assoc.,* 92, 319, 1992.
6. **Parr, R. B., Porter, M. A., and Hodgson, S. C.,** Nutrition knowledge and practices of coaches, trainers, and athletes, *Phys. Sports Med.,* 12, 126, 1984.
7. **Nieman, D. C., Gates, J. R., Butler, J. V., Pollett, L. M., Dietrich, S. J., and Lutz, R. D.,** Supplementation patterns in marathon runners, *J. Am. Diet. Assoc.,* 89, 1615, 1989.
8. **Lamar-Hildebrand, N., Saldanha, L., and Endres, J.,** Dietary and exercise practices of college-aged female bodybuilders, *J. Am. Diet. Assoc.,* 89, 1308, 1989.
9. **Grandjean, A. C.,** Vitamins, diet, and the athlete, *Clin. Sports Med.,* 2, 105, 1983.
10. **Clarkson, P. M.,** Vitamins and trace minerals, in *Ergogenics, Enhancement of Performance in Exercise and Sport,* Lamb, D. R. and Williams, M. H., Eds., Perspectives in Exercise Science and Sports Medicine, Vol. 4, Wm. C. Brown, 1991, 123.
11. **Archdeacon, J. W. and Murlin, J. R.,** The effects of thiamine depletion and restoration of muscular efficiency and endurance, *J. Nutr.,* 28, 241, 1944.
12. **van der Beek, E. J., van Dokkum, W., Schrijver, J., Wedel, M., Gaillard, A. W. K., Wesstra, A., van de Weerd, H., and Hermus, R. J. J.,** Thiamin, riboflavin, and vitamins B-6 and C: impact of combined restricted intake on functional performance in man, *Am. J. Clin. Nutr.,* 48, 1451, 1988.
13. *Recommended Dietary Allowances,* 10th ed., National Academy of Sciences, Washington, D.C., 1989.
14. **Krause, M. V. and Mahan, L. K.,** *Food, Nutrition and Diet Therapy,* 7th ed., W. B. Saunders, Philadelphia, 1984.
15. **Machlin, L. J., Ed.,** *Handbook of Vitamins,* 2nd ed., Marcel Dekker, New York, 1991.
16. **Hunt, S. M. and Groff, J. L.,** *Advanced Nutrition and Human Metabolism,* West, St. Paul, MN, 1990.
17. **Bialecki, M. and Nijakowski, F.,** Influences of physical effort on the blood level of thiamin in tissues and blood, *Acta Physiol. Pol.,* 15, 192, 1964.
18. **Stewart, G. A.,** Drugs, performance and responses to exercise in the racehorse, *Aust. Vet. J.,* 48, 544, 1972.
19. **McNeill, A. W. and Mooney, T. J.,** Relationship among carbohydrate loading, elevated thiamine intake and cardiovascular endurance of conditioned mice, *J. Sports Med.,* 23, 257, 1983.
20. **McCormick, W. J.,** Vitamin B1 and physical endurances, *Med. Rec.,* 152, 439, 2940.
21. **Karpovich, P. V. and Millman, N.,** Vitamin B1 and endurance, *N. Engl. J. Med.,* 226, 881, 1942.
22. **Keys, A., Henschel, A. F., Mickelsen, O., and Brozek, J. M.,** The performance of normal young men on controlled thiamine intakes, *J. Nutr.,* 26, 399, 1943.
23. **Nijakowski, F.,** Assays of some vitamins of the B complex group in human blood in relation to muscular effort, *Acta Physiol. Pol.,* 17, 397, 1966.
24. **Early, R. and Carlson, B.,** Water soluble vitamin therapy on the delay of fatigue from physical activity in hot climatic conditions, *Int. Z. Angew. Physiol.,* 27, 43, 1969.
25. **Haralambie, G.,** Vitamin B2 status in athletes and the influence of riboflavin administration on neuro-muscular irritability, *Nutr. Metab.,* 20, 1, 1976.
26. **Read, M. and McGuffin, S.,** The effect of B complex supplementation on endurance performance, *J. Sports Med. Phys. Fitness,* 23, 178, 1983.
27. **Bonke, D.,** Influence of vitamin B1, B6, and B12 on the control of fine motoric movements, in *Nutrition and Neurobiology,* Sumogyi, J. C. and Hötzel, D., Eds., Biblio. Nutr. Diet (series), 38, 104, 1986.
28. **Caster, W. O. and Mickelsen, O.,** Effect of diet and stress on the thiamin and pyramin excretion of normal young men maintained on controlled intakes of thiamin, *Nutr. Res.,* 11, 549, 1991.
29. **Hunter, K. E. L. and Turkki, P. R.,** Effect of exercise on riboflavin status of rats, *J. Nutr.,* 117, 298, 1987.
30. **Delachaux, A. and Ott, W.,** Quelques observations sur le metabolisme du fer et de vitamines au cours de l'effort physique et de l'entrainement, *Schweiz. Med. Wochenschr.,* 73, 1026, 1943.
31. **Friedemann, T. E., Ivy, A. C., Jung, F. T., and Sheft, B. B.,** Work at high altitudes. IV. Utilization of thiamine and riboflavin at low and high dietary intakes, *Q. Bull. Northwest. Univ. Med. Sch.,* 23, 177, 1949.
32. **Potenza, P.,** Estere fosforica della riboflavina et fatica, *Vitaminologia,* 17, 345, 1959.

33. **Tucker, R. G., Mickelsen, D., and Keys, A.,** The influence of sleep, work, diuresis, heat, acute starvation, thiamine intake and bed rest on human riboflavin excretion, *J. Nutr.*, 72, 251, 1960.

34. **Belko, A. Z., Obarzanek, E., Kalkwarf, H. J., Rotter, M. A., Bogusz, S., Miller, D., Haas, J. D., and Roe, D. A.,** Effects of exercise on riboflavin requirements of young women, *Am. J. Clin. Nutr.*, 37, 509, 1983.

35. **Belko, A. Z., Obarzanek, M. P., Rotter, B. S., Urgan, G., Weinberg, S., and Roe, D. A.,** Effects of aerobic exercise and weight loss on riboflavin requirements of moderately obese, marginally deficient young women, *Am. J. Clin. Nutr.*, 40, 553, 1984.

36. **Belko, A. Z., Meredith, M. P., Kalkwarf, H. J., Obarzanek, E., Weinberg, S., Roach, R., McKeon, G., and Roe, D. A.,** Effects of exercise on riboflavin requirements: biological validation in weight reducing women, *Am. J. Clin. Nutr.*, 41, 270, 1985.

37. **Yoon, J. S., Trebler, L., and Roe, D. A.,** Effect of exercise on the riboflavin requirements of older women, *Fed. Proc.*, 46, 1166, 1987.

38. **Tremblay, A., Boiland, F., Breton, M., Bessette, H., and Roberge, A. G.,** The effects of a riboflavin supplementation on the nutritional status and performance of elite swimmers, *Nutr. Res.*, 4, 201, 1984.

39. **Keith, R. E. and Alt, L. A.,** Riboflavin status of female athletes consuming normal diets, *Nutr. Res.*, 11, 727, 1991.

40. **Lewis, R. D., Yates, C. Y., and Driskell, J. A.,** Riboflavin and thiamin status and birth outcome as a function of maternal aerobic exercise, *Am. J. Clin. Nutr.*, 48, 110, 1988.

41. **Carlson, L. A., Havel, R. J., Ekelund, L. G., and Holmgren, A.,** Effect of nicotinic acid on the turnover rate and oxidation of the free fatty acids of plasma in man during exercise, *Metab. Clin. Exp.*, 12, 837, 1963.

42. **Bergstrom, J., Hultman, E., Jorfeldt, L., Pernow, B., and Wahnen, J.,** Effect of nicotinic acid on physical working capacity and on metabolism of muscle, *J. Appl. Physiol.*, 26, 170, 1969.

43. **Pernow, B. and Saltin, B.,** Availability of substrates and capacity for prolonged heavy exercise, *J. Appl. Physiol.*, 31, 416, 1971.

44. **Lassers, B. W., Wahlqvist, M. L., Kaijser, L., and Carlson, L. A.,** Effect of nicotinic acid on myocardial metabolism in man at rest and during exercise, *J. Appl. Physiol.*, 33, 72, 1972.

45. **Kaijser, L., Nye, E. R., Eklund, B., Olsson, A. G., and Carlson, L. A.,** The relation between carbohydrate extraction by the forearm and arterial free fatty acid concentration in man. I. Forearm work with nicotinic acid, *Scand. J. Clin. Lab. Invest.*, 38, 41, 1978.

46. **Frankau, I.,** Acceleration of co-ordinated muscular effort by nicotinamide, *Br. Med. J.*, 2, 601, 1943.

47. **Hilsendager, D. and Karpovich, P. V.,** Ergogenic effect of glycine and niacin separately and in combination, *Res. Q. Am. Assoc. Health Phys. Educ. Recreat.*, 35, 389, 1964.

48. **Borisov, I. M.,** Niacin allowance of students of a sports college, *Vopr. Pitan.*, 6, 43, 1977.

49. **Jett'e, M., Pelletier, O., Parker, L., and Thoden, J.,** The nutritional and metabolic effects of a carbohydrate-rich diet in a glycogen supercompensation training regimen, *Am. J. Clin. Nutr.*, 31, 2140, 1978.

50. **Yefremov, V. V. and Faburken, Y. M.,** Peculiarities of pyridoxine and nicotinic acid metabolism in experimental animals under the physical stresses of prolonged swimming, *Vopr. Pitan.*, 3, 39, 1973.

51. **Shock, N. W. and Sebrell, W. H.,** The effect of different concentrations of pyridoxine hydrochloride on the work output of perfused frog muscles, *Am. J. Physiol.*, 146, 399, 1946.

52. **Richardson, J. H. and Chenman, M.,** Effect of vitamin B6 on muscle fatigue, *J. Sports Med. Phys. Fitness*, 21, 119, 1981.

53. **McMillan, J., Keith, R. E., and Stone, M. H.,** The effects of supplemental vitamin B6 and exercise on the contractile properties of rat muscle, *Nutr. Res.*, 8, 73, 1988.

54. **Lawrence, J. D., Smith, J. L., Bower, R. C., and Riehl, W. P.,** Effect of alpha-tocopherol (vitamin E) and pyridoxine HCL (vitamin B6) on the swimming endurance of training swimmers, *J. Am. Coll. Health Assoc.*, 23, 219, 1975.

55. **Borisov, I. M.,** Pyridoxine allowance of the students in a sports school, *Vopr. Pitan.*, 3, 48, 1977.

56. **Moretti, C., Fabbri, A., Gnessi, L., Bonifacio, U., Fraioli, F., and Isidori, A.,** Pyridoxine (B6) suppresses the rise in prolactin and increases the rise in growth hormones induced by exercise, *N. Engl. J. Med.*, 307, 444, 1982.

57. **Hatcher, L., Leklem, J., and Campbell, D.,** Altered vitamin B6 metabolism during exercise in man: effect of carbohydrate modified diets and B6 supplements, *Med. Sci. Sports Exercise*, 14, 112, 1982.

58. **deVos, A., Leklem, J., and Campbell, D.,** Carbohydrate loading, vitamin B6 supplementation and fuel metabolism during exercise in man, *Med. Sci. Sports Exercise*, 14, 137, 1982.

59. **Manore, M. M. and Leklem, J. E.,** Effect of carbohydrate and vitamin B6 on fuel substrates during exercise in women, *Med. Sci. Sports Exercise*, 20, 233, 1988.

60. **Leklem, J. E. and Shultz, T. D.,** Increased plasma pyridoxal 5'-phosphate and vitamin B6 in male adolescents after a 4500-meter run, *Am. J. Clin. Nutr.*, 38, 541, 1983.

61. **Hofman, A., Reynolds, R. D., Smoak, B. L., Villanueva, V. G., and Deuster, P. A.,** Plasma pyridoxal and pyridoxal 5'-phosphate concentrations in response to ingestion of water or glucose polymer during a 2-h run, *Am. J. Clin. Nutr.,* 53, 84, 1991.

62. **Dreon, D. M. and Butterfield, G. E.,** Vitamin B6 utilization in active and inactive young men, *Am. J. Clin. Nutr.,* 43, 816, 1986.

63. **Manore, M. M., Leklem, J. E., and Walter, M. C.,** Vitamin B6 metabolism as affected by exercise in trained and untrained women fed diets differing in carbohydrate and vitamin B6 content, *Am. J. Clin. Nutr.,* 46, 995, 1987.

64. **Yates, C. Y., Boylan, L. M., Lewis, R. D., and Driskell, J. A.,** Maternal aerobic exercise and vitamin B6 status, *Am. J. Clin. Nutr.,* 48, 117, 1988.

65. **Shock, N. W. and Sebrell, W. H.,** The effects of changes in concentration of pantothenate on the work output of perfused frog muscle, *Am. J. Physiol.,* 142, 274, 1944.

66. **Ralli, E. P. and Dumm, M. E.,** Relation of pantothenic acid to adrenal cortical function, *Vitam. Horm.,* 11, 133, 1953.

67. **Bialecki, M. and Nijakowski, F.,** Behavior of pantothenic acid in tissues and blood of white rats following short and prolonged physical strain, *Acta Physiol. Pol.,* 18, 25, 1967.

68. **Nice, C., Reeves, A. G., Brinck-Johnsen, T., and Noll, W.,** The effects of pantothenic acid on human exercise capacity, *J. Sports Med.,* 24, 26, 1984.

69. **Litoff, D., Scherzer, H., and Harrison, J.,** Effects of pantothenic acid on human exercise, *Med. Sci. Sports Exercise,* 17, 287, 1985.

70. **Ryan, A.,** Nutritional practices in athletics abroad, *Phys. Sportsmed.,* 5, 33, 1977.

71. **Wetzel, N. C., Hopwood, H. H., Kuechle, M. E., and Grueninger, R. M.,** Growth failure in school children: further studies of vitamin B12 dietary supplements, *J. Clin. Nutr.,* 1, 17, 1952.

72. **Montoye, H. J., Spata, P. J., Pinckney, V., and Barron, L.,** Effects of vitamin B12 supplementation on physical fitness and growth of young boys, *J. Appl. Physiol.,* 7, 589, 1955.

73. **Tin-May-Than, Ma-Win-May, Khin-Sann-Aung, and Mya-Tu, M.,** The effect of vitamin B12 on physical performance capacity, *Br. J. Nutr.,* 40, 269, 1978.

74. **Poston, H. A. and McCartney, T. H.,** Effect of dietary biotin and lipid on growth, stamina, lipid metabolism and biotin-containing enzymes in brook trout (Salvelinus fontinalis), *J. Nutr.,* 104, 315, 1974.

75. **Sieburg, H.,** Redoxon as a tonic for sportsmen, *Duetsch. Med. Wochenschr.,* 13, 11, 1937.

76. **Lemmel, G.,** Vitamin C deficiency and general capacity for work, *Munch. Med. Wochenschr.,* 85, 1381, 1938.

77. **Wiebel, H.,** Studies of dosage with vitamin C in athletic female students, *Duetsch. Med. Wochenschr.,* 65, 60, 1939.

78. **Basu, N. M. and Ray, G. K.,** The effect of vitamin C on the incidence of fatigue in human muscles, *Indian J. Med. Res.,* 28, 419, 1940.

79. **Brunner, H.,** Vitamin C and armessport, *Schweiz. Med. Wochenschr.,* 71, 715, 1941.

80. **DuPain, R. and Loutfi, M.,** Vitamin C et courbatures, *Rev. Med. Suisse Romande,* 63, 640, 1943.

81. **Harper, A. A., MacKay, I. F. S., Raper, H. S., and Camm, G. L.,** Vitamins and physical fitness, *Br. Med. J.,* i, 243, 1943.

82. **Hoitink, A. W.,** Vitamin C and work. Studies on the influence of work and of vitamin C intake on the human organism, *Verh. Nederlands Inst. Praevent. Geneesk,* 4, 176, 1946.

83. **Wachholder, K.,** Rise in the turnover and destruction of ascorbic acid (vitamin C) during muscle work, *Arbeitsphysiologie,* 14, 342, 1951.

84. **Namyslowski, L. and Desperak-Secomska, B.,** The vitamin C content of the blood in a selected group of students during 1952 and 1953, *Rocz. Panstw. Zakl. Hig.,* 6, 289, 1955.

85. **Namyslowski, L.,** Investigations of the vitamin C requirements of athletes during physical exertion, *Rocz. Panstw. Zakl. Hig.,* 7, 97, 1956.

86. **Bacinskij, P. P.,** Effect of physical activity on the vitamin C and B1 supply of the body, *Vopr. Pitan.,* 18, 53, 1959.

87. **Nitzescu, I. I., Marinescu, G., Gardev, M., Ozun, M., Popa, A., and Cavrila, I. M.,** Blood lactic acid and ascorbic acid in cardiac insufficiency, *Z. Gesamte Inn. Med.,* 14, 458, 1959.

88. **Babadzanjan, M. G., Kalnyn, V. R., Koslynn, S. A., and Kostina, E. I.,** Effect of vitamin supplements on some physiological functions of workers in electric locomotive teams, *Vopr. Pitan.,* 19, 18, 1960.

89. **Prokop, L.,** The effect of natural vitamin C on oxygen utilization and metabolic efficiency, *N A F Arzt. Fortbildung,* 49, 448, 1960.

90. **Hoogerwerf, A. and Hoitink, A. W.,** The influence of vitamin C administration on the mechanical efficiency of the human organism, *Int. Z. Angew. Physiol. Arbeitsphysiol.,* 20, 164, 1963.

91. **Margolis, A. M.,** Vitamin C status of miners and some other population groups in the Don basin, *Vopr. Pitan.,* 23, 78, 1964.

92. **Spioch, F., Kobza, R., and Mazur, B.,** Influence of vitamin C upon certain functional changes and the coefficient of mechanical efficiency in humans during physical effort, *Acta Physiol. Pol.,* 17, 204, 1966.
93. **Asano, K.,** The influence of hypoxia and exercise on ascorbic acid metabolism, *Jpn. J. Phys. Sport Med.,* 21, 69, 1972.
94. **Boddy, K., Hume, R., King, P. C., Weyers, E., and Rowan, T.,** Total body, plasma and erythrocyte potassium and leucocyte ascorbic acid in "ultra-fit" subjects, *Clin. Sci. Mol. Med.,* 46, 449, 1974.
95. **Meyer, B. J., deBruin, E. J., Brown, J. M., Bieler, E. U., Meyer, A. C., and Grey, P. C.,** The effect of a predominately fruit diet on athletic performance, *Plant Foods Man,* 1, 223, 1975.
96. **Howald, H., Segesser, B., and Korner, W. F.,** Ascorbic acid and athletic performance, *Ann. N.Y. Acad. Sci.,* 258, 458, 1975.
97. **Van Huss, W.,** What made the Russians run?, *Nutr. Today,* 1, 20, 1966.
98. **Keith, R. E. and Lawson, C. J.,** Effects of dietary ascorbic acid and exercise on plasma ascorbic acid, cortisol, serum enzymes, blood pressure and heartrate response in trained cyclists, *FASEB J.,* 5, A1655, 1991.
99. **Garry, P. J. and Appenzeller, O.,** Vitamins A and C and endurance races, *Ann. Sports Med.,* 1, 82, 1983.
100. **Duthie, G. G., Robertson, J. D., Maughn, R. J., and Morrice, P. C.,** Blood antioxidant status and erythrocyte lipid peroxidation following distance running, *Arch. Biochem. Biophys.,* 282, 78, 1990.
101. **Gleeson, M., Robertson, J. D., and Maughn, R. J.,** Influence of exercise on ascorbic acid status in man, *Clin. Sci.,* 73, 501, 1987.
102. **Fishbaine, B. and Butterfield, G.,** Ascorbic acid status of running and sedentary men, *Int. J. Vitam. Nutr. Res.,* 54, 273, 1984.
103. **Henschel, A., Taylor, H. L., Brozek, J., Mickelsen, O., and Keys, A.,** Vitamin C and the ability to work in hot environments, *Am. J. Trop. Med.,* 24, 259, 1944.
104. **Visagie, M. E., du Plessis, J. P., and Laubscher, N. F.,** Effect of vitamin C supplementation on black mineworkers, *S. Afr. Med. J.,* 49, 889, 1975.
105. **Karnaugh, N.,** Effect of physical work and heat microclimate on the excretion of 17-hydroxycorticosteroids and ascorbic acid, *Vrach. Delo,* 3, 134, 1976.
106. **Strydom, N. B., Kotze, H. F., van der Walt, W. H., and Rogers, G. G.,** Effect of ascorbic acid on rate of heat acclimatization, *J. Appl. Physiol.,* 41, 202, 1976.
107. **Kotze, H. F., van der Walt, W. H., Rogers, G. G., and Strydom, N. B.,** Effects of plasma ascorbic acid levels on heat acclimatization in man, *J. Appl. Physiol.,* 42, 771, 1977.
108. **Akamatsu, A., Whan, Y. W., Yamada, K., and Hosoya, N.,** The effect of high environmental temperature and exercise on the metabolism of ascorbic acid in rats, *Vitamins (Jpn.),* 60, 199, 1986.
109. **Mosonyi, J. and Rigo, L.,** Influence of vitamin C on the gaseous exchange of normal scorbutic guinea pigs, *Z. Physiol. Chem.,* 222, 100, 1933.
110. **Mosonyi, J. and Rigo, L.,** Effect of vitamin C on the basal metabolism of healthy and scorbutic guinea pigs, *Magy. Orv. Arch.,* 34, 64, 1934.
111. **Altenburger, E.,** Relationship of ascorbic acid to the glycogen metabolism of the liver, *Klin. Wochenschr.,* 15, 1129, 1936.
112. **Stojan, B., Pfefferkorn, B., and Schmieder, J.,** Studies on the ascorbic acid content of the adrenals of the rat after muscular work under normal and lowered oxygen partial pressure, *Acta Biol. Med. Ger.,* 18, 369, 1967.
113. **Hughes, R. E., Jones, P. R., Williams, R. S., and Weight, P. F.,** Effect of prolonged swimming on the distribution of ascorbic acid and cholesterol in the tissues of the guinea pig, *Life Sci.,* 10, 661, 1971.
114. **Keith, R. E. and Hicks, V.,** Effects of exercise on ascorbic acid tissue levels in male guinea pigs, *FASEB J.,* 4, A750, 1990.
115. **Bushnel, R. G. and Lehmann, A. G.,** Antagonistic effect of sodium ascorbate on ethanol-induced changes in swimming of mice, *Behav. Brain Res.,* 1, 351, 1980.
116. **Richardson, J. H. and Allen, R. B.,** Dietary supplementation with vitamin C delays onset of fatigue in isolated striated muscle of rats, *Can. J. Appl. Sport Sci.,* 8, 140, 1983.
117. **Basu, N. M. and Biswas, P.,** The influence of ascorbic acid on contractions and the incidence of fatigue of different types of muscles, *Indian J. Med. Res.,* 28, 405, 1940.
118. **Jetzler, A. and Haffler, C.,** Vitamin C-bedarf bei einmaliger sportlicher dauerleistung, *Wein. Med. Wochenschr.,* 89, 332, 1939.
119. **Fox, F. W., Dangerfield, L. F., Gottlich, S. F., and Jokl, E.,** Vitamin C requirements of native mine labourers. An experimental study, *Br. Med. J.,* ii, 143, 1940.
120. **Jokl, E. and Suzman, H.,** A study of the effects of vitamin C upon physical efficiency, *Transvaal Mine Med. Off. Assoc. Proc.,* 19, 292, 1940.
121. **Keys, A. and Henschel, A. F.,** Vitamin supplementation of U.S. Army rations in relation to fatigue and the ability to do muscular work, *J. Nutr.,* 23, 259, 1942.

122. **Jenkins, G. N. and Yudkin, J.,** Vitamins and physiological function, *Br. Med. J.,* ii, 265, 1943.

123. **Staton, W. M.,** The influence of ascorbic acid in minimizing post-exercise muscle soreness in young men, *Res. Q. Am. Assoc. Health Phys. Educ. Recreat.,* 23, 356, 1952.

124. **Vinarickij, R.,** An attempt to improve the efficiency of medium distance runners by large doses of vitamin B1, B2 and C, *Scripta Med.,* 27, 1, 1954.

125. **Rasch, P.,** Effects of vitamin C supplementation on cross country runners, *Sportzarztliche Praxis,* 5, 10, 1962.

126. **Margaria, R., Agheno, P., and Rovelli, E.,** The effect of some drugs on the maximal capacity of athletic performance in man, *Int. Z. Angew. Physiol.,* 20, 281, 1964.

127. **Snigur, O. I.,** Signs of fatigue in school children in different states of ascorbic acid supply, *Gig. Sanit.,* 7, 117, 1966.

128. **Kirchhoff, H. W.,** Effect of vitamin C on energy expenditure and circulatory and ventilatory function in stress studies, *Nutr. Diet,* 11, 184, 1969.

129. **Gey, G. O., Cooper, K. H., and Bottenberg, R. A.,** Effect of ascorbic acid on endurance performance and athletic injury, *JAMA,* 211, 105, 1970.

130. **Bailey, D. A., Carron, A. V., Teece, R. G., and Wehner, H. J.,** Vitamin C supplementation related to physiological response to exercise in smoking and nonsmoking subjects, *Am. J. Clin. Nutr.,* 23, 905, 1970.

131. **Bailey, D. A., Carron, A. V., Teece, R. G., and Wehner, H. J.,** Effect of vitamin C supplementation upon the physiological response to exercise in trained and untrained subjects, *Int. J. Vitam. Res.,* 40, 435, 1970.

132. **Bender, A. E. and Nash, A. H.,** Vitamin C and physical performance, *Plant Foods Man,* 1, 217, 1975.

133. **Horak, J. and Zenisek, A.,** Vitamin C blood level before and after laboratory load and its relation to cardiorespiratory performance parameters in top sportsmen, *Cas. Lek. Cesk.,* 116, 679, 1977.

134. **Keren, G. and Epstein, Y.,** Effect of high dosage vitamin C intake on aerobic and anaerobic capacity, *J. Sports Med. Phys. Fitness,* 20, 145, 1980.

135. **Keith, R. E. and Merrill, E.,** The effects of vitamin C on maximum grip strength and muscular endurance, *J. Sports Med. Phys. Fitness,* 23, 253, 1983.

136. **Keith, R. E. and Driskell, J. A.,** Lung function and treadmill performance of smoking and nonsmoking males receiving ascorbic acid supplements, *Am. J. Clin. Nutr.,* 36, 840, 1982.

137. **Driskell, J. A. and Herbert, W. G.,** Pulmonary function and treadmill performance of males receiving ascorbic acid supplements, *Nutr. Rep. Int.,* 32, 443, 1985.

138. **Fumich, R. M. and Essig, G. W.,** Hypervitaminosis A: case report in an adolescent soccer player, *Am. J. Sports Med.,* 11, 34, 1983.

139. **Wald, G., Brouha, L., and Johnson, R. E.,** Experimental vitamin A deficiency and the ability to perform muscular exercise, *Am. J. Physiol.,* 137, 551, 1942.

140. **Abrams, J. T.,** The effect of dietary vitamin A supplements on the clinical condition and track performance of racehorses, in *Nutritional Aspects of Physical Performance,* Somogyi, J. C. and deWijn, J. F., Eds., Biblio. Nutr. Diet (series), 27, 113, 1979.

141. **Seidl, E. and Hettinger, T.,** Der einfluss von vitamin D-3 auf kraft und leistungsfahigkeit des gesunden erwachsenen, *Int. Z. Angew. Physiol.,* 16, 365, 1957.

142. **Berven, H.,** The physical working capacity of healthy children: seasonal variation and effect of ultraviolet radiation and vitamin D supply, *Acta Paediatr. Scand.* (Suppl.), 148, 1, 1963.

143. **Bikle, D. D., Hagler, L., Lollini, L. O., Hull, S. F., and Herman, R. H.,** Work induced muscle hypertrophy in vitamin D-deficient rats, *Am. J. Clin. Nutr.,* 32, 515, 1979.

144. **Bell, N. H., Godsen, R. N., Henry, D. P., Shary, J., and Epstein, S.,** The effects of muscle-building exercise on vitamin D and mineral metabolism, *J. Bone Miner. Res.,* 3, 369, 1988.

145. **Talbot, D. and Jamieson, J.,** An examination of the effect of vitamin E on the performance of highly trained swimmers, *Can. J. Appl. Sport Sci.,* 2, 67, 1977.

146. **Brunnell, R. H., DeRitter, E., and Rubin, S. H.,** Effect of feeding polyunsaturated fatty acids with a low vitamin E diet on blood levels of tocopherol in men performing hard physical labor, *Am. J. Clin. Nutr.,* 28, 706, 1975.

147. **Sharman, I. M., Down, M. G., and Sen, R. N.,** The effects of vitamin E and training on physiological function and athletic performance in adolescent swimmers, *Br. J. Nutr.,* 26, 265, 1971.

148. **Sharman, I. M., Down, M. G., and Norgan, N. G.,** The effects of vitamin E on physiological function and athletic performance of trained swimmers, *J. Sports Med.,* 16, 215, 1976.

149. **Lawrence, J. D., Bower, R. C., Riehl, W. P., and Smith, J. L.,** Effects of alpha-tocopherol acetate on the swimming endurance of trained swimmers, *Am. J. Clin. Nutr.,* 28, 205, 1975.

150. **Shephard, R. J., Campbell, R., Pimm, P., Stuart, D., and Wright, G. R.,** Vitamin E, exercise and the recovery from physical activity, *Eur. J. Appl. Physiol.,* 33, 119, 1974.

151. **Liang, H., Wang, G., and Li, Z.,** A research of the relationships between vitamin E and motor ability, *Chin. J. Sports Med.,* 2, 33, 1983.

152. **Simon-Schnass, I. and Korniszewski, L.,** The influence of vitamin E on rheological parameters in high altitude mountaineers, *Int. J. Vitam. Nutr. Res.,* 60, 26, 1990.
153. **Watt, T., Romet, T. T., McFarlane, I., McGuey, D., and Allen, C.,** Vitamin E and oxygen consumption, *Lancet,* 2, 354, 1974.
154. **Helgheim, I., Hetland, O., Nilsson, S., Ingjer, F., and Stromme, S. B.,** Effects of vitamin E on serum enzyme levels following heavy exercise, *Eur. J. Appl. Physiol.,* 40, 283, 1979.
155. **Quintanilha, A. T. and Packer, L.,** Vitamin E, physical exercise and tissue oxidative damage, *Ciba Found. Symp.,* 101, 56, 1983.
156. **Brady, P. S., Brady, L. J., and Ullrey, D. E.,** Selenium, vitamin E and the response to swimming stress in the rat, *J. Nutr.,* 109, 1103, 1979.
157. **Dillard, C. J., Liton, R. E., Savin, W. M., Dumelin, E. E., and Tappel, A. L.,** Effects of exercise, vitamin E and ozone on pulmonary function and lipid peroxidation, *J. Appl. Physiol. Respir. Environ. Exercise Physiol.,* 45, 927, 1978.
158. **Gohil, K., Rothfuss, L., Lang, J., and Packer, L.,** Effect of exercise training on tissue vitamin E and ubiquinone content, *J. Appl. Physiol.,* 63, 1638, 1987.
159. **Simon-Schnass, I. and Pabst, H.,** Influence of vitamin E on physical performance, *Int. J. Vitam. Nutr. Res.,* 58, 49, 1988.
160. **Pincemail, J., Deby, C., Camus, G., Pirnay, F., Bouchez, R., Massaux, L., and Goutier, R.,** Tocopherol mobilization during intensive exercise, *Eur. J. Appl. Physiol.,* 57, 189, 1988.
161. **Sumida, S., Tanaka, K., Kitao, H., and Nakadomo, F.,** Exercise-induced lipid peroxidation and leakage of enzymes before and after vitamin E supplementation, *Int. J. Biochem.,* 21, 835, 1989.
162. **Francis, K. T. and Hoobler, T.,** Failure of vitamin E and delayed muscle soreness, *J. Med. Assoc. Alabama,* 55, 15, 1986.

Chapter 9

THE SIGNIFICANCE OF VITAMIN E AND FREE RADICALS IN PHYSICAL EXERCISE

Valerian E. Kagan
Vladimir B. Spirichev
Elena A. Serbinova
Eric Witt
Alexander N. Erin
Lester Packer

CONTENTS

0-8493-7911-3/94/$0.00+$.50
© 1994 by CRC Press, Inc.

I. INTRODUCTION

Vitamin E is an essential fat-soluble vitamin. Vitamin E is a generic name for a group of naturally occurring substances found mainly in plant oils that exhibit vitamin E-like activity. The term vitamin E embraces compounds represented by methyl derivatives of tocol and tocotrienol, possessing the biological activity of α-tocopherol (Figure 1). The term tocopherols is attributed only to derivatives of tocol and, strictly speaking, is not fully identical to the term vitamin E, which also includes tocotrienols. However, because tocopherols are the most abundant forms of vitamin E, we, in common with others in the field, shall use the terms vitamin E and tocopherols as equivalents.

The chemical structure and properties of tocopherols, the biological activity of different forms of vitamin E, main manifestations of vitamin E deficiency, as well as tocopherol content of natural products and body tissues, have been extensively studied. Thus, it is not necessary to present all these data in this chapter and we refer the reader to reviews on the topics.[1-9]

II. MECHANISM OF ACTION OF VITAMIN E

The specific mechanisms of vitamin E action at the molecular and biochemical levels have not yet been completely deciphered and are the subject of intensive investigation.

The more than 65-year history of these investigations has culminated in the polyfunctional hypothesis of the mode of action of vitamin E. A variety of theories concerning the molecular mechanisms of this vitamin have been put forward, and these provide for a more or less complete interpretation of physiological manifestations of vitamin E deficiency.

Vitamin E is important for energy production in mitochondria. It is thought that vitamin E is a link in membrane electron transport chains.[10] In the mitochondria of vitamin E-deficient laboratory animals, reduced respiration is common; it is not a result of blockage of the cytochrome c redox series.[11] Various investigations have shown that blockage of electron flow in vitamin E deficiency occurs at the beginning of the respiratory chain during the transfer of hydrogen from NADH or from succinate to Fe–S proteins in complex I or complex II, respectively. Vitamin E-sensitive enzymes in mitochondria are proteins with labile SH groups. Oxidation of these sulfhydryl groups leads to the loss of the biological activity. It has been demonstrated that vitamin E is localized in the mitochondrial membrane in the immediate vicinity of the enzymes containing SH groups, protecting them from oxidation. In this way, vitamin E plays an important role in electron transport and, thus, in the production of energy. Consequently, a significant influence of vitamin E on energy metabolism can be expected only when performance is accomplished with the help of aerobic energy supply.[12]

Vitamin E also exerts a protective effect on selenium (Se), a component of Se-containing proteins,[13] and plays a key role in regulation of heme synthesis, thus controlling the activity of heme-containing enzymes.[14] Vitamin E has been shown to be an efficient inhibitor of several enzymes involved in the arachidonic acid cascade: phospholipase A_2, cyclooxygenase, and lipoxygenase.[15-17] Additionally, vitamin E is an immunomodulating agent.[2] The fact, that after being incorporated, the bulk of labeled α-tocopherol binds to nonhistone proteins of chromatin has led to a hypothesis that the effect of vitamin E is coupled with the functioning of the genetic mechanism of the cell.[18]

One of the most advanced and well-founded hypotheses which allows for the interpretation of various manifestations of vitamin E deficiency is based on the concept that the biological role of vitamin E is in the stabilization of biological membranes. Evidence for this hypothesis has been obtained in a large number of experiments which have revealed multiple damage of membrane structures during vitamin E deficiency: e.g., increased sensitivity of erythrocytes to hemolytic agents,[19,20] oxidative phosphorylation uncoupling,[21,22] damage of endo-

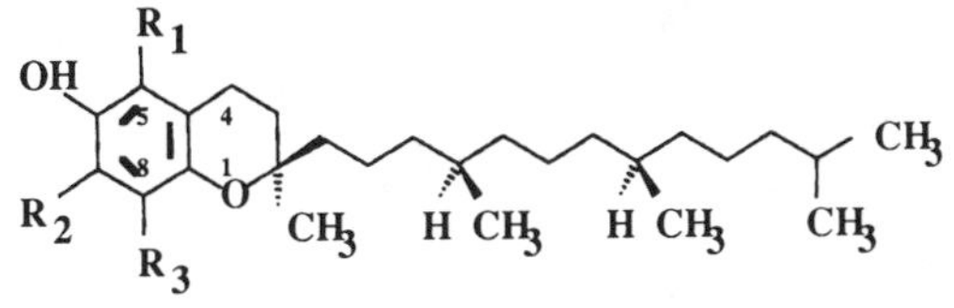

α–Tocopherol
(5,7,8,-trimethyltocol) $R_1 = R_2 = R_3 = CH_3$

β–Tocopherol
(5,8,-dimethyltocol) $R_1 = R_3 = CH_3$ $R_2 = H$

γ–Tocopherol
(7,8,-dimethyltocol) $R_1 = H$ $R_2 = R_3 = CH_3$

δ–Tocopherol
(8-methyltocol) $R_1 = R_2 = H$ $R_3 = CH_3$

FIGURE 1. Structural formulae of tocopherols.

plasmic reticulum enzymes,[23] increased sensitivity of intracellular lysosomal enzymes,[24] impairment of the Ca^{2+} transport function in sarcoplasmic reticulum membranes,[25] and release of intracellular enzymes into the blood.[26] Whatever the nature of these disturbances, they are all caused by the same factor, namely, the changes in the properties of the membrane lipid bilayer. Further on we shall demonstrate that the stabilizing effect of a α-tocopherol on the membrane lipid bilayer is mediated via at least three different mechanisms, i.e., (1) regulation of peroxidation of membrane lipids, (2) interaction with free fatty acids and lysophospholipids, and (3) stabilization of physical properties (microviscosity) of the membrane lipid bilayer. There exists an additional molecular mechanism of biomembrane protection by α-tocopherol. This mechanism is based on the ability of α-tocopherol to interact with singlet molecular oxygen, a potent oxidative damaging agent.[27] However, since the formation of singlet oxygen in biomembranes is, as a rule, coupled with photodynamic conditions unrelated to muscle tissue, no detailed description of the mechanism will be given here.

A. Vitamin E as an Inhibitor of Free-Radical Oxidation of Membrane Lipids

The general concepts of the function of vitamin E as protector of polyunsaturated acyls of biomembrane phospholipids against peroxidation was first formulated by Tappel.[28] Later, this hypothesis was verified experimentally[29,30] and vitamin E is believed to be the major lipid-soluble chain-breaking antioxidant in membranes.

1. Induction of Lipid Peroxidation in Membrane Structures

Polyenoic fatty acid residues of membrane phospholipids undergo oxidative modifications by molecular oxygen and its activated species, which eventually result in marked changes in the structural and functional properties of biomembranes.[31,32] The oxidative process is based on free-radical interactions between the lipids and oxygen.

In the ground state the O_2 molecule is chemically inert and cannot interact effectively with organic substrates. However, the functioning of intracellular enzymatic and nonenzymatic oxidative systems leads to the production of so-called "activated O_2 species".

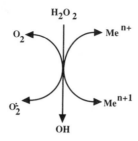

FIGURE 2. Scheme of HO· radical production in the modified Haber–Weiss reaction, Me^{n+}, Me^{n+1} are reduced and oxidized forms of transition metals.

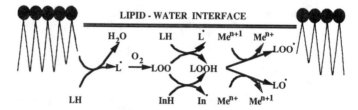

Me^{n+}, Me^{n+1} - REDUCED AND OXIDIZED FORMS OF TRANSITION METALS
LH - OXIDATION SUBSTRATES
InH - INHIBITOR OF FREE - RADICAL OXIDATION
In· - INHIBITOR RADICAL

FIGURE 3. Scheme of the initiation, propagation, and inhibition of free-radical lipid peroxidation. Me^{n+}, Me^{n+1} are reduced and oxidized forms of transition metals; LH, oxidation substrate; L·, LO·, LO_2·, lipid radicals; InH, inhibitor of free radical oxidation; In·, inhibitor radical.

For instance, the products of a stepwise one-electron reduction of O_2 formed in the course of numerous oxidase reactions are superoxide anion radicals (O_2^-) and hydrogen peroxide (H_2O_2).[33,34] Although the reactivity of these compounds is not sufficient to attack membrane lipids, they can interact with one another in the presence of transition metals (the so-called modified Haber–Weiss cycle), thus generating hydroxyl radicals (OH·) which possess a high oxidation potential (Figure 2). These OH· radicals readily interact with biomembrane lipids to produce lipid radicals, i.e., alkyl (L·), alkoxyl (LO·), and alkylperoxy radicals (LO_2·) which are schematically presented in Figure 3. As a result of multiple alternating reactions between lipid radicals (L·, LO·, LO_2·) and nonoxidized lipids (LH) during lipid peroxidation, additional "detachments" of membrane lipids become involved in this process. This is possible largely because lipid hydroperoxides (LOOH), the molecular products formed via lipid radical interactions with nonoxidized lipids, are relatively unstable compounds and are prone to homolytic splitting (especially in the presence of transition metals). This process leads to the formation of new alkoxyl (LO·) or alkylperoxy (LO_2·) radicals. Since the efficiency of lipid radical interaction with LH is directly correlated with the number of double bonds in the nonoxidized lipid molecule, it is clear that the main substrates of the free-radical oxidation in biological membranes are polyenoic fatty acid phospholipid residues containing three to six double bonds. The degradation of hydroperoxides, the recombination and further conversions of lipid radicals give rise to a great number of lipid peroxidation products (for details see Reference 32), of which, besides hydroperoxides, the most important are dialkyl peroxides, carbonyl compounds (including dialdehydes such as malonyl dialdehyde), short-chain volatile hydrocarbons (ethane, pentane, ethylene, etc.), aldehyde acids, oxyranes, etc. (Figure 4). In addition to accumulation of various lipid peroxidation products,

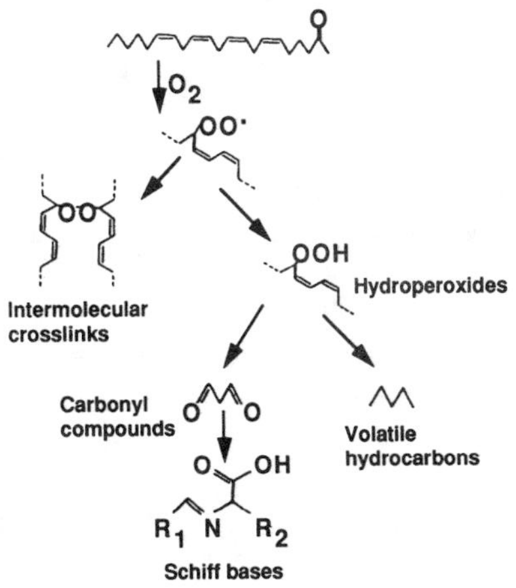

FIGURE 4. Scheme of the formation of some important molecular products of lipid peroxidation.

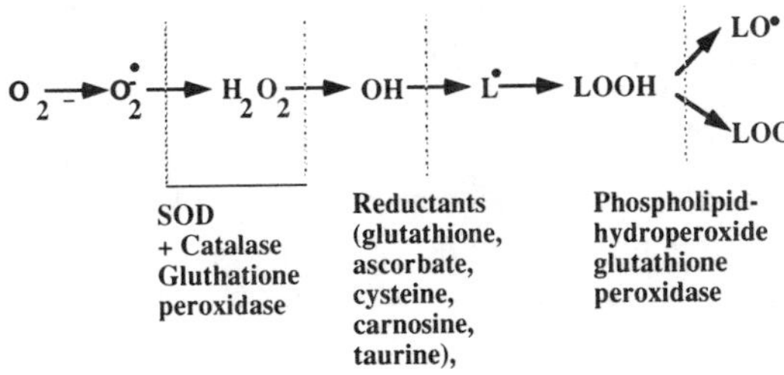

FIGURE 5. Scheme of some important inhibitory systems of lipid peroxidation.

this chain of events also leads to a decrease in the number of polyenoic lipids in the membrane as well as to the aggregation (cross linking) of membrane proteins.

If the concentration of O_2 is high enough, free-radical oxidation may lead to oxidative modifications of the bulk of polyenoic lipids. However, this does not occur in membranes *in vivo*. The reason for this is that special enzymatic and nonenzymatic systems of the cell interfere with the course of free-radical oxidation of membrane lipids and restrict this process. This system of lipid peroxidation regulation is multicomponent and functions both in the aqueous (cytosolic) phase of the cell, where it regulates the generation of activated O_2 species, and in membranes, where it restricts the propagation of free-radical reactions. Figure 5 gives a schematic representation of the main components of this regulation system at the level of lipid peroxidation initiation in the aqueous phase of the cell. The three main enzymes constituting this regulatory system are superoxide dismutase, catalase, and glutathione peroxidase, which prevent the formation of reactive OH· radicals.[35] Because of the exceedingly high chemical activity of hydroxyl radicals (which effectively attack biomolecules of any type) control over their level is mediated not via specific enzymatic mechanisms, but by nonspecific reducing agents, such as glutathione, cysteine, carnosine, taurine, ascorbic acid, etc., whose concentration in the cytosol may be as high as 10 to 20 mM.

The reduction of phospholipid hydroperoxides to stable hydroxy derivatives occurs on the membrane surface and is mediated by specific glutathione peroxidases which utilize phospholipid hydroperoxides as substrates and thus control the rate of lipid radical generation.[36] Finally, the hydrophobic lipid phase of the membrane contains special molecules of lipid antioxidants which, similarly to hydroxyl radical scavengers in the aqueous phase, interact with their hydrophobic analogs in the lipid bilayer (Figure 3). These compounds are often hydrophobic reducing agents, the most common being tocopherols and ubiquinols.[37]

2. Vitamin E as a Free-Radical Scavenger

Tocopherols effectively scavenge lipid radicals. The antioxidant (inhibitor) radical (In·) thus formed possesses a low reactivity and is further converted into molecular products, eventually resulting in the inhibition of lipid peroxidation (Figure 3).[28-30,35,36] Tocopherols are phenolic lipid peroxidation inhibitors which act by donating hydrogen from a readily deprotonated hydroxy group to a peroxyl radical. The efficiency of this reaction determines the potency of the inhibitor, i.e., its antiradical activity.[29,30] The antiradical activity of tocopherols is known to be correlated with their vitamin E activity.[37]

The antioxidant properties of tocopherols have been well documented. Here we shall cite only some works illustrating the prominent antioxidant role of vitamin E. Besides the above-mentioned relationship between vitamin E and antiradical activities, the other aspects of its antioxidant functions deserve special mention.

Tocopherols possess the ability to inhibit lipid peroxidation in a great variety of model systems (both in solutions and in model membranes), as well as in various biological membranes *in vitro*, irrespective of the mode of lipid peroxidation induction.[2,29,30] Some manifestations of vitamin E deficiency can be prevented by the use of synthetic antioxidants — butylhydroxytoluene (BHT; 2,6-di-tertbutyl-4-methylphenol), santoquine (ethoxyquine; 1,2-dihydroxy-6-ethoxy-2,2,4-trimethylquinone), N,N'-diphenyl-p-phenylene diamine, etc. — some of which are used as food additives for preventing the rancidification of fats.[1] Vitamin E exerts a protective effect in some pathological situations (e.g., poisoning with CCl_4 and ozone, ionizing radiation injury, etc.) that are considered to result from lipid peroxidation activation.[2,29] The importance of the antioxidant function of vitamin E is illustrated by the fact that the main α-tocopherol metabolites detected in animals are its dimeric form and tocopheryl-p-quinone, which are the compounds formed in free-radical reactions occurring in model systems.[38] Further evidence for the antioxidant activity of vitamin E is provided by the increase in free-radical concentration in animal tissues at early stages of vitamin E deficiency in experiments employing electron paramagnetic resonance,[39] by the accumulation of lipid peroxidation products in the membrane structures of vitamin E-deficient animals,[40,41] and by the considerable increase of ethane and pentane contents in the air exhaled by vitamin E-deficient animals.[42]

Results obtained in the last decade shed new light on the molecular mechanism of the high antioxidant effectiveness of vitamin E. The concentration of vitamin E in membrane is usually lower than 0.5 to 1.0 nmol/mg of protein, or 0.05 to 0.1 mol% of membrane phospholipids.[1,2] The rate of lipid radical generation dependent on electron transport (e.g., NADPH-dependent lipid peroxidation in liver microsomes) may be as high as 1 to 5 nmol/ mg of protein per minute. It would be expected that rapid vitamin E depletion would occur. Nevertheless, under physiological conditions this low concentration of vitamin E is sufficient to prevent membrane oxidative damage, and the concentration of vitamin E in biomembranes under normal conditions remains relatively constant. Thus, mechanisms of reduction of α-tocopherol radicals (tocopheroxyl radicals), formed during interaction of α-tocopherol with lipid radicals, must exist. Indeed, it has been demonstrated recently that tocopheroxyl radicals can be reduced either nonenzymically (e.g., by ascorbate), or enzymically (e.g., by NADPH-, NADH-, and succinate-dependent electron transport in microsomes and mitochondria), while reduced thiols (glutathione, dihydrolipoate) and ubiquinols synergistically enhance vitamin E regeneration.[43-49] Thus, the well-known synergistic effects of these physiologically important antioxidants (reductants) with vitamin E are probably mediated by their ability to donate electrons for tocopherol recycling in the "vitamin E" cycle (Figure 6).

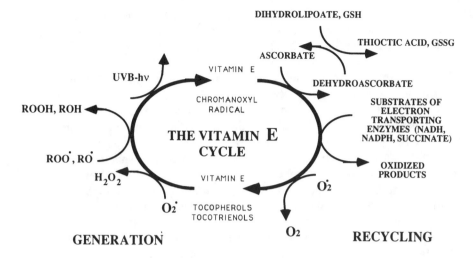

FIGURE 6.   Scheme of vitamin E cycle.

The antioxidant function of vitamin E is due to the hydroxy group of its chromanol nucleus, whereas the role of the isoprenoid (phytol) chain is to orientate the molecule in the membrane lipid bilayer for its strictly complementary interaction with fatty acid residues of membrane phospholipids, which prevents the occurrence of defects in the membrane structure.[50-52] Recent electron spin resonance (ESR) and nuclear magnetic resonance (NMR) studies have demonstrated that the whole α-tocopherol molecule is localized in the hydrophobic region of the lipid bilayer in such a way that its hydroxy group forms a hydrogen bond with the C=O group of the glycerol moiety of phospholipids.[53,54] This location of the chromanol nucleus of vitamin E at the membrane interface affords both efficient interaction with lipid peroxyl radicals and the regeneration of tocopheroxyl radicals.

B. Structural Effects of Vitamin E on Biological Membranes

The hypothesis on the structural effects of α-tocopherol in biological membranes was first postulated by Diplock and Lucy.[55,56] According to this hypothesis, the molecular interactions of α-tocopherol with phospholipids stabilize membranes, due to the London–Van der Waals forces between the methyl groups of the α-tocopherol phytol side chain and the *cis* double bonds of polyunsaturated fatty acid residues of phospholipids.[55,56] The biological significance of this hypothesis lies in the fact that vitamin E influences the microviscosity of the lipid bilayer and the passive permeability of biological membranes.

Compelling evidence in favor of this hypothesis has been forthcoming in the past 15 years. Studies employing different experimental approaches have demonstrated that α-tocopherol increases the microviscosity of model membranes composed of unsaturated lipids and decreases the passive permeability of these membranes to ions, water, and other low-molecular-weight substances.[55,57,58] A similar effect of α-tocopherol on membrane permeability has been reported for erythrocyte, fibroblast, and sarcoplasmic reticulum membranes.[20,58,59]

The effects of α-tocopherol on model membranes formed from saturated lipids is quite opposite: α-tocopherol increases the passive permeability of saturated model membranes and exerts a disordering effect on them, i.e., it decreases their microviscosity.[59,60] Even in the same model membranes, α-tocopherol exhibits two different effects by ordering membrane structure at temperatures above the phase-transitions point and by disordering it at temperatures below this value.[61-65] These results indicate that vitamin E exerts a cholesterol-like effect on biomembranes, i.e., it restores their microviscosity when the latter increases or decreases. One possible reason for fluctuations in the properties of the membrane lipid bilayer, besides lipid peroxidation, is the phospholipid hydrolysis by phospholipases.

C. Protection of Biological Membranes Against the Damaging Action of Phospholipase A_2 and Free Fatty Acids

The hypothesis that vitamin E protects biological membranes against the damaging action of phospholipase A_2 was primarily based on the fact that α-tocopherol prevents the effect of one of the two products of phospholipid hydrolysis by phospholipase A_2 — free fatty acids — on the Ca^{2+} transport system in skeletal muscle sarcoplasmic reticulum.[66] Later, it was demonstrated that α-tocopherol exerts a protective effect against damage induced by the other product of phospholipid hydrolysis by phospholipase A_2, lysophospholipids, as well as by phospholipase A_2 itself, which causes accumulation of both free fatty acids and lysophospholipids in membranes.[67,68] This effect consists in stabilization of the transmembrane potential and microviscosity of biomembranes, as well as protection of membrane proteins (cytochrome P-450, rhodopsin, Ca^{2+}-ATPase) against inactivation induced by either free fatty acids or lysophospholipids. This protective effect is not based on the inhibition of phospholipase A_2, but on the ability of α-tocopherol to form complexes with phospholipid hydrolysis products.[69,70] Biological membranes are protected from the damaging action of phospholipase A_2 by α-tocopherol, but not by its derivative devoid of the phytol chain, 2,2,5,7,8-pentamethyl chromanol.[71]

This mechanism, along with the antiradical activity and effect on the physical properties of the lipid bilayer, plays an important role in the stabilization of biological membranes by vitamin E. This conclusion follows from the observation that in vitamin E-deficient animals, biological membranes become more sensitive to the damaging action of phospholipase A_2, free fatty acids, or lysophospholipids.[72]

III. THE NECESSITY OF VITAMIN E FOR MUSCLE ACTIVITY

A. The State of Muscles in Vitamin E Deficiency

Vitamin E deficiency leads to multiple pathological changes in the organs and tissues of the body, the most common sign of vitamin E deficiency in many animal species, including man, being muscular dystrophy. These changes affect both skeletal and cardiac muscles, although in the myocardium, the pathological changes are less conspicuous.[73-75]

The first morphological studies on vitamin E-deficient rabbits and guinea pigs demonstrated that the onset of general weakness was concomitant with profound changes in skeletal muscles. The degenerative lesions of myofibrils detected in early vitamin E deficiency manifest themselves in a decrease in myofibrillar diameter, loss of transversal striation, granular partial degeneration of muscle fibers, and subsequent necrosis. The myocardium of vitamin E-deficient animals reveals local contractures and necrotic zones.[74,75]

Simultaneous with degenerative and atrophic lesions of muscle fibers, the proliferation of intermuscular connective tissue increases, as evidenced not only by results of histological studies, but also by an anomalous increase in collagen concentration in the muscle. The latter is characterized by a high number of α-chains and a small number of cross links which provide for a greater solubility of collagen.[73-75]

In muscles, this process is accompanied by the accumulation of lipids and the formation of basophilic granules, presumably of calcium origin.[75] The accumulation of Ca^{2+} in the muscles of vitamin E-deficient animals was observed in very early studies and it is especially well pronounced in the mitochondria, nuclei, and sarcoplasm.[73,76]

Electron microscopic data also revealed that the most conspicuous changes in vitamin E deficiency in muscle tissue are observed in myofibrils. These changes consist of the loss of the bulk of myosin protofibrils, as well as the dissociation of actin protofibrils into globules, which can be seen by the disappearance of A-discs and granulation of l-discs. The structure of Z-bands and the loci of tropomyosin are also changed.[73-77]

Structural changes in sarcolemma are either absent or are very insignificant.[73,74] However, biomedical studies show that the number of SH-groups in the sarcolemma of vitamin E-deficient rabbits is decreased by 30 to 40%.[78]

Changes in the structure of skeletal muscle mitochondria during vitamin E deficiency are not so well pronounced and vary in different animal species. In rats with strongly impaired muscle fibers, the changes in mitochondria are confined to insignificant fragmentation.[74,77] However, in vitamin E-deficient rats, strenuous exercise results in increased membrane fragility and a decreased respiratory control ratio of muscle mitochondria. Vitamin E deficiency caused a 40% decrease in running time to exhaustion in untrained animals. Reduced endurance capacity in vitamin E-deficient rats was associated with peroxidative damage to mitochondria.[79]

In rabbits, mitochondrial changes are far more apparent and are manifested as swelling, fragmentation, and enlargement of mitochondrial crysts. In strongly impaired fibers, the mitochondria diminish in size and have the appearance of round structures with single crysts and a low-density matrix.[74]

The sarcoplasmic reticulum of muscle fibers from E-deficient animals is prone to degradation and vacuolization;[77] in rats its ability for energy-dependent uptake of Ca^{2+} is decreased fourfold, whereas that in the myocardium is decreased by 30%.[20,80]

The development of muscular dystrophy during vitamin E deficiency is accompanied by a significant elevation of corresponding organ-specific enzymes in the blood plasma due to their release from the damaged tissue. Muscular dystrophy in guinea pigs, rabbits, rats, and other animals is accompanied by an increased activity in the blood plasma (serum) of alanine and aspartate aminotransferases, lactate dehydrogenase, fructose-1,6-diphosphate aldolase, creatine phosphokinase, and pyruvate kinase.[21,81] The increase in the activity of lactate dehydrogenase in the blood plasma of vitamin E-deficient rabbits is caused by muscle isoenzyme M_4, which points to its release from the damaged muscle.[21]

The elevated activity of muscle enzymes in blood plasma is observed at early stages of vitamin E deficiency, before the changes in muscle tissue are revealed histologically.[81] However, the highest enzyme activity is seen at the stage of dystrophic degeneration of muscle tissue, at which point the activity of alanine aminotransferase in the blood plasma is increased 15-fold, that of fructose-1,6-diphosphate aldolase, 60-fold, and that of creatine phosphokinase, 76-fold.[21,81]

The increase in the activity of these enzymes in the blood plasma is accompanied by their decline in muscle tissue, which correlates with their release from degenerative muscles into the blood.[81] At the early stages preceding necrotic degradation of some muscle fibers this release can be due to membrane damage and to the increased permeability to intracellular enzymes (see below). Recent studies showed that the reduction of creatine phosphokinase activity in rat myocardium is one of the early biochemical changes occurring in this organ prior to the loss of ATP.[82]

Muscular dystrophy in vitamin E deficiency is also associated with a significant increase in the activity of lysosomal enzymes (e.g., aryl sulfatase, 13-glucuronidase, cathepsins, acid phosphatase) in degenerating muscles. As a rule, such an increase is observed in severe vitamin E deficiency and is concomitant with dystrophic changes of the muscles, being more effect than cause. In rats with continuous severe vitamin E deficiency concomitant with a lowered α-tocopherol concentration in the blood plasma (23-fold), the activity of free cathepsin in the myocardium and skeletal muscles is increased 1.5- and 2.5-fold, respectively.[83] In rats kept on a vitamin E-free diet over a period of 2 months the concentration of α-tocopherol in the blood plasma, skeletal muscles, and myocardium decreased by 10-, 5.4-, and 3.4-fold, respectively, while the cathepsin activity (both total and nonsedimenting) in the myocardium was essentially unchanged.[80] In skeletal muscles, the nonsedimenting activity of acid phosphatase and the total activity of cathepsin D are increased by 30 to 40%, but are unaffected in the blood plasma. Immobilization stress causes a 30% elevation of the acid phosphatase activity in the blood plasma of vitamin E-deficient rats; that of cathepsin D appears to be increased twofold. In rats kept on a vitamin E-rich diet the activity of the above enzymes in the blood plasma is unaffected by stress. These findings testify to the fact that stress plays a role in the manifestation of vitamin E deficiency and causes the release of lysosomal enzymes into the blood of animals with vitamin E deficiency. In blood plasma and tissue unaffected by the pathological process, the activity of lysosomal enzymes in vitamin E deficiency does not change significantly.[81,83]

The development of muscular dystrophy in vitamin E deficiency is accompanied by severe disturbances of energy metabolism, such as the decline of high-energy compounds and of oxidative phosphorylation efficiency.[73,84] In rats kept on a vitamin E-free diet for a period of 5 to 10 weeks, the level of creatine phosphate and ATP in limb muscles decreased by 60% and 20%, respectively, ADP increased twofold, and AMP remained constant. Lactate concentrations in the muscles of vitamin E-deficient animals is increased three- to fourfold, whereas that of pyruvate only two- to threefold.[84] These changes are thought to be due to disturbances in the energy supply of skeletal muscles, which is paralleled by a compensatory activation of glycolysis. The latter hypothesis is consistent with the results of earlier studies which demonstrated a decrease in the intramuscular concentration of glycogen during vitamin E deficiency.

The myocardium enjoys a greater protection from avitaminosis E, the former being a more vitally important organ than skeletal muscles. The concentration of vitamin E in the plasma of adult rats kept on a vitamin E-free diet over a period of 2 months decreased from 1.0 to 0.1 mg/100 ml, whereas in the myocardium the adenyl nucleotide concentration was unchanged, while that of creatine phosphate was decreased by 20%.[82] These data indicate that the earliest symptom of vitamin E deficiency in the energy supply system of the muscles, in particular, of the myocardium, is a decrease in the concentration of creatine phosphate, which precedes and exceeds that of ATP. A possible reason for the observed disturbances in the metabolism of high-energy compounds in muscle tissue in vitamin E deficiency is the lowered efficiency of oxidative phosphorylation and the augmented energy expenditure needed for compartmentalization and intracellular transport of Ca^{2+} due to the inability of the sarcoplasmic reticulum membrane to maintain the concentration of Ca^{2+} at a constant level (see below).[20]

What are the mechanisms underlying the biochemical, structural, and physiological changes occurring in muscles in vitamin E deficiency? As stated above, the most likely hypothesis attributes the biological role of α-tocopherol to its stabilizing action on biological membranes, in particular, to its antioxidant effects. This hypothesis also explains the disturbances of vitamin E deficiency as being due to the activation of lipid peroxidation and to the impairment of the structure, permeability, and functioning of cellular and subcellular membranes. Of special interest are results demonstrating the activation of lipid peroxidation and accumulation of lipid peroxidation products in the skeletal muscles and myocardium of vitamin E-deficient animals.

B. Activation of Lipid Peroxidation and its Role in the Impairment of Muscle Contractility in Vitamin E Deficiency

It is well known that in skeletal muscles and, to a lesser degree, in cardiomyocytes, the bulk of membranes are the sarcoplasmic reticulum membranes. Therefore we shall consider

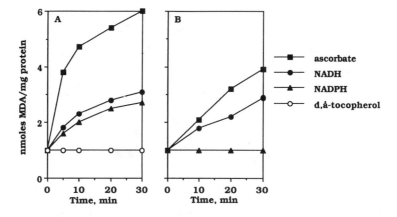

FIGURE 7. Accumulation of lipid peroxidation products in sarcoplasmic reticulum membranes of rat skeletal (A) and cardiac (B) muscles, induced by NADH, NAD(P)H or ascorbate. Incubation medium contained: Tris-HCl buffer, 20 mM; NaCl, 100 mM; pH 7.1 at 37°C; Fe(II), 10 μM; NAP(P)H (ascorbate), 0.5 mM; membranes, 1 mg protein/ml; d-α-tocopherol, 50 μM.

the molecular mechanisms underlying the damaging effects of lipid peroxidation in these membranes. The main function of the sarcoplasmic reticulum is the transformation of the nervous signal transmitted to the sarcolemma into a mechanical and chemical response of contractile proteins.[85,86] This function is accomplished by the alteration of the Ca^{2+} concentration in the sarcoplasm: a rise in this concentration causes muscle contraction, whereas its decrease causes muscle relaxation. The sarcoplasmic reticulum is a continuous membrane-limited system composed of vesicles, tubules and cisterns which form a vast network around the myofibrils. The sarcoplasmic reticulum membrane is rich in phospholipids containing polyenoic fatty acid residues (60 to 70% of the total fatty acid content),[87,88] which are potential substrates of lipid peroxidation.

Sarcoplasmic reticulum membranes of skeletal and cardiac muscles contain enzymatic systems which generate activated O_2 species capable of inducing the accumulation of lipid peroxidation products.[89,90] These systems utilize reduced pyridine nucleotides as a source of reducing equivalents. Curves illustrating the accumulation of lipid peroxidation products (carbonyl compounds of malonyl dialdehyde [MDA] type interacting with 2-thiobarbituric acid [TBARS]) in sarcoplasmic reticulum fragments from skeletal muscle and in the microsomal fraction of cardiac muscle of the rat in the presence of NADPH (or NADH) and Fe^{2+} are shown in Figure 7. For comparison, we present the curves for the accumulation of lipid peroxidation products during nonenzymatic induction of lipid peroxidation by the Fe^{2+}-ascorbate system. Addition of α-tocopherol causes a complete inhibition of lipid peroxidation. Cardiac and skeletal muscles contain the enzymatic systems which afford antioxidant protection (i.e., superoxide dismutase, catalase, glutathione peroxidase), although the activities of these enzymes are comparatively low.[89,90] However, skeletal muscles and myocardium contain high (millimolar) amounts of water-soluble antioxidants — carnosine and taurine.[91] Finally, the α-tocopherol content in sarcoplasmic reticulum membranes of skeletal muscles is as high as 0.2 mol%, i.e., much higher than that in other membrane structures of muscle cells;[90] in cardiomyocyte sarcoplasmic reticulum membranes the level of vitamin E is even higher.[80] Hence, this compound seems to afford the strongest protection of muscle cells against oxidative stress. Evidence for this assumption can be derived from the activation of lipid peroxidation in muscle tissue under vitamin E deficiency. The concentration of ethane and pentane in the air exhaled by vitamin E-deficient animals is considerably elevated[42] as a result of lipid peroxidation. In rats kept on a vitamin E-free diet for 32 weeks, the

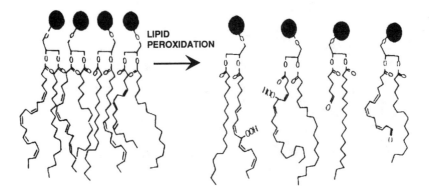

FIGURE 8. Scheme of the changes in the hydrophilic–hydrophobic balance of phospholipid molecules as a result of their oxidation.

concentration of lipid peroxides in myocardial lipids and skeletal muscles is increased 1.5- to 2.0-fold.[92] Lack of vitamin E in the diet of growing rats for a period of 2 months leads to an accumulation of lipid peroxidation products: their content increases 3.9-fold in skeletal muscles and 1.6-fold in the myocardium.[93]

Despite the greater resistance of the myocardium to vitamin E deficiency, lack of this vitamin can result in a significant deterioration of the functional state of this vitally important organ, as well as in reduced resistance to factors causing an arrhythmia and fibrillation.[93,94]

Of special interest are results[95] indicating that in rats kept on a diet including 12.5 mg of *d,l*-α-tocopheryl acetate per kilogram of chow, which provides for the stability of erythrocytes to peroxide hemolysis, the resistance of the myocardium to physical load and to Ca^{2+} excess appears to be significantly reduced, in comparison with animals receiving the optimal dose of vitamin E, i.e., 100 mg/kg of the diet. These results provide an example of the important role of vitamin E in maintaining a high level of functional activity of the myocardium and its resistance to excessive load and damaging influences.

1. Mechanisms of Damage of Muscle Cell Membranes by Lipid Peroxidation

It is well known that lipid peroxidation is a universal mechanism of biomembrane damage capable of modifying the main structural and functional properties of membranes, i.e., their barrier, receptor, and catalytic functions.[31-33] let us now consider the specific molecular mechanisms of biomembrane damage during lipid peroxidation. There are three major mechanisms that cause the damaging effects of molecular oxygen and its activated species on biological membranes:

1. Membrane phospholipids of mammals contain, as a rule, polyunsaturated fatty acid acyls in the second position of the glycerol moiety which is exposed to peroxidation (see Figure 4). The resulting phospholipid peroxidation products (phospholipids carrying polar hydroperoxyl or carbonyl groups in one of their fatty acid residues) are characterized by a marked shift of the hydrophobic–hydrophilic balance towards lower hydrophobicity values (Figure 8).
2. Dialdehydes (e.g., malonyl dialdehyde) formed as a result of lipid peroxidation act as cross-linking bifunctional reagents and cause the polymerization and aggregation of biomolecules (membrane proteins and lipids) as well as the accumulation of lipofuscin-like compounds.
3. Amino acid residues (SH-groups, histidine, tryptophan, etc.) of membrane proteins are oxidized by oxygen and lipid radicals. These residues can include those in the active center of membrane proteins.

These three primary modifying effects of activated O_2 species and lipid radicals provide for a great variety of lipid peroxidation manifestations at the molecular, ultrastructural, and

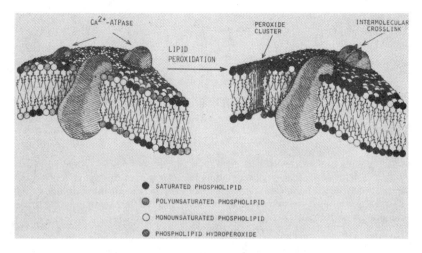

FIGURE 9. Scheme of the "peroxide clusters" formation and of the Ca^{2+}-ATPase damage in the sarcoplasmic reticulum membranes upon lipid peroxidation.

functional levels of biomembrane organization. The most typical are the following: restriction of molecular mobility of phospholipids and the appearance of "peroxide clusters" in the lipid bilayer, reduction in the number of fluid lipids in the microenvironment of membrane proteins, impairment of lipid–protein interactions, disappearance of trans-bilayer asymmetry of phospholipids, decreased thickness of the membrane hydrophobic zone, transmembrane migration of intrinsic proteins, formation of permeability channels for ions and nonelectrolytes, decreased catalytic activity and thermal stability of membrane proteins, decreased electrical stability of membranes (electrical breakdown potential reduction), and membrane disintegration and fragmentation.[31-33]

Here it seems reasonable to consider the effects of lipid peroxidation on the membrane structures of myocytes and on the contractility of muscle fibers with primary emphasis on the membrane systems responsible for the regulation of Ca^{2+} homeostasis. Sarcoplasmic reticulum membranes are known to contain an enzymatic system responsible for Ca^{2+} transport which produces and maintains a more than 1000-fold gradient of these cations.[85,86] The main components of this system are (1) Ca^{2+}-dependent ATPase (Ca^{2+} pump) which is capable of transporting Ca^{2+} from the outer medium to sarcoplasmic reticulum vesicles utilizing the energy of ATP hydrolysis, and (2) the phospholipid matrix of the membrane which possess a low passive permeability for Ca^{2+}. In intact sarcoplasmic reticulum membranes the hydrolysis of one ATP molecule is coupled with the translocation of two Ca^{2+} ions into the sarcoplasmic reticulum vesicles ($Ca^{2+}/ATP = 2$).

Lipid peroxidation in sarcoplasmic reticulum vesicular suspensions causes inhibition of Ca^{2+} transport. The Ca^{2+}/ATP ratio decreases as the concentration of lipid peroxidation products rises, i.e., the efficiency of the Ca^{2+} transport system gradually diminishes. This is due to a sharp increase in the permeability of sarcoplasmic reticulum membranes for Ca^{2+} through so-called "peroxide clusters" (Figure 9). The formation of such clusters may be the cause of excessive accumulation of Ca^{2+} in muscle cell sarcoplasma and the damage to muscle under vitamin E deficiency and at excessive physical load.[96] The loss of the Ca^{2+}-ATPase activity is due to the polyenoic lipid depletion in the enzyme microenvironment as a result of lipid peroxidation, as well as to the formation of intermolecular cross links by dialdehydic secondary products of lipid peroxidation. The essential mechanisms of lipid peroxidation-induced damage of the enzymatic Ca^{2+} transport system are schematically presented in Figure 9.

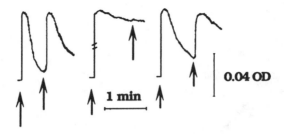

FIGURE 10.. Records of the "contraction–relaxation" cycles in a model system consisting of myofibrils and vesicles of sarcoplasmic reticulum. The changes in the optical density of the system are recorded. Arrows indicate the addition of Ca^{2+} (to a concentration of 10^{-5} M). 1, control; 2, induction of lipid peroxidation; 3, induction of lipid peroxidation in the presence of d,l-α-tocopherol (50 μM).

Vitamin E exerts a stabilizing effect by preventing the damage of the enzymatic system of Ca^{2+} transport induced *in vitro* by the Fe^{2+} + ascorbate system. *In vivo*, the changes in the activity of the enzymatic Ca^{2+} transport system in skeletal muscle sarcoplasmic reticulum similar to those described above are observed under vitamin E deficiency. In this case, too, the accumulation of endogenous lipid peroxidation products in sarcoplasmic reticulum membranes leads to a decrease in efficiency of Ca^{2+} transport (Ca^{2+}/ATP ratio decrease) and, at later stages, to diminution of the Ca^{2+}-ATPase activity.[41]

Since the sarcoplasmic reticulum is the main factor which regulates the level of Ca^{2+} in myocyte sarcoplasm, any damage to the enzymatic system of Ca^{2+} transport should inevitably lead to the excessive accumulation of Ca^{2+} and, eventually, to muscle contractures. This possibility can best be illustrated by experiments with isolated myofibrils and sarcoplasmic reticulum fragments. Typical curves showing the changes in light scattering in this model system are presented in Figure 10. Addition of Ca^{2+} to the incubation medium significantly increases the turbidity of suspension as a result of myofibrillar contraction. In the presence of ATP and Mg^{2+}, the suspension is "cleared up", which points to myofibrillar relaxation due to exogenous Ca^{2+} transport into the sarcoplasmic reticulum vesicles. These "contraction–relaxation" cycles can be reproduced many times. However, lipid peroxidation induction in such a system causes the disappearance of "relaxation" of myofibrils after their contraction in the presence of exogenous Ca^{2+}. One possible explanation of this phenomenon is the inability of the enzymatic Ca^{2+} transport system damaged by lipid peroxidation to accumulate Ca^{2+} in the vesicles and thus decrease the concentration of Ca^{2+} in the incubation medium. These effects of lipid peroxidation may be the molecular mechanism of muscle contracture under various pathological conditions, in particular, in vitamin E deficiency.[96,97] In the presence of α-tocopherol (2×10^{-5} M) lipid peroxidation inducers exert no damaging effect on the enzymatic system of Ca^{2+} transport, and the alternation of the "contraction–relaxation" cycles persists.

2. Activation of Lipid Peroxidation Under Intensive Physical Load

Optimal physical performance capacity is impossible without optimum cellular function. Physical performance always creates situations which subject cellular metabolism to the limits of stress. The supply, turnover, and regeneration of substrates for producing energy are only part of the whole. Effects on the structural components of the cell are also important. Although it is up to the individual, even with optimal training and nutrition, whether to stress his or her body beyond its given limits and to accept possible damage or sacrifice in performance, there is no doubt that targeted nutritional planning in conjunction with optimized training can clearly extend these limits.[98]

During high levels of physical exercise, oxygen consumption may rise several-fold. Analysis of hind limb skeletal muscles of endurance-trained rats demonstrated a twofold increase in the mitochondria and associated enzyme activities. It can be anticipated that trained animals produce higher levels of free radicals than sedentary animals, since mitochondria are increased in amount and activity per unit of muscle weight.[99]

Intensive muscle activity is accompanied by the development of oxidative stress in various body tissues, including muscles, evidenced by a decrease of vitamin E concentration in membranes,[100-102] activation of lipid peroxidation,[42,102-107] a decrease in the level of reduced glutathione, and an increase of its oxidized form.[102,103] These effects are much more pronounced in vitamin E-deficient animals than in normal animals. Lipid peroxidation enhancement due to intensive physical exercise is also demonstrated by a twofold increase in pentane content in the air exhaled by mountain climbers[108] and by a significant increase in the MDA content as well as in the activity of both mitochondrial glutamate–oxalacetate–transaminase (by 65%) and lysosomal glucuronidase (by 23%) in the serum of subjects following exhaustive exercise on a bicycle ergometer.[109]

One may assume that the damage of muscle membranes typical for vitamin E deficiency due to the activation of lipid peroxidation is similar to that observed during intense physical exercise.

What are the mechanisms of lipid peroxidation activation in this case? The specific mechanisms are still to be elucidated, although there are several hypothetical pathways which may contribute to exercise-induced oxidative stress.

It is known that intensive physical load causes damage of erythrocyte and myocyte membranes associated with the liberation of Fe-containing proteins (hemoglobin and myoglobin) which catalyze H_2O_2 degradation, thus giving rise to OH· radicals and lipid peroxidation products.[103] As an example of such a release of heme-containing proteins under exhaustive physical load, we may cite the "anemia of runners" typical of marathon runners.[110,111]

Another source of oxygen radicals and lipid peroxides during intensive physical load is xanthine oxidase, the activity of which is sharply augmented as a result of xanthine dehydrogenase conversion into xanthine oxidase due to the impairment of Ca^{2+} homeostasis, and activation of endogenous proteases.[112,113] With a decrease of the ATP/ADP ratio under physical load the accumulation of purines (hypoxanthine), i.e., substrates for xanthine oxidase, occurs, which may be one mechanism for the generation of O_2 radicals and, consequently, for the activation of lipid peroxidation.

Physical exercise also stimulates oxygen consumption and electron transport in membrane structures. In this way, intensive physical load creates the necessary prerequisites for the increased production of activated O_2 species and lipid peroxides, i.e., the development of oxidative stress.[102,103] One possible source of oxygen radicals is an electron "leak", probably at the ubiquinone–cytochrome *b* level, of the mitochondrial electron transport chain, which produces superoxide radical.[114-116]

During exercise, blood flow is shunted away from many organs and tissues (e.g., kidneys, splanchnic region) to the working muscles, and part or all of these regions may experience hypoxia; in addition, during exercise at or above $\dot{V}O_2$ max, and perhaps at lower intensities, it is certain that fibers within the working muscles undergo hypoxia. At the cessation of exercise, these regions then undergo reoxygenation, and such reoxygenation may lead to the well-known burst of free-radical production that occurs during ischemia-reperfusion.[117,118] ESR techniques have been used to directly demonstrate exercise-induced free-radical production in skeletal muscles and liver of animals.[101,119] The decrease of vitamin E and reduced glutathione levels in animal tissues seems to be one of the most essential reasons for the development of oxidative stress upon exhaustive physical load.[102,103] However, the data available are too scant to allow discrimination between the cause and effect of oxidative stress under intensive physical exercise. There is no doubt that lipid peroxidation products accumulate in the course of exhaustive physical exercise of animals or humans[102-107] in different tissues and in the whole organism. TBARS have been shown to increase in muscles and liver of exercised animals.[101,120] In humans, however, measurements of lipid peroxidation due to exercise are not consistent. An increase in expired pentane has been found during exercise in humans,[121] and ultramarathon runners completing an 80.5-km run had increased levels of plasma lipid peroxidation,[122] but in another study, runners completing a half marathon had no change either in plasma TBARS or conjugated dienes.[123] Viinikka et al.[124] also reported no increase in plasma lipid peroxidation with exercise in highly trained subjects, but Sumida et al.,[125] using a similar exercise protocol but less well-trained subjects, found a slight but significant elevation in serum TBARS. The intensity and duration of exercise also influences the appearance of lipid peroxidation products; in one study, a decrease in plasma lipid peroxidation occurred with exercise at 40 and 70% of $\dot{V}O_2$ max while an increase was observed at 100% $\dot{V}O_2$ max.[126] We have performed experiments in which the level of lipid peroxidation end-products, i.e., volatile lower hydrocarbons, was estimated in the air exhaled by individuals exposed to maximal physical load (Figure 11). The pentane content was measured in the air exhaled by 15 untrained healthy male volunteers aged 20 to 23 years, prior to physical exercise, and 0 and 2 h postexercise (exercising on a cycloergometer, pedaling rate — 60 rpm, physical load up to voluntary exhaustion — 1500 kg/min). The pronounced activation of lipid peroxidation under these conditions was observed 2 h after cessation of the exercise. By stipulating that the rate of respiration increases a great deal during physical exercise, one can presume that the total content of lipid peroxidation products (but not the pentane content in the exhaled air) greatly exceeds that of control.

Thus, the chances of finding evidence for oxidative damage during exercise seem to depend on the intensity of the exercise, the location of the sample site, and the state of training of the subjects. Intense or exhaustive exercise in untrained subjects is more likely to produce oxidative damage, which is more likely to be seen in muscle than in blood.

IV. REQUIREMENTS FOR VITAMIN E AND EFFECT OF INTENSIVE PHYSICAL EXERCISE

Estimation of the requirement of humans for vitamin E is a difficult task, hence there are only a few reports addressing this problem. These difficulties arise from the fact that vitamin E is only one of the constituent components of the antioxidant system of the organism which also includes enzymes (e.g., superoxide dismutase, glutathione peroxidase, catalase) and biologically active substances that partly compensate for vitamin E deficiency, preventing the propagation of free-radical oxidation of membrane lipids. This consideration can be confirmed by the elimination of vitamin E deficiency through administration of synthetic free-radical scavengers.[1]

Recommended daily allowances (RDA) for vitamin E in the U.S., Canada, France, and Russia are 10 mg of α-tocopherol equivalents for young and adult males and 8 mg of α-tocopherol equivalents for young and adult women. In Germany, RDA for vitamin E is higher, constituting 12 mg of α-tocopherol equivalents daily.[127-129]

According to Horwitt,[3] 15 IU/d is the lowest threshold value for humans, whose daily need for this vitamin can be as high as 45 IU. The need for vitamin E can increase with a rise in the consumption of unsaturated lipids. Therefore, some authors suggest that the RDA should be calculated from the concentration of unsaturated fatty acids in the food, using the index of 0.6 mg of α-tocopherol per gram of unsaturated fatty acids as a coefficient.[130]

Opinions still differ as to the amount of vitamin E necessary to overcome its deficit in the organism; the criteria used in various allowance tests aimed at the estimation of the need for this vitamin can be the cause of discrepancies. For instance, myopathy in rats in which ration included 35% lard is eliminated by administration of 0.5 mg of D,L-α-tocopheryl acetate per kilogram of fodder. The optimal dose of the same vitamin necessary to prevent testicular degeneration and to provide for normal growth is 1.5 mg/kg. At the same time, the corresponding dose of vitamin E determined in a spontaneous erythrocyte hemolysis test is equal to 12.5 mg/kg.[131] This dose, however, appears to be too low for the optimal functioning of cardiac muscle.[95]

Of special interest is the question of how excessive physical load influences the requirements of the organism for vitamin E. Experiments with animals clearly demonstrate that the requirement for vitamin E increases significantly with intensive physical exercise. The content of α-tocopherol, at least in the organs involved, sharply decreases in parallel with the development of biochemical and pathophysiological manifestations of vitamin E deficiency which prevention requires exceedingly high doses of this vitamin.[100-102] Aikawa et al.[100] demonstrated that continuous (daily for 9 weeks) intensive physical exercise resulted in a decrease of the α-tocopherol concentration in limb muscles of rats fed a vitamin E-sufficient diet from 7.2 to 0.15 mg/g of tissue wet weight, whereas α-tocopherol in vitamin E-deficient rats decreased from 1.17 mg/g to undetectable values. Experiments by Efremov and Sakaeva[132] showed that swimming (1 h daily) decreased the vitamin E level in the blood sera of young growing rats receiving a daily dose of 1 to 3 mg of tocopherol from 1.01 ± 0.07 to 0.43 ± 0.05 mg/100 ml and augmented daily excretion of creatine in the urine from 0.25 ± 0.12 to 0.80 ± 0.20 mg. These parameters could be brought back to normal by daily administration of 15 IU of vitamin E. An increase in physical load (swimming for 4 h daily for 20 d) brought on the symptoms of vitamin E deficiency, which could be eliminated by administration of 25 mg of α-tocopherol per day.[132] Swimming to exhaustion in vitamin E-fed rats burdened with a weight increased the pentane content in the expired air by 40 to 50%[42] and elevated the malonic dialdehyde concentration in the muscles and liver.[133] These data testify to the intensification of vitamin E-induced lipid peroxidation. Excessive physical exercise has also been shown to be the cause of the changes characteristic of vitamin E deficiency (e.g., myopathy) in pigs.[134]

Information on the need by humans for vitamin E for physical exercise is scant. It has been found, for instance, that after 1 h of training on a bicycle ergometer pentane content in exhaled air considerably increased, which points to the activation of lipid peroxidation. This effect was abolished by the administration of 1200 IU of vitamin E (daily for 2 weeks).[122,135]

At the same time, moderate physical load (exercise therapy, 20 min, three times a week) and daily physical exercise (10 min) over a period of 1 year had no effect on vitamin E content or malonic dialdehyde levels in the plasma, erythrocytes, and platelets of elderly patients (aged 68 to 92 years) with a sufficient level of vitamin E in the blood.[136] The vitamin E concentration in the serum of athletes does not differ significantly from that in nonathlete healthy individuals.[137] In contrast, intensive physical exercise (especially in combination with emotional stress), e.g., in sport competitions, may significantly enhance the need of the human organism for vitamin E and its administration in high doses. Data, however, are lacking.

A. Vitamin E Supply in Humans

The most common method employed for estimating the requirement of human and animal organisms for vitamin E is the measurement of α-tocopherol concentration in the blood serum or plasma. Normally, the concentration of tocopherols in the blood plasma of healthy adult individuals is more than 0.7 mg/100 ml,[1,138] or, according to other authors, 0.8 to 1.2 mg/100 ml.[139] Manifestation of vitamin E deficiency in adult humans, i.e., increased sensitivity of erythrocytes to peroxide hemolysis and their low survival, is observed when α-tocopherol content in the blood plasma decreases to 0.5 mg/100 ml/l, therefore lower α-tocopherol concentrations are considered to be symptomatic of vitamin E deficiency. α-Tocopherol concentrations ranging from 0.5 to 0.7 mg/100 ml are considered as low, those above 0.7 satisfactory.[1,138]

α-Tocopherol concentration in the blood plasma (serum) has been shown to depend in large measure not only on its administration with food, but on the level of α-tocopherol carriers — β-lipoproteins — in the blood. Hence, the elevation of α-tocopherol content in aged individuals and in patients with hyperlipidemias, diabetes, or cardiovascular disturbances normally associated with an elevated cholesterol and triglyceride content, does not imply better provision of the organism with vitamin E, but reflects rather the increase in the concentration of β-lipoproteins.[140] In contrast, the lowering of α-tocopherol level in newborns and especially in premature babies in the case of innate α,β-lipoproteinemia is due to disturbances in vitamin E transport by the blood rather than to its decreased content in the food.[1]

For this reason, some authors recommend using as a criterion of vitamin E content in the organism not the α-tocopherol level in the blood plasma (serum), but the concentration ratio of this vitamin to total lipids, β-lipoproteins, or cholesterol.[140] Thus, it has been demonstrated that in patients receiving food poor in vitamin E over a period of 4 years, the tocopherol/total lipid ratio (mg/g) was below 0.8 mg/g, whereas in patients adequately supplied with vitamin E this value was more than 0.8.[140] Consequently, a tocopherol/total lipid ratio value higher than 0.8 mg/g can be considered as an index of an adequate provision of the organism with vitamin E, while that lower than 0.8 is a sign of deficiency.[1]

Administration of vitamin E in amounts greatly exceeding the norm does not lead to a large increase in its concentration in the blood serum. In healthy subjects receiving 100 to 800 IU of vitamin E daily for 3 years (amounts which exceeded 10 to 50 times the RDA value) the α-tocopherol concentration in the blood serum was 1.32 mg/100 ml on average, i.e., slightly above the normal level.[141] According to the data of Kitagawa and Mino,[142] regular intake of 600 mg (900 IU) of α-tocopherol per day for 12 weeks by male volunteers resulted in a 2.5- to 3.0-fold increase in its plasma concentration after 4 weeks and remained at this level during the following 8 weeks.[142] Noninvasive determinations of vitamin E content in buccal mucosal cells using sensitive high-performance liquid chromatography (HPLC) procedure with an electrochemical detector showed that in healthy male individuals *d*-α-tocopherol concentration was 46.4 ± 21.4 ng/mg of protein and increased two- to threefold after 1 month of daily intake of 600 mg of *d*-α-tocopherol. This correlated with the increase in α-tocopherol content in the plasma and red blood cells in this group.[143]

B. Dietary Intake of Vitamin E in Humans

According to the data of the second national study of the nutritional status and public health in the U.S. (11,658 adults) the average vitamin E intake is 9.6 mg per day for males and 7.0 mg per day for females. Median were 7.3 mg and 5.4 mg of *d*-α-tocopherol equivalents for males and females, respectively. These numbers are significantly lower than the RDA values. As a result, 23% of males and 15% of females had vitamin E/polyunsaturated fatty acid ratios in serum below normal.[144]

Studies carried out in Great Britain in the 1970s[145,146] revealed that dietary vitamin E consumption was 5 mg in half the populations observed and in many cases was even less than 3 mg/d. Nevertheless, in none of the cases investigated was vitamin E deficiency observed: the content of α-tocopherol in blood serum was in all cases higher than 0.5 mg/100 ml). Later studies showed that the average daily ration of a British family, calculated from foodstuff consumption and obtained by interviews of 6832 British families in 1979, included up to 8.3 mg of vitamin E daily per person.[147] In 1986 the average vitamin E consumption in Great Britain was also 8.4 mg of *d*-α-tocopherol equivalents per day.[148]

Vitamin E consumption by agricultural workers in Brazil was, on average, 5.5 ± 3.3 mg/d; its concentration in the blood plasma was 1.14 ± 0.33 mg/100 ml or 2.27 ± 0.53 mg/g as calculated per total lipids. In all cases studied, α-tocopherol concentration in blood plasma was above the lower threshold value, i.e., 0.5 mg/100 ml; in the overwhelming majority of cases (90%) it exceeded the value of 0.7 mg/100 ml, testifying to the satisfactory provision of this vitamin.[149] At the same time, in adult, lower-socioeconomic-class Asian Indians, α-tocopherol content in the blood plasma was 0.39 ± 0.045 mg/100 ml.[150]

Low α-tocopherol levels in the blood plasma was also observed in a limited number of individuals in developed countries. According to reports by Desai, α-tocopherol content in the blood plasma was below 0.5 mg/100 ml in 5.9% of healthy students in Canada.[151]

Thus, although in the majority of certain populations the concentration of dietary vitamin E is high enough to prevent the development of vitamin E deficiency, in a large part of the population of some countries it may be below the optimal level (15 mg); in some cases it can even be too low to maintain the necessary concentration of vitamin E in the blood.

V. VITAMIN E, PHYSICAL ENDURANCE, AND WORKING EFFICIENCY: ADMINISTRATION OF VITAMIN E AND SYNTHETIC ANTIOXIDANTS IN SPORT

The preceding discussion dealt with the important role of vitamin E in the maintenance of normal structure and metabolism of muscle tissue; in particular, in energy supply and Ca^{2+} uptake and release during muscle contraction. Needless to say, vitamin E deficiency has a negative effect on the state of the muscle apparatus and on its efficiency. For instance, as mentioned previously, it has been demonstrated that vitamin E deficiency decreases the endurance of rat muscles by 40%.[101]

The optimal provision of the organism with vitamin E and other vitally important nutrients is a necessary condition for high working efficiency and endurance of any human being, especially athletes. This necessity becomes especially well pronounced in the case of vitamin E deficiency caused by intensive physical exercise. However, questions remain unanswered: the specific body requirement for vitamin E during more or less intensive physical exercise, the true requirement of athletes for this vitamin, effects of additional administration of α-tocopherol on working efficiency and sports competition, and the necessity of additional administration.

Vitamin E-deficient rats exhibit a sixfold increase in expired pentane compared to E-sufficient animals,[152] and vitamin E-deficient rats consistently have shorter times to exhaustion in treadmill running,[101,153,154] but E-deficiency does not alter $\dot{V}O_2$ max.[101] These decrements in performance are accompanied by greater concentrations of stable free radicals and lipid peroxidation products in muscles and liver of the E-deficient compared to E-sufficient animals at rest, as well as disturbances in mitochondrial oxidative function,[101] and a 20-fold increase in erythrocyte hemolysis in the E-deficient animals.[155] Interestingly, neither the ESR free-radical signal nor the concentration of lipid peroxidation products (TBARS) increases in muscle or liver of exhausted E-deficient animals compared to E-sufficient animals.[101] It is possible that membrane function in the muscles and other tissues is sufficiently disrupted at a certain threshold level of lipid peroxidation as to make further exercise at a given level impossible, thus producing exhaustion at that exercise level; E-deficient animals begin exercise with membrane functions already somewhat compromised from oxidative damage, and therefore reach exhaustion earlier. It is unknown which membrane is the limiting factor (e.g., sarcolemma, sarcoplasmic reticulum, mitochondrial), or whether oxidative lipid damage, protein damage, or some interaction between the two is involved. Nonetheless, it is clear that the vitamin E antioxidant function is more important than the intact functioning of the glutathione system in allowing exercise to continue at submaximal levels. Interestingly, rats deficient in vitamin E which were supplemented with vitamin C, on the premise that vitamin C could serve to increase the effectiveness of the vitamin E remaining in the membranes of E-deficient animals through recycling mechanisms, had no greater endurance capacity and did not exhibit less erythrocyte hemolysis than E-deficient animals that were not supplemented with vitamin C.[155]

Most, but not all, studies support the hypothesis that vitamin E supplementation has a protective effect against exercise-induced oxidative damage. In humans taking 600 mg D,L-α-tocopherol three times daily for 2 weeks, a decreased pentane production during graded exercise up to 75% $\dot{V}O_2$ max has been seen,[122] and subjects who ingested vitamin E (300 mg D-α-tocopherol acetate daily for 4 weeks) exhibited a lower exercise-induced increase in plasma lipid peroxidation products after supplementation compared to before.[156] In rats, vitamin E supplementation also reduced exercise-induced liver lipid peroxidation.[157] It has been shown that vitamin E supplementation does not affect the leakage of cytosolic enzymes (creatine kinase and lactate dehydrogenase) into the blood following exercise,[158] but such supplementation has a marked effect in lowering the exercise-induced leakage of enzymes from lysosomes and mitochondria (β-glucuronidase and mitochondrial glutamic–oxaloacetic transaminase),[156] possibly because these membranes, especially the mitochondrial membranes, are more likely to be oxidatively damaged during exercise.

The effects of vitamin E supplementation on physical performance are less clear. Vitamin E-supplemented rats exhibited no greater endurance during treadmill running than rats on normal diet.[159] In humans undergoing progressive exercise to exhaustion, no difference was found in $\dot{V}O_2$ max or exercise time before or after vitamin E supplementation,[156] nor was there any difference in swimming speed between vitamin E-supplemented swimmers and those receiving placebo.[160,161] However, treatment of mice with spin trappers or with vitamin E greatly prolonged time to exhaustion while swimming, compared to time to exhaustion when the mice were untreated, or given saline.[162] Mountain climbers given vitamin E did not exhibit the deterioration in physical performance and increase in breath pentane content seen in unsupplemented climbers.[163] Experiments with rats trained for running along a straight course and rewarded with food at the finish demonstrated that the animals receiving a daily dose of vitamin E of 100 mg finished before rats receiving 1.2 or 50 mg of α-tocopherol.[164] Thus, while studies are in agreement about the protection afforded by supplementation with vitamin E against tissue damage induced by exercise, it is not clear whether such supplementation has an effect on performance.

Interesting results were obtained from the study of 20 prominent long-distance runners.[165] A group of them whose competitive results were essentially the same as those of others, received after competition a daily dose of 300 mg of a α-tocopherol over a period of 44 d. The vitamin E content in the blood sera of these runners amounted to 1.5 to 2.5 mg/100 ml, while in runners receiving a normal ration it was 0.5 to 1.0 mg/100 ml. During cycling, the pulmonary ventilation and O_2 uptake in the experimental group was higher than in the control. The maximal duration of cycling up to exhaustion in cyclists training at sea level and then brought to an altitude of 2700 to 2900 m was considerably decreased in the control group, whereas in the experimental group it was either unchanged or increased. In the group of runners trained at an altitude above 5000 m, better results were obtained in the experimental group than in the control group. The lactate content in the blood of runners in the experimental group measured after the race was lower than in the control. Thus, vitamin E seems to increase the endurance of athletes, especially those training at an altitude above sea level. This is achieved by the enhancement of the efficiency of O_2 utilization due to stimulation of oxidative processes occurring in the mitochondria.[165]

It was reported also that additional administration of high doses of vitamin E prevents or significantly diminishes the biochemical changes occurring under intensive physical load that are seen in avitaminosis E.[135] Thus, an additional administration of 1200 IU of vitamin E daily for 2 weeks prevented the increased production of pentane in expired air as a result of 1 h of exercise on a cycloergometer.[135]

The favorable effect of additional high doses of vitamin E on endurance and sports activities (e.g., in swimmers) was reported.[166,167] It was demonstrated that a short-term administration of vitamin E prior to standard physical tests accelerated the recovery of physical strength of tested subjects after training.

We do not share the view of the authors of the short review on the subjects of vitamin E in athletics who presume that the cause of these discrepancies is the inaccuracy of the methods employed for the investigation of the positive effects of vitamin E.[168] In our opinion, the true reason may be sought in the difference in the initial provision of the tested individuals with α-tocopherol, the intensity and some other parameters of physical load, as well as endurance indices, working efficiency, etc. Presumably, the positive effect of vitamin E can be seen only when a tested individual who was provided with vitamin E was either originally insufficient or became so as a result of intensive physical exercise. Therefore the effect cannot be detected, because of the sufficiently high level of this vitamin in the food or because the physical load is not high enough to cause any further requirement of the body for this vitamin. Besides, not all muscular lesions caused by intensive physical exercise (especially those causing complete muscle exhaustion) are due to lipid peroxidation and the resulting vitamin E deficiency. A prominent role in the degradation of muscle fibers and in muscle enzyme release into the blood can be attributed to other factors. This can serve as a satisfactory explanation of the fact that vitamin E, which causes the reduction of lipid peroxidation (pentane in the exhaled air, MDA in serum) upon physical load,[135] does not prevent the rise in the activity of creatine kinase in the blood.[158]

Finally, one cannot overlook the possibility that the lack of positive effect of vitamin E can, in some cases, be due to its administration at exceedingly high doses. Although vitamin E is one of the most "harmless" vitamins, causing no unfavorable effects in the majority of cases when taken in daily doses as high as 200 IU and even 1000 IU,[144,169,170] in some individuals α-tocopherol may be the cause of gastrointestinal disturbances and weakness.[1]

An interesting effect of super-high doses of vitamin E on rats exposed to exhaustive load (swimming) was reported.[132] When used in a dose of 25 mg per day vitamin E normalized the α-tocopherol level in the blood and creatine excretion by swimming rats, whereas a higher dose (60 mg) of the vitamin caused an opposite effect, i.e., enhanced excretion of creatine.

Studies on the effect of physical exercise of various intensities on the human requirement for vitamin E and on the optimal doses necessary for high working efficiency should be pursued further. The next step is optimizing vitamin E intakes of individuals engaging in intensive physical work or sports. However, the problem is finding the optimal dose of vitamin E in amounts which meet or somewhat exceed the physiological requirement of an individual for α-tocopherol, rather than in the use of this vitamin in super-high doses. In Russia, for example, the recommended requirements of α-tocopherol for athletes whose energy expenditure is 3500 to 4000 kcal exceeds the daily dose recommended for those individuals not involved in sports by 5 mg.[171]

Consideration of the effects caused by additional administration of vitamin E on physical endurance and lipid peroxidation during intensive muscle activity would be incomplete without mentioning the use of synthetic antioxidants. Experiments with male Wistar rats[172] showed that intraperitoneal injections of animals with the free-radical scavenger butylhydroxytoluene (BHT) (20 mg/kg of body weight) daily for 3 d increased the resistance of untrained animals to maximal physical load: this was reflected in a considerable (up to 60%) increase of the maximal duration of treadmill running to exhaustion as well as in a decreased

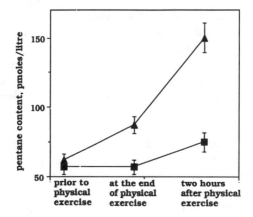

FIGURE 11. Effect of physical exercise (1) and of antioxidants (2) (BHT, 20 mg/kg body weight per 48 h for 15 d) on the pentane content in the air exhaled by sportsmen volunteers.

release of lactate dehydrogenase into the blood plasma after continuous exercise. Simultaneously, the antioxidant prevented the lipid peroxidation activation in skeletal muscles at maximal physical load. Both the damaging effects of exhaustive physical exercise and protective effects of antioxidants become far more pronounced in vitamin E-deficient animals.[173] Similar results on the prevention of lipid peroxidation activation by antioxidants and on the enhancement of endurance to physical load were obtained in experiments with volunteers (see also Figure 11).[104] In animals exposed to continuous training, intensive physical activity causes weaker sequelle of oxidative stress.[103]

Finally, it should be taken into consideration that, whereas in cardiac and skeletal muscles and lungs exhaustive physical exercise causes acceleration of blood flow, in peripheral tissues (intestine, kidneys, spleen) it gives rise to ischemic changes.[174] Cessation of physical activity restores normal circulation. It is well known that ischemia and further restoration of the blood flow may be the cause of severe lesions that are mainly due to excessive activation of lipid peroxidation.[96] These postischemic changes become especially well pronounced in vitamin E-deficient animals.[175] The use of antioxidants for the prophylaxis of these disorders appears to be a highly effective tool for the prevention of lesions resulting from postischemic reoxygenation.[96]

VI. SUMMARY

Vitamin E plays a decisive role in the maintenance of the functional activity of muscle tissues, due to its stabilizing effects on the membrane structures of myocytes. These effects of vitamin E are mainly due to its radical-scavenging activity. Thus, the maintenance of vitamin E in sufficient concentrations is a necessary prerequisite for good health and physical performance.

Vitamin E deficiency induces myodystrophy in animals and might also be the cause of decreased physical endurance in man. Clinical vitamin E deficiency is rarely observed in human beings and the amount of this vitamin in the standard diet is quite enough to ensure normal physical activity. However, increased or even exhausting physical exercise which activates free-radical reactions, results in an increased requirement for vitamin E, i.e., it necessitates an additional supply of vitamin E. This necessity could be even greater when exhaustive physical exercise is combined with stress, which could also contribute to the activation of free-radical reactions. The additional uptake of vitamin E under these conditions will preserve muscle structures, thus increasing physical endurance and capabilities. Daily intake of 15 to 20 mg of vitamin E, which is higher than RDA for adult males, may be sufficient for normal individuals during physical exercises. Since dietary intake of vitamin E in the U.S. and other developed countries on the average does not exceed 8 to 10 mg of α-tocopherol per day, the optimal supplementation with higher dosage of vitamin E should be provided by sports medical nutritionists.

The problem of whether additional regular intake of vitamin E in a dose range as high as 200 to 400 mg daily may be beneficial is a complicated one. Although the data on the effects of high doses of vitamin E on physical performance are contradictory, its ability to prevent the physical exercise-induced enhancement of lipid peroxidation and damage of muscle cell membranes is indisputable. It is not only the physical performance itself but also the "metabolic price" of it that is important for every sportsman, his coaches, and his physicians. Thus, the preventive effects of high vitamin E doses against exhaustive exercise-induced membrane injuries may be reasonable, even if this does not improve the physical performance in trained sportsmen. This raises the question of the safety of the regular intake of high vitamin E doses. The above-mentioned data indicated that long-term (4 to 12 weeks) daily intake of 200 to 1000 IU of vitamin E did not cause any harmful side effects in normal individuals.

Based upon the amount of vitamin E needed to double serum levels of *d*-α-tocopherol,[176] Horwitt et al. suggest that 269 mg/d of *d*-α-tocopherol equivalents (400 IU) should be the maximum for extended periods.[177]

The intake of this high dose of vitamin E during several weeks prior to heavy physical exercise (exhaustive physical practices, competitions) may be safe and useful for trained sportsmen under conditions of physical and emotional stress. Additional research on exercise-induced free-radical reactions, the consequences of harmful products of lipid peroxidation, and the protective role of α-tocopherol is necessary for broader recommendations to use high doses of vitamin E on a long-term basis.

REFERENCES

1. **Machlin, L. J.**, Vitamin E, in *Handbook of Vitamins: Nutritional, Biochemical, and Clinical Aspects*, Machlin, L. J., Ed., Marcel Dekker, New York, 1984, 99.
2. **Machlin, L. J., Ed.**, *Vitamin E*, Marcel Dekker, New York, 1980.
3. **Horwitt, M. K.**, Vitamin E: a reexamination, *Am. J. Clin. Nutr.*, 29, 569, 1976.
4. **Weiser, H. and Vecchi, M.**, Stereoisomers of alpha-tocopheryl acetate. II. Biopotencies of all eight stereoisomers, individually or in mixtures, as determined by rat resorption gestation test, *Int. J. Vitam. Nutr. Res.*, 52, 351, 1982.
5. **Bunnell, R. H., Keating, J., Quaresima, A., and Parman, G. K.**, Alpha-tocopherol content of foods, *Am. J. Clin. Nutr.*, 17, 1, 1965.
6. **Binder, H. J., Hertig, D. C., Hurst, V., Finch, S. C., and Spiro, N. P.**, Tocopherol deficiency in man, *N. Engl. J. Med.*, 273, 1289, 1965.
7. **Gross, S. J. and Landaw, S. A.**, The effect of vitamin E on red cell hemolysis and bilirubinemia, *Ann. N.Y. Acad. Sci.*, 393, 315, 1982.
8. **Stuart, M. J.**, Vitamin E deficiency: its effect on platelet-vascular interaction in various pathologic states, *Ann. N.Y. Acad. Sci.*, 393, 277, 1982.
9. **Horwitt, M. K., Century, B., and Zemen, A. A.**, Erythrocyte survival time and reticulocyte levels after tocopherol depletion in man, *Am. J. Clin. Nutr.*, 12, 99, 1963.
10. **Nason, A. and Lehman, I. R.**, The role of lipids in electron transport. II. Lipid cofactor replaced by tocopherol for enzymatic reduction of cytochrome c, *J. Biol. Chem.*, 222, 511, 1956.
11. **Carabello, F. B.**, Role of tocopherol in the reduction of mitochondrial NAD, *Can. J. Biochem.*, 52, 679, 1974.
12. **Schwartz, K.**, The cellular mechanisms of vitamin E action: direct and indirect effects of alpha-tocopherol on mitochondrial respiration, *Ann. N.Y. Acad. Sci.*, 203, 42, 1972.

13. **Caugill, C. P. J., Lucy, J. A., and Diplock, A. T.,** The effect of vitamin E on the intracellular distribution of the different oxidation states of selenium in rat liver, *Biochem. J.,* 125, 407, 1971.
14. **Nair, P. P.,** Vitamin E and metabolic regulation, *Ann. N.Y. Acad. Sci.,* 203, 53, 1972.
15. **Wu-Wang, C., Craig-Schmidt, M., and Faircloth, S. A.,** Conversion of arachidonate to prostanoids by lung microsomes from rats fed varying amounts of vitamin E, *Prost. Leuc. Med.,* 26, 291, 1987.
16. **Sagamoto, W., Fujie, K., Nishihara, J., Mino, M., Morita, I., and Murota, S. I.,** Inhibition of PGE2 production in macrophages from vitamin E-treated rats, *Prostaglandins Leucotrienes and Essential Fatty Acids,* 44, 89, 1991.
17. **Bakalova, R. A., Nekrasov, A. S., Lankin, V. Z., Kagan, V. E., Stoytchev, T., and Evstigneeva, R. P.,** The mechanism of inhibitory effects of alpha-tocopherol and its synthetic homologues on oxidation of linoleic acid, catalysed by reticulocyte lipoxygenase, *Proc. Natl. Acad. Sci. U.S.S.R.,* 299(4), 1008, 1988.
18. **Patnaik, R. N. and Nair, P. P.,** Studies on the binding of alpha-tocopherol to rat brain liver nuclei, *Arch. Biochem. Biophys.,* 178, 333, 1977.
19. **Tsen, C. C. and Collier, A. B.,** The protective action of tocopherol against hemolysis of rat erythrocytes by dialuric acid, *Can. J. Biochem. Physiol.,* 38, 957, 1960.
20. **Lucy, J. A. and Dingle, J. T.,** Fat-soluble vitamins and biological membranes, *Nature,* 204, 156, 1964.
21. **Corkin, V. Z.,** On the participation of vitamins E, K and related compounds in oxidation and phosphorylation, *Ukran Biochem. J.,* 31, 270, 1959 (in Russian).
22. **Djvczenko, W., Urbanovich, M., and Crabska, L.,** Ultrastructural changes of mitochondria in the rat liver on experimental tocopherol deficiency, *Acta Med. Pol.,* 5, 54, 1971.
23. **McCay, P. B. and Pfeifer, P. M.,** Vitamin E protection of membrane lipids during electron transport function, *Ann. N.Y. Acad. Sci.,* 203, 62, 1971.
24. **Wills, E. D. and Wilkinson, A. E.,** Release of enzymes from lysosomes by irradiation and relation of lipid peroxides formation to enzyme release, *Biochem. J.,* 99, 657, 1966.
25. **Arkhipenko, Yu. V., Gazdarov, A. K., Kozlov, Yu. P., Kagan, V. E., and Spirichev, V. B.,** Lipid peroxidation and inhibition of Ca^{2+}-transport in skeletal muscles sarcoplasmic reticulum membranes of vitamin E-deficient animals, *Biochemistry U.S.S.R.,* 41, 1898, 1976 (in Russian).
26. **Angelini, C., Di Mauro, S., and Margreth, A.,** Relationship of serum enzyme changes to muscle damage in vitamin E deficiency of the rabbit, *Sperimentale,* 118, 349, 1968.
27. **Grams, Y. W. and Eskins, K.,** Dye-sensitized photoperoxidation of tocopherols. Correlation between singlet oxygen reactivity and vitamin E activity, *Biochemistry,* 11, 606, 1972.
28. **Tappel, A. L.,** Vitamin E is the biological lipid antioxidant, *Vitam. Horm. N.Y.,* 20, 493, 1962.
29. **Tappel, A. L.,** Vitamin E and free radical peroxidation of lipids, *Ann. N.Y. Acad. Sci.,* 203, 12, 1972.
30. **Witting, L. A.,** Vitamin E and lipid antioxidants in free radical-initiated reactions, in *Free Radicals in Biology,* Vol. 4, Pryor, W. A., Ed., Academic Press, New York, 1980, 295.
31. **Halliwell, B. and Gutteridge, J. M. C.,** The importance of free radicals and catalytic metal ions in human diseases, *Mol. Aspects Med.,* 8, 89, 1985.
32. **Kagan, V. E., Ed.,** *Lipid Peroxidation in Biomembranes,* CRC Press, Boca Raton, FL, 1988, 1.
33. **Halliwell, B. and Gutteridge, J. M. C.,** Oxygen toxicity oxygen radicals transition metals and disease, *Biochem. J.,* 219, 1, 1984.
34. **Chance, B., Sies, H., and Boveris, A.,** Hydroperoxide metabolism in mammalian organs, *Physiol. Rev.,* 59, 527, 1979.
35. **Ursini, F., Maiorino, M., and Gregolin, C.,** Phospholipid hydroperoxide glutathione peroxidase, *Int. J. Tissue React.,* 8, 99, 1986.
36. **Bieri, J. G. and Evarts, R. P.,** Tocopherols and polyunsaturated fatty acids in human tissues, *Am. J. Clin. Nutr.,* 28, 717, 1975.
37. **Stocks, J. and Dormandy, T. L.,** The autooxidation of human red cells lipids induced by hydrogen peroxide, *Br. J. Haematol.,* 5, 95, 1971.
38. **Csallany, A. S., Draper, H. H., and Chan, S. H.,** Conversion of alpha-tocopherol C14 to tocopherylquinone *in vivo, Arch. Biochem. Biophys.,* 95, 142, 1962.
39. **Gazdarov, A. K., Spirichev, V. J., Saprin, A. N., Barkova, L. V., and Djachkova, L. V.,** Vitamin E and content of free radicals in animal tissues, *Biophysics U.S.S.R.,* 19, 300, 1974 (in Russian).
40. **McCay, P. B. and Poyer, J. L.,** A function for alpha-tocopherol: stabilization of the microsomal membrane from radical attack during TPNH-dependent oxidations, *Lipids,* 6, 297, 1971.
41. **Kagan, V. E., Arkhipenko, Yu. V., Dobrina, S. K., Kozlov, Yu. P., and Ritov, V. B.,** Stabilizing effects of vitamin E on biomembranes exposed to lipid peroxidation, *Biochemistry U.S.S.R.,* 42, 1194, 1977.
42. **Gee, P. L. and Tappel, A. L.,** The effect of exhaustive exercise on expired pentane as a measure of *in vivo* lipid peroxidation in the rat, *Life Sci.,* 28, 2425, 1981.

43. **Kagan, V. E., Serbinova, E. A., and Packer, L.,** Generation and recycling of radicals from phenolic antioxidants, *Arch. Biochem. Biophys.,* 280(1), 33, 1990.
44. **Kagan, V. E., Serbinova, E. A., and Packer, L.,** Recycling and antioxidant activity of tocopherol homologues of differing hydrocarbon chain length in liver microsomes, *Arch. Biochem. Biophys.,* 282, 221, 1990.
45. **Kagan, V., Serbinova, E., and Packer, L.,** Antioxidant effects of ubiquinones in microsomes and mitochondria are mediated by tocopherol recycling, *Biochem. Biophys. Res. Commun.,* 169(3), 851, 1990.
46. **Serbinova, E., Kagan, V., Han, D., and Packer, L.,** Intramembrane mobility and recycling in antioxidant properties of alpha-tocopherol and alpha-tocotrienol, *Free Rad. Biol. Med.,* 10, 263, 1991.
47. **Packer, J. E., Slater, T. F., and Willson, R. L.,** Direct observation of a free radical interaction between vitamin E and vitamin C, *Nature,* 278, 737, 1979.
48. **Niki, E., Tsuchiya, J., Tanimura, R., and Kamiya, Y.,** Regeneration of vitamin E from alpha-chromanoxyl radical by glutathione and vitamin C, *Chem. Lett.,* 89, 792, 1982.
49. **Liebler, D. C., Kling, D. S., and Reed, D. J.,** Antioxidant protection of phospholipid bilayers by alpha tocopherol. Control of alpha-tocopherol states and lipid peroxidation by ascorbic acid and glutathione, *J. Biol. Chem.,* 261, 12114, 1986.
50. **Niki, E., Kawakami, A., Saito, M., Yamamoto, Y., Fsuchiya, J., and Kaniya, T.,** Effects of phytol side chain of vitamin E on its antioxidant activity, *J. Biol. Chem.,* 260, 2191, 1985.
51. **Erin, A. N., Davitashvily, N. Y., Kagan, V. E., Zacharova, E. I., Saricheva, E. I., and Evstigneeva, R. P.,** Mechanisms of stabilization of biological membranes by vitamin E. Role of isoprenoid chain in protection of synaptosomes under activation of lipid peroxidation and action of phospholipase A2, *Biochemistry U.S.S.R.,* 53, 591, 1988.
52. **Viner, R. L., Novikov, K. N., Arkhipenko, Yu. V., Skrypin, V. I., Kozlov, Y. P., Spirichev, V. B., and Kagan, V. E.,** Non-antioxidant mechanism of cytochrome P-450 stabilization by alpha-tocopherol efficiency in vitamin E-deficient animals, *Biochemistry U.S.S.R.,* 51, 1549, 1986 (in Russian).
53. **Lucy, J. A.,** Functional and structural aspects of biological membranes: a suggested structural role for vitamin E in the control of membrane permeability and stability, *Ann. N.Y. Acad. Sci.,* 203, 3, 1972.
54. **Kagan, V. E., Skrypin, V. I., Serbinova, E. A., Rajkova, D. P., Tyurin, V. A., Bushuev, V. N., Erin, A. N., and Stoychev, Ts. S.,** Localization of alpha tocopherol in hydrophobic zone of lipid bilayer, *Dokl. Akad. Nauk U.S.S.R.,* 288, 1242, 1986.
55. **Diplock, A. T. and Lucy, J. A.,** The biochemical models of action of vitamin E and selenium: a hypothesis, *FEBS Lett.,* 29, 205, 1973.
56. **Lucy, J. A.,** Structural interactions between vitamin E and polyunsaturated phospholipids, in *Tocopherol, Oxygen and Biomembranes,* De Duve, C. and Hayaishi, O., Eds., Elsevier, New York, 1978, 109.
57. **Fukuzawa, K., Ikeno, H., Tokumura, A., and Tsukabni, H.,** Effect of alpha tocopherol incorporation on glucose permeability and phase transition of lecithin liposomes, *Chem. Phys. Lipids,* 23, 13, 1979.
58. **Corda, D., Pasthrnak, B., and Shinitzky, H.,** Increase of lipid microviscosity of unilamellar vesicles upon the creation of membrane potential, *J. Membr. Biol.,* 65, 235, 1982.
59. **Skrypin, V. I., Erin, A. N., Bratkovskaya, L. B., and Kagan, V. E.,** Alpha tocopherol as a modifier of the phase state of the lipid bilayer, *Bull. Exp. Biol. Med.,* 98, 673, 1984.
60. **Srivastava, S., Phadke, R. S., Govil, Y., and Rao, C. N. R.,** Fluidity, permeability and antioxidant behavior of model membranes incorporated with alpha tocopherol and vitamin E acetate, *Biochim. Biophys. Acta,* 734, 353, 1983.
61. **Urano, S., Kitahara, M., Kato, Y., Hasegawa, Y., and Matsuo, M.,** Membrane stabilizing effect of vitamin E: existence of a hydrogen bond between alpha-tocopherol and phospholipids in bilayer liposomes, *J. Nutr. Sci. Vitaminol.,* 36(6), 513, 1990.
62. **Ursano, S., Shichita, N., and Matsuo, M.,** Interaction of vitamin E and its model compounds with unsaturated fatty acids in homogeneous solution, *J. Nutr. Sci. Vitaminol.,* 34(2), 189, 1988.
63. **Ursano, S., Yano, K., and Matsuo, M.,** Membrane-stabilizing effect of vitamin E: effect of alpha-tocopherol and its model compounds on fluidity of lecithin liposomes [published erratum appears in *Biochem. Biophys. Res. Commun.,* 151(1), 631, 1988], *Biochem. Biophys. Res. Commun.,* 150(1), 469, 1988.
64. **Ursano, S., Iida, M., Otani, I., and Matsuo, M.,** Membrane stabilization of vitamin E; interactions of alpha-tocopherol with phospholipids in bilayer liposomes, *Biochem. Biophys. Res. Commun.,* 146(3), 1413, 1987.
65. **Wassal, S. R., Thewalt, J. L., Wong, L., Yorrissen, H., and Cushley, R. J.,** Deuterium NMR study of the interaction of alpha-tocopherol with a phospholipid model membranes, *Biochemistry,* 25, 319, 1986.
66. **Tabidze, L. V., Ritov, V. B., Kagan, V. E., and Kozlov, Yu. P.,** Vitamin E protects sarcoplasmic reticulum membranes against damage induced by free fatty acids, *Bull. Exp. Biol. Med.,* 96, 1548, 1983 (in Russian).
67. **Kagan, V. E.,** Tocopherol stabilizes membrane against phospholipases A, free fatty acids and lysophospholipids, *Ann. N.Y. Acad. Sci.,* 570, 121, 1989.

68. **Novikov, K. N. and Kagan, V. E.**, Stabilization of cytochrome P-450 in hepatocytes by free radical scavengers of different nature, *Acta Physiol. Pharmacol. Bulg.*, 11(3), 6169, 1985.
69. **Erin, A. N., Spirin, M. M., Tabidze, L. V., and Kagan, V. E.**, Formation of α-tocopherol complexes with fatty acids. A hypothetical mechanism of stabilization of biomembranes by vitamin E, *Biochim. Biophys. Acta*, 774, 96, 1984.
70. **Erin, A. N., Gorbunov, N. N., Brusovanik, v. L., Tyurin, V. A., and Prilipko, L. L.**, Stabilization of synaptic membranes by α-tocopherol against the damaging action of phospholipases. Possible mechanism of biological action of vitamin E, *Brain Res.*, 398, 85, 1986.
71. **Erin, A. N., Skrypin, V. I., and Kagan, V. E.**, Formation of α-tocopherol complexes with fatty acids. Nature of complexes, *Biochim. Biophys. Acta*, 815, 209, 1985.
72. **Skrypin, V. I., Brusovanik, V. I., Djaparidze, L. M., Erin, A. N., Selisheva, A. A., Prilipko, L. L., Spirichev, V. B., and Kagan, V. E.**, Enhanced damage of brain synaptosomes from vitamin E-deficient rats by free fatty acids, *Bull. Exp. Biol. Med.*, 102, 547, 1986.
73. **Grigorieva, V. A. and Medovar, E. N.**, Ultrastructural organization of muscles in vitamin E-deficient animals, *Vitamins*, 8, 61, 1975 (in Russian).
74. **Van Vleet, J. H., Hall, S. V., and Simon, Y.**, Vitamin E deficiency, *Am. J. Pathol.*, 52, 1067, 1968.
75. **Chan, A. Y. and Hegarty, P. V. J.**, Morphological changes in skeletal muscle in vitamin E-deficient and refed rabbits, *Br. J. Nutr.*, 38, 361, 1977.
76. **Zuckerman, L. and Marquardt, G. H.**, Muscle, erythrocyte and plasma electrolytes and some other muscle constituents of rabbits with nutritional muscular dystrophy, *Proc. Soc. Exp. Biol. Med.*, 112, 609, 1963.
77. **Rumery, R. E. and Hampton, I. C.**, Microscopic and submicroscopic observations on skeletal muscle from vitamin E-deficient rats, *Anat. Rec.*, 133, 1, 1959.
78. **Tugai, V. A. and Litvinenko, O. O.**, Structural changes in sarcolemma upon E avitaminosis dystrophy, *Ukran. Biochem. J.*, 49, 97, 1977 (in Russian).
79. **Davies, K. J. A., Quintanilha, A. T., Brooks, G. A., and Packer, L.**, Free radical tissue damage produced by exercise, *Biochem. Biophys. Res. Commun.*, 107, 1198, 1982.
80. **Arkhipenko, Yu. V., Djaparidze, L. M., Gutkin, Yu. V., Rozhizkaya, I. L., and Spirichev, V. B.**, Vitamin E-deficiency, lipid peroxidation and Ca^{2+}-transport in rat myocardium, *Problems Med. Chem.*, 33, 47, 1987 (in Russian).
81. **Eschraghi, B., Elmadfa, L., and Feldheim, M.**, Einfluss der Tocopherol Ersorgung auf Enzymaktivitaten und Redox Systeme 11. Mitt. Zietlicher Verlauf der Aktivitaten von sechs Enzymen in Plasma, Muskel, Herz und Leber des Meerschweinchens nach Unterbrechung der Tocopherol Zufuhr, *Int. J. Vir. Nutr. Res.*, 44, 32, 1974.
82. **Golubeva, L. Y. and Djaparidze, L. M.**, Vitamin E deficiency and creatin phosphate content in cardiac muscle, *Problems Med. Chem.*, 32, 121, 1986 (in Russian).
83. **Lin, Ch. T. and Chen, L. H.**, Ultrastructural and lysosomal enzyme studies of skeletal muscle and myocardium in rats with long-term vitamin E deficiency, *Pathology*, 14, 375, 1982.
84. **Dhalla, N. S., Fedelesova, M., and Tomer, I.**, Biochemical alterations in the skeletal muscle of vitamin E deficient rats, *Can. J. Biochem.*, 49, 1202, 1971.
85. **Hasselbach, W. and Oelliker, H.**, Energetics and electrogenicity of the sarcoplasmic reticulum calcium pump, *Annu. Rev. Physiol.*, 45, 325, 1983.
86. **Martonosi, J. A.**, The development of sarcoplasmic reticulum membranes, *Annu. Rev. Physiol.*, 44, 337, 1982.
87. **Takagy, A.**, Lipid composition of sarcoplasmic reticulum of human skeletal muscle, *Biochim. Biophys. Acta*, 248, 12, 1971.
88. **Nagatamo, T., Hitori, K., Ikeda, M., and Shimada, K.**, Lipid composition of sarcolemma, mitochondria and sarcoplasmic reticulum from newborn and adult rabbit cardiac muscle, *Biochem. Med.*, 23, 108, 1980.
89. **Shewfelt, R. L. and Hultin, H. O.**, Inhibition of enzymic and non-enzymic lipid peroxidation of flounder muscle sarcoplasmic reticulum by pretreatment with phospholipase A2, *Biochim. Biophys. Acta*, 751, 432, 1983.
90. **Arkhipenko, Yu. V., Pisarev, V. A., and Kagan, V. E.**, Modification of enzymatic system for Ca^{2+} transport in sarcoplasmic reticulum during lipid peroxidation. Systems for generation and regulation of lipid peroxidation in skeletal and heart muscles, *Biochemistry U.S.S.R.*, 48, 1080, 1983.
91. **Boldyrev, A. A.**, On the biological role of histidine dipeptides, *Biochemistry U.S.S.R.*, 51, 1930, 1986.
92. **Sylven, Ch. and Glavind, J.**, Peroxide formation, vitamin E and myocardial damage in the rat, *Int. J. Vitam. Nutr. Res.*, 47, 9, 1977.
93. **Djaparidze, L. M., Ustinova, E. E., Arkhipenko, Yu. V., Spirichev, V. B., and Meerson, F. Z.**, Activation of lipid peroxidation and decrease of the heart fibrillation threshold upon E-avitaminosis, *Probl. Nutr.*, 6, 48, 1986 (in Russian).

94. **Meerson, F. Z., Belkina, L. M., Arkhipenko, Yu. V., Djaparidze, L. M., and Saltykova, V. A.,** Vitamin E-deficiency and appearance of heart arrhythmias in acute ischaemia, *Bull. Exp. Biol. Med.,* 103, 1987, in press.

95. **Djaparidze, L. M., Belkina, L. M., Dosmagambedova, R. S., Spirichev, V. B., and Meerson, F. Z.,** Vitamin E-deficiency and cardiac muscle contractility, *Probl. Nutr.,* 1, 25, 1986 (in Russian).

96. **Meerson, F. Z., Kagan, V. E., Kozlov, Yu. P., Belkina, L. M., and Arkhipenko, Yu. V.,** The role of lipid peroxidation in pathogenesis of ischemic damage and the antioxidant protection of the heart, *Basic Res. Cardiol.,* 77, 465, 1982.

97. **Kagan, V. E., Arkhipenko, Yu. V., Meerson, F. Z., and Kozlov, Yu. P.,** Modification of the enzyme system of Ca^{2+} transport in the sarcoplasmic reticulum during lipid peroxidation. Damage *in vivo* caused by pathological changes, *Biochemistry U.S.S.R.,* 48, 977, 1983.

98. **Keul, J., Jakob, E., Berg, A., Dickhuth, H. H., and Lehmann, M.,** Zur Wirkung von Vitaminen auf die Leistungs- und Erholungsfahigkeit des Menschen, *Pharmazeut Rundschau,* 9, 94, 1987.

99. **Packer, L.,** Vitamin E, physical exercise and tissue damage in animals, *Med. Biol.,* 62, 105, 1984.

100. **Aikawa, K. M., Quintanilha, A. T., de Zumen, B., Brooks, G. A., and Packer, L.,** Exercise endurance training alters vitamin E tissue level and red blood cells hemolysis in rodents, *Biosci. Rep.,* 4, 253, 1984.

101. **Davies, K. Y., Quintanilha, A. T., Brooks, G. A., and Packer, L.,** Free radicals and tissue damage produced by exercise, *Biochem. Biophys. Res. Commun.,* 107, 1198, 1982.

102. **Pyke, S., Lew, H., and Quintanilha, A. T.,** Severe depletion in liver glutathione during physical exercise, *Biochem. Biophys. Res. Commun.,* 139, 926, 1986.

103. **Packer, L.,** Mitochondria, oxygen radicals and animal exercise, in *Membranes and Muscle, Proc. Int. Symp.,* Cape Town, March 18–21, 1985, IRL Press, Oxford, 1985, 135.

104. **Meerson, F. Z., Beresneva, Z. V., Boev, V. M., Kagan, V. E., Orlov, O. N., and Prilipko, L. L.,** The effect of antioxidant on the contractility of the heart muscle and on the resistance to strenuous physical exercise, *Theory Prac. Phys. Cult.,* 8, 14, 1983 (in Russian).

105. **Viinikha, L., Vuori, J., and Ylikorkala, O.,** Lipid peroxides, prostacyclin and thromboxane A2 in runners during acute exercise, *Med. Sci. Sports Exercise,* 16, 275, 1984.

106. **Balke, P. O., Shider, M. T., and Bull, A. P.,** Evidence for lipid peroxidation during moderate exercise in man, *Med. Sci. Sports Exercise,* 16, 181, 1984.

107. **Kanter, M. M., Lesmes, G. R., Nequin, N. D., Kaminsky, L. A., and Saeger, J. M.,** Serum enzyme levels and lipid peroxidation in ultramarathon runners, *Med. Sci. Sports Exercise,* 17, 245, 1985.

108. **Simon-Schnass, I., and Pabsts, H.,** Influence of vitamin E on physical performance, *Int. J. Vitam. Nutr. Res.,* 58, 49, 1988.

109. **Sumida, S., Tanaka, K., Kitao, H., and Nakadomo, F.,** Exercise-induced lipid peroxidation and leakage of enzymes before and after vitamin E supplementation, *Int. J. Biochem.,* 21, 835, 1989.

110. **Hunding, A., Jordal, R., and Poulev, P. E.,** Runner's anemia and iron deficiency, *Acta Med. Scand.,* 209, 315, 1981.

111. **Siegel, A. J., Hennekens, C. H., and Solomon, H. S.,** Exercise related hematuria: findings in a group of marathon runners, *JAMA,* 241, 391, 1979.

112. **Roy, R. S. and McCord, J. M.,** Superoxide and ischaemia: conversion of xanthine dehydrogenase to xanthine oxidase, in *Oxy-radicals and Their Scavenger Systems,* Greenwald, R. A. and Cohen, G., Eds., Elsevier, Amsterdam, 1983, 224.

113. **McCord, J.,** Oxygen-derived free radicals in post-ischemic tissue injury, *N. Engl. J. Med.,* 312, 159, 1985.

114. **Boveris, A. and Chance, B.,** The mitochondrial generation of hydrogen peroxide: general properties and effect of hyperbaric oxygen, *Biochem. J.,* 134, 707, 1973.

115. **Boveris, A. and Cadenas, E.,** Mitochondrial production of superoxide anions and its relationship to the antimycin insensitive respiration, *FEBS Lett.,* 54, 311, 1975.

116. **Cadenas, E., Boveris, A., Ragan, C. I., and Stoppani, A. O. M.,** Production of superoxide radicals and hydrogen peroxide by NADH-ubiquinone reductase and ubiquinol-cytochrome c reductase from beef heart mitochondria, *Arch. Biochem. Biophys.,* 180, 248, 1977.

117. **Kellog, E. W., III and Fridovich, I.,** Superoxide, hydrogen peroxide, and singlet oxygen in lipid peroxidation by a xanthine oxidase system, *J. Biol. Chem.,* 250, 8812, 1975.

118. **Wolbarsht, M. L. and Fridovich, I.,** Hyperoxia during reperfusion is a factor in reperfusion injury, *Free Rad. Biol. Med.,* 6, 61, 1989.

119. **Jackson, M. J., Edwards, R. H. T., and Symons, M. C. R.,** Electron spin resonance studies of intact skeletal muscle, *Biochim. Biophys. Acta,* 847, 185, 1985.

120. **Alessio, H. M., Goldfarb, A. H., and Cutler, R. G.,** MDA content increases in fast- and slow-twitch skeletal muscle with intensity of exercise in a rat, *Am. J. Physiol.,* 251, C874, 1988.

121. **Dillard, C. J., Litov, R. E., Savin, W. M., Dumelin, E. E., and Tappel, A. L.,** Effects of exercise, vitamin E, and ozone on pulmonary function and lipid peroxidation, *J. Appl. Physiol.,* 45, 927, 1978.

122. **Kanter, M. M., Lesmes, G. R., Kaminsky, L. A., Ham-Saeger, J., and Nequin, N. D.,** Serum creatine kinase and lactate dehydrogenase changes following an eighty kilometer race. Relationship to lipid peroxidation, *Eur. J. Appl. Physiol.,* 57, 60, 1988.

123. **Duthie, G. G., Robertson, J. D., Maughan, R. J., and Morrice, P. C.,** Blood antioxidant status and erythrocyte lipid peroxidation following distance running, *Arch. Biochem. Biophys.,* 282, 78, 1990.

124. **Viinikka, L., Vuori, J., and Ylikorkala, O.,** Lipid peroxides, prostacycline, and thromboxane A₂ in runners during acute exercise, *Med. Sci. Sports Exercise,* 16, 275, 1984.

125. **Sumida, S., Tanaka, K., Kitao, H., and Nakamodo, F.,** Exercise-induced lipid peroxidation and leakage of enzymes before and after vitamin E supplementation, *Int. J. Biochem.,* 21, 835, 1989.

126. **Lovlin, R., Cottle, W., Pyke, I., Kavanach, M., and Belkastro, A. N.,** Are inducers of free radical damage related to exercise intensity, *Eur. J. Appl. Physiol.,* 56, 313, 1987.

127. Physiological requirements in nutritional components and dietary energy consumption for different groups of population in Russia. Ministry of Public Health of Russia, Moscow, 1991.

128. Recommended Dietary Allowances, 10th ed., National Academy Press,Washington, D.C., 1989.

129. **Truswell, A. S.,** Recommended Dietary Intakes around the world, *Nutr. Abstr. Rev.,* 53, 1075, 1983.

130. **Harris, P. L. and Embree, N. D.,** Quantitative consideration of the effect of polyunsaturated fatty acid content of the diet upon the requirements for vitamin E, *Am. J. Clin. Nutr.,* 13, 385, 1963.

131. **Jager, F. C.,** Long-test dose-response effects of vitamin E in rats, *Nutr. Metab.,* 14, 1, 1972.

132. **Efremov, V. V. and Sakaeva, E. A.,** Creatine and creatinine urinary excretion in experimental animals exposed to vitamin E-deficiency and physical load, *Probl. Nutr.,* 6, 19, 1974 (in Russian).

133. **Brady, P. S., Brady, L. J., and Ullrey, D. E.,** Selenium, vitamin E and the response to swimming stress in the rat, *J. Nutr.,* 109, 1103, 1979.

134. **Young, L. C., Lumsden, J. H., Lun, A., Claxton, Y., and Edmea des, D. E.,** Influence of dietary levels of vitamin E and selenium on tissue and blood parameters in pigs, *Can. J. Comp. Med.,* 40, 92, 1976.

135. **Tappel, A. L. and Dillard, C. J.,** *In vivo* lipid peroxidation: measurement via exhaled pentane and protection by vitamin E, *Fed. Proc.,* 40, 174, 1981.

136. **Both-Bedenbender, N. and Sierakowski, B.,** Einfluss der massigen physikalischen Training auf Lipidperoxydierung und Vitamin E-Versorgung der alteren Leute, *Akruel, Ernahrllngsmed.,* 11, 173, 1986.

137. **Rokitzki, L., Berg, A., and Keul, J.,** Blood and serum status of water- and fat-soluble vitamins in athletes and non-athletes, *Int. J. Vitam. Nutr. Res. Suppl.,* 30, 192, 1989.

138. **Sauberlich, H. E., Dowdy, R. P., and Skala, J. H.,** Laboratory tests for the assessment of nutritional states, *CRC Crit. Rev. Clin. Lab. Sci.,* 288, 1973.

139. **Gonthea, I. and Nicolan, N.,** Tocopherolemia in healthy human adults, *Nutr. Metab.,* 14, 349, 1972.

140. **Horwitt, M. K., Harvey, C. C., Dahm, D. H., and Searcy, M. T.,** Relationship between tocopherol and serum lipid levels for determination of nutritional adequacy, *Ann. N.Y. Acad. Sci.,* 203, 233, 1972.

141. **Farrell, P. H. and Bicre, L. G.,** Megavitamin E supplementation in man, *Am. J. Clin. Nutr.,* 28, 1381, 1975.

142. **Kitagawa, M. and Mino, M.,** Effect of elevated D-α-R,R,R-tocopherol dosage in man, *J. Nutr. Sci. Vitaminol.,* 35, 133, 1989.

143. **Tamai, H. and Manago, M.,** Determination of alpha-tocopherol in buccal mucosal cells using an electrochemical detector, *Int. J. Vitam. Nutr. Res.,* 58, 202, 1988.

144. **Murphy, S. P., Subar, A. F., and Block, G.,** Vitamin E intakes and sources in the United States, *Am. J. Clin. Nutr.,* 53, 361, 1990.

145. **Losowsky, M. S., Kelleher, Y., Walker, B. E., Davies, T., and Smith, C. I.,** Intake and absorption of tocopherol, *Ann. N.Y. Acad. Sci.,* 203, 212, 1972.

146. **Smith, C. L., Kelleher, J., Losowsky, M. S., and Morrish, N.,** The content of vitamin E in British diets, *Br. J. Nutr.,* 26, 89, 1971.

147. **Bull, N. L. and Buss, D. H.,** Biotin, pantothenic acid and vitamin E in British household food supply, *Hum. Nutr. Appl.,* 36, 190, 1982.

148. **Lewis, J. and Buss, D. H.,** Trace nutrients. 5 Minerals and vitamins in the British household food supply, *Br. J. Nutr.,* 60, 413, 1988.

149. **Desai, I. D., Swann, M. A., Garcia, M. L., Dutra de Oliveira, B. S., Duarte, F. A. M., and Dutra de Oliveira, I. A.,** Vitamin E states of agricultural migrant workers in Southern Brazil, *Am. J. Clin. Nutr.,* 33, 2668, 1980.

150. **Nadiger, H. A.,** Studies on interrelationship between vitamins E and B-complex, *Nutr. Metab.,* 24, 352, 1980.

151. **Desai, I. D.,** Plasma tocopherol levels on normal adults, *Can. J. Physiol. Pharmacol.,* 46, 819, 1968.

152. **Dillard, C. J., Litov, R. E., and Tappel, A. L.,** Effects of dietary vitamin E, selenium, and polyunsaturated fats on in vivo lipid peroxidation in the rat as measured by pentane production, *Lipids,* 13, 396, 1978.

153. **Ji, L. L., Stratman, F. W., and Lardy, H. A.,** Antioxidant enzyme systems in rat liver and skeletal muscle: influences of selenium deficiency, chronic training, and acute exercise, *Arch. Biochem. Biophys.,* 263, 150, 1988.

154. **Lang, J. K., Gohil, K., Packer, L., and Burk, R. F.,** Selenium deficiency, endurance exercise capacity, and antioxidant status in rats, *J. Appl. Physiol.,* 63, 2532, 1987.

155. **Gohil, K., Packer, L., De Lumen, B., Brooks, G. A., and Terblanshe, S. E.,** Vitamin E deficiency and vitamin C supplements: exercise and mitochondrial oxidation, *J. Appl. Physiol.,* 60, 1986, 1986.

156. **Sumida, S., Tanaka, K., Kitao, H., and Nakadomo, F.,** Exercise-induced lipid peroxidation and leakage of enzymes before and after vitamin E supplementation, *Int. J. Biochem.,* 21, 835, 1989.

157. **Brady, P. S., Brady, L. J., and Ulrey, D. E.,** Selenium, vitamin E, and the response to swimming stress in the rat, *J. Nutr.,* 10, 1103, 1979.

158. **Helgheim, I., Hetland, O., Nilsson, S., Inger, F., and Stromme, S. B.,** The effects of vitamin E on serum enzyme levels following heavy exercise, *Eur. J. Appl. Physiol.,* 40, 283, 1979.

159. **Mehlhorn, R. J., Sumida, S., and Packer, L.,** Tocopheroxyl radical persistence and tocopherol consumption in liposomes and in vitamin E-enriched rat liver mitochondria and microsomes. *J. Biol. Chem.,* 261, 13, 448, 1989.

160. **Shephard, R. J., Campbell, R., Pimm, P., Stuart, D., and Wright, G. R.,** Vitamin E, exercise and the recovery from physical activity, *Eur. J. Appl. Physiol.,* 33, 119, 1974.

161. **Lawrence, J. D., Bower, R. C., Riehl, W. P., and Smith, J. L.,** Effects of alpha tocopherol acetate on the swimming endurance of trained swimmers, *Am. J. Clin. Nutr.,* 28, 205, 1975.

162. **Novelli, G. P., Bracciotti, G., and Falsini, S.,** Spin-trappers and vitamin E prolong endurance to muscle fatigue in mice, *Free Rad. Biol. Med.,* 8, 9, 1990.

163. **Simon-Schnass, I. and Pabst, H.,** Influence of vitamin E on physical performance, *Int. J. Vitam. Nutr. Res.,* 58, 49, 1988.

164. **Rosen, A. Y., Cohen, M. E., and Pieken, L.,** DL-alpha tocopherol acetate and instrumental conditioning in the rat, *Nutr. Rep. Int.,* 6, 181, 1972.

165. **Tatsuo, N., Hiroshi, K., Yunichiro, A., Takershi, M., and Kiniko, S.,** The effect of vitamin E on endurance, *Asian Med. J.,* 11, 619, 1968.

166. **Cureton, T. K.,** Influence of wheat germ oil as a dietary supplement in a program of conditioning exercises with middle aged subjects. *Res. Q. Am. Assoc. Health Phys. Educ. Recreat.,* 26, 391, 1955.

167. **Von Prokop, L.,** Die Wirkung von naturlichem Vitamin E auf Sauerstoffverbrauch und Sauerstoffschuld, *Sportarzt. Prax.,* 1, 19, 1960.

168. **Anon, P.,** Vitamin E in Athletics, *Br. Med. J.,* 251, 1971.

169. **Bendich, A. and Machlin, L.,** Safety of oral vitamin E, *Am. J. Clin. Nutr.,* 48, 612, 1988.

170. **Machlin, L.,** Use and safety of elevated dosage of vitamin E in adults, *Int. J. Vitam. Nutr. Res.,* 30, 56, 1989.

171. **Pokrovsky, A. A., Ed.,** *A Recommended Dietary Allowance for Sportsmen,* Medizina Publishing House, Moscow, 1975 (in Russian).

172. **Meerson, F. Z., Krasikov, S. I., Boev, V. M., and Kagan, V. E.,** Effect of an antioxidant on the untrained body resistance to maximal exercise, *Bull. Exp. Biol. Med.,* 94, 17, 1982.

173. **Salminen, A., Kainulainen, H., Arstila, A. U., and Vihko, V.,** Vitamin E deficiency and the susceptibility to lipid peroxidation of mouse cardiac and skeletal muscles, *Acta Physiol. Scand.,* 122, 565, 1984.

174. **Basson, A. B. K., Terblanche, S. E., and Oelofsen, W.,** A comparative study of the effects of aging and training on the levels of lipofuscin in various tissues of the rat, *Comp. Biochem. Physiol.,* 71A, 369, 1982.

175. **Jackson, M. J., Jones, D. A., and Edwards, R. H.,** Vitamin E and skeletal muscle, in *Biology of Vitamin E,* Proc. Ciba Found. Symp. 7–10 March, 1983, Vol. 101, Pitman Medical, London, 1983, 224.

176. **Horwitt, M. K., Elliott, W. H., Kanjananggulpan, P., and Fitch, C. D.,** Serum concentrations of α-tocopherol after ingestion of various vitamin E preparations, *Am. J. Clin. Nutr.,* 40, 240, 1984.

177. **Horwitt, M. K.,** Data supporting supplementation of humans with vitamin E, *J. Nutr.,* 121, 424, 1991.

Chapter 10

BONE AND CALCIUM IN EXERCISE AND SPORT

Ira Wolinsky
James F. Hickson, Jr.
Sara B. Arnaud

CONTENTS

0-8493-7911-3/94/$0.00+$.50
© 1994 by CRC Press, Inc.

I. INTRODUCTION

Skeletal load-bearing ability is determined by the mass, mechanical and material properties, and architecture of the component bones. Mechanical forces exert an influence on bone structure. Bone elements place or displace themselves in the direction of functional forces and increase or decrease their mass to reflect the amount of the forces, i.e., bone is dynamically responsive to the functional demand placed on it — Wolff's law.[1-4] Skeletal elements are normally aligned so as to provide maximum strength and to resist compressive and longitudinal tensile stresses encountered in gravity. These elements can realign themselves in the direction of functional forces and change their mass to adapt to modified environmental forces. Functional forces may include mechanical loading and exercise or the lack thereof.

II. INACTIVITY AND WEIGHTLESSNESS

Weightlessness and immobilization may be considered extreme forms of inactivity. The consequence of muscle atrophy from inactivity induced by bed rest, immobilization, or space flight is a decrease in the mechanical stimuli to bone and reduced bone mass. Reduced formation and loss of bone mineral is localized to the unloaded bone(s).[5,6] After 9 months of bed rest the decrease in bone mineral in the *os calcis* was 25 to 45% of pre-bed-rest levels.[7] Other sites vulnerable to mineral loss, assessed by dual photon absorptiometry in six men after 17 weeks of horizontal bed rest, are the trochanter, femoral neck, lumbar spine, and proximal tibia, with losses amounting to 4.5, 3.6, 3.9, and 2.2% of pre-bed-rest levels.[8] Decreases in total body calcium were modest (1.4 ± 0.8%), a phenomenon due to either redistribution of bone mineral or deposition of newly acquired mineral in the upper skeleton. Head-down tilt bed rest flight simulation models show this gravitational effect on bone mineral density in the adult skeleton after only 4 weeks.[9]

Bone loss and negative calcium balance are potentially the most serious of physiological changes occurring during flights into space; it may prove to be a serious limiting factor for the duration of space flight. Astronauts and cosmonauts routinely use exercise countermeasures to prevent bone mineral losses.[10,11] However, the types of exercise needed to prevent loss of bone from the weight-bearing bones and to restore it following disuse are not clearly defined. Restoration of mineral density following disuse from a variety of causes generally proceeds more slowly than its loss, with rates differing in each bone and in individuals.[12] It seems logical that the time needed for restoration of muscle strength must precede recovery of bone mineral losses.[13] Because other factors may account for individual variations in bone loss and the delays in repair, the effects of diet and drugs have been tested.[14] High levels of dietary calcium and phosphorus, and diphosphonate, did not alter bone mineral density, but improved negative calcium balance.

In spite of adequate diets, negative calcium balance is regularly reported in association with prolonged inactivity.[15] The loss of calcium occurs through increases in urinary excretion and reduced intestinal absorption. Its magnitude is variable in individuals, ranging from 50 to 200 mg/d.[7] In bed rest, there is a prompt increase in urinary calcium associated with urinary sodium excretion.[16] This naturesis from fluid shifts subsides but calcium excretion remains elevated, decreasing gradually to near basal levels after 4 months.[14] Initially, fecal calcium does not contribute to negative balance, but accounts for 50% of the negative balance after 2 months when intestinal absorption is reduced.

The response of the calcium endocrine system secondary to the mobilization of calcium from bone during inactivity may partially explain the associated negative balance. Suppression of the parathyroid–1,25-dihydroxyvitamin D axis could account for both the increase in excretion of urinary calcium and depressed intestinal absorption.[17] Decreased parathyroid hormone would act to reduce the renal tubular reabsorption of calcium and the vitamin D hormone, its intestinal absorption. This response to inactivity seems to be an appropriate adaptation to a reduced requirement for bone mineral. However, the failure of renal and intestinal hormone responses to restore calcium balance during bed rest or space flight suggests that other elements in either diet or the endocrine system may be involved.

III. EXERCISE AND SPORTS

A. Bone Mass

Evidence has accumulated that exercise and sport can result in increased bone mass. These studies have included both men and women (both pre- and postmenopause), athletes and nonathletes, younger and older individuals. Because of the increasing interest and participation of females in physical fitness activities and competitive sports, a growing number of these studies involved women subjects.

Data suggesting that important increments in skeletal mass may result from physical activity during childhood have been reported by Slemenda et al.[18] A group of 118 children (5.3 to 14 years old) were studied. Consistent positive associations were observed between bone mineral densities (single or dual photon absorptiometry) in the radius, spine, and hip and most self-reported exercise/sport activities. Total hours of vigorous, weight-bearing activity per day was significantly related to bone mineral densities in the radius and hip, independent of age or gender effects. Meleski et al.[19] measured bone dimensions of the second metacarpal in 280 male ice hockey players 10 to 12 years old compared with nonathletic youth control data from other studies. For the same stature, the hockey players had a larger periosteal diameter, cortical thickness, and cortical area. Among the hockey players, defensemen had the largest cortical bone dimensions followed by forwards and the goalkeepers. After correcting, by statistical procedures, for the effects of height, weight, chronological and skeletal age, players at the forward position had larger cortical bone dimensions than defensemen or goalies. Cortical bone of the second metacarpal was used by this research group as a reasonable index of skeletal mineralization. However, it must be realized that cortical bone in children is influenced by normal growth and hence it is difficult to separate out effects of exercise from those changes associated with normal growth and maturation. It is tempting to attribute differences in cortical bone dimensions within the hockey group to different activity levels inherent in the different hockey positions.

There have been only relatively few studies of bone mass in children and the studies cited above are two of only several studies reporting on the influence of activity on bone mass. It is difficult to assess exercise in childhood and to obtain accurate information from very young children.

Stillman et al.[20] investigated the relationship between level of physical activity and bone mineral content in adult females aged 30 to 85 years. Assessment of level of physical activity was made on the basis of an activity profile questionnaire covering past and present recreational and athletic pursuits; anthropometric measurements were also used to detect body composition differences that might reflect different activity levels. Percent fat and skinfold measurements indicated that the high physical activity group was leaner than those assigned by questionnaire evaluation to the low physical activity group. Bone mineral content at midshaft of the radius and ulna was measured by direct single photon absorptiometry. When adjusted for both age and menstrual status, mean bone mineral content divided by bone width (BMC/BW ($g \cdot cm^{-2}$) increased from 0.622 for the low activity group to 0.679 for the high activity group ($p < 0.05$).

Menopause, regardless of the age or condition of the woman, influences bone mineral content, causing lower average bone mineral content.[21-26] Smith and colleagues[21] tested the hypothesis that physical activity could slow bone loss and/or increased bone mineral content in females, aged 69 to 95 years (mean age about 82 years). The subject population was from a nursing home and groups were matched on the basis of age, weight, and degree of ambulation. The control group made no change in their daily activities. The physical activity group regularly participated in light to mild exercise while sitting in a chair. Bone mineral content of the nondominant arm was determined by photon absorptiometry. The bone mineral content of the control group decreased about 3.3% while during the same 3-year period the exercise group showed an increase of about 2.3%. The researchers suggest that the increased physical stress on the bone of the more active group seemed to be the cause of the increased bone mineral content. An exercise training program for elderly women (mean age 72 years) had a positive effect on bone mineral content after a 10-month training period, as reported by Rundgren et al.[27] If physical inactivity or aging can cause bone loss, the physical exercise can be used as a nonpharmacologic strategy to slow bone loss or even result in bone accretion. However, from their observations on the association between weight-bearing exercise and lumbar bone mineral content (quantitative computed tomography) in a cross-sectional study of 78 male and female subjects older than 50 years, Michel et al.[28] warn that whereas moderate weight-bearing exercise may increase lumbar bone density, extremely vigorous exercise may actually be detrimental to bone density.

Specificity of bone density increase in relation to activity mode was demonstrated by Jacobson et al.[29] Bone density (single or double dual photon densitometry) at several sites was measured in adult women college athletes and older athletic women. Women varsity athletes (aged 18 to 22 years) included tennis players and swimmers. The adult group of athletic women (aged 22 to 70 years) was comprised of individuals who exercised regularly for at least 3 years prior to the study. Although their exercise program included some intense physical activity, it was not at the level required for varsity athletes. Most of this group were avid tennis players, but also included swimmers, weightlifters, golfers, and aerobic exercisers. Control subjects were age-matched normal women whose exercise program did not qualify them as athletic women. Bone mineral content of the radius and metatarsus of the intercollegiate athletes was significantly above control values. Lumbar spine density was significantly higher only in the tennis players, indicating the potential role of weight-bearing activities in bone mass accretion. Bone density for adult athletic women was greater than in age-matched controls; the largest increase occurred in the oldest group of athletic women (55 to 75 years). Body weights were not measured in this study, a factor which could alter interpretation of these results. Running is associated with increased bone mineral. Lane et al.[30] measured bone mineral content (computed tomographic scan of first lumbar vertebra) of matched (age, sex, occupation, exercise level) long-distance runners, 50 to 72 years old. No information on menstrual history before menopause was provided in this study. Both male and female runners had significantly higher (40%) bone density that matched controls. Brewer and co-workers[31] compared the skeletal status of two groups of premenopausal 30- to 49-year-old women of different physical activity levels. The exercise group was composed of women with a history (at least 2 years) of running exercise and in training for a marathon at the time of the study; the control group was of a similar age who had not participated in regular exercise or sport for the two previous years. Bone mineralization was determined by X-ray densitometry (phalanx V-2 and *os calcis*) and single photon absorptiometry (radius). Bone mineral content as well as bone density were significantly greater ($p < .05$) in the runners at the midshaft radius and the middle phalanx of the small finger. The mean density of the os calcis was higher ($p < .001$) in the control group of women than in the runners. The control group subjects weighed, on average, about 14% more than the runners and the os calcis measurement may be weight dependent and should have been corrected for subjects' weights. Marcus et al.[32] observed higher lumbar spine density in elite women distance runners than in sedentary women of similar ages. Radial densities of these women, however, were not significantly different.

Granhed et al.[33] measured the loads on the lumbar spine (L3 vertebra) in eight champion male power lifters when they performed extremely heavy lifts (212 to 335 kg). L3 vertebra bone mineral content (dual photon absorptionmetry) of an age- and weight-matched group of 39 controls averaged 5.18, whereas the powerlifters averaged 7.07 g·cm^{-1}. When L3 bone mineral content of the lifters was related to their estimated annually lifted weight (300 to 5000 tons) a close correlation was found between the two parameters, indicating a relationship between training intensity and bone mineral content. Weight training (resistance training exercise to increase muscular strength) may be a useful exercise for maintaining, or increasing, lumbar bone mineral density in early postmenopausal women.[26] This 9-month weight-training program did not result in significant differences for the following variables related to bone metabolism: osteocalcin, alkaline phosphatase, 25-hydroxyvitamin D, para-thyroid hormone, and urinary hydroxyproline: creatinine. The research of Hickson et al.[34] on untrained, young-adult college men, suggests that the positive relationship between body-building weight-training exercise and bone density is not achieved through decreased urinary excretion facilitating positive calcium balance.

In addition to gravity, loads generated from high-intensity muscular activity may stimulate bone density increase.[26,35-37] Nine 20- to 30-year-old women (mean age 24.5 years) who supplemented aerobic exercise with muscle-building activity for a minimum of 1 h a week had greater spinal bone densities (dual photon absorptiometry) than women who were sedentary or performed aerobic exercises only.[37] For all 27 women in this cross-sectional study, body mass index kg·m^{-2}) was the single best predictor of lumbar bone mineral density; hours in muscle-building exercise conferred an additive effect. Swimming is considered a non-weight-bearing activity, but it may contribute to bone mineral density by virtue of muscular pull creating loads on the bone.[35,36] At both radial and vertebral sites, adult male, but not female, swimmers had greater bone mineral density (single photon absorptiometry) than nonexercising controls.[36] Muscle strength was not measured. In a study executed by Block and co-workers,[35] a group of young males (18 to 30 years) engaged in a strenuous non-weight-bearing form of activity (water polo) and another population engaged in rigorous weight training were examined for differences in bone density at the spine (quantitative computed tomography) and hip (dual photon absorptiometry). There were no significant differences in bone density at these sites between these two groups of athletes; both had generally higher bone density than a control group of less active nonexercisers. Suggestive statistical correlations were found between the variations in bone densities and the paraspinous muscle area.

The studies cited above demonstrate, in the main, that physical activity has a beneficial effect on bone mineral maintenance and that bone mineral content is greater in active individuals and athletes than in more sedentary individuals. The relationship between calcium physical inactivity, and bone demineralization in aging, osteoporosis, and amenorrhea is discussed elsewhere in this volume. More studies using appropriate instrumentation are needed to gauge the effectiveness of specific types, durations, frequencies, and intensities of physical activity and sport on the skeleton. More information on the effect of weight-bearing vs. non-weight-bearing exercise could also be useful, for example, more studies of swimmers where the gravitational aspects of exercise are largely reduced. Unanswered is the question whether the quality of bone changes following prolonged exercise, i.e., are there attenuated changes in its composition and mechanical properties? Virtually all the studies that we have access to in the literature are basically cross-sectional ones in which a group of sedentary or low physical activity or nonathletes is compared to a higher activity or athlete group. Longitudinal studies, in which the same individuals are first observed in low or moderate activity and then later observed when they perform considerably increased physical activity, are needed before the beneficial effects of physical activity on bone mass can be established with reasonable certainty. Longitudinal prospective studies will help to eliminate possible effects of different dietary intakes, stature, menstrual status, body weight and composition, skeletal and muscle mass, and lifestyle variables such as smoking, parity, and caffeine ingestion.

B. Dietary Calcium Intake of Athletes

Recent studies have examined the dietary intake of athletes.[38-47] In a continuing series of studies by Hickson and colleagues,[39,40,42,46] exercise-induced, self-selected food intake in high school and intercollegiate athletes undergoing daily training, conditioning, or competition was measured. In 13 women basketball athletes and 9 gymnasts, the mean intake of calcium closely approximated the U.S. recommended dietary allowances (1980 RDA).[48] In 18 male soccer players, the mean intake of calcium exceeded the 1980 RDA and was significantly higher during preseason conditioning (302% 1980 RDA ± 32%) than during the fall competitive season (213% 1980 RDA ± 25%). Increased intakes of energy and other nutrients were also observed during preseason conditioning, likely due to prolonged scrimmage situations. In 11 male football athletes during the winter stage of conditioning, overall mean intakes for calcium exceeded 165% of the 1980 RDA. In these studies, there were individual instances of marginal intakes (<70% of 1980 RDA). However, calcium intakes below 70% of 1980 RDA may be adequate for some individuals because of built-in safety factors included in the formulation of the RDA recommendations. In 1989[48] the RDA was increased from 800 mg calcium per day to 1200 mg calcium per day for the 19- to 24-year-old age group in order to promote full bone mineral deposition, since peak bone mass is probably not attained before the age of 25. Reexamination of calcium intakes reported by Hickson et al.[39,40,42] in light of the 1989 RDA[48] would possibly show less athletes achieving the recommended intake for calcium.

C. Calcium Requirements and Supplementation

In the U.S., no specific standards exist for athletes for most nutrients. With the evidence at hand[48] this seems warranted for calcium. Probably because there are no ergogenic qualities attributed to its use, calcium supplementation to increase physical performance does not seem to be practiced widely by the athletic community.[49] Amenorrheic athletes may require extra daily calcium for calcium balance to accommodate their lower estrogen levels and decreased calcium absorption.[50] A calcium supplement in this case may be indicated if they cannot meet their calcium needs with proper food choices.

IV. SUMMARY

Scientific evidence has accumulated to indicate that physical activity and sport can result in increased bone mass, a result of slowing of bone loss and/or an increase in bone mineral content. Longitudinal studies to define the effectiveness of specific types (e.g., weight-bearing vs. non-weight-bearing) and duration, frequency, and intensity of physical activity and sport on the phenomenon need to be performed, as well as intervention studies where the effects of an imposed exercise program on bone mass are monitored. Currently, there is no indication that in the presence of an adequate dietary calcium intake, increased calcium consumption from food or supplements have a beneficial effect on physical performance or that a specific dietary calcium standard for athletes is warranted.

REFERENCES

1. **Woo, S. L.-Y., Kuei, S. C., Amiel, D., Gomez, M. A., Hayer, E. C., White, F. C., and Akeson, W. H.,** The effects of prolonged physical training on the properties of long bone: a study of Wolff's law, *J. Bone Jt. Surg.,* 63, 780, 1981.
2. **Greenleaf, J. E.,** Physiological responses to prolonged bed rest and fluid immersion in humans, *J. Appl. Physiol.,* 57, 619, 1984.
3. **Simon, M. E., Holmes, K. R., and Olson, A. M.,** Bone mineral content of limb bones of male weanling rats subjected to 30 and 60 days of simulated increases in body weight, *Acta Anat.,* 121, 7, 1985.
4. **Whedon, G. D.,** The influence of activity on calcium metabolism, *J. Nutr. Sci. Vitaminol.,* 31 (Suppl.), S41, 1985.
5. **Dalen, N. and Olson, K. E.,** Bone mineral content and physical activity, *Acta Orthop. Scand.,* 45, 170, 1974.
6. **Whedon, G. D.,** Disuse osteoporosis: physical aspects, *Calcif. Tissue Int.,* 36, S146, 1984.
7. **Donaldson, C. L., Hulley, S. B., Vogel, J. M., Hattner, R. S., Boyers, J. H., and McMillan, D. E.,** Effect of prolonged bed rest on bone mineral, *Metabolism,* 19, 1071, 1970.
8. **LeBlanc, A. D., Schneider, V. S., Evans, H. J., Engelbretson, D. A., and Krebs, J. M.,** Bone mineral loss and recovery after 17 weeks of bed rest, *J. Bone Miner. Res.,* 5, 843, 1990.
9. **Arnaud, S. B. and Morey-Holton, E.,** Gravity, calcium and bone: update, 1989, *Physiologist,* 33, S65, 1990.
10. **Thornton, W. E. and Rummel, J. A.,** Muscular deconditioning and its prevention in space flight, in *Biomedical Results from Skylab,* Johnston, R. S. and Dietlein, L. F., Eds., NASA SP-377, National Aeronautics and Space Administration, Washington, D.C., 1977, 191.
11. **Stepantsov, V. I., Eremin, A. V., and Tikhonov, M. A.,** Means and methods of human physical training during long term space flight, in *Weightlessness,* Parin, V. V., Ed., Medicina, Moscow, 1974, 298.
12. **LeBlanc, A. and Schneider, V.,** Can the adult skeleton recover lost bone?, *Exp. Gerontol.,* 26, 189, 1991.
13. **Ellis, K. J. and Cohn, S. H.,** Correlation between skeletal calcium mass and muscle mass in man, *J. Appl. Physiol.,* 38, 455, 1975.
14. **Schneider, V. S. and McDonald, J.,** Skeletal calcium homeostasis and countermeasures to prevent disuse osteoporosis, *Calcif. Tissue Int.,* 36, S151, 1984.
15. **Dietrik, J. E., Whedon, G. D., and Shorr, E.,** Effects of immobilization upon various metabolic and physiologic functions in normal men, *Am. J. Med.,* 4, 3, 1948.
16. **Arnaud, S. B., Sherrard, D. J., Maloney, N., Whalen, R. T., and Fung, P.,** Effect of 1-week head-down tilt bed rest on bone formation and the calcium endocrine system, *Aviat. Space Environ. Med.,* 63, 14, 1992.
17. **Stewart, A. F., Adler, M., Byers, C. M., Segre, G. V., and Broadus, A. E.,** Calcium homeostasis in immobilization: an example of resorptive hypercalciuria, *N. Engl. J. Med.,* 306, 1136, 1982.
18. **Slemenda, C. W., Miller, J. Z., Hui, S. L., Reister, T. K., and Johnston, C. C. Jr.,** Role of physical activity in the development of skeletal mass in children, *J. Bone Miner. Res.,* 6, 1227, 1991.
19. **Meleski, B. W., Malina, R. M., and Bouchard, C.,** Corticol bone, body size, and skeletal maturity in ice hockey players 10 to 12 years of age, *Can. J. Appl. Sport Sci.,* 6, 212, 1981.
20. **Stillman, R. J., Lohman, T. G., Slaughter, M. H., and Massey, B. H.,** Physical activity and bone mineral contents in women aged 30 to 85 years, *Med. Sci. Sports Exercise,* 18, 576, 1986.
21. **Smith, E. L., Reddan, W., and Smith, P. E.,** Physical activity and calcium modalities for bone mineral increase in aged women, *Med. Sci. Sports Exercise,* 13, 60, 1981.
22. **Drinkwater, B. L., Nilson, K., Chesnut, C. H., III, Bremmer, W. J., Shainholtz, S., and Southworth, M. B.,** Bone mineral content of amenorrheic and eumenorrheic athletes, *N. Engl. J. Med.,* 311, 277, 1984.
23. **White, M. K., Martin, R. B., Yeater, R. A., Butcher, R. L., and Radin, E. L.,** The effects of exercise on the bones of postmenopausal women, *Int. Orthop.,* 7, 209, 1984.
24. **Lloyd, T., Buchanan, J. R., Bitzer, S., Woldman, C. J., Meyers, C., and Ford, B. G.,** Interrelationships of diet, athletic activity, menstrual status, and bone density in collegiate women, *Am. J. Clin. Nutr.,* 46, 681, 1987.
25. **Snow-Harter, C. and Marcus, R.,** Exercise, bone mineral density, and osteoporosis, *Exercise Sport Sci. Rev.,* 19, 351, 1991.
26. **Pruitt, L. A., Jackson, R. D., Bartels, R. L., and Lehnhard, H. J.,** Weight-training effects on bone mineral density in early postmenopausal women, *J. Bone Miner. Res.,* 7, 179, 1992.
27. **Rundgren, A., Aniansson, A., Ljungberg, P., and Wetterquist, H.,** Effects of a training programme for elderly people on mineral content of the heel bone, *Arch. Gerontol. Geriatr.,* 3, 243, 1984.
28. **Michel, B. A., Bloch, D. A., and Fries, J. F.,** Weight-bearing exercise, overexercise, and lumbar bone density over age 50 years, *Arch. Intern. Med.,* 149, 2325, 1989.

29. **Jacobson, P. C., Beaver, W., Grubb, S. A., Taft, T. N., and Talmage, R. V.,** Bone density in women: college athletes and older athletic women, *J. Orthop. Res.,* 2, 328, 1984.

30. **Lane, N. E., Bloch, D. A., Jones, H. H., Marshall, W. H., Wood, P. D., and Fries, J. F.,** Long-distance running, bone density and osteoarthritis, *JAMA,* 225, 1147, 1986.

31. **Brewer, V., Meyer, B. M., Keele, M. S., Upton, S. J., and Hagan, R. D.,** Role of exercise in prevention of involutional bone loss, *Med. Sci. Sports Exercise,* 15, 445, 1983.

32. **Marcus, R., Cann, C., Madvig, P., Minkoff, J., Goddard, M., Bayer, M., Martin, M., Gaudiani, L., Haskell, W., and Genant, H.,** Menstrual function and bone mass in elite women distance runners: endocrine metabolic features, *Ann. Intern. Med.,* 102, 158, 1985.

33. **Granhed, H., Jonson, R., and Hansson, T.,** The loads on the lumbar spine during extreme weight lifting, *Spine,* 12, 146, 1987.

34. **Hickson, J. F., Jr., Vogel, J. J., Wolinsky, I., Pivarnik, J. M., and Tramposch, T.,** Urinary calcium and bodybuilding exercise, *Nutr. Rep. Int.,* 38, 1049, 1988.

35. **Block, J. E., Friedlander, A. L., Brooks, G. A., Steiger, P., Stubbs, H. A., and Genant, H. K.,** Determinants of bone density among athletes engaged in weight-bearing and non-weight-bearing activity, *J. Appl. Physiol.,* 67, 1100, 1989.

36. **Orwell, E. S., Ferar, J., Oviatt, S. K., McClung, M. R., and Huntington, K.,** The relationship of swimming exercise to bone mass in men and women, *Arch. Intern. Med.,* 149, 2197, 1989.

37. **Davee, A. M., Rosen, C. J., and Adler, R. A.,** Exercise patterns and trabecular bone density in college women, *J. Bone Miner. Res.,* 5, 245, 1990.

38. **Moffatt, R. J.,** Dietary status of elite female high school gymnasts: inadequacy of vitamin and mineral intake, *J. Am. Diet. Assoc.,* 84, 1361, 1984.

39. **Hickson, J. F., Schrader, J., Pivarnik, J. M., and Stockton, J. E.,** Nutritional intake from food sources of soccer athletes during two stages of training, *Nutr. Rep. Int.,* 34, 85, 1986.

40. **Hickson, J. F., Schrader, J., and Trischler, L. C.,** Dietary intakes of female basketball and gymnastics athletes, *J. Am. Diet. Assoc.,* 86, 251, 1986.

41. **Faber, M. and Benade, A. J. S.,** Nutrient intake and dieting supplementation in body builders, *S. Afr. Med. J.,* 72, 831, 1987.

42. **Hickson, J. F., Jr., Wolinsky, I., Pivarnik, J. M., Neuman, E. A., Itak, J. F., and Stockton, J. E.,** Nutritional profile of football athletes eating from a training table, *Nutr. Res.,* 7, 27, 1987.

43. **Keith, R. E., O'Keeffe, K. A., Alt, L. A., and Young, K. L.,** Dietary status of trained female cyclists, *J. Am. Diet. Assoc.,* 89, 1620, 1989.

44. **Lamar-Hildebrand, N., Saldanha, L., and Endres, J.,** Dietary and exercise practices of college-aged female bodybuilders, *J. Am. Diet. Assoc.,* 89, 1308, 1989.

45. **Tilgner, S. A. and Schiller, M. R.,** Dietary intakes of female college athletes: the need for nutrition education, *J. Am. Diet. Assoc.,* 89, 967, 1989.

46. **Hickson, J. F., Jr., Coleman, A. E., Wolinsky, I., and Buck, B.,** Preseason nutritional profile of high school basketball athletes, *J. Appl. Sport Sci. Res.,* 4, 131, 1990.

47. **Kleiner, S. M., Bazzarre, T. L., and Litchford, M. D.,** Metabolic profiles, diet, and health practices of championship male and female bodybuilders, *J. Am. Diet. Assoc.,* 90, 962, 1990.

48. **Food and Nutrition Board,** Recommended Dietary Allowances, National Academy of Sciences, Washington, D.C., 1980; 1989.

49. **Short, S. H. and Short, W. R.,** Four-year study of university athletes' dietary intake, *J. Am. Diet. Assoc.,* 82, 632, 1983.

50. **Heaney, R. D.,** Nutritional factors and estrogen in age-related bone loss, *Clin. Invest. Med.,* 5, 147, 1982.

Chapter 11

TRACE MINERALS AND EXERCISE

———————— Emily M. Haymes

CONTENTS

0-8493-7911-3/94/$0.00+$.50
© 1994 by CRC Press, Inc.

I. INTRODUCTION

Trace minerals are defined as those minerals essential for life found in the body in quantities less than 5 g. Although there is some disagreement about the need for some of the trace minerals, the following minerals are considered to be essential: iron, iodine, zinc, copper, chromium, selenium, manganese, fluoride, cobalt, silicon, nickel, molybdenum, vanadium, and arsenic. Very little information is available relative to exercise for most of the trace minerals. On the other hand, the role of iron in exercise has been thoroughly investigated. Recent research has focused on zinc, copper, and chromium metabolism during exercise. The following discussion will be limited to those trace minerals that have been studied in exercising individuals.

II. IRON

Iron is the trace mineral found in the body in greatest amounts. Distribution of iron in the body and avenues of excretion are illustrated in Figure 1. Because two thirds of the iron is found in hemoglobin, its presence or absence greatly affects oxygen transport in the blood. Small amounts of iron are found in the muscles as myoglobin and iron-containing enzymes in the mitochondria, including the cytochromes. Iron is stored primarily in the bone marrow as ferritin and hemosiderin. The average man will store about 1000 mg of iron, but the average woman will only have about 300 mg of stored iron.

A. Iron Requirements

Iron is lost from the body through desquamation of cells from the skin, through the gastrointestinal tract, and through the urinary tract (see Figure 1). Daily iron loss by adult men is 1.0 mg and by adult women who are not menstruating is 0.8 mg.[1] Women who are menstruating lose additional iron through the menses which averages 0.6 mg/d and increases the requirement to 1.4 mg/d. Iron loss through the menses will exceed 1.4 mg/d in about 10% of adult women and increase the requirement to more than 2.2 mg/d.[2] During pregnancy, women need additional iron for expanding their red cell volume (450 mg), for the fetus (290 mg), and for the placenta (25 mg). Because cessation of the menses saves about 270 mg of iron, pregnant women will need an additional 500 mg or 2 mg/d during pregnancy.[3]

Children and adolescents require iron to support the growth of tissues and the expansion of blood volume, in addition to replacing iron losses. Children up to 10 years of age will require 1.0 mg/d. Boys will need more iron (0.2 mg/d) during the adolescent growth spurt (ages 11 to 18 years). Once menarche occurs, girls will need even more iron to replace blood lost through the menses. Adolescent girls (ages 12 to 16 years) require approximately 1.7 mg/d.[4]

Based on an average iron absorption of 10%, the recommended dietary allowance (RDA) for iron is 10 mg/d for men aged 19 and older, women after menopause, and children 4 to 10 years of age. The RDA for boys 11 to 18 years is 12 mg/d, while the RDA for girls 11 to 18 years and nonpregnant women ages 19 to menopause is 15 mg/d.[5] During pregnancy, a supplement providing 30 to 60 mg iron per day is recommended in addition to the normal recommendation for nonpregnant women.

The amount of iron absorbed from food varies considerably and averages about 10% under normal circumstances. Iron absorption is increased when iron stores are depleted and may exceed 20% in iron-deficient persons. Two forms of food iron, heme and nonheme iron, are absorbed through the walls of the small intestine by different mechanisms. About 40% of the iron found in meat, fish, and poultry is heme iron. Heme iron is more easily absorbed (about 23%) and is not affected by other foods in a meal. Nonheme iron is the form found in vegetables and grains and makes up the remaining 60% of the iron in meat, fish, and poultry. Absorption of nonheme iron varies from 3 to 8%, depending on the

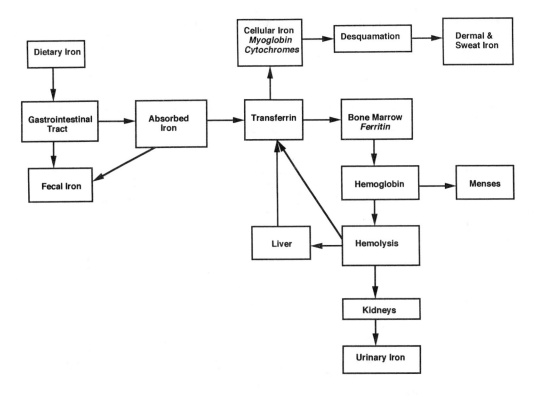

FIGURE 1. Metabolism of iron in the human body, including pathways for excretion.

presence of enhancing and inhibiting factors in the meal and the amount of iron stored in the body.[6] The presence of meat, fish, and poultry in a meal enhances the absorption of nonheme iron. Ascorbic acid (vitamin C) also increases nonheme iron absorption. Tannic acid (found in tea), phytic acid (found in whole grains), and bran are inhibitors of nonheme iron absorption. Large quantities of calcium, phosphate, and zinc, as might be found in a mineral supplement, will interact and inhibit absorption of nonheme iron.[3]

B. Iron Deficiency

If a person consumes and absorbs less iron than she/he loses, the negative iron balance will eventually drain the iron stores of the body. There are three stages of iron deficiency: iron depletion, iron-deficient erythropoiesis, and iron-deficiency anemia. The first stage, iron depletion, develops as the body's stores are depleted. Depletion of the bone marrow iron stores can be detected by the absence of, or only traces of, iron in a bone marrow biopsy. Plasma ferritin concentration is closely correlated with the amount of iron stored and is a more practical method of detecting iron depletion. Plasma ferritin concentrations of 12 µg/l or less are an indication that iron stores are depleted.[7]

As iron stores are depleted, iron absorption increases. Depletion of iron stores reduces the amount of iron available for hemoglobin formation. Because less hemoglobin is formed, protoporphyrin used to form heme is released into the blood. This is known as free erythrocyte protoporphyrin (FEP). Transferrin, a plasma protein that transports iron in the blood, is produced in greater quantities. If the total quantity of iron in the blood does not increase proportionately, the saturation of transferrin with iron decreases. When the FEP concentration exceeds 100 µg/dl red blood cells (RBC) and the transferrin saturation falls below 16%, the second stage of iron-deficient erythropoiesis has developed.

TABLE 1 Prevalence of Iron Deficiency Among Athletes

Study	Sport	Gender	Low[a] ferritin (%)	Iron[b] deficiency (%)	Anemia[c] (%)
Balaban et al.[11]	Runners	Women	25		5.4
		Men	8		5.7
Colt and Heyman[13]	Runners	Women	28		0
		Men	3.5		1.2
Deuster et al.[15]	Runners	Women	35		
Haymes and Spillman[16]	Runners	Women	30	9	0
Pate et al.[18]	Runners	Women	20		2.8
Nickerson et al.[17]	Runners	Girls		34	5.7
		Boys		8	
Clement et al.[21]	Skiers	Women	21		7
		Men	13		0
Haymes et al.[22]	Skiers	Women	20	20	0
		Men	11	0	0
Rowland and Kelleher[25]	Swimmers	Girls	47		0
		Boys	0		6.7
Risser et al.[24]	Variety	Women	31	18	7
Brown et al.[12]	Track	Girls	44		12.5
U.S. Population[8-10]		Girls	24.5	14.2	5.9
		Women	21.1	9.6	5.8
		Boys	11.9	0.1	2.6
		Men	1.7	0.6	2.9

[a] Ferritin <12 μg/l.
[b] Ferritin <12 μg/l and transferrin saturation <16%.
[c] Hemoglobin <12 g/dl for women and <13 g/dl for men.

Hemoglobin concentration remains within the normal range until the third stage develops. Anemia is defined as a hemoglobin concentration of less than 12 g/dl for women, less than 13 g/dl for men, and less than 11 g/dl during pregnancy.[3] Iron-deficiency anemia is characterized not only by low hemoglobin and ferritin concentrations, low transferrin saturation, and elevated FEP concentrations, but also by erythrocytes that are microcytic (smaller than normal) and hypochromic (low in iron).

In one recent study, iron-deficient erythropoiesis in the U.S. population was found to be most common in adolescent girls aged 15 to 19 years (14%), adolescent boys aged 11 to 14 years (12%), and nonpregnant women aged 20 to 44 years (9.6%).[8] The prevalence of iron-deficient erythropoiesis in women aged 45 to 64 years, adolescent girls aged 11 to 14 years, and children aged 3 to 10 years ranged from 4 to 6%. Less than 2% of the men and boys over 14 years old were classified with iron-deficient erythropoiesis. Another study reported that low ferritin concentrations indicative of iron depletion were found in more than 20% of the adolescent girls aged 12 to 18 years and women aged 18 to 45 years, 15% of the children aged 5 to 11 years, and 10% of the adolescent boys aged 12 to 18 years.[9] Iron-deficiency anemia was found in approximately 6% of the women and adolescent girls.[10]

C. Iron Deficiency in Athletes

Low ferritin concentrations and depleted bone marrow iron stores have been found in both men and women runners.[11-19] Poor iron status has also been observed in women athletes competing in other sports, including field hockey, cross-country skiing, crew, basketball, and softball (Table 1).[20-26] The questions are: (1) Is the proportion of athletes who are iron depleted greater than that found in the general population? (2) Do low ferritin concentrations mean that the iron stores are depleted?

In the case of men distance runners the answer to the first question is probably yes. Low plasma ferritin in men is very rare in the normal population. Because many of the studies of women runners have not used a plasma ferritin <12 µg/l as a criterion for iron depletion, it is more difficult to compare the incidence of iron depletion in runners with the normal population. Several recent studies reported no significant differences in plasma ferritin between women distance runners and control groups matched for age.[11,16,18] Some of the variation in ferritin concentration among studies could be due to recent strenuous exercise. Lampe and colleagues[27] observed significantly increased serum ferritin concentrations for 3 days following a marathon. Transferrin saturation has been observed to increase during heavy training and decrease during periods of relative rest.[28] Elevation of either ferritin or transferrin saturation by intense exercise bouts could mask iron depletion and iron-deficient erythropoiesis in an athlete. Plasma ferritin is also increased by infection and inflammation, which would mask depleted iron stores. Immediately following prolonged exercise (e.g., triathlon), serum iron was significantly decreased but plasma ferritin was elevated for 48 h after the race.[29] Taylor and colleagues suggested changes in ferritin and iron were likely due to an acute-phase response to inflammation.[29]

Under normal circumstances low ferritin concentrations and reduced bone marrow iron are adequate evidence of iron depletion. Eichner[30] has suggested that low plasma ferritin in athletes is due to an expanded plasma volume. However, this explanation does not appear to be valid in the case of elite male distance runners, who were found to have a mean serum ferritin of 32 µg/l.[31] Because the median serum ferritin for adult males is 94 µg/l,[9] this would require a threefold expansion of the plasma volume, which is highly unlikely. An expanded plasma volume has been observed in some distance runners, but the 15% difference in plasma volume could not explain the 78% reduction in serum ferritin.[32] Magnusson and colleagues found that all of the runners with low serum ferritin had at least traces of hemosiderin in their bone marrow and normal FEP concentrations and concluded that none was truly iron deficient.[32]

Several studies have examined whether iron status changes during training. Significant reductions in ferritin have been observed in some studies,[20,33,34] but not in others.[22,27] Transient reductions in hemoglobin concentration have been observed at the beginning of training that may be due to RBC destruction and/or an expansion of plasma volume. Hemoglobin is restored to normal concentrations after a few weeks of training, accompanied by significant increases in FEP and transferrin.[35] Increases in FEP would be expected if inadequate iron was available to support hemoglobin formation, while increases in transferrin occur when iron stores are depleted. The restoration of hemoglobin during training puts an added strain on the iron stores.

Many athletes have hemoglobin concentrations that are in the lower part of the normal range.[36-38] However, the incidence of iron-deficiency anemia is relatively low and appears to be no more prevalent than in the normal population. Low hemoglobin concentration in some athletes may be due to plasma volume expansion.[39,40] Pate has described low hemoglobin concentration as suboptimal and suggests it may be detrimental to performance.[41] Because most of the oxygen transported in the blood is bound to hemoglobin, a reduction in hemoglobin concentration necessitates an increase in cardiac output to maintain oxygen delivery to the tissues.[42] On the other hand, increased plasma volume could be beneficial because of decreased resistance to blood flow, improved sweating, and a larger stroke volume.[30,40] Red cell mass may also increase during training; however, the results of studies are equivocal.[36,40,43,44]

Reduced hemoglobin concentration in athletes may also be due to increased RBC destruction. Evidence of red cell destruction includes reduced haptoglobin concentration, increased plasma hemoglobin concentration, and the presence of hemoglobin in the urine

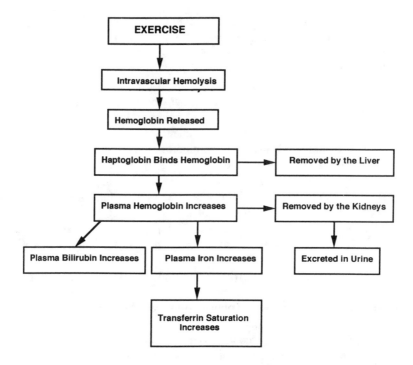

FIGURE 2.   Exercise-induced intravascular hemolysis and the fate of heme iron.

(hemoglobinuria). When RBC are destroyed in the blood vessels (intravascular hemolysis), the hemoglobin is released and picked up by haptoglobin (Figure 2). The haptoglobin is then removed from the blood as it passes through the liver and the haptoglobin concentration decreases. If more hemoglobin is released than can be bound to haptoglobin, the hemoglobin concentration in the plasma rises. Excess plasma hemoglobin will be removed in the kidneys and excreted in the urine. Several studies have reported evidence of intravascular hemolysis in runners and swimmers;[45-50] however, other studies did not find any evidence of hemo-lysis.[36,51] If anemia is due to intravascular hemolysis, the red cell volume will be increased (macrocytic) rather than decreased (microcytic). Magnusson and colleagues suggested that heme iron removed from haptoglobin by hepatocytes may be stored in the liver.[47] Plasma ferritin reflects iron storage in the bone marrow. Even though plasma ferritin was low, hemoglobin synthesis would not be impaired because iron could be transported from the liver to the bone marrow by transferrin.

D. Negative Iron Balance in Athletes
The most likely causes of iron depletion in women athletes are (1) inadequate iron intake, (2) reduced iron absorption due to diets with low bioavailability, (3) excessive iron loss through the menses, (4) excessive iron loss through sweating, (5) gastrointestinal blood loss, and (6) excretion of iron in the urine. One of the most likely causes of iron depletion among women is low iron intake. Approximately 50% of all women and girls over the age of 11 years in the U.S. consume less than 10 mg of iron per day. Low iron intake may also contribute to iron depletion in adolescent boys and children. About 50% of all children under the age of 11 years have less than adequate iron intakes. Average dietary iron intake is 6 mg/1000 kcal.

Women runners typically consume 2000 to 2500 kcal/d or about 12 to 15 mg of iron per day.[16,52,53] If they lose 1.5 mg of iron daily through desquamation and the menses, assuming

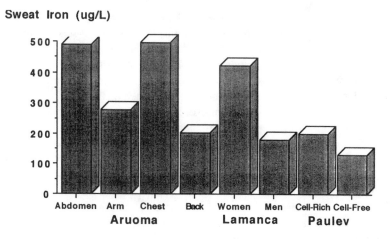

FIGURE 3. Sweat iron concentration during exercise measured at various sites,[57] from the arm,[56] and from the back.[55]

that 10% of the iron is absorbed would result in negative iron balance for some of these women (1.2 − 1.5 mg = −.3 mg). Many women runners consume diets low in meat and high in fiber, which reduces iron bioavailability to less than 10%.[16,52,53] Women runners with a bioavailable iron intake of 0.9 mg/d are more likely to be in negative iron balance than women with a bioavailable iron intake of 1.5 mg/d.

Iron loss through the menses averages 0.6 mg/d.[4] Approximately 25% of menstruating women lose 0.9 mg of iron or more through the menses.[4] These women would be more likely to be in negative iron balance and become iron deficient.[2] Many of the women athletes who are iron depleted may have greater blood losses through the menses. Some women athletes are amenorrheic (three or fewer menses per year) and lose very little iron through the menses. Deuster and colleagues found no significant difference in serum ferritin concentrations of eumenorrheic and amenorrheic women distance runners.[54] However, a greater percentage of the amenorrheic runners (46%) were iron depleted compared to eumenorrheic runners (31%).

Excretion of iron through sweating is a potential cause of negative iron balance in both women and men. Sweat iron concentrations of 0.13 to 0.50 mg/l have been reported for men and women during exercise (Figure 3).[55-57] Higher sweat iron concentrations have been reported for men and women resting in hot environments (0.17 to 1.6 mg/l).[58-63] Athletes training in hot environments may lose 1 to 2 l of sweat per hour. An athlete sweating at a rate of 1 l/h for several hours of training could lose a substantial amount of iron. However, part of the iron excreted in the sweat may come from desquamated skin cells that are normally lost each day. Recent evidence suggests that the amount of iron excreted in the sweat may be overestimated if only the first sweat excreted is sampled.[64] Subsequent sweat samples were found to have a much lower iron concentration.[64] Sweat iron concentration during exercise has also been found to decrease over time.[55] This is consistent with the theory that the initial sweat is contaminated with iron from cellular debris and the environment.

Distance runners may lose some iron through gastrointestinal bleeding. The incidence of gastrointestinal bleeding reported among runners ranges from 8 to 85%.[65-70] Both qualitative and quantitative techniques have been used to detect blood in the feces. When a quantitative method, HemoQuant, was used, the average amounts of hemoglobin lost in races ranging from 10 km through a marathon were 1.5 mg/g and 2.25 mg/g of stool, respectively.[68,69] This would be about 1.0 to 1.5 mg of iron per day or about twice the normal rate of iron loss through the feces. Presence of blood in the feces was more frequent when running at faster speeds in one study,[67] but not in two others.[70,71] Bleeding into the gastrointestinal tract may be due to vasoconstriction of splanchnic vessels during heavy exercise.[69] In an ultramarathon race, symptoms of lower gastrointestinal tract distress were significantly related to the presence of fecal blood.[70] Use of aspirin or nonsteroidal anti-inflammatory drugs by exercising persons may increase bleeding and the amount of iron lost through the gastrointestinal tract;[68] however, two recent studies reported that runners with gastrointestinal bleeding were not more likely to use nonsteroidal anti-inflammatory drugs.[70,71]

The amount of iron lost in the urine of runners was 0.18 mg/d or about twice the normal rate of 0.1 mg/d.[32] Possible sources of this iron are hemosiderin, transferrin, hemoglobin, and red blood cells. Following distance runs increased red cell counts were found in the urine of most runners.[72] Transferrin has also been found in the urine of distance runners.[73] Evidence of hematuria has been observed in 17 to 18% of runners following marathon runs.[74,75] One possible cause of hematuria is trauma to the bladder wall during running.[76] Because the amount of iron found in the urine is relatively small, it is unlikely that this is a major source of iron loss in most exercising individuals.

E. Iron Deficiency and Performance

There is ample evidence that iron-deficiency anemia has a significant negative effect on physical work capacity and maximal oxygen uptake.[77-79] When hemoglobin concentration is low, the amount of oxygen transported by the blood is reduced. During maximal exercise, cardiac output cannot increase to compensate for the lower oxygen transport. The question is, does iron deficiency without anemia have a negative effect on physical performance?

Theoretically iron depletion could have an adverse effect on the amounts of myoglobin, cytochromes, and iron-containing enzymes in muscle. Animal studies in which rats with iron-deficiency anemia were transfused to restore hemoglobin concentration showed they still had reduced endurance capacities in comparison to nonanemic rats.[80-82] Iron-deficient rats have significantly lower concentrations of cytochromes *c*, *b*, and *a*, and the activities of cytochrome oxidase, pyruvate-malate oxidase, succinate dehydrogenase, and NADH dehydrogenase are significantly lower than in skeletal muscle of normal rats.[83,84] Iron repletion restores maximal oxygen uptake and hemoglobin concentration faster than muscle enzyme activity and endurance, which follow similar patterns.[83]

Men and women who are iron deficient but have hemoglobin concentrations that are borderline for anemia (approximately 12 g/dl) have significantly lower heart rates during exercise after only 2 d of iron therapy.[85] Iron-deficient adults also have higher blood lactate concentrations following maximal exercise than subjects with normal hemoglobin concentrations.[26,85] Celsing and associates attempted to simulate the animal studies with men by doing repeated phlebotomies to deplete the iron stores over a 9-week period.[77] Following transfusion that restored normal hemoglobin levels, maximal oxygen uptake, endurance time, and blood lactate returned to prephlebotomy levels.[77] Because no significant impairment in muscle enzyme activity was observed during this study, the length of the iron-deficiency period may have been too short to deplete the tissue iron.

F. Iron Supplementation

Because many women are iron depleted or iron deficient, there has been much interest in the use of iron supplements. It is well established that iron therapy is beneficial in increasing iron concentration and physical work capacity and reducing exercise heart rate and lactate in persons with iron-deficiency anemia.[86,87] The question is whether iron supplements would be beneficial to athletes or physically active persons who are not anemic.

Several studies have examined changes in hematologic status of athletes taking iron supplements during training. The results of these studies are summarized in Table 2. Most

TABLE 2 Iron Supplementation during Training

Study	Sport	Amount of iron (mg)	Increased hemoglobin	Increased ferritin
Cooter and Mowbray[88]	Basketball	18	No	—
Haymes et al.[22]	Cross-country skiing	18	No	No
Pate et al.[89]	Variety	50	No	—
Matter et al.[90]	Running	50	No	Yes
Nickerson and Tripp[91]	Running	60	Yes	Yes
Hunding et al.[38]	Running	60	Yes	—
Yoshida et al.[97]	Running	60	No	Yes
Lamanca and Haymes[92]	Endurance	100	Yes	Yes
Newhouse et al.[93]	Running	100	No	Yes
Clement et al.[94]	Running	100	No	Yes
	Running	200	Yes	Yes
Plowman and McSwegin[95]	Running	234	Yes	—
Schoene et al.[26]	Variety	270	Yes	Yes
Rowland et al.[96]	Running	300	No	Yes

of the studies that did not observe any significant changes in hemoglobin or iron status used low dosages of iron (18 mg/d) and athletes who were not iron deficient.[22,88,89] When supplements containing larger dosages of iron (50 mg/d or more) have been given to iron-deficient athletes, significant improvements in iron status have been observed.[26,90-97] Use of iron supplements may also be beneficial in preventing iron depletion from developing in some girl and women athletes during prolonged endurance training.[22,34]

Most studies of iron supplementation have not found improved exercise performance in nonanemic iron-deficient women athletes.[26,90,92,93] Only one study found that adolescent girl runners improved in endurance after 4 weeks of iron supplementation.[96] Competitive women runners could also run 3000 m faster after 8 weeks of iron supplementation.[97] However, use of iron supplements by women athletes has been found to reduce blood lactate concentrations following heavy exercise[26,92] and to increase the running velocity at which the onset of blood lactate accumulation (OBLA) occurred.[97] Reduction in blood lactate could be due to an improvement in aerobic metabolism in the muscles.

Indiscriminate use of iron supplements with dosages of 75 mg or more by athletes is not advised, because of the possibility of iron toxicity. Some individuals have a genetic disorder called hemochromatosis that causes them to absorb and store large amounts of iron which can damage the liver. Intake of large iron dosages may also interfere with the absorption of zinc.[3] It is preferable to screen athletes for iron deficiency at the annual physical examination. Those athletes with low iron status should be given iron supplements. Some girls and women may choose to take a low-dosage iron supplement (15 mg/d) to ensure an adequately daily iron intake.

III. ZINC

Another essential mineral in many metabolic pathways is zinc. Zinc is a part of many enzymes, including lactate dehydrogenase, carbonic anhydrase, alkaline phosphatase, alcohol dehydrogenase, and superoxide dismutase. Approximately 2 g of zinc is stored in the body, primarily in the muscles and bones. Bone zinc is not metabolized during negative zinc balance; however, muscle catabolism is accompanied by the release of zinc into the plasma.[98] Zinc in blood is found primarily in erythrocytes, with much smaller amounts found in plasma. It is thought that plasma zinc is a part of the exchangeable zinc pool which can be mobilized during stress and is useful as an index of zinc deficiency.[99] Zinc deficiency

TABLE 3 Mean Food Zinc and Copper Intakes of Athletes

Study	Sport	Sex	Zinc (mg/d)	Copper (mg/d)
Deuster et al.[113]	Runners	Women	10.3	
	Untrained	Women	10.0	
Singh et al.[106]	Marathon	Women	13.1	2.1
	Untrained	Women	9.9	1.5
Lukaski et al.[120]	Swimmers	Women	10.4	1.3
	Control	Women	9.8	1.2
	Swimmers	Men	15.6	1.6
	Control	Men	15.2	1.8
Hackman and Keen[123]	Runners	Men	7.4	
	Untrained	Men	5.7	
Benson et al.[102]	Dancers	Girls	7.6	
U.S. Population[101]		Girls	10.1	0.8
		Boys	15.8	1.2
		Women	9.7	0.9
		Men	16.4	1.2

results in growth retardation, delayed sexual maturation, anorexia, loss of taste acuity, and impaired wound healing.

A. Zinc Intake

Foods that contribute the greatest amount of zinc to the diet are meats, seafood, and poultry. Plants containing phytate and dietary fiber are not good sources, because they inhibit zinc absorption. The RDA for zinc is 15 mg/d for men and 12 mg/d for women.[5] Mean dietary zinc density is 5 mg/1000 kcal, with the average woman consuming 10 mg/d and the average man consuming 16 mg/d.[100,101] Some female athletes have zinc intakes that are below the RDA.[15,102,103] For example, Deuster and colleagues found that more than 40% of the elite women marathon runners they studied consumed less than 10 mg/d.[15] Mean zinc intake for several athletic groups is reported in Table 3.

B. Zinc Depletion in Athletes

Several recent studies have reported that plasma zinc concentration is below the normal range (80 to 130 μg/dl) in many athletes. Dressendorfer and Sockolov found that 23% of the men runners they examined had less than 65 μg zinc/dl serum.[104] The runners had significantly lower serum zinc concentrations than a group of nonrunning men. Haralambie also found 23% of the men and 43% of the women athletes examined had serum zinc below the normal range.[105] Women marathon runners have plasma zinc concentrations that are near the lower limit of the normal range and 22% were below the normal range.[15,106] On the other hand, no significant difference in plasma zinc was found between varsity men athletes and nonathletes, but both groups were at the lower end of the normal range.[107]

There are several possible reasons for low plasma zinc concentrations in athletes, including low dietary zinc intake, excessive zinc loss during exercise, expansion of the plasma volume during training, which dilutes the zinc concentration, and redistribution of plasma zinc to other tissues. Although some athletes have low zinc intakes, Deuster and colleagues found a low correlation between zinc intake and plasma zinc.[15] They did find, however, that zinc intake was significantly correlated with erythrocyte zinc ($r = 0.35$). Plasma zinc concentration declines when dietary zinc is restricted to less than 4 mg/d.[99] Therefore, low zinc intake could be a contributing factor in zinc depletion for some athletes.

Sweat Zinc (ug/L)

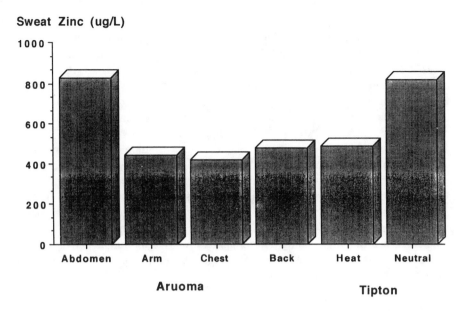

FIGURE 4. Sweat zinc concentration during exercise measured at various sites[57] and from the arm in different environments.[110]

Zinc is excreted in the urine, sweat, and feces. Normal loss through the skin for sedentary men has been estimated to be 0.76 mg/d.[108] Zinc concentration of the sweat has been reported to be as high as 1.15 mg/l of sweat.[61] Men and women exposed to a hot environment for 1 week have significantly decreased serum zinc concentrations.[109] It is quite possible that individuals who exercise or are heat exposed lose more zinc through the sweat than estimated for sedentary individuals. Results of two studies that examined sweat zinc during exercise are presented in Figure 4.[57,110] Increased excretion of zinc through the urine has also been observed following exercise.[111,112] Highly trained women runners excreted more zinc in the urine than untrained women.[113] The combination of increased zinc excretion and low zinc intake could be responsible for the low plasma zinc concentration observed in many athletes.

Expansion of the plasma volume during training could also dilute the plasma zinc concentration. About 75% of the plasma zinc is bound to albumin and the remainder is bound to α-macroglobulin. During training, the concentration of α-macroglobulin increases and the relative decrease in albumin is much less than the increase in plasma volume.[105] It would seem less likely that plasma volume expansion was the cause of the low plasma zinc concentrations, although it may be a contributing factor.

There is also evidence that zinc may be redistributed within the body during and following exercise. Some studies have reported an increase in plasma zinc concentration immediately following short, intense exercise bouts,[99,112,114,115] other studies reported no increase after distance runs but significant decreases 2 to 4 h postexercise.[111,112] The increase in plasma zinc immediately following intense exercise bouts is reduced following endurance training.[115] It has been suggested that increased plasma zinc could be due to muscle catabolism during exercise. On the other hand, decreased erythrocyte zinc concentration is seen after exercise, accompanied by a decrease in carbonic anhydrase I concentration in the erythrocyte.[114] Both plasma and erythrocyte zinc returned to normal 30 min postexercise. The increase in plasma zinc is probably due to a shift from the erythrocyte.

Stresses, including exercise, stimulate the uptake of zinc by the liver and synthesis of metallothionen and are accompanied by a reduction in plasma zinc.[116] Stress stimulates an acute-phase response, which is associated with significant decreases in plasma zinc and iron. U.S. Navy SEAL trainees undergoing the physical and psychological stresses of "Hell Week" (5 d) had significantly lower plasma zinc concentrations but no increase in urinary zinc loss.[117] The results are consistent with zinc removal by other tissues. Plasma zinc also decreased in soldiers during field exercises lasting 34 d; however, urinary zinc loss increased.[118] Because the soldiers lost weight during the field exercises, Miyamura and colleagues suggested that muscle catabolism may have been responsible for increasing zinc excretion.[118]

Low plasma zinc during training may be due to a redistribution of zinc to the erythrocyte or liver. Elite women marathon runners have significantly higher erythrocyte zinc and slightly lower plasma zinc concentrations than untrained women.[106] Ten weeks of running training increased erythrocyte zinc concentration and, specifically, carbonic anhydrase I-derived zinc and reduced albumin-bound plasma zinc.[115] No significant changes in α-macroglobulin-bound plasma zinc occurred with training. Plasma zinc decreased significantly after 5 months of middle-distance running training and remained low over the remainder of the 9-month training season.[119] On the other hand, no changes in plasma zinc were observed over a 6-month competitive swimming season.[120]

C. Zinc Supplementation

Zinc supplements are used by some athletes to improve their zinc status. Singh et al. found 21% of the elite marathon runners they studied took zinc supplements.[106] Because zinc is a part of lactate dehydrogenase, a zinc deficiency could potentially affect anaerobic muscle performance. Some evidence has been reported that zinc supplements increase muscle endurance in rats[121] and humans.[122] Krotkiewski and colleagues used a large zinc supplement (135 mg/d) and found that isometric endurance but not isokinetic endurance was increased.[122] Lukaski and colleagues found no relationship between $\dot{V}O_2$ max and either plasma or erythrocyte zinc of trained athletes.[107] In a subsequent study, neither a low zinc intake (3.6 mg/d) for 120 d nor a diet supplemented with zinc (33.6 mg/d) for 30 d significantly changed $\dot{V}O_2$ max.[99]

Zinc supplements should be used with caution. Copper absorption is inhibited by zinc supplements containing 22.5 mg.[123] Larger zinc supplements (160 mg/d) reduce high-density lipoprotein (HDL) cholesterol concentration.[124] Because HDLs are beneficial in removing cholesterol, they are antiatherogenic. A lower HDL cholesterol suggests that large zinc supplements may be atherogenic. There is evidence that zinc supplements may reverse the positive effect of exercise in increasing HDL cholesterol.[125] Zinc supplements containing less than 30 mg do not appear to affect HDL cholesterol.[126] Supplementing the diet with more than 15 mg of zinc per day is not recommended.

IV. COPPER

Copper is another trace mineral that has attracted the attention of exercise physiologists because it is part of cytochrome oxidase, the final step in the electron transport system. In the plasma protein, ceruloplasmin, it is involved in the transfer of iron from ferritin to transferrin for transport to the tissues. Copper is also part of superoxide dismutase, a free radical scavenger that protects tissues from peroxidation.

A. Copper Intake

There is no RDA for copper; however, the recommended safe and adequate copper intake is 1.5 to 3 mg/d.[5] The best sources of copper are shellfish, organ meats, legumes, and nuts. Copper bioavailability is reduced by zinc intakes that are 1.5 RDA or more and by diets that are high in fructose.[5] One recent study reported that men consumed about one half the

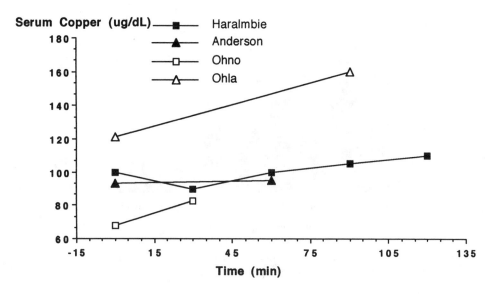

FIGURE 5. Changes in serum copper during exercise. (Data from Anderson et al.,[111] Haralambie,[127] Ohla et al.,[131] and Ohno et al.[132])

recommended amount (1.2 mg/d) and women consumed even less (0.9 mg/d).[101] Women and men athletes appear to consume slightly more copper than the average adult (Table 3).

B. Copper Status and Exercise

Copper is found in the blood in both the plasma and erythrocytes. Copper in the plasma includes that bound to ceruloplasmin, a protein important in iron metabolism, and that carried by albumin. Erythrocyte copper includes that bound to superoxide dismutase. Although plasma copper is frequently used as an indicator of copper status, the erythrocyte superoxide dismutase may be a better indication of copper status.[5]

Several studies have examined plasma copper in athletes and reported mixed results. Lukaski and colleagues[107] and Haralambie[127] reported significantly higher plasma copper in male athletes compared to controls. Resina and colleagues[128] found significantly lower plasma copper in distance runners than controls, but no difference in plasma copper between professional soccer players and controls.[129] Decreases in plasma copper and ceruloplasmin were observed after several months of competitive swim training in one study.[130] In another study no significant change in plasma copper or ceruloplasmin concentration was found in women or men swimmers over a 6-month competitive swimming season.[120] However, erythrocyte superoxide dismutase activity increased during swim training.[120] Superoxide dismutase (SOD) contains both copper and zinc, but the activity of this enzyme depends on copper. SOD is an important enzyme that protects tissues from free radicals by converting superoxide anions to peroxides.

Plasma copper and ceruloplasmin concentrations increase during prolonged exercise[127,131,132] or remain relatively constant (Figure 5).[111] Ohla and colleagues also found significant increases in plasma copper during graded exercise that were greater for trained than untrained subjects.[131] Haralambie observed a decrease in plasma copper but not ceruloplasmin during the early minutes of exercise and suggested that copper might be mobilized from the ceruloplasmin.[127] Plasma copper was inversely correlated with the catecholamines dopamine, norepinephrine, and epinephrine after 30 min of recovery from exercise, but not immediately following exercise.[132]

Excessive loss of copper through sweating could be responsible for the lower plasma copper observed in some studies. Prolonged heat exposure led to a reduction in plasma

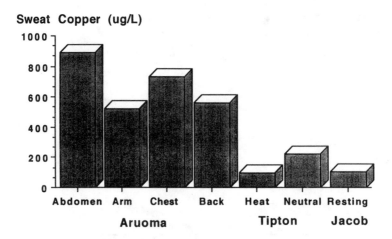

FIGURE 6. Sweat copper concentration measured during exercise at various sites,[57] from the arm in different environments,[110] and during rest in a sauna, from the arm.[108]

copper, but not ceruloplasmin.[109] Sweat copper concentration in resting men is approximately 0.11 mg/l and sedentary men lose 0.41 mg/d through the skin.[108] The copper content of the sweat during exercise varies according to the site (Figure 6).[57] Sweat copper concentration was higher during exercise in a thermoneutral environment than in a hot environment.[110] Although heavy sweating during exercise could lead to excessive loss of copper, the increased caloric intake of exercising individuals may prevent a negative copper balance from occurring.

V. CHROMIUM

Chromium is of interest because it enhances glucose tolerance and affects lipid metabolism. Increased chromium concentration may decrease the amount of insulin needed for glucose uptake by the tissues.[133] Non-insulin-dependent diabetics had lower fasting blood glucose concentrations after 6 weeks of chromium supplementation.[134] Supplementing the diet with chromium picolinate has been found to decrease total and low-density lipoprotein (LDL) cholesterol and increase HDL cholesterol.[134]

A. Chromium and the Diet

Although there is no RDA for chromium, the recommended intake is 50 to 200 μg/d. The amount of chromium in the U.S. diet is quite small (5 to 150 μg/d), probably due to the highly refined nature of many foods consumed. Best sources of chromium in the diet are meats, whole grains, brewer's yeast, nuts, cheese, and molasses.[133]

Foods that are high in simple sugars, especially glucose, stimulate an increased insulin response.[135] In subjects with the greatest insulin responses, >718 pmol/l, there was no relationship between the insulin response and chromium excretion in the urine.[135] However, in subjects with smaller insulin responses to carbohydrates, increases in chromium excretion were related to the increase in insulin.[135]

B. Exercise and Chromium

Recent studies have examined the effects of exercise on serum and urine chromium concentrations. Increases in serum chromium, glucose, and insulin have been observed immediately after a run, but 2 h after the run only chromium was still elevated.[136] Urinary chromium excretion was doubled following exercise, which suggests that physically active people may have a greater need for chromium.[111] The amount of chromium excreted in response to exercise appears to be related to the individual's fitness level. Trained runners had lower basal urinary chromium losses and greater increases in urinary chromium in response to exercise than untrained men.[137] Anderson and colleagues suggested that lower basal urinary chromium in trained subjects may be due to excessive chromium losses during training leading to chromium depletion.[137] Studies of chromium losses during training are needed to test this hypothesis.

Dietary intake prior to exercise affects the amount of chromium excreted during exercise. Carbohydrate loading for 3 d prior to exercise resulted in significantly lower urinary chromium excretion following exercise compared to a normal mixed diet.[138] Serum cortisol concentrations were also significantly lower postexercise following carbohydrate loading and there was a significant positive correlation between serum cortisol and urinary chromium. Because serum cortisol is considered a valid indicator of stress, the reduction in urinary chromium following carbohydrate loading could be due to a reduction in stress.[138]

Chromium picolinate is included in ergogenic products that are being advertised as beneficial to athletes. Most of the research support for these claims has come from two studies by Evans.[134] In the first study students enrolled in a weight-training class were given chromium picolinate (200 μg Cr) for 40 d. Subjects receiving chromium significantly increased their lean body mass, while those receiving a placebo had only a slight increase in lean body mass. The second study involved football players who were given the same chromium picolinate supplement for 6 weeks during a weight-training program. Football players receiving chromium had greater increases in lean body mass than those receiving the placebo. Evans suggested that additional chromium was needed for insulin to regulate fat utilization and muscle development.[134] Hasten and colleagues attempted to replicate Evans' study on weight lifting.[139] Both men and women students enrolled in a 12-week weight-lifting program were given either chromium picolinate (200 μg Cr) or a placebo. Significantly greater increases in lean body mass were observed only in the women on the chromium supplement. No significant differences in muscle strength gains were observed between the treatments. Clarkson concluded from her review of the research on chromium that further well-controlled studies are required before recommending chromium supplements as an aid to increasing muscle mass.[140]

VI. SELENIUM

Interest in selenium has evolved because of its presence in the enzyme glutathione peroxidase. Glutathione peroxidase is one of the antioxidant enzymes that helps to remove hydrogen peroxide or other organic hydroperoxides by combining it with glutathione to form oxidized glutathione, which can then be reduced by glutathione reductase.[141]

A. Selenium Intake

In 1989 the Food and Nutrition Board of the National Research Council established recommended dietary allowances for selenium for the first time. The RDA for men was set at 70 μg/d and for women at 55 μg/d.[5] Rich sources of selenium include seafood, liver, kidney, and other meats. The selenium content of grains depends primarily on the soil selenium content in which the grains are grown. According to one recent study of dietary intake in the U.S., the average man 25 to 30 years old consumes 100 μg of selenium per day and the average 25- to 30-year-old woman consumes 70 μg/d.[101] Selenium intake of athletes is unknown at present, but it is unlikely that athletes are deficient in this mineral. Because selenium can be toxic, selenium supplementation is not recommended.

B. Selenium and Exercise

There has been very little research to date on the relationship of selenium to exercise performance. Because free radicals are produced during exercise, glutathione peroxidase may be an important antioxidant enzyme protecting tissues from destruction. Two studies have examined the effects of a selenium-deficient diet on endurance and antioxidant status of rats.[141,142] Lang and colleagues found that selenium deficiency reduced the glutathione peroxidase activity in muscle and liver by 80%.[142] Ji and colleagues reported glutathione peroxidase decreased more than 90% in the liver and more than 75% in skeletal muscle of selenium-deficient rats.[141] Endurance was not affected by selenium deficiency and there appeared to be no difference in oxidized glutathione postexercise between deficient and control rats.[142] Evidence of increased lipid peroxidation in skeletal muscle mitochondria was observed following exercise in selenium-deficient rats.[141]

In assessing selenium status in humans, erythrocyte selenium content is an indicator of long-term selenium status, while plasma selenium concentration is affected by shifts among different body pools.[5] The combined physical and psychological stresses of "Hell Week" significantly decreased plasma selenium but had no significant effect on erythrocyte selenium or urinary selenium excretion.[117] Singh and colleagues suggested that the decline in plasma selenium may be due to its use by other tissues in protecting against oxidants.[117] Further research is needed on the role of selenium in humans during exercise.

VII. SUMMARY

Iron is the trace mineral that has been studied most extensively with respect to exercise. Iron depletion is relatively common among women athletes, but the prevalence among athletes does not appear to be greater than among age-matched peers in the U.S. population. Possible causes of iron depletion in women athletes include inadequate intake of iron and iron loss through the menses, sweat, and gastrointestinal bleeding. Iron-deficiency anemia reduces physical work capacity and endurance. The effects of iron depletion without anemia on performance are more variable. Iron supplements (50 mg/d or more) are effective in increasing plasma ferritin of iron-depleted athletes, but should be used cautiously and only after iron depletion has been verified.

Low serum zinc concentrations in athletes have been reported in several studies. Elevated zinc excretion through the urine and sweat, coupled with a low zinc intake, is a possible cause of hypozincemia. Zinc is redistributed among the tissues during exercise and low plasma zinc during training may be due to increased uptake by the liver and skeletal muscles. Zinc supplements in excess of the RDA are not recommended, because of its inhibition of copper absorption.

Plasma copper and ceruloplasmin increase during exercise, but decreases or does not change with training. The copper-containing enzyme, superoxide dismutase, increases with training. Excretion of copper in sweat is a possible cause of lower plasma copper. Chromium excretion in the urine following exercise is greater than at rest and is higher when the carbohydrate content of the diet of low. Supplementation of the diet with chromium needs further research. Very little research on selenium and exercise has been conducted. Selenium supplements are not recommended because of toxicity.

REFERENCES

1. **Hallberg, L.,** Iron, in *Nutrition Reviews' Present Knowledge in Nutrition,* 5th ed., The Nutrition Foundation, Washington, D.C., 1984, chap. 32.
2. **Hallberg, L., Hogdahl, A. M., Nilsson, L., and Rybo, G.,** Menstrual blood loss and iron deficiency, *Acta Med. Scand.,* 180, 639, 1966.
3. **Herbert, V.,** Recommended dietary intakes (RDI) of iron in humans, *Am. J. Clin. Nutr.,* 45, 679, 1987.

4. **Hallberg, L. and Rossander-Hulten, L.,** Iron requirements in menstruating women, *Am. J. Clin. Nutr.,* 54, 1047, 1991.
5. **Food and Nutrition Board,** National Research Council, *Recommended Dietary Allowances,* 10th ed., National Academy Press, Washington, D.C., 1989.
6. **Monsen, E. R., Hallberg, L., Layrisse, M., Hegsted, D. M., Cook, J. D., Mertz, W., and Finch, C. A.,** Estimation of available dietary iron, *Am. J. Clin. Nutr.,* 31, 134, 1978.
7. **Cook, J. D. and Finch, C. A.,** Assessing iron status of a population, *Am. J. Clin. Nutr.,* 32, 2115, 1979.
8. **Expert Scientific Working Group,** Summary of a report on assessment of the iron nutritional status of the United States population, *Am. J. Clin. Nutr.,* 42, 1318, 1985.
9. **Cook, J. D., Finch, C. A., and Smith, N. J.,** Evaluation of the iron status of a population, *Blood,* 48, 449, 1976.
10. **Dallman, P., Yip, R., and Johnson, C.,** Prevalence and causes of anemia in the United States, 1976 to 1980, *Am. J. Clin. Nutr.,* 39, 437, 1984.
11. **Balaban, E. P., Cox, J. V., Snell, P., Vaughan, R. H., and Frenkel, E. P.,** The frequency of anemia and iron deficiency in the runner, *Med. Sci. Sports Exercise,* 21, 643, 1989.
12. **Brown, R. T., McIntosh, S. M., Seabolt, V. R., and Daniel, W. A.,** Iron status of adolescent female athletes, *J. Adolesc. Health Care,* 6, 349, 1985.
13. **Colt, E. and Heyman, B.,** Low ferritin in runners, *J. Sports Med. Phys. Fitness,* 24, 13, 1989.
14. **Ehn, L., Carlmark, B., and Hoglund, S.,** Iron status in athletes involved in intense physical activity, *Med. Sci. Sports Exercise,* 12, 61, 1980.
15. **Deuster, P. A., Dyle, S. B., Moser, P. B., Vigersky, R. A., Singh, A., and Schoomaker, E. B.,** Nutritional survey of highly trained women runners, *Am. J. Clin. Nutr.,* 45,. 954, 1986.
16. **Haymes, E. M. and Spillman, D. M.,** Iron status of women distance runners, *Int. J. Sports Med.,* 10, 430, 1989.
17. **Nickerson, H. J., Holubets, M. C., Weller, B. R., Haas, R. G., Schwartz, S., and Ellefson, M. E.,** Causes of iron deficiency in adolescent athletes, *J. Pediatr.,* 114, 657, 1989.
18. **Pate, R. R., Dover, V., Goodyear, L., Jun-Zong, P., and Lambert, M.,** Iron storage in female distance runners, in *Sport, Health, and Nutrition,* Katch, F. I., Ed., Human Kinetics, Champaign, 1986, chap. 9.
19. **Wishnitzer, R., Vorst, E., and Berrebi, A.,** Bone marrow iron depression in competitive distance runners, *Int. J. Sports Med.,* 4, 27, 1983.
20. **Diehl, D. M., Lohman, T. G., Smith, S. C., and Kertzer, R.,** Effects of physical training and competition on the iron status of female field hockey players, *Int. J. Sports Med.,* 7, 264, 1986.
21. **Clement, D. B., Lloyd-Smith, D. R., MacIntyre, J. G., Matheson, G. O., Brock, R., and DuPont, M.,** Iron status in winter Olympic sports, *J. Sports Sci.,* 5, 261, 1987.
22. **Haymes, E. M., Puhl, J. L., and Temples, T. E.,** Training for cross-country skiing and iron status, *Med. Sci. Sports Exercise,* 18, 162, 1986.
23. **Parr, R. B., Bachman, L. A., and Moss, R. A.,** Iron deficiency in female athletes, *Phys. Sportsmed.,* 12(4), 81, 1984.
24. **Risser, W. L., Lee, E. J., Poindexter, H. B. W., West, M. S., Pivarnik, J. M., Risser, J. M. H., and Hickson, J. F.,** Iron deficiency in female athletes: its prevalence and impact on performance, *Med. Sci. Sports Exercise,* 20, 116, 1988.
25. **Rowland, T. W. and Kelleher, J. F.,** Iron deficiency in athletes: insights from high school swimmers, *Am. J. Dis. Child.,* 142, 197, 1989.
26. **Schoene, R. B., Escourrou, P., Robertson, H. T., Nilson, K. L., Parsons, J. R., and Smith, N. J.,** Iron repletion decreases maximal exercise lactate concentrations in female athletes with minimal iron-deficiency anemia, *J. Lab. Clin. Med.,* 102, 306, 1983.
27. **Lampe, J. W., Slavin, J. L., and Apple, F. S.,** Poor iron status of women runners training for a marathon, *Int. J. Sports Med.,* 7, 111, 1986.
28. **Banister, E. W. and Hamilton, C. L.,** Variation in iron status with fatigue modelled from training in female distance runners, *Eur. J. Appl. Physiol.,* 54, 16, 1985.
29. **Taylor, C., Rogers, G., Goodman, C., Baynes, R. D., Bothwell, T. H., Bexwoda, W. R., Kramer, F., and Hattingh, J.,** Hematologic, iron-related, and acute-phase protein response to sustained strenuous exercise, *J. Appl. Physiol.,* 62, 464, 1987.
30. **Eichner, E. R.,** The anemias of athletes, *Phys. Sportsmed.,* 14, 122, 1986.
31. **Martin, D., Vroom, D. H., May, D. F., and Pilbeam, S. P.,** Physiological changes in elite male distance runners training for Olympic competition, *Phys. Sportsmed.,* 14(1), 152, 1986.
32. **Magnusson, B., Hallberg, L., Rossander, L., and Swolin, B.,** Iron metabolism and "sports anemia". I. A study of several iron parameters in elite runners with differences in iron status, *Acta Med. Scand.,* 216, 149, 1984.
33. **Blum, S. M., Sherman, A. R., and Boileau, R. A.,** The effects of fitness-type exercise on iron status in adult women, *Am. J. Clin. Nutr.,* 43, 456, 1986.

34. **Nickerson, H. J., Holubets, M., Tripp, A. D., and Pierce, W. E.,** Decreased iron stores in high school female runners, *Am. J. Dis. Child.,* 139, 1115, 1985.

35. **Frederickson, L. A., Puhl, J. L., and Runyan, W. S.,** Effects of training on indices of iron status of young female cross-country runners, *Med. Sci. Sports Exercise,* 15, 271, 1983.

36. **Brotherhood, J., Brozovic, B., and Pugh, L.,** Hematological status of middle and long distance runners, *Clin. Sci.,* 48, 135, 1975.

37. **Clement, D. B., Asmundson, R. C., and Medhurst, C. W.,** Hemoglobin values: comparative survey of the 1976 Canadian Olympic team, *Can. Med. Assoc. J.,* 117, 614, 1977.

38. **Hunding, A., Jordal, R., and Paulev, P. E.,** Runner's anemia and iron deficiency, *Acta Med. Scand.,* 209, 315, 1981.

39. **Convertino, V. A., Brock, P. J., Kell, L. C., Bernauer, E. M., and Greenleaf, J. E.,** Exercise training-induced hypervolemia: role of plasma albumin, renin, and vasopressin, *J. Appl. Physiol.,* 48, 665, 1980.

40. **Dill, D. B., Braithwaite, K., Adams, W. C., and Bernauer, E. M.,** Blood volume of middle-distance runners: effect of 2300-m altitude and comparison with non-athletes, *Med. Sci. Sport,* 6, 1, 1974.

41. **Pate, R. R.,** Sports anemia: a review of the current research literature, *Phys. Sportsmed.,* 11(2), 115, 1983.

42. **Freedson, P. S.,** The influence of hemoglobin concentration on exercise cardiac output, *Int. J. Sports Med.,* 2, 81, 1981.

43. **Glass, H. L., Edwards, R. H. T., DeGarreta, A. C., and Clark, J. C.,** [11]CO red cell labeling for blood volume and total hemoglobin in athletes: effect of training, *J. Appl. Physiol.,* 26, 131, 1969.

44. **Holmgren, A., Mossfeldt, F., Sjostrand, T., and Strom, S.,** Effect of training on work capacity, total hemoglobin, blood volume, heart volume and pulse rate in recumbent and upright positions, *Acta Physiol. Scand.,* 50, 72, 1960.

45. **Dufaux, B., Hoedegrath, S., Streitberger, I., Hollman, W., and Assmann, G.,** Serum ferritin, transferrin, haptoglobin, and iron in middle- and long-distance runners, elite rowers, and professional racing cyclists, *Int. J. Sports Med.,* 2, 43, 1981.

46. **Weight, L. M., Byrnes, M. J., and Jacobs, P.,** Haemolytic effects of exercise, *Clin. Sci.,* 81, 147, 1991.

47. **Magnusson, B., Hallberg, L., Rossander, L., and Swolin, B.,** Iron metabolism and "sports anemia". II. A hematological comparison of elite runners and control subjects, *Acta Med. Scand.,* 216, 156, 1984.

48. **Miller, B. J., Pate, R. R., and Burgess, W.,** Foot impact force and intravascular hemolysis during distance running, *Int. J. Sports Med.,* 9, 56, 1988.

49. **Puhl, J. L., Runyon, W. S., and Kruse, S. J.,** Erythrocyte changes during training in high school women cross-country runners, *R. Q. Exercise Sport,* 52, 484, 1981.

50. **Selby, G. B. and Eichner, E. R.,** Endurance swimming, intravascular hemolysis, anemia, and iron depletion, *Am. J. Med.,* 81, 791, 1986.

51. **Steenkamp, I., Fuller, C., Graves, J., Noakes, T. D., and Jacobs, P.,** Marathon running fails to influence RBC survival rates in iron-replete women, *Phys. Sportsmed.,* 14, 89, 1986.

52. **Manore, M. M., Besenfelder, P. D., Wells, C. L., Carroll, S. S., and Hooker, S. P.,** Nutrient intakes and iron status in female long-distance runners during training, *J. Am. Diet. Assoc.,* 89, 257, 1989.

53. **Snyder, A. C., Dvorak, L. L., and Roepke, J. B.,** Influence of dietary iron source on measures of iron status among female runners, *Med. Sci. Sports Exer.,* 21, 7, 1989.

54. **Deuster, P. A., Kyle, S. B., Moser, P. B., Vigersky, R. A., Singh, A., and Schoonmaker, E. B.,** Nutritional intakes and status of highly trained amenorrheic and eumenorrheic women runners, *Fertil. Steril.,* 46, 636, 1986.

55. **Paulev, P. E., Jordal, R., and Pedersen, N. S.,** Dermal excretion of iron in intensely training athletes, *Clin. Chim. Acta,* 127, 19, 1983.

56. **Lamanca, J. J., Haymes, E. M., Daly, J. A., Moffatt, R. J., and Waller, M. F.,** Sweat iron loss of male and female runners during exercise, *Int. J. Sports Med.,* 9, 52, 1988.

57. **Aruoma, O. I., Reilly, T., MacLaren, D., and Halliwell, B.,** Iron, copper and zinc concentrations in human sweat and plasma; the effect of exercise, *Clin. Chim. Acta,* 177, 81, 1988.

58. **Coltman, C. A. and Rowe, N. J.,** The iron content of sweat in normal adults, *Am. J. Clin. Nutr.,* 18, 270, 1966.

59. **Consolazio, C. F., Matoush, L. O., Nelson, R. A., Harding, R. S., and Canham, J. E.,** Excretion of sodium, potassium, magnesium and iron in human sweat and the relation of each to balance and requirements, *J. Nutr.,* 79, 407, 1963.

60. **Hussein, R. and Patwardhan, V. N.,** Iron content of thermal sweat in iron-deficiency anemia, *Lancet,* 1, 1073, 1959.

61. **Prasad, A. S., Schulert, A. R., Sandstead, H. H., and Miale, A.,** Zinc, iron, and nitrogen content of sweat in normal and deficient subjects, *J. Lab. Clin. Med.,* 62, 84, 1963.

62. **Vellar, O. D.,** Studies on sweat losses of nutrients. I. Iron content of whole body sweat and its association with other sweat constituents, serum iron levels, hematological indices, body surface area, and sweat rate, *Scand. J. Clin. Lab. Invest.,* 21, 157, 1968.

63. **Wheeler, E. F., El-Neil, H., Wilson, J. O., and Weiner, J. S.,** The effect of work level and dietary intake on water balance and the excretion of sodium, potassium and iron in a hot climate, *Br. J. Nutr.,* 30, 127, 1973.

64. **Brune, M., Magnusson, B., Persson, H., and Hallberg, L.,** Iron losses in sweat, *Am. J. Clin. Nutr.,* 43, 438, 1986.

65. **Porter, A. M. W.,** Do some marathon runners bleed into the gut?, *Br. Med. J.,* 287, 1427, 1983.

66. **McCabe, M. E., Peura, D. A., Kadakia, S. C., Bocek, Z., and Johnson, L. F.,** Gastrointestinal blood loss associated with running a marathon, *Dig. Dis. Sci.,* 31, 1229, 1986.

67. **McMahon, L. F., Ryan, M. J., Larson, D., and Fisher, R. L.,** Occult gastrointestinal blood loss in marathon runners, *Ann. Intern. Med.,* 100, 846, 1984.

68. **Robertson, J. D., Maughan, R. J., and Davidson, R. J. L.,** Fecal blood loss in response to exercise, *Br. Med. J.,* 295, 303, 1987.

69. **Stewart, J. G., Ahlquist, D. A., McGill, D. B., Ilstrup, D. M., and Schwartz, S.,** Gastrointestinal blood loss and anemia in runners, *Ann. Intern. Med.,* 100, 843, 1984.

70. **Baska, R. S., Moses, F. M., Graeber, G., and Kearney, G.,** Gastrointestinal bleeding during an ultra-marathon, *Dig. Dis. Sci.,* 35, 276, 1990.

71. **Lampe, J. W., Slavin, J. L., and Apple, F. S.,** Iron status of active women and the effect of running a marathon on bowel function and gastrointestinal blood loss, *Int. J. Sports Med.,* 12, 173, 1991.

72. **Fassett, R. G., Owen, J. E., Fairley, J., Birch, D. F., and Fairley, K. F.,** Urinary red-cell morphology during exercise, *Br. Med. J.,* 285, 1455, 1982.

73. **Poortmans, J. R.,** Exercise and renal function, *Sports Med.,* 1, 125, 1984.

74. **Boileau, M., Fuchs, E., Barry, J. M., and Hodges, C. V.,** Stress hematuria: athletic pseudonephritis in marathoners, *Urology,* 15, 471, 1980.

75. **Siegal, A. J., Hennekens, C. H., Solomon, H. S., and Van Boekel, B.,** Exercise-related hematuria: findings in a group of marathon runners, *JAMA,* 241, 391, 1979.

76. **Blacklock, N. J.,** Bladder trauma in the long-distance runner, *Br. J. Urol.,* 49, 129, 1977.

77. **Celsing, F., Blomstrand, E., Werner, B., Pihlstedt, P., and Ekblom, B.,** Effects of iron deficiency on endurance and muscle enzyme activity in man, *Med. Sci. Sports Exercise,* 18, 156, 1986.

78. **Edgerton, V. R., Ohira, Y., Hettiarachchi, J., Senewiratne, B., Gardner, G. W., and Barnard, R. J.,** Elevation of hemoglobin and work tolerance in iron deficient subjects, *J. Nutr. Sci. Vitam.,* 27, 77, 1981.

79. **Gardner, G. W., Edgerton, V. R., Senewiratne, B., Barnard, R. J., and Ohira, Y.,** Physical work capacity and metabolic stress in subjects with iron deficiency anemia, *Am. J. Clin. Nutr.,* 30, 910, 1977.

80. **Davies, K. J. A., Donovan, C. M., Refino, C. J., Brooks, G. A., Packer, L., and Dallman, P. R.,** Distinguishing effects of anemia and muscle iron deficiency on exercise bioenergetics in the rat, *Am. J. Physiol.,* 246, E535, 1984.

81. **Finch, C. A., Miller, L. R., Inamdar, A. R., Person, R., Seiler, K., and Mackler, B.,** Iron deficiency in the rat: physiological and biochemical studies of muscle dysfunction, *J. Clin. Invest.,* 58, 447, 1976.

82. **Finch, C. A., Gollnick, P. D., Hlastala, M. P., Miller, L. R., Dillmann, E., and Mackler, B.,** Lactic acidosis as a result of iron deficiency, *J. Clin. Invest.,* 64, 129, 1979.

83. **Davies, K. J. A., Maguire, J. J., Brooks, G. A., Dallman, P. R., and Packer, L.,** Muscle mitochondrial bioenergetics, oxygen supply, and work capacity during dietary iron deficiency and repletion, *Am. J. Physiol.,* 242, E418, 1982.

84. **McLane, J. A., Fell, R. D., McKay, R. H., Winder, W. W., Brown, E. B., and Holloszy, J. O.,** Physiological and biochemical effects of iron deficiency on rat skeletal muscle, *Am. J. Physiol.,* 241, C47, 1981.

85. **Ohira, Y, Edgerton, V. R., Gardner, G. W., Gunawardena, K. A., Senewiratne, B., and Ikawa, S.,** Work capacity after iron treatment as a function of hemoglobin and iron deficiency, *J. Nutr. Sci. Vitam.,* 27, 87, 1981.

86. **Gardner, G. W., Edgerton, V. R., Barnard, R. J., and Bernauer, E. M.,** Cardiorespiratory, hematological and physical performance responses of anemia subjects to iron treatment, *Am. J. Clin. Nutr.,* 28, 982, 1975.

87. **Ohira, Y., Edgerton, V. R., Gardner, G. W., Senewiratne, B., Barnard, R. J., and Simpson, D. R.,** Work capacity, heart rate and blood lactate responses to iron treatment, *Br. J. Haematol.,* 41, 365, 1979.

88. **Cooter, G. R. and Mowbray, K.,** Effects of iron supplementation and activity on serum iron depletion and hemoglobin levels in female athletes, *Res. Q.,* 49, 114, 1978.

89. **Pate, R. R., Maguire, M., and Van Wyk, J.,** Dietary supplementation in women athletes, *Phys. Sportsmed.,* 7(9), 81, 1979.

90. **Matter, M., Stittfall, T., Graves, J., Myburgh, K., Adams, B., Jacobs, P., and Noakes, T. D.**, The effect of iron and folate therapy on maximal exercise performance in female marathon runners with iron and folate deficiency, *Clin. Sci.*, 72, 415, 1987.

91. **Nickerson, H. J. and Tripp, A. D.**, Iron deficiency in adolescent cross-country runners, *Phys. Sportsmed.*, 11, 60, 1983.

92. **Lamanca, J. J. and Haymes, E. M.**, Effects of dietary iron supplementation on endurance, *Med. Sci. Sports Exercise*, 21, S77, 1989.

93. **Newhouse, I. J., Clement, D. B., Taunton, J. E., and McKenzie, D. C.**, The effects of prelatent/latent iron deficiency on work capacity, *Med. Sci. Sports Exercise*, 21, 263, 1989.

94. **Clement, D. B., Taunton, J. E., McKenzie, D. C., Sawchuk, L. L., and Wiley, J. P.**, High- and low-dosage iron-supplementation in iron-deficient, endurance trained females, in *Sport, Health, and Nutrition*, Katch, F. I., Ed., Human Kinetics, Champaign, 1986, chap. 6.

95. **Plowman, S. A. and McSwegin, P. C.**, The effects of iron supplementation on female cross-country runners, *J. Sports Med. Phys. Fitness*, 21, 407, 1981.

96. **Rowland, T. W., Deisroth, M. B., Green, G. M., and Kelleher, J. F.**, The effect of iron therapy on exercise capacity of nonanemic iron-deficient adolescent runners, *Am. J. Dis. Child.*, 142, 165, 1988.

97. **Yoshida, T., Udo, M., Chida, M., Ichioka, M., and Makiguchi, K.**, Dietary iron supplement during severe physical training in competitive distance runners, *Sports Training Med. Rehab.*, 1, 279, 1990.

98. **Sandstead, H. H. and Evans, G. W.**, Zinc, in *Nutrition Reviews' Present Knowledge in Nutrition*, 5th ed., The Nutrition Foundation, Washington, D.C., 1984, chap. 33.

99. **Lukaski, H. C., Bolonchuk, W. W., Klevay, L. M., Milne, D. B., and Sandstead, H. H.**, Changes in plasma zinc content after exercise in men fed a low-zinc diet, *Am. J. Physiol.*, 247, E88, 1984.

100. **Patterson, K. Y., Holbrook, J. T., Bodner, J. E., Kelsay, J. L., Smith, J. C., and Veilon, C.**, Zinc, copper, and manganese intake and balance for adults consuming self-selected diets, *Am. J. Clin. Nutr.*, 40, 1397, 1984.

101. **Pennington, J. A. T., Young, B. E., and Wilson, D. B.**, Nutritional elements in U.S. diets: results from the total diet study, 1982 to 1986, *J. Am. Diet. Assoc.*, 89, 659, 1989.

102. **Benson, J., Gillien, D. M., Bourdet, K., and Loosli, A. R.**, Inadequate nutrition and chronic calorie restriction in adolescent ballerinas, *Phys. Sportsmed.*, 13(10), 79, 1985.

103. **Loosli, A. R., Benson, J., Gillien, D. M., and Bourdet, K.**, Nutrition habits and knowledge in competitive adolescent female gymnasts, *Phys. Sports Med.*, 14(8), 118, 1986.

104. **Dressendorfer, R. H. and Sockolov, R.**, Hypozincemia in runners, *Phys. Sportsmed.*, 8(4), 97, 1980.

105. **Haralambie, G.**, Serum zinc in athletes in training, *Int. J. Sports Med.*, 2, 135, 1981.

106. **Singh, A., Deuster, P. A., and Moser, P. B.**, Zinc and copper status of women by physical activity and menstrual status, *J. Sports Med. Phys. Fitness*, 30, 29, 1990.

107. **Lukaski, H. C., Bolonchuk, W. W., Klevay, L. M., Milne, D. B., and Sandstead, H. H.**, Maximum oxygen consumption as related to magnesium, copper, and zinc nutriture, *Am. J. Clin. Nutr.*, 37, 407, 1983.

108. **Jacob, R. A., Sandstead, H. H., Munoz, J. M., Klevay, L. M., and Milne, D. B.**, Whole body surface loss of trace metals in normal males, *Am. J. Clin. Nutr.*, 34, 1379, 1981.

109. **Uhari, M., Pakarinen, A., Hietala, J., Nurmi, T., and Kouvalainen, K.**, Serum iron, copper, zinc, ferritin, and ceruloplasmin after intense heat exposure, *Eur. J. Appl. Physiol.*, 51, 331, 1983.

110. **Tipton, K., Green, N. R., Waller, M., and Haymes, E. M.**, Mineral losses from sweat in athletes exercising at two different temperatures, *FASEB J.*, 6, A768, 1991.

111. **Anderson, R. A., Plansky, M. M., and Bryden, N. A.**, Strenuous running: acute effects on chromium, copper, zinc, and selected clinical variables in urine and serum of male runners, *Biol. Trace Elem. Res.*, 6, 327, 1984.

112. **Van Rij, A. M., Hall, M. T., Dohm, G. L., Bray, J., and Pories, W. J.**, Changes in zinc metabolism following exercise in human subjects, *Biol. Trace Elem. Res.*, 10, 99, 1986.

113. **Deuster, P. A., Day, B. A., Singh, A., Douglass, L., and Moser-Veillon, P. B.**, Zinc status of highly trained women runners and untrained women, *Am. J. Clin. Nutr.*, 49, 1295, 1989.

114. **Ohno, H., Yamashita, K., Doi, R., Yamamura, K., Kondo, T., and Taniguchi, N.**, Exercise-induced changes in blood zinc and related proteins in humans, *J. Appl. Physiol.*, 58, 1453, 1985.

115. **Ohno, H., Sato, Y., Ishikawa, M., Yahata, T., Gasa, S., Doi, R., Yamamura, K., and Taniguchi, N.**, Training effects on blood zinc levels in humans, *J. Sports Med. Phys. Fitness*, 30, 247, 1990.

116. **Oh, S. H., Deagen, J. T., Whanger, P. D., and Weswig, P. H.**, Biological function of metallothionein. V. Its induction in rats by various stresses, *Am. J. Physiol.*, 234, E282, 1978.

117. **Singh, A., Smoak, B. L., Patterson, K. Y., LeMay, L. G., Veillon, C., and Deuster, P. A.**, Biochemical indices of selected trace minerals in men: effect of stress, *Am. J. Clin. Nutr.*, 53, 126, 1991.

118. **Miyamura, J. B., McNutt, S. W., Lichton, I. J., and Wenkam, N. S.**, Altered zinc status of soldiers under field conditions, *J. Am. Diet. Assoc.*, 87, 595, 1987.

119. **Couzy, F., Lafarue, P., and Guezennec, C. Y.,** Zinc metabolism in the athlete: influence of training, nutrition and other factors, *Int. J. Sports Med.,* 11, 263, 1990.

120. **Lukaski, H. C., Hoverson, B. S., Gallagher, S. K., and Bolonchuk, W. W.,** Physical training and copper, iron, and zinc status of swimmers, *Am. J. Clin. Nutr.,* 51, 1093, 1990.

121. **Richardson, J. H. and Drake, P. D.,** The effects of zinc on fatigue of striated muscle, *J. Sports Med. Phys. Fitness,* 19, 133, 1979.

122. **Krotkiewski, M., Gudmundsson, M., Backstrom, P., and Mandroukas, K.,** Zinc and muscle strength and endurance, *Acta Physiol. Scand.,* 116, 309, 1982.

123. **Hackman, R. M. and Keen, C. L.,** Changes in serum zinc and copper levels after zinc supplementation in running and nonrunning men, in *Sport, Health, and Nutrition,* Katch, F. I., Ed., Human Kinetics, Champaign, 1986, chap. 8.

124. **Hooper, P. L., Visconti, L., Garry, P. J., and Johnson, G. E.,** Zinc lowers high-density lipoprotein-cholesterol levels, *JAMA,* 244, 1960, 1980.

125. **Goodwin, J. S., Hunt, W. C., Hooper, P., and Garry, P. J.,** Relationship between zinc intake, physical activity, and blood levels of high-density lipoprotein cholesterol in a healthy elderly population, *Metabolism,* 34, 519, 1985.

126. **Crouse, S. F., Hooper, P. L., Atterbom, H. A., and Papenfuss, R. L.,** Zinc ingestion and lipoprotein values in sedentary and endurance trained men, *JAMA,* 252, 785, 1984.

127. **Haralambie, G.,** Changes in electrolytes and trace elements during long-lasting exercise, in *Metabolic Adaptations to Prolonged Physical Exercise,* Howald, H. and Poortmans, J., Eds., Birkhauser Verlag, Basel, 1975, 340.

128. **Resina, A., Fedi, S., Gatteschi, L., Rubenni, M. G., Giamberardino, M. A., Trabassi, E., and Imreh, F.,** Comparison of some serum copper parameters in trained runners and control subjects, *Int. J. Sports Med.,* 11, 58, 1990.

129. **Resina, A., Gatteschi, L., Rubenni, M. G., Giamberardino, M. A., and Imreh, F.,** Comparison of some serum copper parameters in trained professional soccer players and control subjects, *J. Sports Med. Phys. Fitness,* 31, 413, 1991.

130. **Dowdy, R. P. and Burt, J.,** Effect of intensive long-term training on copper and iron nutriture in man, *Fed. Proc.,* 39, 786, 1980.

131. **Ohla, A. E., Klissouras, V., Sullivan, J. D., and Skoryna, S. C.,** Effect of exercise on concentration of elements in the serum, *J. Sports Med. Phys. Fitness,* 22, 414, 1982.

132. **Ohno, H., Yahata, T., Hirata, F., Yamamura, K., Doi, R., Harada, M., and Taniguchi, N.,** Changes in dopamine-β-hydroxylase, and copper, and catecholamine concentrations in human plasma with physical exercise, *J. Sports Med. Phys. Fitness,* 24, 315, 1984.

133. **Pi-Sunyer, F. X. and Offenbacher, E. G.,** Chromium, in *Nutrition Review's Present Knowledge in Nutrition,* 5th ed., The Nutrition Foundation, Washington, D.C., 1984, chap. 40.

134. **Evans, G. W.,** The effect of chromium picolinate on insulin controlled parameters in humans, *Int. J. Biosocial Med. Res.,* 11, 163, 1989.

135. **Anderson, R. A., Bryden, N. A., Polansky, M. M., and Reiser, S.,** Urinary chromium excretion and insulinogenic properties of carbohydrates, *Am. J. Clin. Nutr.,* 51, 864, 1990.

136. **Anderson, R. A., Polansky, M. M., Bryden, N. A., and Guttman, H. N.,** Strenuous exercise may increase dietary needs for chromium and zinc, in *Sport, Health, and Nutrition,* Katch, F. I., Ed., Human Kinetics, Champaign, 1986, chap. 7.

137. **Anderson, R. A., Bryden, N. A., Polansky, M. M., and Deuster, P. A.,** Exercise effects on chromium excretion of trained and untrained men consuming a constant diet, *J. Appl. Physiol.,* 64, 249, 1988.

138. **Anderson, R. A., Bryden, N. A., Polansky, M. M., and Thorp, J. W.,** Effects of carbohyrate loading and underwater exercise on circulating cortisol, insulin and urinary losses of chromium and zinc, *Eur. J. Appl. Physiol.,* 63, 146, 1991.

139. **Hasten, D. L., Rome, E. P., Franks, B. D., and Hegsted, M.,** Anabolic effects of chromium picolinate on beginning weight training students, *Int. J. Sport. Nutr.,* 2, 343, 1993.

140. **Clarkson, P. M.,** Nutritional ergogenic aids: chromium, exercise, and muscle mass, *Int. J. Sport Nutr.,* 1, 289, 1991.

141. **Ji, L. L., Stratman, F. W., and Lardy, H. A.,** Antioxidant enzyme systems in rat liver and skeletal muscle: influences of selenium deficiency, chronic training, and acute exercise, *Arch. Biochem. Biophys.,* 263, 150, 1988.

142. **Lang, J. K., Gohil, K., Packer, L., and Burk, R. F.,** Selenium deficiency, endurance exercise capacity, and antioxidant status in rats, *J. Appl. Physiol.,* 63, 2532, 1987.

Chapter 12

WATER AND ELECTROLYTE BALANCE DURING REST AND EXERCISE

James M. Pivarnik
Robert A. Palmer

CONTENTS

0-8493-7911-3/94/$0.00+$.50
© 1994 by CRC Press, Inc.

I. INTRODUCTION

This chapter deals with the principles and mechanisms involved in the proper balance of body water and electrolytes. Of particular importance are the potential consequences of pushing these regulatory mechanisms to their limits, such as during endurance exercise in hot, humid environments. We will discuss the basic concepts behind water and electrolyte balance, physiological adaptations of exercise training that relate to fluid balance, and various behavioral adaptations to exercise sessions in hot environments. In the following discussions (unless otherwise noted), values given will assume an average body weight of 70 kg for men (154 lbs) and 55 kg for women (121 lbs).

II. PHYSIOLOGICAL IMPORTANCE OF WATER AND ELECTROLYTES

Nearly all of the many chemical reactions that occur in body cells depend on fluid (water) and electrolyte balance. Beyond the fact that this intricate balance is important to maintain life, several specific areas relate directly to exercise performance. All communications between muscles and nerves depend on the flow of electric current within each cell.[1] The skeletal muscles are "turned on" in response to a signal from their associated nerves. Information about the end result of a particular movement is then sent back to the brain where it is interpreted. As a result, new signals to move may be given to the same or additional muscles. This elaborate movement/feedback system depends on a precise balance of concentrations of electrically charged particles (electrolytes). The concentrations of electrolytes both inside and outside the cells must be maintained within relatively narrow limits for nervous transmission and resulting muscular contractions to occur. Nowhere is this more critical than in the heart muscle, where electrolyte imbalances can lead to dangerous arrhythmias and possibly even death.[2]

During exercise, an increase in cardiac output is necessary for the transport of oxygen toward, and carbon dioxide away from, the working muscles. Adequate cardiac output during exercise is a function of the hydrostatic pressure that propels the blood through the arteries. This is largely dependent on an adequate blood volume, which is obviously related to the total amount of water in the body.

Heat removal is also of prime importance during exercise. When muscles contract, approximately 75 to 80% of the energy that is used is converted to heat.[3] Without an efficient cooling system, body temperature would rise dramatically in a matter of minutes, resulting in death from heat injury. The regulation and removal of body heat (thermoregulation) depends on an adequate supply of body water for sweat production.[4] Physical properties such as conductance (for heat transfer from the core of the body), heat of vaporization (for heat removal via evaporation of sweat), and specific heat of water illustrate its value in temperature regulation.

Although water is not often thought of as a nutrient, our survival depends more on this fluid than any energy substrate or other metabolic cofactors that we might ingest. While humans may live for months without food, death occurs in a matter of days if we are unable to obtain water. Major functions of water include (1) dissolving a majority of the substances that we ingest or produce, (2) transporting dissolved molecules to nearly every location in the body, (3) regulating body temperature through the conservation or liberation of heat, and (4) shock absorbing and lubricating various body compartments and joints.

Water makes up a small or large part of every cell, depending on the function of the cell. Likewise, specific quantities of salts are dissolved both in the intracellular and extracellular water.[5] When a salt such as sodium chloride enters the body, it almost completely dissociates into positively charged sodium (Na^+) and negatively charged chloride (Cl^-) ions. Other examples are potassium (K^+), magnesium (Mg^{2+}), and calcium (Ca^{2+}) salts. Since these dissolved ions possess positive and negative charges, they conduct electricity, i.e., are

**TABLE 1 Distribution of Water in
Various Tissues**

Tissue	% Water
Blood	83.0
Kidneys	82.7
Heart	79.2
Lungs	79.0
Spleen	75.8
Muscle	75.6
Brain	74.8
Intestine	74.5
Skin	72.0
Liver	68.3
Skeleton	22.0
Adipose	10.0

electrolytes. Salts that tend to dissociate almost completely are known as strong electrolytes (e.g., sodium and chloride) and those that dissociate to a lesser extent are weak electrolytes (e.g., calcium). These electrolytes function to control the activity within, and communication between, each cell in the body. They are also involved in regulating total body water and maintaining proper acid–base balance which enables the cells to function properly.

Both water and electrolyte concentrations are fairly tightly controlled; even in cases of extreme variations in nutrient intakes, environmental temperatures, and physical activity. Nature has provided several methods of response to the various and dynamic stresses placed on the maintenance of water and electrolyte balance (homeostasis).

III. BODY-WATER COMPARTMENTS

Although direct measurement of body-water compartments is difficult in humans, some reasonable approximations can be made. Fat-free mass (such as muscle) is made up of approximately 73% water.[6] This figure represents an average of all tissues and varies from one body part to another (Table 1). For example, you would intuitively suspect that blood contains a higher percentage of water (83%) than does bone (22%). If we assume that there is only a small amount of water in fat cells (estimates range from 0 to 10%), the greatest difference in total body water between individuals of the same weight would be due to a difference in body fat content. Let us take an example of two individuals who both weigh 70 kg; one has 10% (7 kg) body fat and the other has 30% (21 kg) body fat. The individual with 10% fat would have 63 kg of fat-free mass which would contain 46 kg of water (63 × 0.73), while the individual with 30% fat would have 49 kg of fat-free mass containing 35.8 kg of water (49 × 0.73). Females tend to have a larger percentage of body fat than males.[7] This has been shown in total body water estimates of 60 to 65% body weight in males and approximately 10% less in females.

Although individual water molecules can easily pass from one area to another, it is useful to divide the body into separate fluid compartments.[5] These are (1) intracellular, (2) extracellular, and (3) transcellular. Approximately 60% of the total body water is intracellular, i.e., inside individual cells surround by membranes. Due to the diversity of cells in the human body, this percentage may vary from cell to cell.

Extracellular water is located outside the cells and comprises approximately 30% of total water stores. It is further subdivided into fluid located between the tissues (interstitial) and water located in the blood vessels in the plasma portion of the blood (intravascular). The plasma water should not be, but often is, confused with water contained inside the red blood cells, which by definition is considered intracellular fluid. Approximately 75% of extra-

**TABLE 2 Total Body Water and
Various Compartment Volumes**

	Male	Female
Body weight	70.0 kg	55.0 kg
Total body water	42.0 l	28.0 l
Intracellular	26.0 l	17.0 l
Extracellular	13.0 l	9.0 l
(Interstitial)	(10.0 l)	(6.5 l)
(Plasma)	(3.0 l)	(2.5 l)
Transcellular	3.0 l	2.0 l

cellular water is contained in the interstitial spaces and 25% in the plasma. Interstitial fluid is the most difficult to isolate and measure accurately, and is the least understood of the body fluids. Although it is in intimate contact with the intravascular fluid, via the capillaries, its makeup is thought to be quite different. Guyton et al.[8] have proposed that interstitial fluid is a part of a highly complex gel-like material which is located between tissues throughout the body.

Transcellular fluid is rarely considered when dealing with water balance and exercise. Examples include fluid in the joints, eyeballs, and spinal cord. Digestive secretions are also included in transcellular fluid, but these are not usually significant during exercise, since digestion tends to be inhibited during physical activity.

Table 2 is a summary of total body water contents divided into its various compartments in the average male and female. One must remember that these are only estimates and are no better or worse than the methods used to obtain them. For instance, intracellular water is not measured directly, but is calculated from the difference between total body water and extracellular water. Any errors in either of these two measures will be reflected in a less accurate calculation of intracellular water volume. However, although absolute values reported for the various body water compartments may be incorrect, it is still useful to think of these divisions and relative proportions of fluid contained in each.

IV. ELECTROLYTE COMPOSITION OF BODY FLUIDS

Although it is relatively straightforward to consider body water in terms of its mass or volume, concentrations of electrolytes are a bit more difficult to calculate. They are usually discussed in terms of chemical equivalents.[5] This is necessary since different electrolytes do not all weigh the same. For example, one equivalent of a monovalent (one + or − charge) electrolyte such as Na^+ contains 6.023×10^{23} sodium molecules and weighs 23 g. This is known as the gram equivalent weight of sodium. One equivalent of Cl^- also contains 6.023×10^{23} chloride molecules, but weighs 35.5 g. With such large numbers of small molecules, it is easy to see why the term equivalent is used. Divalent electrolytes (two + or − charges) contain half the number of molecules per equivalent. An example is Ca^{2+}, which contains 3.012×10^{23} molecules and weighs 20 g. The concentrations of electrolytes in body fluids are frequently discussed in terms of milliequivalents (meq, 1/1000 of an equivalent). The reason is quite simple: the numbers are easier to deal with. For example, the concentrations of Cl^- in the plasma is 103 meq/l of plasma which is the same as 0.103 equivalents/l. A milliequivalent of a monovalent electrolyte contains 6.023×10^{20} molecules ($10^{23}/1000 = 10^{20}$).

The electrolyte concentrations in the plasma and interstitial fluid are approximately the same. Sodium (Na^+, 142 meq/l) and chloride (Cl^-, 103 meq/l) are the major extracellular electrolytes, with potassium (K^+, 4 meq/l), calcium (Ca^{2+}, 5 meq/l), and magnesium (Mg^{2+}, 3 meq/l) present in smaller concentrations. The situation is much different inside the cells.

TABLE 3 Average Daily Water Intake and Output in a Nonexercising Man

Intake (ml)		Output (ml)	
Liquids	1500	Kidneys	1500
Food	1000	Lungs	350
Metabolic water	300	Feces	200
		Skin	750

Although it is difficult to determine exact values, the major intracellular electrolytes are K^+ (160 meq/l) and Mg^{2+} (35 meq/l), with Na^+ (10 meq/l) and Cl^- (2 meq/l) concentrations being much lower. Activities such as nervous transmission and muscular contraction (including the heart) specifically depend on these concentration differences. It has been estimated that approximately one third of all resting energy is involved in the maintenance of these electrolyte concentration differences.[9] This is accomplished by an adenosine triphosphate (ATP)-driven system that "pumps" out (or in) electrolytes that have managed to diffuse through highly selective cell membranes.

Although the ionic makeup of the intra- and extracellular fluids are different, there are approximately the same total *number* of the various molecules dissolved both inside and outside the cells. The total number of dissolved particles is described in terms of the osmotic pressure that the fluid exerts. For example, assume that two equal volumes of fluid are separated by a barrier that allows water to pass through, but nothing else (semipermeable membrane). Then dissolve 100 molecules of a certain electrolyte on one side of the barrier and 50 molecules on the other side. The osmotic pressure on the side with the 100 electrolyte molecules is twice that of the other. Water will quickly pass through the membrane from the side with the lower osmotic pressure until the concentration of molecules becomes equal on both sides. This situation exists within and between the various body-water compartments with the osmolarity being measured in milliosmoles per liter of water (mosm/l). For accounting purposes, each milliequivalent represents one milliosmole. Total osmolarity represents the total of all of the osmotically active particles in a particular body fluid compartment. A typical osmolarity is approximately 290 mosm/l. In the plasma, Na^+ and Cl^- contribute significantly to the osmolarity, while K^+ and Mg^{2+} are more important in the maintenance of intracellular osmolarity. Osmolarity is regulated very closely by the body in an effort to maintain fluid and electrolyte equilibrium.

V. RESTING WATER AND ELECTROLYTE BALANCE

Intake of water is solely from ingestion of liquids and foods. This amounts to approximately 2 l of fluid per day in a nonexercising sedentary individual. The amount of electrolytes contained in foods and liquids is usually more than adequate to meet an individual's needs, particularly if the diet is reasonably well balanced. In fact, it is not uncommon for the kidneys to remove several grams of salt per day due to excess intake.

An often-overlooked source of water is that which is metabolically produced as a result of the oxidation of energy substrates such as carbohydrates and fats. This amounts to approximately 250 ml/d. While this amount may be relatively insignificant in humans, certain animals, such as the desert rodent, survive with little or no water intake, and rely almost exclusively on metabolic water production for their fluid replacement. As you might imagine, these animals have rather impressive urine-concentrating capabilities!

As can be seen in Table 3, most of our water output occurs via the kidneys. Typically, urine production is 1 ml/min. Obviously, this can change due to alterations in fluid intake and/or behavior patterns, and this will be discussed later. Suffice it to say that the kidneys are the most important organs for long-term water and electrolyte balance. Some water is also lost through respiration, since expired air passes through warm, moist bronchioles and is totally saturated when it leaves the body. Although only small amounts of water and electrolytes are typically lost in the feces, this could become a major problem if an individual has severe diarrhea. Finally, approximately 0.75 l of water is excreted through the skin on a daily basis. This is accomplished through both diffusion of fluid through the epidermis (insensible water loss) and perspiration through sweat gland activity.

VI. PLASMA SHIFTS DURING EXERCISE

A series of "snapshots" of the body water balance taken at any time would likely result in very similar pictures. However, one should not overlook the fact that there is tremendous activity in the capillaries, including diffusion of oxygen, carbon dioxide, and small molecules such as electrolytes and glucose, to say nothing of the water moving back and forth from the vascular volume to the interstitium. As mentioned earlier, a combination of opposing forces is responsible for maintenance of the vascular volume. Fluid is forced out of the capillaries due to the hydrostatic pressure that drives the blood through the vascular system. Additionally, osmotic pressure in the interstitial fluid tends to "pull" water out of the capillaries. These two forces are opposed by the osmotic pressure present in the capillaries and the tissue pressure surrounding the capillaries. These are termed "Starling forces", named for the man who first described this intricate balance.[10] At rest, nearly equal amounts of water leave the capillaries which adjoin the arterioles and return almost immediately via the capillaries which adjoin the venules.[11] Over the course of 24 h, the result is a slight loss of fluid (1 to 2 l) which is continuously returned to the circulatory system via the lymphatic vessels.

During cardiovascular exercise, an individual's blood pressure is significantly elevated so that adequate blood flow will reach the working muscles. This results in an increase in the hydrostatic pressure which drives fluid out of the capillaries and into the interstitium. There is also an increased osmotic pressure in the muscle cells (due to their increased activity) which tends to "pull" water out of the interstitial fluid and capillaries. In most cases, the vascular fluid comes from the plasma portion of the blood, as red blood cells tend to maintain their volume during exercise. In experiments done with cycling exercise, the amount of plasma that leaves the vascular volume depends on the intensity of exercise.[12] That is, the greater the exercise intensity, the greater the reduction of plasma volume. This makes intuitive sense since arterial blood pressure also increases as a function of exercise intensity. While different studies have yielded slightly different results, it appears that the maximum plasma volume loss that will occur during exercise is approximately 20%.[13,14] Although experimental results obtained using the cycle ergometer are fairly consistent, the same cannot be said about treadmill exercise. The results appear to conflict, with some investigators showing losses,[15-17] and others gains[15,18,19] in plasma volume during treadmill running and walking. A few other modes of exercise have been examined, with some amount of plasma volume loss usually occurring.[20-22] Some differences that have been found in the amount (if any) of plasma volume that leaves the vascular space during exercise may be due to differences in plasma protein dynamics.[12] These proteins are much larger and occupy a much greater volume than the electrolytes which are dissolved in the blood. Because of this significant size difference, the proteins possess a greater capacity to osmotically "hold" water in the vascular space. This is known as protein "oncotic" (from the Greek, meaning "to swell") pressure. Depending on the exercise setting, training state of the individual, ambient temperature, and various other factors, the amount of protein in the plasma may either increase (via addition from the lymphatic vessels),[18] decrease (through the capillaries of the active muscles),[23] or remain the same.[24] The point is, protein concentration in the plasma appears to be negatively related to the amount of fluid which leaves the vascular volume during exercise.

Although the term "loss" of plasma is frequently used, it is usually only a temporary situation since the vascular volume typically returns on preexercise levels within minutes after exercise is completed. The Starling forces simply return to preexercise conditions.

While at first glance it may appear that acute reductions in plasma volume would be deleterious to exercise performance, shift of plasma from the blood results in an increase in hemoglobin concentration. This translates into enhanced oxygen-carrying capacity per unit of blood. During exercise, water that leaves the vascular volume is likely sequestered in the interstitial spaces surrounding the active muscles.[12] This can either be the space in direct contact with the muscles or possibly the subcutaneous spaces that seem to be highly compliant (they can hold a great deal of fluid without a major change in the interstitial pressure). Long-term plasma volume deficits only appear to occur if the exercise has been lengthy and/or performed in the heat and combined with a great deal of sweating.[12]

It should be noted that long-term plasma volume expansion has been shown to occur after strenuous exercise such as marathon running. This appears most common in mild to moderate environmental conditions. While fluid has been shown to shift out of the vascular spaces during the activity, protein movement has been implicated in long-lasting plasma volume expansion during recovery (22 h to 6 d postexercise).[25-27]

VII. WATER AND ELECTROLYTE BALANCE DURING EXERCISE

During a bout of endurance exercise, there are significant changes in the volume of water being added to or lost from the body. For the moment, ignore the activity of drinking during exercise. Without ingestion of water, two sources (often overlooked) may be considered to add to the total body water supply.

The first source is an increase in the previously discussed metabolic water production, which is a function of energy expenditure.[28] That is, as exercise intensity increases, so too does the metabolic water that is produced. If we consider a man who is expending energy during a run at a rate of 15 kcal/min, we would find that metabolic water production would amount to approximately 100 g/h.

The second source of water during exercise is that which is liberated when muscle glycogen is utilized as an energy substrate during exercise. Each gram of glycogen is stored with approximately 3 to 4 g of water, which is released during glycogenolysis (splitting of glycogen for energy production).[29] If we assume that glycogen has accounted for approximately 80% of the energy expended by the runner (who is exercising at a rate of 15 kcal/min), approximately 500 g of water will be released per hour.

During 1 h of exercise, the runner has just "added" 600 g of water to his total body fluid stores without even taking a drink. In reality, he has not added anything "new" into his body. In one case the water was formed from hydrogen and oxygen during metabolism, and the other was simply an addition of previously "bound" water to the total body water pool. Although the quantity of this water is not adequate for total fluid replacement needs during lengthy exercise in a hot environment, its importance should not be totally ignored.[18,30]

On the negative side of the water balance ledger there is an increase in respiratory water loss during exercise. Much like metabolic water production, respiratory water loss is directly related to energy expenditure.[31] The 15-kcal/min runner will lose approximately 75 g of water per hour through respiration. While respiration increases during exercise, the amount of water lost via the kidneys will likely decrease and should not amount to more than 50 g/h.

The largest and potentially most serious alteration in body fluid status during exercise is related to increased sweat production for temperature regulation. Only 20 to 25% of the energy that we utilize during exercise results in actual mechanical work from muscle contractions.[3] The remainder is released in the form of heat. Let us continue to discuss the 70-kg man who is using energy at a rate of 15 kcal/min during his run. Using a mechanical efficiency estimate of 20%, he will add approximately 720 kcal of heat to his body in the course of a 1-h run. If this heat is not removed, his body temperature would be raised approximately 12°C! Clearly, this does not happen, as core temperature typically increases only 1 to 2°C after an hour of exercise.[32] Under cool, breezy conditions, a great deal of metabolically generated heat is removed via convection and radiation.[4,33] The body effectively accomplishes this task by diverting a portion of the cardiac output to the peripheral blood vessels, which results in an increased skin temperature. Effective convection and radiation depend primarily on increasing the temperature gradient between the two mediums of heat transfer, in this case the skin and the air.[4,33] As air temperature increases and exercise intensity increases, body heat can no longer be removed quickly enough via convection and radiation. At this point, sweat evaporation becomes the only means of heat removal that can potentially keep up with the pace of heat production. Basically, fluid diffuses into the sweat glands from the interstitial spaces surrounding the skin capillaries. As sweat is secreted onto the skin, heat is removed if the water is evaporated into the surrounding air. The amount of heat that can be removed via evaporation is approximately 580 kcal for every liter (kg) of sweat that is evaporated.[34] In the case of the runner, he could potentially remove all of the metabolically produced heat (720 kcal) if he produced 1.25 l of sweat during the hour-long run and it all evaporated. This is well within the maximal sweat rate of average individuals (approximately 1.5 l/h).[34] Although sweat rate may be affected by many factors, including ambient temperature, the volume of sweat produced during exercise is largely related to duration and intensity of activity. It should be noted that heat removal via evaporation also occurs with respiratory water loss, but this is far less effective in humans than in several other animal species.

It is important to emphasize that it is sweat *evaporation,* not merely sweat production, that results in heat removal. Heat is removed from the body when water changes from a liquid to a gaseous state on the surface of the skin. Any sweat that merely drips or rolls off the skin is virtually no help in the thermoregulatory process. The ideal situation for maximal heat removal would be to have an infinitely thin layer of sweat continuously form (and immediately evaporate) over the entire surface of the body. If the air is dry, most, if not all, sweat produced will be evaporated. However, very humid air contains a significant amount of water and very little can be added. Consequently, evaporation will be compromised. We will discuss how this can lead to potentially fatal consequences during severe exercise in extreme environmental conditions.

Although difficult to determine precisely, it appears that fluid for sweat comes mainly from intracellular water and the interstitial spaces of the extracellular fluid compartment.[35,36] In many instances, plasma volume has been found to be only slightly reduced, even after exercise in which body weight decreased as much as 8% (a total body water decrease of 12 to 15%).[37] This helps explain why the cardiac output of some runners can remain fairly constant during a marathon even though sweat output may exceed 5 to 7 l. However, this is not the case for all runners (or other athletes) after such dehydration. Although the mechanism is not clear, it appears that defense of the plasma volume is critical to maintaining endurance performance in the face of significant body water losses.[12]

Although sweat is mainly composed of water, it also contains a significant amount of electrolytes.[35] Table 4 shows the ionic composition of sweat in relation to that of blood plasma and muscle tissue. Electrolyte concentrations found in the muscle cells are similar to those found in many other cells of the body. As can be seen in Table 4, sweat is hypotonic to the plasma (and all other body fluid compartments for that matter). That is, the electrolyte concentration of sweat is lower than that of the body fluids. You can see that Na^+ and Cl^-

TABLE 4 Electrolyte Concentrations of Selected Body Fluids

	Na^+ (meq/l)	Cl^- (meq/l)	K^+ (meq/l)	Mg^{2+} (meq/l)	Osm (mosm/l)
Sweat	40–60	30–50	3–4	1–5	80–150
Plasma	140	101	4	1–2	290
Muscle	9	6	162	31	290

make up the majority of electrolytes found in sweat in concentrations approximately one third to one half of those found in plasma. In contrast, K^+ and Mg^{2+} add little to the osmolarity of sweat even though the total body stores of these electrolytes are large. (Remember, intracellular ions are largely prevented from leaving the cells due to the ATP pump.) Therefore, sweat losses will deplete the total body stores of Na^+ and Cl^- to a much greater extent than any other electrolytes.

VIII. PHYSIOLOGICAL CONFLICT DURING EXERCISE

Although the thermoregulatory system operates fairly effectively during moderate exercise in cool, dry conditions, problems can arise in more extreme environments.[38] Take an example of a reasonably trained individual who is competing in a marathon that may take from 3 to 3.5 h to complete. Like most racers, our subject is planning to run the race at the fastest possible pace that he can maintain for an extended period of time. This will require a significant elevation of his cardiac output, with the largest fraction going to working muscles to provide them with an adequate supply of oxygen. Environmental conditions during the race are hot and humid. Heat removal via convection and radiation will require a large increase in skin temperature, since ambient air temperature is high. This can be accomplished if a significant amount of blood flow is diverted to the peripheral vessels of the skin. You can see the conflict arising. Cardiac output is not sufficient to adequately perfuse both working muscles for oxygen delivery and skin for heat removal.[39] It would be helpful if the thermoregulatory demand could elicit an increase in total blood flow, but unfortunately, it is exercise intensity and not environmental temperature that determines the rise in cardiac output. The result of this conflict will be inadequate heat removal and a slight decrease in the blood flow (oxygen delivery) to the muscles.

As the race progresses, core temperature will continue to rise (since heat has been stored and not adequately removed) and sweat production will increase. If the air were dry, then it might be possible for heat removal via evaporation to keep pace with heat gained from exercise. However, since humidity is high, the air is nearly saturated with water and a large volume of sweat will simply drip off the skin. The result is inadequate heat removal coupled with a significant (15 to 20%) loss of body water. Also, peripheral blood vessels are vasodilated during exercise in the heat and the skin acts as a reservoir for the blood (i.e., the blood is pumped into the skin faster than it is pumped out). The result will likely be a decrease in blood pressure and diminished cardiac output. Since the runner is determined to maintain his pace despite these adverse circumstances, his body will respond by elevating the heart rate (since stroke volume has likely decreased due to decreased return of blood to the heart) and shutting down a portion of the blood vessels to the skin (vasoconstriction). The result will be an even greater increase in the heat that is stored in the body rather than dissipated into the environment. As you might suspect, this conflict cannot continue indefinitely and something will eventually have to "give". Hopefully, the runner will realize his physical distress and either slow his pace or drop out of the race. Unfortunately, the result may also be serious heat illness, injury, or death.

At the very least, there is usually a decrement in endurance performance in the heat. Decreased performance can result from as little as a 2% loss in body weight.[37,40] This would occur in a 70-kg man if he produced 1.5 l of sweat in 1 h without replacement. Significantly greater weight losses usually occur during a race such as a marathon.[35]

Another physiological conflict worth mentioning briefly is dry mouth, a common malady that can occur prior to, during, and after exercise. More than one road racer has blamed his or her poor finish on this phenomenon. Studies have shown decreased saliva production after submaximal and supramaximal exercise.[41] Several factors may play a role in decreased saliva production, including decreased blood flow to the salivary glands. Other factors include dehydration, vigorous mouth breathing, and increased salivary viscosity.[41] Other than fully hydrating prior to an athletic event, there appears to be little to prevent dry mouth in susceptible individuals.

IX. FLUID REPLACEMENT DURING EXERCISE

The best advice that can be given regarding exercise in the heat is to drink fluids before, during, and after the session. In humans, this is largely a behavioral rather than a physiological adaptation. In some species, the thirst mechanism is extremely finely tuned. Dogs have been shown to have the seemingly innate ability to drink the appropriate amount of water when it is presented in order to maintain proper body fluid levels and electrolyte concentrations.[5] They seem to know exactly when to stop drinking so as not to overhydrate. This is an amazing phenomenon since the ingested water has not yet entered the circulation when drinking ceases. In man, the thirst response is less developed. By the time we are thirsty during exercise, we have already become at least partially dehydrated. Also, unless a conscious effort to rehydrate is made, thirst alone will be responsible for only a fraction of the drinking needed for sufficient fluid replacement.[42]

How much should one drink during exercise? Since little to no absorption of water occurs in the stomach, the answer is directly related to the speed of gastric emptying of fluid into the gut.[43] Costill[44] has studied this extensively, and it appears that water can be absorbed at a maximal rate of slightly less than 1 l/h. This occurs only under ideal circumstances when maximal fluid absorption is possible. Fluids that are hyperosmotic (greater than 280 to 290 mosm/l) to the plasma are absorbed more slowly. In other words, the fluid should not contain large concentrations of sugar and/or electrolytes. The ability of the body to absorb water in order to maintain body fluid levels is a limiting factor in exercise performance. Remember, individuals with only average maximal sweat rates can produce from 1.0 to 2.0 l of sweat per hour. Therefore, even with adequate fluid intake during exercise in a hot environment, it is not possible to keep pace with the body water that is lost through sweat and respiration. More detailed information concerning the pros and cons of various sports drinks can be found in another chapter of this text.

Although it may not be possible to prevent body water losses during exercise, it is much easier to maintain a reasonable electrolyte balance. In Table 4, it was seen that sweat is hypoosmotic (hypotonic) to the plasma and other body fluids. Water is lost in greater proportion than either Na^+ or Cl^-, which are the two major electrolytes contained in sweat. The result is an increase in the electrolyte concentration (and osmolarity) of fluid that remains in the body. Therefore, one must replace only a fraction of water lost via sweating to return the electrolyte concentrations to normal.

To illustrate the previous point, let us take an example of a 70-kg man with 42 l of total body water and a preexercise osmolarity of 286 mosm/l. This means that there are approximately 12,012 osmotically active particles contained in the total body fluids (286 mosm/l × 42 l = 12,012 mosm). During a 2-h run, he will produce 3 l of sweat with an osmolarity of 120 mosm/l (360 mosm). The result is a reduction of both total body water to 39 l (i.e., 42 − 3 l) and total osmotically active particles to 11,652 mosm (12,012 − 360 mosm). Therefore, the osmolarity of the remaining body fluids has become 299 mosm/l (11,652 mosm/39 l). If the subject drinks and absorbs 1.7 l of pure water, the osmolarity of his body fluids will return to 286 mosm/l (11,640 mosm/40.7 l). This is an important concept since an increase in plasma osmolarity during exercise has been shown to be related to the inhibition of the sweating response.[45-46] Clearly, although an individual may still be somewhat volume depleted, even partial rehydration during exercise will be of benefit to performance.

It should now seem apparent that water, rather than electrolyte replacement, is of primary importance *during* an exercise bout. In some cases, serious electrolyte losses or imbalances are much less frequent than dehydration due to water deficit. Exceptions might be repeated exposures to exercise or work in the heat, or ultradistance events where individuals compete for several hours. Typically, problems begin to occur in events lasting over 4 h, and become more common as activity time approaches or even exceeds 8 h. Recently, the most commonly reported electrolyte imbalance is hyponatremia, or water intoxication where plasma Na^+ levels become diluted. Hiller et al.[47] reported 27% of athletes they studied that required medical treatment after the 1984 Hawaii Ironman Triathlon were hyponatremic following the race.

Controversy exists concerning the reason for the dilute $[Na^+]$ in the plasma. Some investigators feel that hyponatremia is due to copious losses of Na^+ in the sweat.[47-50] Others believe that it is due to overconsumption of fluids during the exercise or work bout.[30,51,52] It appears that environmental conditions are key to resolving this issue. Studies that support the role of Na^+ loss in hyponatremia have been primarily conducted in extreme conditions of heat and humidity. Conversely, data that implicate overhydration have been collected in mild to moderate environments. While hyponatremia is certainly a medical concern, it should be noted that the subjects in the above-mentioned papers represented a small percentage of the total number of participants in the ultradistance events studied.

While the issue of hyponatremia is not resolved, it would seem prudent to include 1 g of salt per liter of water (scant 1/4 tsp. per quart) drunk during events lasting greater than 4 h, particularly when environmental conditions are hot and humid. Guidelines for fluid replacement in the heat have been included in a document published in 1985 by the American College of Sports Medicine concerning prevention of thermal injuries during road races.[53]

Although plasma K^+ levels are known to be critical to muscle (including the heart) function, the total amount of K^+ lost in sweat is rather small in proportion to total body stores.[35,54] While some serious complications have been noted in the past,[55] many experts now believe that sweat losses of K^+ should not ordinarily affect an individual's performance or health.[35,54] More recently, a tragic fatality resulted in a marathon race due to elevated plasma $[K^+]$ in a highly trained, apparently healthy male runner.[56] While the reasons for this individual's dramatically elevated $[K^+]$ are not totally obvious, it is possible that muscle tissue breakdown (due to the excessive stress of the marathon) played a significant role. Severe dehydration and excessive K^+ intake during the event may have exacerbated this individual's electrolyte imbalance, but it appears that some individuals may be genetically predisposed to this type of muscular trauma.[57]

In events lasting under 4 h, the more logical time for electrolyte replacement is *after* the competition is over. Food intake is encouraged at this time not only for its electrolyte value, but also because it has been shown to increase fluid consumption and thereby aid the rehydration process.[58] In most cases, the daily diet of most Americans will contain sufficient quantities of electrolytes to adequately replace those lost in the sweat. Sprinkling food with table salt might be beneficial to those who are usually very conservative in their salt intake, or have lost a great deal of sweat. Electrolyte replacement drinks may be of some value here as well.

If hydration status is a key to exercise performance in the heat, how might performance be affected by either hyper- or hypohydrating before physical activity? A summary of the literature concerning hydration status and exercise performance was recently written by Sawka and co-workers.[46] They found that hypohydration resulted in greater heat storage during exercise. This was attributed to a decrease in sweat rate and skin blood flow which would compromise evaporation as well as convective and radiative heat loss. This problem was alluded to earlier in the discussion of our hot-weather marathoner.

Hyperhydration, however, has not been found to offer any advantage during exercise sessions in the heat except for the fact that it may delay the onset of problems related to sweat loss. Also, it is difficult for an individual to hyperhydrate significantly by ingesting large quantities of fluid prior to competition. The same mechanisms which protect against hypohydration (see following section) are equally effective at decreasing body water to a given level. Any rapid increase in fluid is interpreted as an increase in blood pressure and the kidneys respond accordingly.[59] However, it should be noted that Lyons et al. have demonstrated significant hyperhydration for up to 4 h in individuals who were administered glycerol, a natural metabolite, along with large volumes of water prior to exercise.[60] During moderate exercise in the heat, subjects exhibited elevated sweat rates and lower rectal temperatures. Although thermoregulation was enhanced, no conclusions could be drawn concerning improved performance.

X. THE ROLE OF THE KIDNEYS

The involvement of the kidneys in water and electrolyte balance intensifies during an endurance exercise session. However, they are typically thought of more in terms of maintaining long-term balance between exercise bouts. The most basic response (and unique feature) of the kidney is its intrinsic ability to regulate the volume of blood that is filtered through each nephron (smallest functional unit of the kidney).[59] Briefly stated, if blood pressure progressively decreases during endurance exercise (due to a large sweat loss) the vessels leading to the nephrons will vasoconstrict and reduce the blood flow through them. Even if nothing else changes, a decrease in the volume of blood filtered by the kidney would result in a reduced urine volume.

Other body fluid and electrolyte adjustments by the kidneys are under hormonal control.[59] One such hormone is vasopressin, which is more commonly known as antidiuretic hormone (ADH). As its name implies, the action of this hormone results in a conservation of body water via the kidney. Vasopressin is produced and secreted from the posterior pituitary gland of the brain. It is released as a response to (1) a decrease in blood pressure via receptors located in the atria of the heart (baroreceptors); and (2) an increase in osmolarity of the blood via osmoreceptors located in the hypothalamus of the brain. This is advantageous during endurance exercise in the heat when plasma volume decreases and plasma osmolarity increases as a result of sweat losses.

The action of ADH is to increase the reabsorption of water in the collecting tubule of the nephron, which results in a concentration of urine.[59] A word of caution should be mentioned here for those who feel that beer or other alcoholic beverages are the most suitable "fluid replacement drinks". Ethyl alcohol is known to be a diuretic, since it is an inhibitor of ADH. While some individuals feel that beer is just the thing to drink after a long run, the result could be a retarding of the water balance effort by the kidneys.

Aldosterone is another hormone that acts on the kidney to maintain electrolyte (specifically Na^+) balance.[59] It is produced in the cortex of the adrenal gland in response to a chain of events occurring in the blood known as the renin–angiotensin system. The renin–angiotensin system is stimulated by a decrease of Na^+ passing by a group of specialized cells in the kidney. The result is an increase in the reabsorption of Na^+ in the distal tubule of the nephron. It should be pointed out that as Na^+ goes, so goes Cl^-. Therefore, as Na^+ is reabsorbed in the kidney via the action of aldosterone, so too is Cl^-. This process is of benefit during exercise since Na^+ and Cl^- are the main electrolytes contained in sweat. Although aldosterone production is mainly related to Na^+ retention, another indirect benefit is that a significant amount of water is reabsorbed in the same process (this is unrelated to water reabsorption due to ADH).

XI. HEAT ACCLIMATIZATION

On the first hot day of summer, or when an individual travels to a warm environment, he or she may experience difficulty when performing what seems to be a typical exercise session. Heart rate is elevated, legs feel heavy, and one might feel exceptionally tired from a seemingly moderate workout. Almost everyone has experienced this phenomenon at one time or another. However, after several days of exercise in the heat, we begin to "get used to it". This adaptation process is known as heat acclimatization. The body can be "trained" to perform more effectively in the heat simply by exercising in the heat. Researchers have studied this phenomenon for years,[22,61] with some of the most notable work occurring at the onset of World War II when American soldiers were faced with the task of fighting in the deserts of North Africa.[42]

Actually, we receive partial heat acclimatization simply by performing aerobic exercise on a regular basis in any environment, even the cold. Simply stated, those who are endurance trained have fewer problems adjusting to hot conditions than do untrained individuals. Individuals who become aerobically fit through endurance training develop a decreased threshold for sweating.[62] A part of the brain, the hypothalamus, acts much like a thermostat in the body.[63] When it heats up (increased core temperature) the sweating mechanism is turned on, much like an air conditioner. Aerobically trained individuals simply have a more finely tuned thermostat (hypothalamus) that initiates the sweating response at a lower core temperature. Anecdotal evidence for this phenomenon is shared by individuals who say that they "break out in a sweat" sooner if they have been training regularly.

One can also receive partial heat acclimatization simply by being exposed to, but not exercising in, the heat (30 to 40°C or more) for extended periods of time.[62] This can occur as a result of simply sitting or standing outdoors in a hot climate or by sitting in a sauna or steam room. Adaptation to this passive acclimatization procedure results in an increase in sweat sensitivity (sweat rate). While the sweat rates of unacclimatized individuals may be 1 to 1.5 l/h, short-term (1 to 2 h) sweat rates may increase to as much as 3 to 4 l/h during exercise performed in hot, humid conditions after acclimatization.[64,65] All other things being equal, an individual who has doubled his or her sweat rate, has potentially doubled the amount of heat that can be removed from the body.

In order to achieve "total" heat acclimatization, an individual must perform endurance exercise in a hot environment. It is difficult to say exactly how much (and how intense) exercise is needed and how hot the temperature must be during daily activities or sports practice sessions to achieve optimum heat acclimatization. Most research on this topic has been conducted in laboratories with climate-controlled environmental chambers. It has been found that 7 to 14 d of repeated exposure to 35 to 45°C with subjects performing 60 to 90 min of treadmill walking seems to be adequate for total adaptation to the heat.[66] Others have used different intensities and environmental temperatures with similar results. Suffice it to say, the hotter the environment, the less exercise intensity is required. Strictly speaking, we must term these artificially induced heat adaptations as acclimation rather than acclimatization (which denotes natural heat adaptation). Whatever the method, it is only the end result of increased exercise performance in the heat that counts.

During a standard test for heat acclimation, a subject performs endurance exercise in the heat at a given temperature and exercise intensity. The exercise heart rate and rectal temperature should be lower after, as compared to before, the acclimation period. There may also be an increase in sweat rate during the test, but this does not always occur. Another result of heat training is an increase in skin conductance and a more efficient use of the sweat glands.[67] Remember that it is evaporation of sweat that is crucial to the heat removal process. If the body can make better use of all its sweat glands, a greater percentage of sweat will be evaporated for a given output. The result will be a decrease in core temperature.

Men and women do not respond to heat acclimatization in quite the same fashion. While untrained women seem to have more difficulty performing in the heat, once they are acclimatized they tend to be more efficient sweaters and hence have potentially fewer problems with heat injury. At a given exercise intensity, heat-acclimatized men tend to produce more sweat than women, but achieve similar results in heat removal.[68]

Total body water and, in particular, plasma volume have been shown to expand after endurance training in the heat.[12] Plasma volume expansion may or may not be accompanied by equivalent increase in the number of red blood cells (RBCs). This seems to be dependent on the intensity of the exercise-training sessions (greater intensity, greater increase in RBCs).[12] In any case, an expanded plasma volume facilitates the maintenance of cardiac output during exercise in the heat, as more water can be lost from the vasculature before the circulation is compromised. Effects of acute plasma volume expansion on performance have been studied by Coyle et al.[69] The authors showed that plasma volume expansion of 200 to 300 ml can increase an individual's aerobic capacity as stroke volume enhancement is proportionally greater than the resulting hemodilution. However, plasma volume expansion of greater than 300 to 400 ml leads to excessive hemodilution, and hence, decreased oxygen-carrying capacity of the blood.

Some investigators feel that NaCl content of the sweat may be reduced as a result of heat acclimatization.[70] Kirby and Convertino[71] found a 59% decrease in sweat sodium excretion after 10 d of heat acclimation despite an increase in total sweat rate. Although this phenomenon has not been found by everyone[72] and may be related to dietary Na^+ intake,[73] a conservation of salt by the kidney via increased hormonal action seems to occur.[71]

Although no one would argue against endurance training in the heat to gain heat adaptation, an acclimatized person should remain cautious when exercising in the heat. Trained individuals can perform exercise at greater intensities and for longer periods of time in hot environments because they can dissipate heat more effectively. However, this also means that they have the ability to push themselves closer to potentially serious heat injury. Still, top finishes of road races are not usually affected by heat problems (maybe they are not out there long enough!). Also, individuals who are not highly trained but are well aware of their lack of fitness seem to fare reasonably well, since they do not push themselves. It may be that an individual in the most potential danger is someone moderately trained who attempts a personal best time (fast pace, no water stops) in hot conditions. It is important to realize that when the internal air conditioner shuts down, it is often too late to fix it.

XII. BEHAVIORAL ADAPTATIONS

Endurance training and heat acclimatization have been shown to be of prime importance in temperature regulation during exercise in the heat. There are also several behavioral modifications that can help maximize performance in the heat, while obviously protecting against life-threatening heat injuries.

We have already discussed the effects of heat and humidity on exercise tolerance. The bottom line is to minimize heat gain, while maximizing heat loss, during exercise. A combination of air temperature, relative humidity, and solar radiation presents the most complete picture of potential environmental heat hazards. Dry bulb (index of ambient temperature), wet bulb (index of relative humidity), and black globe (index of radiation)

TABLE 5 Wet Bulb Globe Temperatures

Less than 80° F   **ALL**
Activities may be performed by most individuals without a risk of
heat problems.
80 to 85°F   **CAUTION**
Frequent water breaks should be given to the participants. This
should alert the coach or trainer to look for signs of heat illnesses
(dizziness, rapid heart rate, nausea, decreased coordination, etc.).
85 to 88°F   **LIMITED**
Activity for unconditioned and unacclimatized individuals should
be suspended and frequent water breaks should be given to those
who are still exercising.
Greater than 88°F   **SUSPEND**
This means what it says. All activities should be suspended or be
moved indoors to a cooler environment.

temperatures are combined into a single factor known as the wet bulb globe temperature (WBGT).[53,74] The formula used to calculate WBGT is as follows:

$$WBGT = 0.7 \text{ (wet bulb)} + 0.2 \text{ (black globe)} + 0.1 \text{ (dry bulb)}$$

You can see that the "everyday" dry bulb temperature plays the least significant role (only 10%) in a composite heat stress index. For example, it is possible that a "hot" day with little sun or humidity can be less potentially dangerous than a seemingly cooler day that is very humid. Table 5 gives the various WBGT ranges and the precautions that need to be taken. The various temperatures can be determined individually or one can purchase a WBGT thermometer commercially. It is a must for coaches or trainers who deal with athletes in hot environments.

Although many individual exercisers may not have access to a WBGT thermometer, a little knowledge will allow the proper adjustments to be made. For instance, when exercising in the heat, we are often faced with low temperatures but high humidity in the morning or high temperature combined with high solar radiation but less humidity in the afternoon or early evening. It would seem prudent to possibly wait until night to exercise since radiative heat gain will be reduced. The temperature may be hotter than in the morning, but it is likely that the humidity will be somewhat less.

Another wise precaution when exercising in the heat is to reduce the exercise intensity. This can easily be done by simply monitoring heat rate during exercise sessions. Since heart rate is higher at a given exercise intensity in the heat (due to a large skin blood flow and a decreased stroke volume), exercise intensity at a given heart rate will decrease as WBGT increases. Following this precaution may be difficult, but necessary, for an individual who wants to maintain the habit of running a certain distance at a prescribed pace.

XIII. SUMMARY

Body water and electrolyte balance in the resting human are maintained in a well-regulated, tightly controlled fashion. During mild exercise, cardiac output is adequately maintained and body temperature is regulated via minor fluid compartment shifts and hormonal changes. However, during intense endurance exercise in the heat, acute physiological adjustments are pushed to their limits, resulting in decreased exercise tolerance and the possibility of heat illness. Behavioral adaptations, such as increasing fluid intake and decreasing exercise intensity in extreme environmental conditions, are necessary if an individual hopes to maintain high-level performance.

REFERENCES

1. **Guyton, A. E., Ed.,** *Human Physiology and Mechanisms of Disease,* W. B. Saunders, Philadelphia, 1982, 400.
2. **Marriott, H. J. L. and Myerburg, R. J.,** Cardiac arrhythmias and conduction disturbances, in *The Heart,* Hurst, J. W. and Logue, R. B., Eds., McGraw-Hill, New York, 1970, 489.
3. **Fox, E. L., Bowers, R. W., and Foss, M. L., Eds.,** *The Physiological Basis of Physical Education and Athletics,* 4th ed., W. B. Saunders, Philadelphia, 1988, 74.
4. **Kerslake, D. McK., Ed.,** *The Stress of Hot Environments,* Cambridge University Press, London, 1972, chaps. 1, 2.
5. **Pitts, R. F., Ed.,** *Physiology of the Kidney and Body Fluids,* 3rd ed., Year Book Medical Publishers, Chicago, 1974, chaps. 2, 12.
6. **Pace, N. and Rathburn, E. N.,** Studies of body composition. III. The body water and chemically combined nitrogen content in relation to fat content, *J. Biol. Chem.,* 158, 685, 1945.
7. **Schloerb, P. R., Friis-Hansen, B. J., Edelman, I. S., Solomon, A. K., and Moore, F. D.,** The measurement of total body water in the human subject by deuterium oxide dilution with consideration of the dynamics of deuterium distribution, *J. Clin. Invest.,* 29, 1296, 1950.
8. **Guyton, A. C., Taylor, A. E., and Granger, H. J., Eds.,** *Circulatory Physiology. II. Dynamics and Control of the Body Fluids,* W. B. Saunders, Philadelphia, 1975, chap. 2.
9. **Vander, A. J., Sherman, J. H., and Luciano, D. S., Eds.,** *Human Physiology. The Mechanisms of Body Function,* 3rd ed., McGraw-Hill, New York, 1980, chap. 6.
10. **Starling, E. H.,** Physiological factors involved in the causation of dropsy, *Lancet,* 1, 1405, 1896.
11. **Pappenheimer, J. R.,** Passage of molecules through capillary walls, *Physiol. Rev.,* 33, 387, 1953.
12. **Senay, L. C., Jr. and Pivarnik, J. M.,** Fluid shifts during exercise, in *Exercise and Sports Sciences Reviews,* Vol. 13, Terjung, R. L., Ed., MacMillan, New York, 1985, 335.
13. **Harrison, M. H.,** Effects of thermal stress and exercise on blood volume in humans, *Physiol. Rev.,* 65, 149, 1985.
14. **Sejersted, O. M., Vollestad, N. K., and Medbo, J. I.,** Muscle fluid and electrolyte balance during and following exercise, *Acta Physiol. Scand.,* 128(Suppl. 556), 119, 1986.
15. **Galbo, H. J., Holst, J., and Christensen, N. J.,** Glucagon and plasma catecholamine responses to graded and prolonged exercise in man, *J. Appl. Physiol.,* 38, 70, 1975.
16. **Senay, L. C., Jr., Rogers, G., and Jooste, P.,** Changes in blood plasma during progressive treadmill and cycle exercise, *J. Appl. Physiol.,* 49, 59, 1980.
17. **Wilkerson, J. E., Gutin, B., and Horvath, S. M.,** Exercise-induced changes in blood, red cell, and plasma volumes in man, *Med. Sci. Sports,* 9, 155, 1977.
18. **Pivarnik, J. M., Leeds, E. M., and Wilkerson, J. E.,** Effects of endurance exercise on metabolic water production and plasma volume, *J. Appl. Physiol.,* 56, 613, 1984.
19. **Sawka, M. N., Francesconi, R. P., Pimental, N. A., and Pandolf, K. B.,** Hydration and vascular fluid shifts during exercise in the heat, *J. Appl. Physiol.,* 56, 91, 1984.
20. **Astrand, P.-O. and Saltin, B.,** Plasma and red cell volume after prolonged severe exercise, *J. Appl. Physiol.,* 19, 829, 1964.
21. **McMurray, R. G.,** Plasma volume changes during submaximal swimming, *Eur. J. Appl. Physiol.,* 51, 347, 1983.
22. **Senay, L. C., Jr. and Kok, R.,** Body fluid response of heat-tolerant and intolerant men to work in a hot, wet environment, *J. Appl. Physiol.,* 40, 55, 1976.
23. **Harrison, M. H., Edwards, R. J., and Leitch, D. R.,** Effect of exercise and thermal stress on plasma volume, *J. Appl. Physiol.,* 39, 925, 1975.
24. **Ekblom, B.,** Effect of physical training on circulation during prolonged severe exercise, *Acta Physiol. Scand.,* 78, 145, 1970.
25. **Altenkirch, H. U., Gerzer, R., Kirsch, K. A. et al.,** Effect of prolonged physical exercise on fluid regulating hormones, *Eur. J. Appl. Physiol.,* 61, 209, 1990.
26. **Irving, R. A., Noakes, T. D., Burger, S. C., Myburgh, K. H., Querido, D., and Van Zyl Smit, R.,** Plasma volume and renal function during and after ultramarathon running, *Med. Sci. Sports Exercise,* 22, 581, 1990.
27. **Rocker, L., Kirsch, K. A., Heyduck, B., and Altenkirch, H. U.,** Influence of prolonged physical exercise on plasma volume, plasma proteins, electrolytes, and fluid regulating hormones, *Int. J. Sports Med.,* 10, 270, 1989.
28. **Consolazio, F. C., Johnson, R. E., and Pecora, L. J., Eds.,** *Physiological Measurements of Metabolic Functions in Man,* McGraw-Hill, New York, 1963, 313.
29. **Olsson, K. E. and Saltin, B.,** Variation in total body water with muscle glycogen changes in man, *Acta Physiol. Scand.,* 80, 11, 1970.

30. **Noakes, T. D., Adams, B. A., Myburgh, K. H., Greeff, C., Lotz, T., and Nathan, M.,** The danger of an inadequate water intake during prolonged exercise. A novel concept re-visited, *Eur. J. Appl. Physiol.,* 57, 210, 1988.

31. **Mitchell, J. W., Nadel, E. R., and Stolwijk, J. A. J.,** Respiratory weight losses during exercise, *J. Appl. Physiol.,* 32, 474, 1972.

32. **Gisolfi, C. V. and Wenger, C. B.,** Temperature regulation during exercise: old concepts, new ideas, in *Exercise and Sport Sciences Reviews,* Vol. 12, Terjung, R. L., Ed., Collamore Press, Lexington, MA, 1984, 339.

33. **Hardy, J. D.,** Heat transfer, in *Physiology of Heat Regulation and the Science of Clothing,* Newburgh, L. H., Ed., W. B. Saunders, Philadelphia, 1949, 79.

34. **Brooks, G. A. and Fahey, T. D., Eds.,** *Exercise Physiology,* John Wiley & Sons, New York, 1984, 451.

35. **Costill, D. L.,** Sweating: its composition and effects on body fluids, in *The Marathon: Physiological, Medical, Epidemiological, and Psychological Studies,* Vol. 301, Milvey, P., Ed., New York Academy of Sciences, New York, 1977, 160.

36. **Kozlowski, C. and Saltin, B.,** Effects of sweat loss on body fluids, *J. Appl. Physiol.,* 19, 1119, 1964.

37. **Costilll, D. L.,** Physiology of marathon running, *JAMA,* 221, 1024, 1972.

38. **Lind, A. R.,** A physiological criterion for setting thermal environmental limits for everyday work, *J. Appl. Physiol.,* 18, 51, 1963.

39. **Nadel, E. R.,** Circulatory and thermal regulations during exercise, *Fed. Proc.,* 39, 1491, 1980.

40. **Armstrong, L. E., Costill, D. L., and Fink, W. J.,** Influence of diuretic-induced dehydration on competitive running performance, *Med. Sci. Sports Exercise,* 17, 456, 1985.

41. **Ben-Aryeh, H., Roll, N., Lahav, M. et al.,** Effects of exercise on salivary composition and cortisol in serum and saliva in man, *J. Dent. Res.,* 68, 1495, 1989.

42. **Adolf, E. F. and Associates, Eds.,** *Physiology of Man in the Desert,* Interscience, New York, 1947.

43. **Costill, D. L. and Saltin, B.,** Factors limiting gastric emptying during rest and exercise, *J. Appl. Physiol.,* 37, 679, 1974.

44. **Costill, D. L.,** Fluids for athletic performance: why and what should you drink during prolonged exercise?, in *The New Runners Diet,* World Publication, Mountain View, CA, 1977, 130.

45. **Nielsen, B.,** Temperature regulation; effects of sweat loss during prolonged exercise, *Acta Physiol. Scand.,* 128(Suppl. 556), 105, 1986.

46. **Sawka, M. N., Francesconi, R. P., Young, A. J., and Pandolf, K. B.,** Influence of hydration level and body fluids on exercise performance in the heat, *JAMA,* 252, 1165, 1984.

47. **Hiller, W. D. B., O'Toole, M. L., Fortess, E. E., Laird, R. H., Imbert, P. C., and Sisk, T. D.,** Medical and physiological considerations in triathlons, *Am. J. Sports Med.,* 15, 164, 1987.

48. **Frizzell, R. T., Lang, G. H., Lowance, D. C., and Lathan, S. R.,** Hyponatremia and ultramarathon running, *JAMA,* 255, 772, 1986.

49. **Hiller, W. D. B.,** Dehydration and hyponatremia during triathlons, *Med. Sci. Sports Exercise,* 21(Suppl.), S219, 1989.

50. **Hiller, W. D. B., O'Toole, M. L., Laird, R. H. et al.,** Electrolyte and glucose changes in endurance and ultraendurance exercise: results and medical implications (Abstract), *Med. Sci. Sports Exercise,* 18(Suppl.), S62, 1986.

51. **Irving, R. A., Noakes, T. D., Buck, R. et al.,** Evaluation of renal function and fluid homeostasis during recovery from exercise-induced hyponatremia, *J. Appl. Physiol.,* 70, 342, 1991.

52. **Noakes, T. D., Goodwin, N., Rayner, B. L., Branken, T., and Taylor, R. K. N.,** Water intoxication: a possible complication during endurance exercise, *Med. Sci. Sports Exercise,* 17, 370, 1985.

53. **American College of Sports Medicine,** Position Stand on Prevention of Thermal Injuries During Distance Running, Indianapolis, 1985.

54. **Costill, D.,** Muscle metabolism and electrolyte balance during heat acclimation, *Acta Physiol. Scand.,* 128(Suppl. 556), 111, 1986.

55. **Knochel, J. P.,** Potassium deficiency during training in the heat, in *The Marathon: Physiological, Medical, Epidemiological, and Psychological Studies,* Vol. 301, Milvey, P., Ed., New York Academy of Sciences, New York, 1977, 175.

56. **Dennis, K. and Renney, K.,** Marathon tragedy raises questions, *Inside Texas Running,* 16(3), 7, 1992.

57. **Jardon, O. M.,** Physiologic stress, heatstroke, malignant hyperthermia — a perspective, *Milit. Med.,* 147, 8, 1982.

58. **Szlyk, P. C., Sils, I. V., Francesconi, R. P., and Hubbard, R. W.,** Patterns of human drinking: effects of exercise, water temperature, and food consumption, *Aviat. Space Environ. Med.,* 61, 43, 1990.

59. **Vander, A. J., Ed.,** *Renal Physiology,* 2nd ed., McGraw-Hill, New York, 1980, chaps. 2, 7.

60. **Lyons, T. P., Riedesel, M. L., Meuli, L. E., and Chick, T. W.,** Effects of glycerol-induced hyperhydration prior to exercise in the heat on sweating and core temperature, *Med. Sci. Sports Exercise,* 22, 477, 1990.

61. **Wyndham, C. H.,** The physiology of exercise under heat stress, *Annu. Rev. Physiol.,* 35, 193, 1973.

62. **Nadel, E. R., Pandolf, K. B., Roberts, M. F., and Stolwijk, J. A. J.,** Mechanisms of thermal acclimation to exercise and heat, *J. Appl. Physiol.,* 37, 515, 1974.
63. **Hammel, H. T.,** Regulation of internal body temperature, *Annu. Rev. Physiol.,* 30, 641, 1968.
64. **Eichna, L. W., Ashe, W. F., Bean, W. B., and Shelley, W. B.,** The upper limits of environmental heat and humidity tolerated by acclimatized men working in hot environments, *J. Ind. Hyg. Toxicol.,* 27, 59, 1945.
65. **Robinson, S., Dill, D. B., Wilson, J. W., and Nielsen, M.,** Adaptations of white men and negroes to prolonged work in humid heat, *Am. J. Trop. Med.,* 21, 261, 1941.
66. **Lind, A. R.,** Human tolerance to hot climates, in *Handbook of Physiology,* Section 9: *Reaction to Environmental Agents,* Lee, D. H. K., Ed., American Physiological Society, Bethesda, MD, 1977, 93.
67. **Hofler, W.,** Changes in regional distribution of sweating during acclimatization to heat, *J. Appl. Physiol.,* 25, 503, 1968.
68. **Wyndham, C. H., Rogers, G. C., Senay, L. C., Jr., and Mitchell, D.,** Acclimatization in a hot, humid, environment: cardiovascular adjustments, *J. Appl. Physiol.,* 40, 779, 1976.
69. **Coyle, E. F., Hopper, M. K., and Coggan, A. R.,** Maximal oxygen uptake relative to plasma volume expansion, *Int. J. Sports Med.,* 11, 116, 1990.
70. **Locke, W., Talbot, N., Jones, H., and Worcester, J.,** Studies on the combined use of measurements of sweat electrolyte composition and rate of sweating as an index of adrenocortical activity, *J. Clin. Invest.,* 30, 325, 1971.
71. **Kirby, C. R. and Convertino, V. A.,** Plasma aldosterone and sweat sodium concentrations after exercise and heat acclimation, *J. Appl. Physiol.,* 61, 967, 1986.
72. **Robinson, S., Maletich, R. T., Robinson, W. S., Rohrer, B. B., and Kunz, A. L.,** Output of NaCl by sweat glands and kidneys in relation to dehydration and to salt depletion, *J. Appl. Physiol.,* 8, 615, 1956.
73. **Armstrong, L. E., Costill, D. L., and Fink, W. J.,** Changes in body water and electrolytes during heat acclimation: effects of dietary sodium, *Aviat. Space Environ. Med.,* 58, 143, 1987.
74. **Minard, D., Belding, H. S., and Kingston, J. R.,** Prevention of heat casualties, *JAMA,* 165, 1813, 1957.

Chapter 13

NUTRIENT BEVERAGES FOR EXERCISE AND SPORT

Susan M. Puhl
Elsworth R. Buskirk

CONTENTS

0-8493-7911-3/94/$0.00+$.50
© 1994 by CRC Press, Inc.

I. INTRODUCTION

Solutions containing various amounts and types of electrolytes and/or nutrients such as carbohydrates have been and continue to be used by athletes in an effort to enhance physical performance. There are currently dozens of such nutrient solutions commercially available. The "athletes" consuming such beverages include both those involved in organized amateur and professional competition and those who participate recreationally in activities for fun or fitness. Several authors have reviewed topics of interest in the area of nutritional supplements ingested before, during, or after physical performance. Table 1[1-14] provides a listing of such reviews. The reader is encouraged to secure those of interest; all are well written and informative about the topic indicated.

A bout of exercise results in changes which affect the homeostasis of the exercising individual. The beneficial effects of electrolyte/carbohydrate beverages are attained if use of such products minimizes or ameliorates the exercise-induced changes which could detrimentally affect performance. Homeostatic disturbances that may result in decreased physical performance during exercise include, but are not limited to, decreased plasma volume, increased deep body or core temperature, plasma and muscle electrolyte alterations, and decreased nutrient fuel availability to the working skeletal muscle. The degree to which each of these disturbances results in a decrease in physical performance is a function of both the magnitude of the disturbance and the concomitant alterations in other homeostatic conditions. Reviews of the effects resulting from such homeostatic disturbances are widely available; the salient features of each will be described briefly.

A. Homeostatic Disturbances During Exercise
1. Plasma Volume

During exercise, plasma volume decreases as a consequence of both an increase in sweating and a net movement of water from the vascular to the interstitial compartment. The loss of plasma volume via sweating is increased if the exercise is performed in a hot environment. The decrease in plasma volume has been estimated to be approximately 2.4% for each 1% loss of body weight occurring through acute dehydration.[15] Movement of water out of the vascular space during exercise is due to the combination of an increased cardiac output, increased arterial pressures, increased capillary hydrostatic pressure, a relative increase in postcapillary resistance, and an increased interstitial oncotic pressure secondary to movement of protein out of the vascular compartment.[16] The shift of water from the plasma to the interstitial space is observable within 1 min of the onset of intense exercise, and tends to become somewhat stable approximately 5 min into exercise.[17] The body attempts to minimize

TABLE 1 Reviews of Carbohydrate Metabolism and Nutritional Beverage Ingestion During Physical Performance

Reference	Information reviewed
Coggan and Coyle, 1991[1]	Carbohydrate use during prolonged exercise
Consolazio and Johnson, 1972[2]	Carbohydrate use at rest and during exercise
Costill, 1985[3]	Carbohydrate ingestion before, during, and after activities of various durations and intensities
Costill, 1988[4]	Carbohydrate use during, and glycogen resynthesis following, intense exercise
Costill and Hargreaves, 1992[5]	Carbohydrates and fatigue
Coyle, 1991[6]	Carbohydrate metabolism and fatigue
Coyle and Coggan, 1984[7]	Carbohydrate ingestion during prolonged exercise
Ivy, 1991[8]	Muscle glycogen synthesis before and after exercise
Lamb and Brodowicz, 1986[9]	Carbohydrate/electrolyte beverages before, during, and after exercise
Maughan and Noakes, 1991[10]	Fluid replacement during exercise
Powers and Dodd, 1985[11]	Caffeine and endurance exercise
Stanley and Connett, 1991[12]	Muscle carbohydrate metabolism during exercise
Valeriani, 1991[13]	Carbohydrate needs during exercise
Wasserman and Cherrington, 1991[14]	Hepatic fuel metabolism during exercise

the loss of circulating blood volume by mobilizing fluid from the intracellular fluid.[18] Thus, intracellular as well as extracellular fluid decreases during endurance exercise.

Hypohydration, defined as a volume of body fluid below normal, and its concomitant decrease in plasma volume, have been shown to result in a decrease in physical performance. Loss of as little as 3% of body water results in detectable changes in physiological function.[19] These changes in function lead to decreases in the performance of anaerobic arm and leg exercise,[20] long- and short-distance running,[21] and maximal aerobic power.[22] In each of these investigations, hypohydration was assessed via changes in hematocrit and blood volume, a method which some have suggested may not be the best indicator of hydration status.[23]

One method by which a decrease in plasma volume may affect performance is by decreasing blood flow to the working muscle. Some investigators have shown that hypohydration results in a decrease in cardiac output and arm blood flow.[24] As a result, the maximal aerobic power ($\dot{V}O_2$ max) of an individual exercising in a hypohydrated state may be less than that obtained from the same individual exercising in a euhydrated state.[25,26] Thus, loss of body water, and particularly of plasma volume, appears to have a significant effect on maximal aerobic performance. While loss of plasma volume is largely a function of loss of body weight, regardless of method of dehydration,[27] some investigators suggest that the method of dehydration may affect subsequent performance.[22] The changes in plasma volume associated with a loss of body mass, and its subsequent consequences, may also be different for men and women.[28-30]

Hypervolemia, whether achieved through short-term exercise (a few minutes)[31] or albumin-induced volume expansion,[32] does not appear to induce increases in endurance performance. However, hypervolemia may result in lowered thermal and cardiovascular stress during subsequent performance by delaying the dehydration process.[32,33] Attempts to rehydrate individuals following exercise/thermal dehydration may not be adequate to allow complete cardiovascular recovery.[34]

Several authors have prepared well-written reviews of the relationship between exercise and plasma volume.[35,36] The interested reader is encouraged to study them.

2. Body Core Temperature

Among the homeostatic functions that are compromised by the loss of plasma volume associated with exercise is the ability to dissipate body heat. As plasma volume decreases, the temperature-related threshold for increased blood flow to the skin is increased.[37,38] Thus, a greater increase in core temperature must occur in a hypohydrated state, as compared to a euhydrated state, before skin blood flow increases. Hypohydration may result in a decrease of up to 50% in maximal arm blood flow,[24] which may hamper passive heat exchange. A decreased plasma volume also results in an increase in the temperature-related threshold for the onset of sweating.[38] The alterations in the thresholds for both an increase in skin blood flow and sweating threshold may lead to an increase in core temperature at any exercise intensity in a hypohydrated, as compared to a euhydrated, state.

Hypohydration also increases the risk of thermoregulatory disorders. Loss of 5% of body water may lead to heat exhaustion; loss of 7% may lead to hallucinations; loss of 10% may lead to heat stroke and death.[19] These complications may well be manifested to a greater extent among the overweight, those in poorer physical condition, and those who are un-acclimatized to exercise in warm or hot environments.

3. Electrolytes

In addition to changes in the volume of fluid in the vascular compartment, exercise may also lead to alterations in the electrolyte composition of the blood. Because sweat is a hypotonic solution when compared to plasma, the greater loss of water than sodium or chloride in sweat leads to an increase in the plasma concentrations of these electrolytes.[15] There are, however, individual athletes who lose significant amounts of sodium and/or chloride during ultraendurance events,[39-41] due largely to the considerable volume of sweat that is lost during such events.

Additional electrolytes excreted in sweat include potassium, chromium, zinc, copper, magnesium, iron, and phosphorous.[42,43] There is also a shift of plasma magnesium to the red blood cells during high-intensity anaerobic exercise, thereby further lowering plasma concentration of this mineral during very intense exercise.[44] Such changes in plasma magnesium concentrations, as well as relative increases in plasma sodium and potassium, have been implicated in the development of muscle cramps. Additionally, it has been proposed that the increase in blood osmolality, in conjunction with the loss of plasma volume resulting from a prolonged exercise bout, may be of significance in the development of thermo-regulatory complications during long-endurance events.[37,38]

Electrolyte concentrations in not only plasma, but also skeletal muscle may be affected by exercise-induced hypohydration. Skeletal muscle magnesium decreases with hypohydra-tion.[15] Muscle potassium increases slightly with hypohydration[15] and with ultraendurance exercise,[39,40] but decreases with short-term moderate, maximal, and supramaximal exercise.[45,46] In contrast, the amount of sodium and chloride in skeletal muscle, when expressed per unit of dry weight, is not changed as a consequence of hypohydration.[15] The relative changes in the electrolyte concentrations, particularly calcium, about the muscle cell membrane have been implicated in local muscle fatigue.[46]

4. Fuel Stores

Another avenue through which prolonged exercise may adversely affect the body's ability to engage in optimal performance is in its depletion of readily available energy stores. The degree to which such energy stores are depleted or unable to keep up with energy demands depends on the type, duration, and intensity of the exercise. Moderate exercise (60 to 75% $\dot{V}O_2$ max) continued for longer than 90 min without appropriate energy replacement may lead to a failure for hepatic glucose producton to keep up with muscle glucose uptake, resulting in a significant decrease in plasma glucose.[7,47] In contrast, if exercise intensity is increased during an exercise bout by the addition of arm to leg exercise, mobilization of hepatic glucose may exceed peripheral uptake.[48] Muscle glycogen may be measurably reduced after 45 min of moderate-intensity exercise, with the rate of decline increasing as the intensity of the exercise increases. Muscle and liver carbohydrate depletion is a significant factor in the development of fatigue during endurance events.[49] Since blood glucose contributes an increasing proportion of the carbohydrate oxidized as duration of high-intensity activity increases,[6,50,51] optimizing blood glucose concentration is important in ensuring continued high-intensity performance during endurance events.[6,7,13,52]

B. Role of Replacement Beverages

In light of the exercise-induced alterations in homeostasis discussed above, the possibility that ingestion of an appropriate carbohydrate/electrolyte solution may enhance physical performance is indeed welcome. However, the benefit of any such beverage comes only if it is capable of diminishing the detrimental effects of changes in plasma volume, blood and muscle electrolyte concentrations, body core temperature, and/or energy stores. If such diminishment is possible, then it can be expected that judicious use of appropriate carbohydrate/electrolyte beverages may lead to enhanced performance, i.e., support an increase in speed of movement or an extension of effort.

II. GENERAL CONSIDERATIONS FOR NUTRIENT BEVERAGE UPTAKE
A. Gastric Emptying

The efficacy of any ingested solution in maintaining plasma volume, electrolyte balance, or blood glucose during exercise is dependent on the ability of the ingested solution to traverse the stomach and be absorbed in the intestines. Relatively little is absorbed directly from the stomach; the small intestine is the primary site of nutrient absorption. Water is absorbed readily once it reaches the small intestine, and various nutrients are absorbed from the intestine at different rates.[53] Since nutrients are not absorbed from the stomach, the rate at which they empty into the intestines is an important limit to the benefit of any carbohydrate/electrolyte solution. Several excellent reviews of factors affecting gastric emptying/intestinal absorption have been written.[53-56]

Gastric emptying of water is due primarily to the pressure gradient between the stomach and duodenum.[54,55] Thus, a larger volume will empty faster than a smaller volume.[57] However, volumes greater than 600 ml do not appear to result in additional increases in emptying rate. Cool water, at a temperature of from 5 to 15°C empties more quickly than warmer solutions.[57-60]

The addition of carbohydrates and/or other nutrients to a beverage slows gastric emptying in proportion to the caloric content of the solution.[55,61-63] Once in the duodenum, nutrients act through neural feedback mechanisms to affect the rate of subsequent gastric emptying, resulting in a rate of gastric emptying which is approximately isocaloric regardless of the nature of the gastric contents.[54,61,64] Carbohydrate solutions empty in relative proportion to the solute concentration,[60,65,66] but such differences are not observed when the concentration differences are small (e.g., from 5 to 7%). The effect of osmolality on rate of gastric emptying has not yet been definitively demonstrated, with some authors reporting a slowing of gastric emptying as osmolality increases above isotonic,[54,55,65] while others show no effect of osmolality aside from its association with calorie-laden nutrients.[63,67,86]

An essential element to the discussion of nutrient beverages is the effect which differences in gastric emptying rates of various beverages may have on actual performance. As discussed above, there is ample evidence to show that the composition of a beverage may affect the rate at which the beverage empties from the stomach. However, a direct effect of such differences on eventual exercise performance has not been demonstrated.

In summary, gastric emptying is largely a function of the volume and caloric content of the beverage ingested. Cool beverages, which increase gastric motility, empty more quickly than warmer beverages. Cool beverages have the added advantage of increased palatability.[58] The addition of carbohydrates to a beverage slows its emptying in proportion to the caloric content. Osmolality itself, in the absence of the caloric influence, may not be an important determinant of gastric emptying. Finally, while beverage content may alter gastric emptying, the effects of such alterations on performance have not been demonstrated.

B. Fluid and Nutrient Uptake From The Intestines

Absorption of water, carbohydrates, and electrolytes occurs largely in the duodenum and jejunum of the small intestine. Net absorption of water is increased via the active transport of glucose and sodium.[69-71] The capacity for water absorption is apparently unlimited, so long as there exists an osmotic gradient which favors movement of water out of the intestinal lumen.[56] The introduction of hypertonic solutions into the intestines rapidly draws water into the intestinal lumen.[55,61] Thus, ingestion of hypertonic solutions, which empty from the stomach into the intestine with no significant alteration in osmolality, may result in decreases in plasma volume.[55]

Carbohydrates are absorbed primarily as monosaccharides along the duodenal and jejunal epithelia.[53] Sodium is essential for operation of the facilitated glucose transport system in the intestine.[69] Indeed, sodium-dependent transport is the rate-limiting step in glucose uptake.[53] Thus, the addition of small amounts of sodium to a carbohydrate solution would appear to enhance availability of the glucose. However, just as was noted in the discussion of gastric emptying, the observed differences in rate of intestinal absorption for various nutrient solutions have not been demonstrated to result in differences in physical performance.

C. Exercise Intensity

Most investigations of the gastric emptying and/or intestinal absorption characteristics of nutrient beverages have been conducted on individuals at rest. The extent to which physical activity may modify those characteristics is important to athletes consuming such beverages in an attempt to ameliorate the effects of exercise. Moderate-intensity exercise (up to 70% $\dot{V}O_2$ max) does not hinder gastric emptying of water or hypotonic nutrient beverages,[57,60,72-74] even when the exercise continues for up to 3 h.[75] Intestinal absorption of water, glucose, and/or electrolytes is, likewise, unaffected by moderate cycling or running exercise.[71,72,76] Indeed, physical activities such as running may aid gastric emptying due to mechanical movement of the fluids or increases in intragastric pressure.[60,74] However, addition of heat and/or hypohydration stress during an exercise bout may impair gastric emptying,[73,77] probably because of the marked reduction in splanchnic blood flow.

D. Metabolic Availability of Ingested Carbohydrates

The degree to which ingested glucose or other carbohydrates are made available for metabolic activity will determine the efficacy of the use of such beverages as a fuel replacement source. Several investigators have shown that a significant portion of ingested carbohydrate is oxidized during exercise. Up to 93% of glucose and glucose polymers ingested during prolonged moderate-intensity exercise is metabolized, as demonstrated using labeled carbon.[78-80] Indeed, exercise increases the rate of oxidation of exogenous carbohydrate.[76] The amount of exogenous carbohydrate oxidized during prolonged, moderate-intensity exercise is relatively independent of time of ingestion[79] or beverage osmolality.[78] However, the type of carbohydrate ingested may affect metabolic availability, with ingested fructose less available for oxidation than glucose.[80] There is, though, no metabolic advantage to the ingestion of glucose polymers over glucose.[80]

III. PREEXERCISE INGESTION OF NUTRIENT BEVERAGES
A. Rationale

Carbohydrate/electrolyte beverages may be ingested prior to exercise in an attempt to prevent or delay the detrimental homeostatic disturbances which can accompany exercise. Pre-event use of such beverages seeks to accomplish two things. First, fluid is ingested in an attempt to ensure adequate plasma volume at the onset of exercise, and to provide a small "reservoir" of fluid in the gastrointestinal lumen which will be absorbed during the early phases of the exercise bout. Net movement of water out of the vascular space and the concomitant increase in plasma osmolality which normally occur during exercise may thereby be reduced. The desired result is an increase in performance time prior to hypohydration-induced compromises in cardiovascular and thermoregulatory functions. A second reason for the preexercise use of nutrient beverages is to optimize circulating blood glucose concentrations by providing carbohydrates. Optimizing blood glucose may enhance performance by increasing carbohydrate oxidation in the latter stages of endurance exercise, thereby increasing time to exhaustion in prolonged moderate- and high-intensity exercise. Table 2[81-101] presents an overview of the efficacy of preexercise use of various nutrient beverages in enhancing physiological status and exercise performance.

B. Preexercise Carbohydrate Ingestion
1. Effect of Time of Ingestion

The time prior to the onset of exercise at which carbohydrate is ingested may affect subsequent performance by altering blood glucose profiles during the exercise bout. At rest, ingestion of glucose results in an initial rise in blood glucose, peaking approximately 30 to 45 min after ingestion.[85,89,90,99,100] Subsequent insulin-dependent uptake of the glucose may cause the blood glucose to fall below normal resting levels. However, the effect which these alterations in blood glucose may have on subsequent performance is not so clear.

Glucose or glucose polymers ingested 5 min to immediately prior to exercise result in a prolonged period of maintenance of blood glucose during moderate- to high-intensity exercise to exhaustion.[4,81,82] However, performance time to exhaustion may[82] or may not[81] be increased.

Ingestion of glucose in the period of from 1 h to 30 min prior to exercise results in the expected initial elevation of plasma glucose and is followed by a fall in plasma glucose during the early stages of exercise.[83-86,88,90,92,100] However, serum glucose returns to normal concentrations within approximately 30 min of the onset of exercise in such glucose ingestion regimens.[84,89] Some investigators have indicated that during moderately high-intensity exercise (75 to 85% $\dot{V}O_2$ max), muscle glycogen utilization was greater[87] and endurance time was decreased[84,86,95] following glucose ingestion during the 60- to 30-min preexercise period. However, others have shown that muscle glycogen utilization during the first 30 min of exercise[83,86] or during prolonged exercise[86,88,89] is not affected by glucose ingested 30 min to 1 h prior to exercise. Time to exhaustion[85] and total carbohydrate oxidation during prolonged exercise are not affected by preexercise ingestion of glucose during this time period.[86] Plasma free fatty acid concentration is decreased during the exercise when glucose is ingested from 1 h to 30 min prior to exercise.[84,85,89,90,92]

Glucose ingested 3 to 4 h prior to exercise results in the initial elevation and subsequent drop in blood glucose discussed above.[99-101] However, subsequent low- (45% $\dot{V}O_2$ max)[99]

TABLE 2 Efficacy of Preexercise Ingestion of Nutrient Beverages

Time of ingestion (min preexercise)	Nutrients ingested	Exercise	Results	Ref.
0	Glucose (90 g)	Cycling, intermittent to exhaustion, 74% $\dot{V}O_2$ max	a. No difference in time to exhaustion b. Increased blood glucose early but not later in exercise	81
5	Mixed carbohydrate (150 g)	Cycling to exhaustion, 68% $\dot{V}O_2$ max	a. Increased time to exhaustion b. Increased plasma glucose throughout exercise	82
30	a. Glucose (75 g) b. Fructose (75 g)	Running, 30 min, 70% $\dot{V}O_2$ max	a. Increased initial blood glucose with glucose b. No change in blood glucose with fructose c. No difference in rate of muscle glycogen use	83
30	a. Glucose (75 g) b. Liquid mixed meal	Cycling to exhaustion, 80% $\dot{V}O_2$ max	a. Decreased time to exhaustion with glucose b. Increased initial blood glucose with glucose c. Decreased serum FFA with glucose	84
45	a. Glucose (1 g/kg) b. Glycerol (1 g/kg)	Cycling to exhaustion, 73% $\dot{V}O_2$ max	a. Increased initial blood glucose with glucose b. Increased carbohydrate oxidation with glucose c. No change in blood glucose during exercise with glucose	85
45	a. Glucose (75 g) b. Fructose (75 g)	Cycling to exhaustion, 75% $\dot{V}O_2$ max	a. No difference in time to exhaustion b. Increased initial blood glucose with glucose c. No difference (as compared to control) in blood glucose with fructose d. No difference in muscle glycogen utilization with glucose or fructose	86
45	a. Glucose (50 g) b. Fructose (50 g)	Cycling 30 min, 75% $\dot{V}O_2$ max	a. Increased initial blood glucose with glucose b. No change in blood glucose with fructose c. No difference in muscle glycogen use (as compared to placebo) with fructose d. Increased muscle glycogen use with glucose	87

TABLE 2 (continued) Efficacy of Preexercise Ingestion of Nutrient Beverages

Time of ingestion (min preexercise)	Nutrients ingested	Exercise	Results	Ref.
45	a. Glucose (0.75 g/ kg) b. Fructose (0.75 g/ kg)	Cycling 4 h, 50% $\dot{V}O_2$ max	a. Increased initial blood glucose with glucose b. No difference in muscle glycogen use	88
45	a. Glucose (75 g) b. Fructose (75 g)	Cycling 2 h, 55% $\dot{V}O_2$ max	a. Increased initial blood glucose with glucose b. No difference in glycogen use with glucose or fructose c. Decreased plasma FFA with fructose	89
45	a. Glucose (75 g) b. Fructose (75 g)	Cycling 30 min, 75% $\dot{V}O_2$ max	a. Increased initial blood glucose with glucose b. Decreased blood glucose during exercise with glucose c. Attenuated blood glucose response with fructose d. Decreased plasma FFA with glucose or fructose	90
45	a. Glucose (75 g) b. Fructose (75 g)	Running 30 min, 75% $\dot{V}O_2$ max	a. Increased initial blood glucose with glucose b. Decreased muscle glycogen utilization with fructose	91
45	a. Glucose (100 g) b. Fructose (100 g)	Running to exhaustion, 80% $\dot{V}O_2$ max	a. Increased time to exhaustion with glucose or fructose b. Increased carbohydrate oxidation with glucose or fructose	92
60	a. Fructose (1 g/kg) b. Caffeine (5 mg/ kg)	Cycling 90 min, 70% $\dot{V}O_2$ max	a. Increased muscle glycogen use with caffeine b. Increased plasma FFA with caffeine or fructose	93
60	Caffeine (9 mg/kg)	Running Cycling to exhaustion, 85% $\dot{V}O_2$ max	a. Increased time to exhaustion b. No change in plasma FFA at rest or during exercise	94
60	Glucose (100 g)	Cycling, intermittent, to exhaustion, 85% $\dot{V}O_2$ max	a. Decreased time to exhaustion with glucose b. Increased initial blood glucose with glucose	95
60	Fructose (60 g, 85 g)	Cycling to exhaustion, 60–80% $\dot{V}O_2$ max	a. Increased time to exhaustion with fructose b. No change in blood glucose with fructose	96

TABLE 2 (continued) Efficacy of Preexercise Ingestion of Nutrient Beverages

Time of ingestion (min preexercise)	Nutrients ingested	Exercise	Results	Ref.
60	a. Sucrose (45 g) b. Caffeine (300 mg)	Running to exhaustion, 80% $\dot{V}O_2$ max	a. Increased time to exhaustion with sucrose or caffeine b. Increased carbohydrate use with sucrose c. Increased FFA use with caffeine	97
60	Caffeine (6 mg/kg)	Running 90 min, 70% $\dot{V}O_2$ max	a. Increased plasma FFA b. No change in plasma glucose or respiratory exchange ratio	98
180	Glucose (100 g) (labeled)	Walking 4 h, 45% $\dot{V}O_2$ max	Exogenous glucose accounted for 68 of the 253 g of carbohydrate used during the exercise	99
180	Mixed carbohydrate (5 g/kg) (glucose polymers and sucrose)	Cycling to exhaustion, 70% $\dot{V}O_2$ max	a. Increased time to exhaustion b. Increased rate of carbohydrate use	100
240	a. Mixed carbohydrate (45 g) b. Mixed carbohydrate (156 g) c. Mixed carbohydrate (312 g)	Cycling, intermittent, 70% $\dot{V}O_2$ max	a. Increased performance with 312 g carbohydrate (as compared to placebo) b. Greater carbohydrate oxidation with 312 g carbohydrate c. Maintenance of blood glucose with 312 g carbohydrate	101

or moderate- (70% $\dot{V}O_2$ max)[100] intensity exercise is enhanced following ingestion of glucose, as compared to the same exercise following placebo. The ingested glucose presumably acts as a readily available energy source during the exercise bout.

2. Effect of Type of Carbohydrate

The rate at which specific carbohydrates are digested and absorbed varies.[53] Likewise, different carbohydrates are associated with different glycemic indices.[102] The effects of preexercise ingestion of carbohydrates on blood glucose and eventual performance may differ, therefore, for the different carbohydrates.

Fructose has often been suggested as an alternative to glucose in nutritional beverages since it results in smaller alterations in both blood glucose and plasma insulin.[103] Several investigators have shown that ingestion of a fructose beverage 1 h to 30 min prior to moderate-intensity exercise (55 to 75% $\dot{V}O_2$ max) does not produce the blood glucose transients associated with glucose ingestion.[83,86-91,96,104] However, no differences in total glycogen use[83,86-89] or time to exhaustion[86,105] are observed when comparing preexercise fructose ingestion to glucose ingestion. Ingestion of fructose, however, has been associated with an increase in gastric distress relative to ingestion of glucose,[93] although such distress may be highly individual.

Results of preexercise ingestion of mixed carbohydrates (sucrose, fructose, and glucose combinations) have varied. Some investigators have shown increased time to performance of moderate-intensity endurance exercise[97] and increased carbohydrate oxidation during exercise,[106] while others have shown no effect of the ingested nutrients on endurance times or total carbohydrate oxidation during exercise.[107]

C. Preexercise Ingestion of Noncarbohydrate Nutrients
1. Glycerol
Ingestion of glycerol 45 min before high-intensity cycling exercise results in a decrease in time to exhaustion and decreased glucose oxidation when compared to glucose ingestion.[85] It has been suggested that the rate at which glycerol is used as a gluconeogenic substrate is not fast enough to allow it to serve as a significant energy source during exercise. Its main effect may simply be associated with temporary expansion and/or maintenance of plasma volume.

2. Caffeine
Ingestion of caffeine may enhance performance by altering endogenous energy supplies, principally by increasing lipolysis.[11] Investigations of the effect of preexercise ingestion of caffeine on subsequent plasma free fatty acids (FFA) and eventual exercise performance are varied. Some investigators have shown an advantage resulting from preexercise ingestion of caffeine[94] while others have shown little or no such advantage.[93,97,98]

3. Sodium Bicarbonate
Ingestion of sodium bicarbonate approximately 1 h prior to short-duration (1 to 2 min), very high-intensity exercise results in increased blood pH and bicarbonate concentration. Significant improvements in time to exhaustion of bicycle sprinting and time to run a fixed distance have been observed.[108,109] The increased performance is most probably associated with an increased buffering capacity of the blood. One side effect of the ingestion of sodium bicarbonate prior to an exercise bout is the development of diarrhea in approximately 50% of subjects.[109] The use of sodium citrate as a substitute for sodium bicarbonate apparently results in similar performance benefits without the gastric distress associated with sodium bicarbonate.[110]

IV. INGESTION OF NUTRIENT BEVERAGES DURING EXERCISE
Alterations in plasma volume, plasma electrolytes, and nutrient fuels which may occur during a bout of exercise can eventually modify physical performance. Athletes may ingest nutrient beverages in an effort to prevent or delay the exercise-induced alterations in homeostasis and consequent decline in performance. Attempts to evaluate the effectiveness of nutrient beverages ingested during exercise are hampered by the lack of consistency in investigations of such beverages. Varying exercise durations and intensities, solution volumes, feeding frequencies, and environmental conditions preclude definitive statements as to the global efficacy of specific nutrient solutions in enhancing physical performance. Additionally, appropriate comparisons among the various commercially available nutrient beverages is difficult owing to the various investigative protocols. There are, though, characteristics of both the exercise and the nutrient beverage which may be examined to determine the best use of such beverages during exercise.

A. Exercise Considerations
1. Duration
Labeled carbon from exogenous glucose appears in the expired air within 7 min of ingestion,[76] indicating the metabolic availability of the carbohydrate during even short-

duration events. However, while the ingested carbohydrate may be available for use, it may be of little or no benefit to the performance of short-duration events,[3] presumably because endogenous glycogen stores will not be depleted in most individuals during events that are of less than 2 h in duration. In contrast, during events lasting longer than 2 h, there may be a failure of hepatic glucose production to keep up with muscle glucose uptake.[7] Plasma glucose may, in fact, measurably decrease after 90 min of moderate exercise.[47] Most investigations of the effect of ingested carbohydrates during low- and moderate-intensity exercise have demonstrated a delay in fatigue and improved performance.[47,100,111-119] However, other investigators have shown no increase in time to fatigue when subjects consumed carbohydrate drinks vs. placebo.[120-123]

Ingestion of carbohydrate during endurance exercise results in maintenance of blood glucose levels and a concomitant increase in the rate of carbohydrate oxidation during the later stages of the exercise.[100,111-114,116-121,123-126,128-130] This, rather than a sparing of muscle glycogen, appears to be the mechanism by which ingestion of carbohydrate-containing beverages during endurance exercise enhances performance, since carbohydrate ingestion does not decrease the rate of muscle glycogen use.[6,112,115,121,131] Carbohydrate ingestion does, however, reduce liver glycogen depletion.[132]

2. Intensity

Ingestion of nutrient beverages has been shown to enhance performance of low- (below 60% $\dot{V}O_2$ max),[116,133] moderate- (60 to 80% $\dot{V}O_2$ max),[47,100,111,112,117-119] and high-intensity (greater than 80%, as a sprint task at the end of moderate-intensity exercise)[115,125] exercise. Thus, it appears that duration, rather than intensity, is the more important element in determining whether or not ingested nutrient beverages will result in improved performance.

B. Beverage Considerations
1. Voluntary Fluid Ingestion

Laboratory-based investigations of nutrient beverage consumption have the advantage of allowing control of the volume of fluid ingested. However, during exercise bouts in "the real world", athletes are free to consume as much, or as little, as they desire. Consequently, characteristics of a beverage which influence voluntary consumption may affect eventual performance. As with preexercise nutrient beverage ingestion, the temperature of a beverage is important in determining the total quantity of beverage consumed. Cool beverages are voluntarily consumed in greater quantities than are warm beverages during exercise.[58,59] Flavoring the beverage further enhances voluntary ingestion.[59,124,134] When flavor is indistinguishable between beverages, no difference exists in voluntary ingestion of isotonic vs. hypotonic beverages.[135]

2. Carbohydrates

Because the various carbohydrates vary in their gastric emptying and intestinal absorption characteristics, they may vary in their effectiveness in ameliorating exercise-induced changes in homeostasis. Table 3 (from References 79, 80, 113, 123, 136–141), Table 4 (References 47, 80, 100, 111, 112, 114, 116, 117, 119, 121–123, 126, 127, 129, 130, 139, 140, 142–144), and Table 5 (References 100, 113, 115, 117, 120, 121, 123–125, 144–147) present the results of studies investigating the effects of glucose, glucose polymers, fructose, and mixed carbohydrates on exercise performance.

Glucose

The hyper- followed by hypoglycemic response often observed with preexercise ingestion of glucose has not been demonstrated with glucose feedings during exercise.[4] The major

TABLE 3 Efficacy of Glucose-Containing Beverages Consumed During Prolonged Exercise

Nutrients ingested[a]	Time/volume	Exercise	Results	Ref.
a. Glucose/electrolyte, isosmotic, acidic b. Glucose/electrolyte, isosmotic, neutral c. Water	After 1-h, 10-min intervals, 120 ml	Cycling, intermittent, 3 h, 90 W	a. Maintenance of plasma volume with water and acid beverage b. Increased plasma volume with neutral beverage c. No difference in plasma osmolality with acidic vs. neutral beverage	136
a. Glucose/electrolyte (2.5% glucose, Na, K) b. Mixed CHO/electrolyte[b] (2% glucose, 4% sucrose, Na, K)	20-min intervals, 275 ml	Cycling, timed performance	a. Decreased time to perform task with high CHO b. Increased blood glucose with high CHO c. Increased respiratory exchange ratio with high CHO	113
a. Glucose/electrolyte (13 g/l glucose, Na, K) b. Water	20-min intervals to replace water loss	Cycling, intermittent, 160 min, 50% $\dot{V}O_2$ max	a. No difference in plasma volume, heart rate, or core temperature b. No difference in losses of Na or K	137
a. Glucose infusion b. Water ingestion	20-min intervals a. to maintain euglycemia b. to replace water loss	Cycling 2 h, 70% $\dot{V}O_2$ max	a. Maintenance of cardiac output, heart rate, and $\dot{V}O_2$ during exercise with glucose b. Attenuation of decreased cardiac output and stroke volume with water	138
Glucose (100 g)	a. 15 min b. 120 min	Walking 4 h, 45% $\dot{V}O_2$ max	a. 55% of endogenous glucose was oxidized b. No difference in glucose oxidation based on time of ingestion	79
a. Glucose (1.33 g/kg) b. Glucose polymer (1.33 g/kg) c. Fructose (1.33 g/kg)	20-min intervals, about 234 ml	Cycling 120 min, 53% $\dot{V}O_2$ max	a. Increased oxidation of endogenous glucose and glucose polymer as compared to fructose b. Increased initial blood glucose with glucose c. Decreased plasma FFA, but not FFA use, with all CHO beverages	80
a. Glucose/electrolyte b. Glucose polymer	10-min intervals, 100 ml	Cycling 60 min, 68% $\dot{V}O_2$ max	a. No difference in blood glucose or CHO oxidation b. Decreased plasma volume with glucose polymer	139

TABLE 3 (continued) Efficacy of Glucose-Containing Beverages Consumed During Prolonged Exercise

Nutrients ingested[a]	Time/volume	Exercise	Results	Ref.
a. Glucose (26 g/h) b. Glucose (52 g/h) c. Glucose (78 g/h)	15-min intervals	Cycling 2 h, 65–75% $\dot{V}O_2$ max, then timed 4.8 km	a. Decreased time to complete 4.8 km with all CHO beverages b. Increased plasma glucose with all CHO beverages c. Decreased plasma FFA with all CHO beverages	118
a. Glucose (10%) b. Glucose polymer (10%) c. Water	20-min intervals, 200 ml	Running 2 h, 65% $\dot{V}O_2$ max	a. Increased plasma glucose with glucose or glucose polymer b. No differences in loss of plasma volume	140
a. Glucose/electrolyte (0.93 g glucose/dl, Na, K, Cl) b. Caffeine (5 mg/kg)	Initial 400 ml, 2.5-mile intervals, 100 ml	Running 20 miles	a. No difference in plasma FFA b. Increased $\dot{V}O_2$ during exercise with caffeine c. Increased respiratory exchange ratio with caffeine	141
a. Glucose polymer with glucose (50 g) b. Glucose polymer with fructose (50 g) c. Water	5-km intervals, 150 ml	Running 30 km, as fast as possible	a. No difference in running time b. Maintenance of blood glucose with either CHO beverages	123

[a] All investigations included a placebo.
[b] CHO, carbohydrate.
[c] GP, glucose polymer.

effect of ingestion of glucose beverages during prolonged exercise of low[80] or moderate[113,118,123,140] intensity appears to be a maintenance of blood glucose in the later stages of the exercise, although some investigators have shown no difference in blood glucose when comparing carbohydrate beverages to placebo.[139] Along with the increase in blood glucose is an increased oxidation of carbohydrate.[80,113] Maintenance of blood glucose, and the concomitant increase in carbohydrate oxidation, late in prolonged exercise appears to be the means by which carbohydrate ingestion enhances performance. It must be noted, however, that maintenance of blood glucose merely delays, rather than prevents, fatigue. Fatigue, usually defined as the inability to continue a prescribed intensity of exercise, occurs even though blood glucose may be well within normal limits.

An additional benefit of the ingestion of glucose beverages during prolonged, moderate-intensity exercise is the maintenance of plasma volume and/or cardiac output.[136,138] The enhanced hydration status occurs, presumably, through an enhanced uptake of fluid in the intestine.

Glucose Polymers

There has been much interest in the past decade in the use of glucose polymers in nutrient beverages. Glucose polymers have the advantage of increasing the carbohydrate content of a solution with less increase in osmolality than would result from addition of the same

TABLE 4 Efficacy of Glucose Polymer-Containing Beverages Consumed During Exercise

Nutrients ingested[a]	Time/volume	Exercise	Results	Ref.
Glucose polymer (3 g/kg)	At 135 min	Cycling to exhaustion, 70% $\dot{V}O_2$ max	a. Increased time to exhaustion b. Increased plasma glucose following CHO ingestion[b] c. Increased respiratory exchange ratio following CHO ingestion	111
Glucose polymer (2 g/kg, then 0.4 g/kg)	20-min intervals	Cycling to exhaustion, 71% $\dot{V}O_2$ max	a. Increased time to exhaustion b. Maintenance of blood glucose c. Maintenance of CHO use d. No difference in rate of muscle glycogen use	112
Glucose polymer (1 g/kg, then 0.25 g/kg)	20, then 60, 90, 120 min, 300 ml	Cycling to exhaustion, 74% $\dot{V}O_2$ max	a. Increased time to exhaustion b. Decreased loss of plasma volume	47
Glucose polymer (7%) with electrolytes	6 rest periods, 170 ml	Football scrimmage	a. No difference in change in plasma electrolytes b. Increased loss of plasma volume with glucose polymer	142
a. Glucose polymer b. Glucose polymer with fructose	25-min intervals	Cycling 55.2 miles	a. Decreased time to finish with either CHO beverage b. Increased blood glucose with either CHO beverage	114
a. Glucose polymer (5%) with fructose (5%) b. Glucose polymer (7.7%) with fructose (2.3%) c. Glucose polymer (3%) with glucose (2%)	20-min intervals, 150 ml	Cycling 2 h, 90 rpm isokinetic	a. No difference in work b. Increased blood glucose with all CHO beverages c. No difference in muscle glycogen use	121
a. Glucose polymer (90 g) b. Caffeine (500 mg)	15-min intervals, 25 ml	Cycling 2 h, 80 rpm isokinetic	a. Increased work and $\dot{V}O_2$ with caffeine vs. placebo b. Increased blood glucose with glucose polymer c. No difference in CHO use d. Increased FFA use during later stages of exercise with caffeine	143

TABLE 4 (continued) Efficacy of Glucose Polymer-Containing Beverages Consumed During Exercise

Nutrients ingested[a]	Time/volume	Exercise	Results	Ref.
Glucose polymer (120 g total)	60, 90, 120, 150 min	Walking to exhaustion, 45% $\dot{V}O_2$ max	a. Increased time to exhaustion b. Increased CHO use c. Increased blood glucose during exercise	116
Glucose polymer (10%)	20-min intervals, 200 ml	Cycling 160 min, 65% $\dot{V}O_2$ max	a. Increased blood glucose and respiratory exchange ratio (as compared to control) b. No difference in plasma volume change	126
Glucose polymer (6.5%)	*ad libitum*	Cycling 270 km, 25 kg/h	a. Longer maintenance of blood glucose with glucose polymer b. Increased respiratory exchange ratio with glucose polymer	127
a. Glucose (1.33 g/kg) b. Glucose polymer (1.33 g/kg) c. Fructose (1.33 g/kg)	20-min intervals, about 234 ml	Cycling 120 min, 53% $\dot{V}O_2$ max	a. Increased oxidation of endogenous glucose and GP[c] as compared to fructose b. Increased initial blood glucose with glucose c. Decreased plasma FFA, but not FFA use, with all CHO beverages	80
a. Glucose/electrolyte b. Glucose polymer	10-min intervals, 100 ml	Cycling 60 min, 68% $\dot{V}O_2$ max	a. No difference in blood glucose or CHO oxidation. b. Decreased plasma volume with glucose polymer	139
Carbohydrate/electrolyte (5% glucose polymer, 2% fructose, Na, K, Cl)	Post-swim, 8-km intervals cycle, 3.2-km intervals, run, 2 ml/kg	Triathlon 1.5-km swim, 40-km cycle, 10-km run	a. Decreased time to complete task with CHO beverage b. Increased blood glucose with CHO beverage c. Increased respiratory exchange ratio with CHO beverage	117
a. Glucose polymer (5%) b. Glucose polymer (5%), with fructose (2%) c. Glucose (2%), with sucrose (4%)	15-min (approx.) intervals, 2 ml/kg	Cycling, intermittent, 140 min, 55 or 65% $\dot{V}O_2$ max	a. Increased plasma glucose with all CHO beverages b. No difference in plasma volume change, plasma electrolytes, or respiratory exchange ratio	144
a. Glucose (10%) b. Glucose polymer (10%) c. Water	20-min intervals, 200 ml	Running 2 h, 65% $\dot{V}O_2$ max	a. Increased plasma glucose with glucose or glucose polymer b. No differences in loss of plasma volume	140

TABLE 4 (continued) Efficacy of Glucose Polymer-Containing Beverages Consumed During Exercise

Nutrients ingested[a]	Time/volume	Exercise	Results	Ref.
a. Glucose polymer with electrolytes b. Electrolytes c. Water	15-min intervals	Cycling to exhaustion, 85% $\dot{V}O_2$ max	a. No difference in time to exhaustion b. No difference in blood electrolytes	122
a. Glucose polymer (7.2%) with electrolytes b. Water	a. *ad libitum* b. 1000 ml/5 km	Walking, intermittent, 30 km, 5 km/h	a. Increased blood glucose with glucose polymer b. No differences in plasma osmolality c. Increased plasma FFA with water	129
Glucose polymer	15-min intervals, 125 ml	Running to exhaustion, 80% $\dot{V}O_2$ max	a. Increased time to exhaustion b. Increased plasma glucose c. Increased respiratory exchange ratio	119
a. Glucose polymer with glucose (50 g) b. Glucose polymer with fructose (50 g) c. Water	5-km intervals, 150 ml	Running 30 km as fast as possible	a. No difference in running time b. Maintenance of blood glucose with either CHO beverage	123
Mixed carbohydrates (5% glucose polymer, 3% fructose)	20-min intervals, 2 g CHO/kg	Cycling to exhaustion, 70% $\dot{V}O_2$ max	a. Increased time to exhaustion b. Increased CHO use	100
a. Glucose polymer (2%) b. Glucose polymer (8.5%)	15-min intervals, 3 ml/kg	Cycling 2 h, 49% $\dot{V}O_2$ max	a. Increased blood glucose with 8.5% solution b. Increased CHO oxidation with 8.5% solution	130

[a] All investigations included a placebo.
[b] CHO, carbohydrate.
[c] GP, glucose polymer.

amount of carbohydrate in the form of glucose or other monosaccharides. Since beverage osmolality may affect gastric emptying,[54,55,65] the use of a carbohydrate source that minimizes alterations in osmolality was thought to be advantageous. While the rate of gastric emptying of solutions containing glucose polymers may exceed that of solutions containing similar amounts of glucose,[65] there appears to be no physiological or performance advantage to the addition of glucose polymers, rather than glucose, to a nutrient beverage.[80,139,140,144]

Just as with ingestion of glucose, ingestion of glucose polymer during prolonged low-[130,144] or moderate-[111,112,114,116,117,119,121,123,126,127,129,130,140,143,144] intensity exercise maintains blood glucose during the exercise. Carbohydrate oxidation is thus maintained at a higher level during the exercise.[80,100,111,112,116,117,119,126,127,130] The result is an increase in performance of prolonged, moderate-intensity exercise.[47,100,111,112,114,116,117,119]

Fructose

Fructose empties from the stomach more quickly than a similar amount of glucose.[60] Additionally, the inclusion of fructose in a nutrient beverage prevents the glycemic responses

TABLE 5 Efficacy of Beverages Containing Fructose, Sucrose, and Mixed Carbohydrates Consumed During Exercise

Nutrients ingested[a]	Time/volume	Exercise	Results	Ref.
Carbohydrate/electrolyte a. 6.6% CHO,[b] 316 mOsmol/l b. 6% CHO, 113 mOsmol/l c. 2.5% CHO, 187 mOsmol/l d. 0% CHO, 16 mOsmol/l	20-min intervals, 250 ml	Cycling to exhaustion, 74% $\dot{V}O_2$ max	a. No difference in time to exhaustion, plasma volume change, or plasma electrolytes b. Increased plasma glucose with 6 or 6.6% CHO	120
Mixed CHO/electrolyte (4.8% glucose polymer, 2.6% fructose, Na, K, Ca, Cl)	*ad libitum*	Cycling 3 h, 60% $\dot{V}O_2$ max	a. Increased plasma volume and plasma electrolytes b. Increased plasma glucose c. Increased voluntary ingestion	124
a. Glucose/electrolyte (2.5% glucose, Na, K) b. Mixed CHO/electrolyte (2% glucose, 4% sucrose, Na, K)	20-min intervals, 275 ml	Cycling, timed performance	a. Decreased time to perform task with high CHO b. Increased blood glucose with high CHO c. Increased respiratory exchange ratio with high CHO	113
Carbohydrate/electrolyte (7% CHO)	30-min intervals, 200 ml	Running 2 h, 60–65% $\dot{V}O_2$ max	a. No difference in plasma electrolytes b. Decreased plasma FFA	145
a. Sucrose (10.75 g) b. Sucrose (21.5 g)	a. 30-min intervals, 200 ml b. 1-h intervals, 400 ml	Cycling, intermittent, 4 h, 50–100% $\dot{V}O_2$ max	a. No difference in muscle glycogen use with CHO b. Improved blood glucose with CHO c. Increased respiratory exchange ratio with CHO d. Improved performance on end-test maximal sprint with CEO	115
a. Glucose polymer (5%) with fructose (5%) b. Glucose polymer (7.7%) with fructose (2.3%) c. Glucose polymer (3%) with glucose (2%)	20-min intervals, 150 ml	Cycling 2 h, 90 rpm isokinetic	a. No difference in work b. Increased blood glucose with all CHO beverages c. No difference in muscle glycogen use	121
Sucrose (43 g)	1-h intervals, 400 ml	Cycling, intermittent, 4 h, 50–100% $\dot{V}O_2$ max	a. Decreased muscle glycogen with CHO b. Increased blood glucose with CHO	125

TABLE 5 (continued) Efficacy of Beverages Containing Fructose, Sucrose, and Mixed Carbohydrates Consumed During Exercise

Nutrients ingested[a]	Time/volume	Exercise	Results	Ref.
			c. Increased respiratory exchange ratio with CHO	
			d. Increased performance in end-test maximal sprint with CHO	
Carbohydrate/electrolyte (5% glucose polymer, 2% fructose, Na, K, Cl)	Post-swim, 8-km interval cycle, 3.2-km interval run, 2 ml/kg	Triathlon, 1.5 km swim, 40-km cycle, 10-km run	a. Decreased time to complete task with CHO beverage b. Increased blood glucose with CHO beverage c. Increased respiratory exchange ratio with CHO beverage	117
a. Glucose/electrolyte (6% glucose, Na, K, Cl) b. Glycerol (10%) c. Glucose/electrolyte (as in a.), with glycerol (4%)	15-min intervals to 60 min, 3 ml/kg	Cycling, 90 min, 50% $\dot{V}O_2$ max	a. Increased plasma osmolality with glycerol b. Increased gastrointestinal distress with glycerol c. No difference in core temperature or sweat rate	146
a. Glucose polymer (5%) b. Glucose polymer (5%) with fructose (2%) c. Glucose (2%) with sucrose (4%)	15-min (approx.) intervals, 2 ml/kg	Cycling, intermittent, 140 min, 55 or 65% $\dot{V}O_2$ max	a. Increased plasma glucose with all CHO beverages b. No difference in plasma volume change, plasma electrolytes, or respiratory exchange ratio	144
a. Glucose (6%) b. Fructose (6%) c. Sucrose (6%)	15-min (approx.) intervals, 3 ml/kg	Cycling, intermittent, 115 min, 65–80% $\dot{V}O_2$ max	a. No difference in CHO use b. Decreased plasma glucose and volume with fructose c. Decreased speed with fructose d. Increased plasma FFA and gastric distress with fructose	147
a. Glucose polymer with glucose (50 g) b. Glucose polymer with fructose (50 g) c. Water	5-km intervals, 150 ml	Running 30 km, as fast as possible	a. No difference in running time b. Maintenance of blood glucose with either CHO beverage	123
Mixed carbohydrates (5% glucose polymer, 3% fructose)	20-min intervals, 2 g CHO/kg	Cycling to exhaustion, 70% $\dot{V}O_2$ max	a. Increased time to exhaustion b. Increased CHO use	100

[a] All investigations included a placebo.
[b] CHO, carbohydrate.

associated with glucose ingestion.[103] For these reasons, the inclusion of fructose in nutrient beverages ingested during exercise has been proposed as a means of minimizing the glucose-induced alterations in blood glucose which occur during the early stages of exercise. While preexercise ingestion of fructose does reduce the glucose transients associated with glucose ingestion,[29,86-89,91,96,104,121] there appears to be no such advantage to fructose ingested during exercise.[114,121,144] Neither does ingestion of fructose result in an increase in performance whem compared to the ingestion of glucose or glucose polymers.[114,121,123,147] However, just as with glucose and glucose polymers, ingestion of fructose may improve prolonged moderate-intensity exercise performance when compared to placebo.[100,114,117] One potential disadvantage to the inclusion of fructose in a nutrient beverage is a potential increase in gastric distress.[93,147]

Mixed Carbohydrate Sources

Nutrient beverages that contain a mixture of carbohydrates may offer advantages over solutions containing a single carbohydrate.[93] Such solutions may capitalize on any advantages incurred in either gastric emptying or maintenance of blood glucose offered by single carbohydrates while minimizing disadvantages such as gastric distress. Investigations of the efficacy of mixed carbohydrate beverages in enhancing prolonged, moderate-intensity exercise performance have indicated no differences when using mixed carbohydrates as compared to single carbohydrate solutions.[120,121,123] However, as with single carbohydrate beverages, mixed carbohydrate beverages maintain blood glucose during prolonged moderate-intensity exercise[113,115,117,120,121,123-125,144] which may result in improved performance when compared to placebo.[10,113,115,117,125]

3. Noncarbohydrate Nutrients

Electrolytes

Ingestion of a glucose/electrolyte solution during exercise may result in a maintenance[120,136] or increase[124,136,137,148,149] in plasma volume. Plasma osmolality during exercise may[120,124,136,149] or may not[122,129,133,137,142,145,148] be enhanced during exercise following ingestion of isotonic electrolyte solutions. Table 6 presents the results of investigations of the efficacy of electrolyte beverages ingested during exercise.

Caffeine

Ingestion of caffeine during prolonged intense exercise may result in an increase in total work performed,[143] an increase in free fatty acid utilization[143] or serum free fatty acid concentrations,[150] and an increase in $\dot{V}O_2$ during prolonged, intense exercise.[141] However, caffeine ingestion by itself has no significant effect on performance during endurance events when compared to ingestion of glucose/electrolyte solutions during exercise.[141,150]

C. Summary

Several factors affect the influence which ingestion of nutrient beverages may have during exercise. Of most significance among these are the duration of the exercise and the composition of the beverage. For exercise lasting less than 90 min, addition of carbohydrates to a nutrient beverage is of little consequence to performance. However, during events lasting 2 h or more, carbohydrate ingestion delays fatigue by maintaining adequate blood glucose levels and thereby a high rate of carbohydrate oxidation during the later stages of the exercise. While carbohydrate solutions do not appear to affect the rate of muscle glycogen use, liver glycogen reserves may be spared.

Ingestion of carbohydrate during exercise does not result in the hypoglycemic response associated with some preexercise regimens of carbohydrate ingestion. While the form of

TABLE 6 Efficacy of Electrolyte Beverages Consumed During Exercise

Nutrients ingested[a]	Time/volume	Exercise	Results	Ref.
a. Saline (25 mmol/l) b. Water	15-min intervals, to replace water loss	Cycling, intermittent up to 6 h, 55% $\dot{V}O_2$ max	a. Increased performance time with saline or water b. No difference in plasma Na with saline vs. water	133
a. Glucose/electrolyte, isosmotic, acidic b. Glucose/electrolyte, isosmotic, neutral c. Water	After 1 h, 10-min intervals, 120 ml	Cycling, intermittent, 3 h, 90 W	a. Maintenance of plasma volume with water and acid beverage b. Increased plasma volume with neutral beverage c. No difference in plasma osmolality with acid vs. neutral beverage	136
Carbohydrate/electrolyte a. 6.6% CHO,[b] 316 mOsmol/l b. 6% CHO, 113 mOsmol/l c. 2.5% CHO, 187 mOsmol/l d. 0% CHO, 16 mOsmol/l	20-min intervals, 250 ml	Cycling to exhaustion, 74% $\dot{V}O_2$ max	a. No difference in time to exhaustion, plasma volume change, or plasma electrolytes b. Increased plasma glucose with 6 or 6.6% CHO	120
a. Hypertonic b. Isotonic c. Hypotonic d. Water	10-min intervals, after 70 min, 1/18 of total water loss during control	Cycling, intermittent 4 h, 50% of W needed to achieve heart rate of 170	a. Increased plasma volume with isotonic b. Decreased plasma osmolality with water	149
Mixed CHO/electrolyte (4.8% glucose polymer, 2.6% fructose, Na, K, Ca, Cl)	*ad libitum*	Cycling 3 h, 60% $\dot{V}O_2$ max	a. Increased plasma volume and plasma electrolytes b. Increased plasma glucose c. Increased voluntary ingestion	124
Glucose polymer (7%) with electrolytes	6 rest periods, 170 ml	Football scrimmage	a. No difference in change in plasma electrolytes b. Increased loss of plasma volume with glucose polymer	142
a. Glucose/electrolyte (2.5% glucose, Na, K) b. Mixed CHO/electrolyte (2% glucose, 4% sucrose, Na, K)	20-min intervals, 275 ml	Cycling, timed performance	a. Decreased time to perform task with high CHO b. Increased blood glucose with high CHO c. Increased respiratory exchange ratio with high CHO	113

TABLE 6 (continued) Efficacy of Electrolyte Beverages Consumed During Exercise

Nutrients ingested[a]	Time/volume	Exercise	Results	Ref.
Carbohydrate/electrolyte (7% CHO)	30-min intervals, 200 ml	Running 2 h, 60–65% $\dot{V}O_2$ max	a. No difference in plasma electrolytes b. Decreased plasma FFA	145
a. Glucose/electrolyte (13 g/l glucose, Na, K) b. Water	20-min intervals, to replace water loss	Cycling, intermittent, 160 min, 50% $\dot{V}O_2$ max	a. No difference in plasma volume, heart rate, or core temperature b. No difference in losses of Na or K	137
Carbohydrate/electrolyte (5% glucose polymer, 2% fructose, Na, K, Cl)	Post-swim, 8-km interval cycle, 3.2-km interval run, 2 ml/kg	Triathlon, 1.5-km swim, 40-km cycle, 10-km run	a. Decreased time to complete task with CHO beverage b. Increased blood glucose with CHO beverage c. Increased respiratory exchange ratio with CHO beverage	117
a. Glucose/electrolyte (6% glucose, Na, K, Cl) b. Glycerol (10%) c. Glucose/electrolyte (as in a.), with glycerol (4%)	15-min intervals to 60 min, 3 ml/kg	Cycling 90 min, 50% $\dot{V}O_2$ max	a. Increased plasma osmolality with glycerol b. Increased gastrointestinal distress with glycerol c. No difference in core temperature or sweat rate	146
a. Glucose polymer with electrolytes b. Electrolytes c. Water	15-min intervals	Cycling to exhaustion, 85% $\dot{V}O_2$ max	a. No difference in time to exhaustion b. No difference in blood electrolytes	122
a. Glucose polymer (7.2%) with electrolytes b. Water	a. *ad libitum* b. 1000 ml/5 km	Walking, intermittent, 30 km, 5 km/h	a. Increased blood glucose with glucose polymer b. No differences in plasma osmolality c. Increased plasma FFA with water	129
a. Glucose/electrolyte (0.93 g glucose/dl, Na, K, Cl) b. Caffeine (5 mg/kg)	Initial 400 ml, 2.5-mile intervals, 100 ml	Running 20 miles	a. No difference in plasma FFA b. Increased $\dot{V}O_2$ during exercise with caffeine c. Increased respiratory exchange ratio with caffeine	141

[a] All investigations included a placebo.
[b] CHO, carbohydrate.

carbohydrate ingested may lead to different plasma glucose responses, muscle glycogen use and performance may be the same regardless of the type of carbohydrate ingested. Ingestion of carbohydrate solutions of glucose, fructose, sucrose, and/or glucose polymer all seem to result in increased plasma glucose, when compared to water ingestion, during prolonged moderate-intensity exercise. Except for those individual athletes subject to hyponatremia, addition of electrolytes to nutrient beverages is not justified on the basis of the small changes which occur in blood osmolality. However, the addition of sodium to a beverage aids fluid and glucose absorption in the intestine, and may thus be a beneficial component of a nutrient beverage solution. In regards to the electrolyte composition of nutrient beverages, hypotonic solutions are probably best for most endurance athletes.

While ingestion of appropriate nutrient beverages during exercise may delay fatigue, it is important to note that it does not prevent fatigue. Fatigue occurs in spite of the maintenance of plasma volume and blood glucose brought about through appropriate nutrient beverage ingestion.

V. INGESTION OF NUTRIENT BEVERAGES FOLLOWING EXERCISE
A. Rationale
The benefit of postexercise ingestion of nutrient beverages comes if such beverages improve the recovery of plasma volume, electrolytes, and/or fuel stores following the exercise stress. Unfortunately, the use of nutrient beverages to enhance recovery from exercise has not been addressed to the same extent as has the use of such beverages to enhance performance during exercise. The advantage of quick recovery from a prolonged bout of exercise, can readily be seen for athletes competing in tournaments, in which a performer is expected to participate in several endurance activities within one or very few days time. However, an increased rate of recovery will also be beneficial to the athlete who engages in moderate-to high-intensity exercise on a daily basis. This enhanced rate of recovery may be greater than that brought about through adjustments in normal meal consumption.

B. Effects of Postexercise Consumption of Carbohydrate/Electrolyte Beverages
The effects of postexercise ingestion of various nutrient beverages are presented in Table 7.[124,151-157] Muscle glycogen resynthesis is enhanced if carbohydrate beverages are ingested immediately following an exercise bout.[151,153,154,157] The rate of glycogen resynthesis is dependent on the amount of carbohydrate in the ingested beverage.[151,153] Replenishment of muscle glycogen is greater when glucose or sucrose, rather than fructose, is included in the beverage.[151] Glucose added to postexercise beverages may result in more rapid recovery of plasma volume through enhanced voluntary fluid ingestion.[124] The addition of sodium to carbohydrate solutions results in increased replenishment of muscle glycogen.[155] Sodium may also act to enhance the rehydration process by maintaining a slightly hypertonic plasma and thereby enhancing dipsogenic stimuli.[155,156]

VI. SUMMARY
Nutrient beverages are ingested before, during, and/or after exercise in an attempt to ameliorate the exercise-induced changes which may affect homeostasis and thereby diminish performance. The homeostatic disturbances associated with exercise include a decrease in plasma volume, an increase in deep body or core temperature, an increase in plasma osmolality, and a decrease in nutrient fuels available to the muscle. Each of these changes may be affected through judicious use of beverages containing various amounts and types of nutrients. Since the homeostatic disturbances, and consequent alteration in performance, vary with the intensity, duration, and type of exercise, no one nutrient beverage is best for all exercise situations. Rather, the informed exerciser should evaluate the different beverages in terms of the desired outcome of beverage ingestion.

In exercise bouts lasting less than 90 min, the availability of nutrient fuels to the working muscles is usually adequate to meet the demands of the exercise for most athletes consuming a well-balanced diet. In such exercise sessions, prevention of hypohydration and thermal stress through maintenance of plasma volume and osmolality, rather than enhancement of nutrient stores, would appear to be the important consideration. Ensuring optimal hydration

TABLE 7 Efficacy of Nutrient Beverages Consumed Following Exercise

Nutrients ingested[a]	Time/volume	Exercise	Results	Ref.
As a 30% solution: a. Glucose (0.35 g/kg) b. Glucose (0.7 g/kg) c. Glucose (1.4 g/kg) d. Sucrose (0.7 g/kg) e. Fructose (0.7 g/kg)	Immediately post, 2 h, 4 h	Cycling, intermittent to exhaustion, 75% $\dot{V}O_2$ max	a. Increased muscle glycogen synthesis with glucose or sucrose vs. fructose b. Increased muscle glycogen synthesis with higher glucose beverages	151
Carbohydrate/electrolyte (4.85% glucose polymer, 2.65% fructose, Na, K, Ca, Mg, Cl)	*ad libitum* 3 h	Cycling 3 h, 60% $\dot{V}O_2$ max	a. Increased voluntary ingestion of CHO[b] beverage b. Increased plasma volume, osmolality, and glucose with CHO beverage c. Increased body weight gain with CHO	124
a. Glucose/electrolyte (13 g glucose, Na, K, Cl) b. Water	*ad libitum* 5 d	Cycling daily, until loss of 3% body weight, 55–60% $\dot{V}O_2$ max	a. No difference in electrolyte balance b. Increased extracellular fluid with water	152
a. Simple sugars (glucose, fructose, sucrose) b. Complex carbohydrates (starches) c. Low CHO (188 g/d) d. Mixed CHO (375 g/d) e. High CHO (525 g/d)		Running 16.1 km, 80% $\dot{V}O_2$ max	a. No difference in muscle glycogen resynthesis 24 h post, simple vs. complex CHO b. Increased muscle glycogen 48 h post with complex CHO c. Increased muscle glycogen resynthesis 24 h post with increased CHO	153
Glucose, 400 g	15 h a. Following rehydration b. With no rehydration	Cycle, intermittent, 2 h, 40–80% $\dot{V}O_2$ max	a. No difference in muscle glycogen resynthesis b. Increased muscle water with rehydration	154
a. High K (2.5% glucose, 51 mmol K/l) b. High Na (2.5% glucose, 128 mmol NaCl/l) c. High CHO (9%)	15-min intervals, 2 h, 300 ml	Cycling 2 h, 50% $\dot{V}O_2$ max	a. Increased plasma volume with high Na beverage b. Increased intracellular rehydration with high K and high CHO beverages	155
NaCl (capsules, 0.45 g/100 ml)	After 60 min, *ad libitum* for 3 h	Cycling 90–110 min, 40% $\dot{V}O_2$ max	a. Increased restoration of water loss with NaCl b. Increased plasma osmolality (and therefore dipsogenic stimulation) with NaCl	156

TABLE 7 (continued) Efficacy of Nutrient Beverages Consumed Following Exercise

Nutrients ingested[a]	Time/volume	Exercise	Results	Ref.
a. Liquid CHO	a. At 0 and 2 h	Cycling 2 h	a. No difference in muscle glycogen resynthesis	157
b. Solid CHO	b. At 0 and 2 h			
c. CHO infusion	c. Constant from 0 to 235 min		b. Increased blood glucose with infusion	

[a] All investigations included a placebo.
[b] CHO, carbohydrate.

is best accomplished through ingestion of cool, flavored beverages. Cool (5 to 15°C) beverages enhance gastric emptying by increasing gastric motility. Adding a flavoring agent, including carbohydrate and electrolytes, to the cool beverage results in increased voluntary consumption of the beverage. Additionally, active transport of sodium and glucose in the intestine increases the net absorption of water. However, since the caloric and perhaps osmotic characteristics of a beverage do affect the rate at which the fluid is emptied from the stomach, limiting the addition of carbohydrates and/or electrolytes would most beneficially affect hydration status. Volumes of fluid up to approximately 600 ml are emptied from the stomach in proportion to the volume. Since volumes greater than this do not add any gastric-emptying benefit, it would appear that volumes of 600 ml, with some adjustment for body size, would be the most beneficial in optimizing fluid maintenance during exercise.

During exercise events lasting longer than 90 min, blood glucose and muscle glycogen stores may be inadequate to meet the demands of the exercising tissues. Appropriate ingestion of carbohydrate may enhance performance of prolonged exercise of moderate to high intensity by maintaining blood glucose concentrations and thereby delaying, but not preventing, fatigue. Cool, flavored beverages, which are voluntarily consumed in greater quantities than are warm, unflavored beverages, are again the most beneficial in meeting the needs of the exercise. This is particularly important in ultra-endurance events, during which substantial loss of water may occur. Since blood glucose falls during prolonged exercise, the addition of carbohydrates in concentrations of 4 to 8% to the nutrient beverage will serve a useful purpose. Addition of carbohydrates within this concentration range has been shown to maintain blood glucose during the later stages of the exercise, and thereby increase endurance time during exhaustive efforts.

The nutrients added to the ingested beverage may affect the efficacy of the solution in optimizing performance. Addition of carbohydrate to a beverage may delay the gastric emptying and intestinal absorption of the nutrients in proportion to the carbohydrate concentration. However, there has been no evidence to suggest that such differences in emptying and absorption characteristics adversely affect performance. Addition of glucose, glucose polymers, sucrose, fructose, or mixed carbohydrates to a nutrient solution results in equally effective maintenance of blood glucose during prolonged exercise. Addition of fructose, however, may result in increased gastric distress in susceptible individuals. Small quantities of sodium in a nutrient solution enhance absorption of the carbohydrate component, and would thus be beneficial. Caffeine may or may not increase the availability of nutrient fuels to working muscle. Consequently, its effectiveness in enhancing exercise performance, based on its ability to increase availability of nutrient fuels, is questionable.

Time of ingestion of a nutrient beverage has been shown to affect blood glucose and insulin. Ingestion of carbohydrate solutions, especially those which contain glucose, more than 30 min prior to an exercise bout may result in a transient increase in plasma glucose and insulin during the early stages of the exercise. However, plasma glucose normalizes within the first hour of exercise; eventual performance time is not adversely affected.

Following exercise, appropriate use of nutrient beverages may enhance the recovery of plasma volume, plasma osmolality, and muscle glycogen stores. Ingestion of a carbohydrate solution immediately following exercise leads to an increase in muscle glycogen resynthesis proportional to the amount of carbohydrate in the beverage. Glucose or sucrose is more effective than fructose in enhancing muscle glycogen resynthesis. Sodium increases the uptake of both the carbohydrate and water, and thus is a beneficial addition to the postexercise nutrient beverage.

In summary, the following guidelines are offered for the selection of an appropriate nutrient beverage.

1. Cool (5 to 15°C), flavored water is voluntarily ingested in greater quantities than is plain, warm water. Therefore, for most exercise and sporting events, cool, flavored water is the optimal beverage for consumption, both before and during the event.
2. Volumes of water of approximately 600 ml are most beneficial in terms of gastric emptying.
3. Addition of small amounts of glucose and sodium (30 to 50 mmol/l) to a nutrient beverage increases the net water absorption and thereby helps to maintain plasma volume and osmolality.
4. Carbohydrates (750 to 1250 ml/h of a 4 to 8% solution) added to a beverage consumed during prolonged exercise help to maintain blood glucose and thereby delay fatigue in exhaustive efforts.
5. The type of carbohydrate added to a beverage consumed prior to or during exercise does not affect exercise performance. However, addition of fructose to a nutrient beverage may increase gastric distress in some individuals.
6. Postexercise consumption of a beverage containing both carbohydrate (glucose rather than fructose) and electrolytes speeds the recovery of plasma volume, plasma osmolality, and muscle glycogen.

REFERENCES

1. **Coggan, A. R. and Coyle, E. F.,** Carbohydrate ingestion during prolonged exercise: effects on metabolism and performance, in *Exercise and Sport Sciences Reviews,* Vol. 19, Holloszy, J. O., Ed., Williams & Wilkins, Baltimore, 1991, chap. 1.
2. **Consolazio, C. F. and Johnson, H. L.,** Dietary carbohydrate and work capacity, *Am. J. Clin. Nutr.,* 25, 85, 1972.
3. **Costill, D. L.,** Carbohydrate nutrition before, during, and after exercise, *Fed. Proc.,* 44, 364, 1985.
4. **Costill, D. L.,** Carbohydrates for exercise: dietary demands for optimal performance, *Int. J. Sports Med.,* 9, 1, 1988.
5. **Costill, D. L. and Hargreaves, M.,** Carbohydrate nutrition and fatigue, *Sports Med.,* 13, 86, 1992.
6. **Coyle, E. F.,** Carbohydrate metabolism and fatigue, in *Muscle Fatigue: Biochemical and Physiological Aspects,* Atlan, G., Beliveau, L., and Bouissou, P., Eds., Masson, Paris, 1991, 153.
7. **Coyle, E. F. and Coggan, A. R.,** Effectiveness of carbohydrate feeding in delaying fatigue during prolonged exercise, *Sports Med.,* 1, 446, 1984.
8. **Ivy, J. L.,** Muscle glycogen synthesis before and after exercise, *Sports Med.,* 11, 6, 1991.
9. **Lamb, D. R. and Brodowicz, G. R.,** Optimal use of fluids of varying formulations to minimize exercise-induced disturbances in homeostasis, *Sports Med.,* 3, 247, 1986.
10. **Maughan, R. J. and Noakes, T. D.,** Fluid replacement and exercise stress, *Sports Med.,* 12, 16, 1991.
11. **Powers, S. K. and Dodd, S.,** Caffeine and endurance performance, *Sports Med.,* 2, 165, 1985.
12. **Stanley, W. C. and Connett, R. J.,** Regulation of muscle carbohydrate metabolism during exercise, *FASEB J.,* 5, 2155, 1991.
13. **Valeriani, A.,** The need for carbohydrate intake during endurance exercise, *Sports Med.,* 12, 349, 1991.
14. **Wasserman, D. H. and Cherrington, A. D.,** Hepatic fuel metabolism during muscular work: role and regulation, *Am. J. Physiol.,* 260, E811, 1991.
15. **Costill, D. L., Coté, R., and Fink, W.,** Muscle water and electrolytes following varied levels of dehydration in man, *J. Appl. Physiol.,* 40, 6, 1976.
16. **Senay, L. C., Jr. and Pivarnik, J. M.,** Fluid shifts during exercise, *Exercise Sport Sci. Rev.,* 13, 335, 1985.

17. **Pivarnik, J. M., Goetting, M. P., and Senay, L. C., Jr.,** The effects of body position and exercise on plasma volume dynamics, *Eur. J. Appl. Physiol.,* 55, 450, 1986.
18. **Nose, H., Mack, G. W., Shi, X., and Nadel, E. R.,** Shift in body fluid compartments after dehydration in humans, *J. Appl. Physiol.,* 65, 318, 1988.
19. National Academy of Sciences-National Research Council, Water deprivation and performance of athletes, *Nutr. Rev.,* 32, 314, 1974.
20. **Corrigan, D. L., Heinsman, K. M., and Bauer, T. J.,** The effects of dehydration and rehydration on anaerobic exercise performance (Abstract), *Med. Sci. Sports Exercise,* 16, 112, 1984.
21. **Armstrong, L. E., Costill, D. L., and Fink, W. J.,** Influence of diuretic-induced dehydration on competitive running performance, *Med. Sci. Sports Exercise,* 17, 456, 1985.
22. **Caldwell, J. E., Ahonen, E., and Nousiainen, U.,** Differential effects of sauna-, diuretic-, and exercise-induced hypohydration, *J. Appl. Physiol. Respir. Environ. Exercise Physiol.,* 57, 1018, 1984.
23. **Francesconi, R. P., Hubbard, R. W., Szlyk, P. C., Schnakenberg, D., Carlson, D., Leva, N., Sils, I., Hubbard, L., Pease, V., Young, J., and Moore, D.,** Urinary and hematologic indexes of hypohydration, *J. Appl. Phys.,* 62, 1271, 1987.
24. **Nadel, E. R., Fortney, S. M., and Wenger, C. B.,** Effect of hydration state on circulatory and thermal regulations, *J. Appl. Physiol. Respir. Environ. Exercise Physiol.,* 49, 715, 1980.
25. **Buskirk, E. R., Iampietro, P. F., and Bass, D. E.,** Work performance after dehydration: effects of physical conditioning and acclimatization, *J. Appl. Physiol.,* 12, 189, 1958.
26. **Sawka, M. N., Francesconi, R. P., Young, A. J., and Pandolf, K. B.,** Influence of hydration level and body fluids on exercise performance in the heat, *JAMA,* 252, 1165, 1984.
27. **Costill, D. L. and Fink, W. J.,** Plasma volume changes following exercise and thermal dehydration, *J. Appl. Physiol.,* 37, 521, 1974.
28. **Grucza, R., Lecroart, J.-L., Carette, G., Hauser, J.-J., and Houdas, Y.,** Effect of voluntary dehydration on thermoregulatory responses to heat in men and women, *Eur. J. Appl. Physiol.,* 56, 317, 1987.
29. **Kolka, M. A. and Stephenson, L. A.,** Plasma volume loss during maximal exercise in females, *Physiologist,* 33, A73, 1990.
30. **Sawka, M. N., Toner, M. N., Francesconi, R. P., and Pandolf, K. B.,** Hypohydration and exercise: effects of heat acclimation, gender and environment, *J. Appl. Physiol. Respir. Environ. Exercise Physiol.,* 55, 1147, 1983.
31. **Jones, L. L., Green, H. J., Hughson, R. L., Painter, D. C., and Farrance, B. W.,** Maximal exercise response following hypervolemia induced by short term exercise (Abstract), *Med. Sci. Sports Exercise,* 16, 112, 1984.
32. **Fortney, S. M., Nadel, E. R., Wenger, C. B., and Bove, J. R.,** Effect of blood volume on sweating rate and body fluids in exercising humans, *J. Appl. Physiol. Respir. Environ. Exercise Physiol.,* 51, 1594, 1981.
33. **Moroff, S. V. and Bass, D. E.,** Effects of overhydration on man's physiological responses to work in the heat, *J. Appl. Physiol.,* 20, 267, 1965.
34. **Singh, M. V., Rawal, S. B., Pichan, G., Tyagi, A. K., and Gupta, A. K.,** Changes in plasma volume during hypohydration and rehydration in subjects from the tropics, *Eur. J. Appl. Physiol.,* 61, 258, 1990.
35. **Harrison, M. H.,** Heat and exercise: effects on blood volume, *Sports Med.,* 3, 214, 1986.
36. **Candas, V. and Bothorel, B.,** Exercise, performance and hydro-electrolyte balance, in *Muscle Fatigue: Biochemical and Physiological Aspects,* Atlan, G., Beliveau, L., and Bouissou, P., Eds., Masson, Paris, 1991, 184.
37. **Fortney, S. M., Vroman, N. B., Beckett, W. S., Permutt, S., and LaFrance, N. D.,** Effect of exercise hemoconcentration and hyperosmolality on exercise responses, *J. Appl. Physiol.,* 65, 519, 1988.
38. **Fortney, S. M., Wenger, C. B., Bove, J. R., and Nadel, E. R.,** Effect of hyperosmolality on control of blood flow and sweating, *J. Appl. Physiol. Respir. Environ. Exercise Physiol.,* 57, 1688, 1984.
39. **Hiller, W. D. B., O'Toole, M. L., Massimino, F., Hiller, R. E., and Laird, R. H.,** Plasma electrolyte and glucose changes during the Hawaiian ironman triathlon (Abstract), *Med. Sci. Sports Exercise,* 17, 218, 1985.
40. **Noakes, T. D., Goodwin, N., Rayner, B. L., Branken, R., and Taylor, R. K. N.,** Water intoxication: a possible complication during endurance exercise, *Med. Sci. Sports Exercise,* 17, 370, 1985.
41. **Noakes, T. D., Norman, R. J., Buck, R. H., Godlonton, J., Stevenson, K., and Pittaway, D.,** The incidence of hyponatremia during prolonged ultraendurance exercise, *Med. Sci. Sports Exercise,* 22, 165, 1990.
42. **Campbell, W. W. and Anderson, R. A.,** Effects of aerobic exercise and training on the trace minerals chromium, zinc and copper, *Sports Med.,* 4, 9, 1987.
43. **Consolazio, C. F., Matoush, L. O., Nelson, R. A., Harding, R. S., and Canham, J. E.,** Excretion of sodium, potassium, magnesium and iron in human sweat and the relation of each to balance and requirements, *J. Nutr.,* 79, 407, 1963.

44. **Deuster, P. A., Dolev, E., Kyle, S. B., Anderson, R. A., and Schoomaker, E. B.,** Magnesium homeostasis during high-intensity anaerobic exercise in men, *J. Appl. Physiol.,* 62, 545, 1987.

45. **Lindinger, M. I. and Sjøgaard, G.,** Potassium regulation during exercise and recovery, *Sports Med.,* 11, 382, 1991.

46. **Sjøgaard, G.,** Electrolytes in slow and fast muscle fibers of humans at rest and with dynamic exercise, *Am. J. Physiol.,* 245, R25, 1983.

47. **Coyle, E. F., Hagberg, J. M., Hurley, B. F., Martin, W. H., Ehsani, A. A., and Holloszy, J. O.,** Carbohydrate feeding during prolonged strenuous exercise can delay fatigue, *J. Appl. Physiol. Respir. Environ. Exercise Physiol.,* 55, 230, 1983.

48. **Kjaer, M., Kiens, B., Hargreaves, M., and Richter, E. A.,** Influence of active muscle mass on glucose homeostasis during exercise in humans, *J. Appl. Physiol.,* 71, 552, 1991.

49. **Callow, M., Morton, A., and Guppy M.,** Marathon fatigue: the role of plasma fatty acids, muscle glycogen and blood glucose, *Eur. J. Appl. Physiol.,* 55, 654, 1986.

50. **Katz, A., Sahlin, K., and Broberg, S.,** Regulation of glucose utilization in human skeletal muscle during moderate dynamic exercise, *Am. J. Physiol.,* 260, E411, 1991.

51. **Stein, T. R., Hoyt, R. W., O'Toole, M., Leskiw, M. J., Schluter, M. D., Wolfe, R. R., and Hiller, W. D. B.,** Protein and energy metabolism during prolonged exercise in trained athletes, *Int. J. Sports Med.,* 10, 311, 1989.

52. **Wahren, J., Felig, P., Ahlborg, G. et al.,** Glucose metabolism during exercise in man, *J. Clin. Invest.,* 50, 2715, 1971.

53. **Caspary, W. F.,** Physiology and pathophysiology of intestinal absorption, *Am. J. Clin. Nutr.,* 55, 299S, 1992.

54. **Burks, T. F., Galligan, J. J., Porreca, F., and Barber, W. D.,** Regulation of gastric emptying, *Fed. Proc.,* 44, 2897, 1985.

55. **Minami, H. and McCallum, R. W.,** The physiology and pathophysiology of gastric emptying in humans, *Gastroenterology,* 86, 1592, 1984.

56. **Murray, R.,** The effects of consuming carbohydrate-electrolyte beverages on gastric emptying and fluid absorption during and following exercise, *Sports Med.,* 4, 322, 1987.

57. **Costill, D. L. and Saltin, B.,** Factors limiting gastric emptying during rest and exercise, *J. Appl. Physiol.,* 37, 679, 1974.

58. **Armstrong, L. E., Hubbard, R. W., Szlyk, P. C., Matthew, W. T., and Sils, I. V.,** Voluntary dehydration and electrolyte losses during prolonged exercise in the heat, *Aviat. Space Environ. Med.,* 56, 765, 1985.

59. **Hubbard, R. W., Sandick, B. L., Matthew, W. T., Francesconi, R. P., Sampson, J. B., Durkot, M. J., Maller, O., and Engell, D. B.,** Voluntary dehydration and alliesthesia for water, *J. Appl. Physiol. Respir. Environ. Exercise Physiol.,* 57, 868, 1984.

60. **Neufer, P. D., Costill, D. L., Fink, W. J., Kirwan, J. P., Fielding, R. A., and Flynn, M. G.,** Effects of exercise and carbohydrate composition on gastric emptying, *Med. Sci. Sports Exercise,* 13, 658, 1986.

61. **Brener, W., Hendrix, T. R., and McHugh, P. R.,** Regulation of the gastric emptying of glucose, *Gastroenterology,* 85, 76, 1983.

62. **Rehrer, N. J., Wagenmakers, A. J. M., Beckers, E. J., Halliday, D., Leiper, J. B., Brouns, F., Maughan, R. J., Westerterp, K., and Saris, W. H. M.,** Gastric emptying, absorption, and carbohydrate oxidation during prolonged exercise, *J. Appl. Physiol.,* 72, 468, 1992.

63. **Shafer, R. B., Levine, A. S., Marlette, J. M., and Morley, J. E.,** Do calories, osmolality, or calcium determine gastric emptying?, *Am. J. Physiol.,* 17, R479, 1985.

64. **Hunt, J. N. and Stubbs, D. F.,** The volume and energy content of meals as determinants of gastric emptying, *J. Physiol. (London),* 215, 209, 1975.

65. **Foster, C., Costill, D. L., and Fink, W. J.,** Gastric emptying characteristics of glucose and glucose polymer solutions, *Res. Q. Exercise Sport,* 51, 299, 1980.

66. **Rehrer, N. J., Beckers, E. J., Brouns, F., Hoor, F. T., and Saris, W. H. M.,** Exercise and training effects on gastric emptying of carbohydrate beverages, *Med. Sci. Sports Exercise,* 21, 540, 1989.

67. **Fink, W. J., Costill, D. L., and Steven, C. F.,** Gastric-emptying characteristics of complete nutritional liquids, in *Nutrient Utilization During Exercise,* Fox, E. Ed., Ross Laboratories, Columbus, OH, 1983, 112.

68. **McHugh, P. R. and Moran, T. H.,** Calories and gastric emptying: a regulatory capacity with implications for feeding, *Am. J. Physiol.,* 236, R254, 1979.

69. **Ferrannini, E., Barrett, E., Bevilacqua, S., Dupre, J., and Defronzo, R. A.,** Sodium elevates the plasma glucose response to glucose ingestion in man, *J. Clin. Endocrinol. Metab.,* 54, 455, 1982.

70. **Gisolfi, C. V.,** Exercise, intestinal absorption, and rehydration, in *Sports Science Exchange,* Vol. 4, Sports Physiology/Biochemistry, Gatorade Sports Science Institute, Chicago, 1991, no. 32.

71. **Gisolfi, C. V., Spranger, K. J., Summers, R. W., Schedl, H. P., and Bleiler, T. L.,** Effects of cycle exercise on intestinal absorption in humans, *J. Appl. Physiol.,* 71, 2518, 1991.

72. **Fordtran, J. S. and Saltin, B.,** Gastric emptying and intestinal absorption during prolonged severe exercise, *J. Appl. Physiol.,* 23, 331, 1967.

73. **Neufer, P. D., Young, A. J., and Sawka, M. N.,** Gastric emptying during exercise: effects of heat stress and hypohydration, *Eur. J. Appl. Physiol.,* 58, 433, 1989.

74. **Neufer, P. D., Young, A. J., and Sawka, M. N.,** Gastric emptying during walking and running: effects of varied exercise intensity, *Eur. J. Appl. Physiol.,* 58, 440, 1989.

75. **Ryan, A. J., Bleiler, T. L., Carter, J. E., and Gisolfi, C. V.,** Gastric emptying during prolonged cycling exercise in the heat, *Med. Sci. Sports Exercise,* 21, 51, 1989.

76. **Costill, D. L., Bennett, A., Branam, G., and Eddy, D.,** Glucose ingestion at rest and during prolonged exercise, *J. Appl. Physiol.,* 34, 764, 1973.

77. **Rehrer, N. J., Beckers, E. J., Brouns, F., Hoor, F. T., and Saris, W. H. M.,** Effects of dehydration on gastric emptying and gastrointestinal distress while running, *Med. Sci. Sports Exercise,* 22, 790, 1990.

78. **Jandrain, B. J., Pirnay, F., Lacroix, M., Mosora, F., Scheen, A. J., and Lefebvre, P. J.,** Effect of osmolality on availability of glucose ingested during prolonged exercise in humans, *J. Appl. Physiol.,* 6, 76, 1989.

79. **Krzentowski, G., Jandrain, B., Pirnay, F., Mosora, F., Lacroix, M., Luyckx, A. S., and Lefebvre, P. J.,** Availability of glucose given orally during exercise, *J. Appl. Physiol. Respir. Environ. Exercise Physiol.,* 56, 315, 1984.

80. **Massicotte, D., Peronnet, F., Brisson, G., Bakkouch, K., and Hillaire-Marcel, C.,** Oxidation of a glucose polymer during exercise: comparison with glucose and fructose, *J. Appl. Physiol.,* 66, 179, 1989.

81. **Segal, K., Nyman, A., Kral, J. G., Bjorntorp, P., Kotler, D. P., and Pi-Sunyer, F. X.,** Effects of glucose ingestion on submaximal intermittent exercise (Abstract), *Med. Sci. Sports Exercise,* 17, 205, 1985.

82. **Snyder, A. C., Lamb, D. R., Baur, T., Connors, D., and Brodowicz, G.,** Maltodextrin feeding immediately before prolonged cycling at 62% VO$_2$ max increases time to exhaustion, *Med. Sci. Sports Exercise,* 15, 126, 1983.

83. **Fielding, R. A., Costill, D. L., Fink, W. J., King, D. S., Kovaleski, J. E., and Kirwan, J. P.,** Effects of pre-exercise carbohydrate feedings on muscle glycogen use during exercise in well-trained runners, *Eur. J. Appl. Physiol.,* 56, 225, 1987.

84. **Foster, C., Costill, D. L., and Fink, W. J.,** Effects of preexercise feedings on endurance performance, *Med. Sci. Sports,* 11, 1, 1979.

85. **Gleeson, M., Maughan, R. J., and Greenhaff, P. L.,** Comparison of the effects of pre-exercise feeding of glucose, glycerol and placebo on endurance and fuel homeostasis in man, *Eur. J. Appl. Physiol.,* 55, 645, 1986.

86. **Hargreaves, M., Costill, D. L., Fink, W. J., King, D. S., and Fielding, R. A.,** Effect of pre-exercise carbohydrate feedings on endurance cycling performance, *Med. Sci. Sports Exercise,* 19, 33, 1987.

87. **Hargreaves, M., Costill, D. L., Katz, A., and Fink, W. J.,** Effect of fructose ingestion on muscle glycogen usage during exercise, *Med. Sci. Sports Exercise,* 17, 360, 1985.

88. **Hughes, V. A., Edwards, J. E., Meredith, C. N., Evans, W. J., Martin, R., and Young, V. R.,** Muscle glycogen utilization during low intensity endurance exercise following glucose or fructose ingestion (Abstract), *Med. Sci. Sports Exercise,* 16, 190, 1984.

89. **Koivisto, V. A., Harkonen, M., Karonen, S.-L., Groop, P. H., Elovainio, R., Ferrannini, E., Sacca, and Defronzo, R. A.,** Glycogen depletion during prolonged exercise: influence of glucose, fructose, or placebo, *J. Appl. Physiol.,* 58, 731, 1985.

90. **Koivisto, V. A., Karonen, S.-L., and Nikkila, E. A.,** Carbohydrate ingestion before exercise: comparison of glucose, fructose, and sweet placebo, *J. Appl. Physiol. Respir. Environ. Exercise Physiol.,* 51, 783, 1981.

91. **Levine, L., Evans, W. J., Cadarette, B. S., Fisher, E. C., and Bullen, B. A.,** Fructose and glucose ingestion and muscle glycogen use during submaximal exercise, *J. Appl. Physiol. Respir. Environ. Exercise Physiol.,* 55, 1767, 1983.

92. **McMurray, R. G., Wilson, J. R., and Kitchell, B. S.,** The effects of fructose and glucose on high intensity endurance performance, *Res. Q. Exercise Sport,* 54, 156, 1983.

93. **Erickson, M. A., Schwarzkopf, R. J., and McKenzie, R. D.,** Effects of caffeine, fructose, and glucose ingestion on muscle glycogen utilization during exercise, *Med. Sci. Sports Exercise,* 19, 579, 1987.

94. **Graham, T. E. and Spriet, L. L.,** Performance and metabolic responses to a high caffeine dose during prolonged exercise, *J. Appl. Physiol.,* 71, 2292, 1991.

95. **Keller, K. and Schwarzkopf, R.,** Preexercise snacks may decrease exercise performance, *Physician Sportsmed.,* 12, 89, 1984.

96. **Okano, G., Takeda, H., Morita, I., Katoh, M., Mu, Z., and Miyake, S.,** Effect of pre-exercise fructose ingestion on endurance performance in fed men, *Med. Sci. Sports Exercise,* 20, 105, 1988.

97. **Sasaki, H., Maeda, J., Usui, S., and Ishiko, T.,** Effect of sucrose and caffeine ingestion on performance of prolonged strenuous running, *Int. J. Sports Med.,* 8, 261, 1987.

98. **Tarnopolsky, M. A., Atkinson, S. A., MacDougall, J. D., Sutton, J., and Sale, D. G.,** Caffeine as a potential ergogenic aid in endurance running, *Can. J. Sports Sci.,* 13, 89P, 1988.

99. **Jandrain, B., Krzentowski, G., Pirnay, F., Mosora, F., Lacroix, M., Luyckx, A., and Lefebvre, P.,** Metabolic availability of glucose ingested 3 h before prolonged exercise in humans, *J. Appl. Physiol. Respir. Environ. Exercise Physiol.,* 56, 1314, 1984.

100. **Wright, D. A., Sherman, W. M., and Dernbach, A. R.,** Carbohydrate feedings before, during, or in combination improve cycling performance, *J. Appl. Physiol.,* 71, 1082, 1991.

101. **Sherman, W. M., Brodowicz, G., Wright, D. A., Simonsen, J., and Dernbach, A.,** Effects of 4 h preexercise carbohydrate feedings on cycling performance, *Med. Sci. Sports Exercise,* 21, 598, 1989.

102. **Thomas, D. E., Brotherhood, J. R., and Brand, J. C.,** Carbohydrate feeding before exercise: effect of glycemic index, *Int. J. Sports Med.,* 12, 180, 1991.

103. **Bohannon, N. V., Karam, J. H., and Forsham, P. H.,** Endocrine responses to sugar ingestion in man, *J. Am. Diet. Assoc.,* 76, 555, 1980.

104. **Geske, B. B. and Sharp, R. L.,** Pre-exercise ingestion of glucose and fructose: effects on exercise performance when exercise is begun at predetermined time of peak blood concentration of the sugar (Abstract), *Med. Sci. Sports Exercise,* 16, 190, 1984.

105. **Calles-Escandon, J., Devlin, J. T., Whitcomb, W., and Horton, E. S.,** Pre-exercise feeding does not affect endurance cycle exercise but attenuates post-exercise starvation-like response, *Med. Sci. Sports Exercise,* 23, 818, 1991.

106. **Coyle, E. F., Coggan, A. R., Hemmert, M. K., Lowe, R. C., and Walters, T. J.,** Substrate usage during prolonged exercise following a preexercise meal, *J. Appl. Physiol.,* 59, 429, 1985.

107. **Devlin, J. T., Calles-Escandon, J., and Horton, E. S.,** Effects of preexercise snack feeding on endurance cycle exercise, *J. Appl. Physiol.,* 60, 980, 1986.

108. **Costill, D. L., Verstappen, F., Kuipers, H., Janssen, E., and Fink, W.,** Acid-base balance during repeated bouts of exercice: influence of HOC_3, *Int. J. Sports Med.,* 5, 228, 1984.

109. **Wilkes, D., Gledhill, N., and Smyth, R.,** Effect of acute induced metabolic alkalosis on 800-m racing time, *Med. Sci. Sports Exercise,* 15, 277, 1983.

110. **McNaughton, L. R.,** Sodium citrate and anaerobic performance: implications of dosage, *Eur. J. Appl. Physiol.,* 61, 392, 1990.

111. **Coggan, A. R. and Coyle, E. F.,** Metabolism and performance following carbohydrate ingestion late in exercise, *Med. Sci. Sports Exercise,* 21, 59, 1989.

112. **Coyle, E. F., Coggan, A. R., Hemmert, M. K., and Ivy, J. L.,** Muscle glycogen utilization during prolonged strenuous exercise when fed carbohydrate, *J. Appl. Physiol.,* 61, 165, 1986.

113. **Davis, J. M., Lamb, D. R., Pate, R. R., Slentz, C. A., Burgess, W. A., and Bartoli, W. P.,** Carbohydrate-electrolyte drinks: effects on endurance cycling in the heat, *Am. J. Clin. Nutr.,* 48, 1023, 1988.

114. **Edwards, T. L., Jr. and Santeusanio, D. M.,** Field test of the effects of carbohydrate solutions on endurance performance, selected blood serum chemistries, perceived exertion, and fatigue in world class cyclists (Abstract), *Med. Sci. Sports Exercise,* 16, 190, 1984.

115. **Fielding, R. A., Costill, D. L., Fink, W. J., King, D. S., Hargreaves, M., and Kovaleski, J. E.,** Effect of carbohydrate feeding frequencies and dosage on muscle glycogen use during exercise, *Med. Sci. Sports Exercise,* 17, 472, 1985.

116. **Ivy, J. L., Miller, W., Dover, V., Goodyear, L. G., Sherman, W. M., Farrell, S., and Williams, H.,** Endurance improved by ingestion of a glucose polymer supplement, *Med. Sci. Sports Exercise,* 15, 466, 1983.

117. **Millard-Stafford, M., Sparling, P. B., Rosskopf, L. B., Hinson, B. T., and Dicarlo, L. J.,** Carbohydrate-electrolyte replacement during a simulated triathlon in the heat, *Med. Sci. Sports Exercise,* 22, 621, 1990.

118. **Murray, R., Paul, G. L., Seifert, J. G., and Eddy, D. E.,** Responses to varying rates of carbohydrate ingestion during exercise, *Med. Sci. Sports Exercise,* 23, 713, 1991.

119. **Wilber, R. L. and Moffatt, R. J.,** Influence of glucose polymer ingestion on plasma glucose concentration and performance in male distance runners (Abstract), *Int. J. Sports Med.,* 12, 251, 1991.

120. **Brodowicz, G. R., Lamb, D. R., Baur, T. S., and Connors, D. F.,** Efficacy of various drink formulations for fluid replenishment during cycling exercise in the heat (Abstract), *Med. Sci. Sports Exercise,* 16, 138, 1984.

121. **Flynn, M. G., Costill, D. L., Hawley, J. A., Fink, W. J., Neufer, P. D., Fielding, R. A., and Sleeper, M. D.,** Influence of selected carbohydrate drinks on cycling performance and glycogen use, *Med. Sci. Sports Exercise,* 19, 37, 1987.

122. **Powers, S. K., Lawler, J., Dodd, S., Tulley, R., Landry, G., and Wheeler, K.,** Fluid replacement drinks during high intensity exercise: effects on minimizing exercise-induced disturbances in homeostasis, *Eur. J. Appl. Physiol.,* 60, 54, 1990.

123. **Williams, C., Nute, M. G., Broadbank, L., and Vinall, S.,** Influence of fluid intake on endurance running performance: a comparison between water, glucose, and fructose solutions, *Eur. J. Appl. Physiol.,* 60, 112, 1990.

124. **Carter, J. E. and Gisolfi, C. V.,** Fluid replacement during and after exercise in the heat, *Med. Sci. Sports Exercise,* 21, 523, 1989.

125. **Hargreaves, M., Costill, D. L., Coggan, A., Fink, W. J., and Nishibata, I.,** Effect of carbohydrate feedings on muscle glycogen utilization and exercise performance, *Med. Sci. Sports Exercise,* 16, 219, 1984.

126. **Kingwell, B., McKenna, M. J., Sandstrom, E. R., and Hargreaves, M.,** Effect of glucose polymer ingestion on energy and fluid balance during exercise, *J. Sports Sci.,* 7, 3, 1989.

127. **Langenfeld, M. E.,** Glucose polymer ingestion during ultraendurance bicycling, *Res. Q. Exercise Sport,* 54, 411, 1983.

128. **Owen, M. D., Kregel, K. C., Wall, P. T., and Gisolfi, C. V.,** Effects of ingesting carbohydrate beverages during exercise in the heat, *Med. Sci. Sports Exercise,* 18, 568, 1986.

129. **Seidman, D. S., Ashkenazi, I., Arnon, R., Shapiro, Y., and Epstein, Y.,** The effects of glucose polymer beverage ingestion during prolonged outdoor exercise in the heat, *Med. Sci. Sports Exercise,* 23, 458, 1991.

130. **Yaspelkis, B. B., III and Ivy, J. L.,** Effect of carbohydrate supplements and water on exercise metabolism in the heat, *J. Appl. Physiol.,* 71, 680, 1991.

131. **Hargreaves, M. and Briggs, C. A.,** Effect of carbohydrate ingestion on exercise metabolism, *J. Appl. Physiol.,* 65, 1553, 1988.

132. **Bosch, A. N., Noakes, T. D., and Dennis, S.,** Carbohydrate ingestion during prolonged exercise: a liver glycogen sparing effect in glycogen loaded subjects (Abstract), *Med. Sci. Sports Exercise,* 23, S152, 1991.

133. **Barr, S. I., Costill, D. L., and Fink, W. J.,** Fluid replacement during prolonged exercise: effects of water, saline, or no fluid, *Med. Sci. Sports Exercise,* 23, 811, 1991.

134. **Johnson, H. L., Nelson, R. A., and Consolazio, C. F.,** Effects of electrolyte and nutrient solutions on performance and metabolic balance, *Med. Sci. Sports Exercise,* 20, 26, 1988.

135. **Decombaz, J., Gmunder, G., Daget, N., Munoz-Box, R., and Howald, H.,** Acceptance of isotonic and hypotonic rehydrating beverages by athletes during training, *Int. J. Sports Med.,* 13, 40, 1992.

136. **Bothorel, B., Follenius, M., Gissinger, R., and Candas, V.,** Physiological effects of dehydration and rehydration with water and acidic or neutral carbohydrate electrolyte solutions, *Eur. J. Appl. Physiol.,* 60, 209, 1990.

137. **Francis, K. T.,** Effect of water and electrolyte replacement during exercise in the heat on biochemical indices of stress and performance, *Aviat. Space Environ. Med.,* 50, 115, 1979.

138. **Hamilton, M. T., Gonzalez-Alonso, J., Montain, S. J., and Coyle, E. F.,** Fluid replacement and glucose infusion during exercise prevent cardiovascular drift, *J. Appl. Physiol.,* 71, 871, 1991.

139. **Maughan, R. J., Fenn, C. E., Gleeson, M., and Leiper, J. B.,** Metabolic and circulatory responses to the ingestion of glucose polymer and glucose/electrolyte solutions during exercise in man, *Eur. J. Appl. Physiol.,* 56, 356, 1987.

140. **Owen, M. D., Kregel, K. C., Wall, P. T., and Gisolfi, C. V.,** Effects of carbohydrate ingestion on thermoregulation, gastric emptying and plasma volume during exercise in the heat (Abstract), *Med. Sci. Sports Exercise,* 17, 185, 1985.

141. **Wells, C. L., Schrader, T. A., Stern, J. R., and Krahenbuhl, G. S.,** Physiological responses to a 20-mile run under three fluid replacement treatments, *Med. Sci. Sports Exercise,* 17, 364, 1985.

142. **Criswell, D., Powers, S., Lawler, J., Tew, J., Dodd, S., Iryiboz, Y., Tulley, R., and Wheeler, K.,** Influence of a carbohydrate-electrolyte beverage on blood homeostasis during football (Abstract), *Physiologist,* 33, A73, 1990.

143. **Ivy, J. L., Costill, D. L., Fink, W. J., and Lower, R. W.,** Influence of caffeine and carbohydrate feedings on endurance performance, *Med. Sci. Sports Exercise,* 11, 6, 1979.

144. **Murray, R., Eddy, D. E., Murray, T. W., Seifert, J. G., Paul, G. L., and Halaby, G. A.,** The effect of fluid and carbohydrate feedings during intermittent cycling exercise, *Med. Sci. Sports Exercise,* 19, 597, 1987.

145. **Deuster, P. A., Singh, A., Hofmann, A., Moses, F. M., and Chrousos, C.,** Hormonal responses to ingesting water or a carbohydrate beverage during a 2 h run, *Med. Sci. Sports Exercise,* 24, 72, 1992.

146. **Murray, R., Eddy, D. E., Paul, G. L., Seifert, J. G., and Halaby, G. A.,** Physiological responses to glycerol ingestion during exercise, *J. Appl. Physiol.,* 71, 144, 1991.

147. **Murray, R., Paul, G. L., Seifert, J. G., Eddy, D. E., and Halaby, G. A.,** The effect of glucose, fructose, and sucrose ingestion during exercise, *Med. Sci. Sports Exercise,* 21, 275, 1989.

148. **Brandenberger, G., Candas, V., Follenius, M., Libert, J. P., and Kahn, J. M.,** Vascular fluid shifts and endocrine responses to exercise in the heat: effect of rehydration, *Eur. J. Appl. Physiol.,* 55, 123, 1986.

149. **Candas, V., Libert, J. P., Brandenberger, G., Sagot, J. C., Amoros, C., and Kahn, J. M.,** Hydration during exercise: effects on thermal and cardiovascular adjustments, *Eur. J. Appl. Physiol.,* 55, 113, 1986.

150. **Giles, D. and Maclaren, D.,** Effects of caffeine and glucose ingestion on metabolic and respiratory functions during prolonged exercise, *J. Sports Sci.,* 2, 35, 1984.

151. **Blom, P. C. S., Høstmark, A. T., Vaage, O., Kardel, K. R., and Maehlum, S.,** Effect of different post-exercise sugar diets on the rate of muscle glycogen synthesis, *Med. Sci. Sports Exercise,.* 19, 491, 1987.

152. **Costill, D. L., Coté, R., Miller, E., Miller, T., and Wynder, S.,** Water and electrolyte replacement during repeated days of work in the heat, *Aviat. Space Environ. Med.,* 46, 795, 1975.

153. **Costill, D. L., Sherman, W. M., Fink, W. J., Maresh, C., Witten, M., and Miller, J. M.,** The role of dietary carbohydrates in muscle glycogen resynthesis after strenuous running, *Am. J. Clin. Nutr.,* 34, 1831, 1981.

154. **Neufer, P. D., Sawka, M. N., Young, A. J., Quigley, M. D., Latzka, W. A., and Levine, L.,** Hypohydration does not impair skeletal muscle glycogen resynthesis after exercise, *J. Appl. Physiol.,* 70, 1490, 1991.

155. **Nielsen, B., Sjøgaard, G., Ugelvig, J., Knudsen, B., and Dohlmann, B.,** Fluid balance in exercise dehydration and rehydration with different glucose-electrolyte drinks, *Eur. J. Appl. Physiol.,* 55, 318, 1986.

156. **Nose, H., Mack, G. W., Shi, X., and Nadel, E. R.,** Role of osmolality and plasma volume during rehydration in humans, *J. Appl. Physiol.,* 65, 325, 1988.

157. **Reed, M. J., Brozinick, J. T., Jr., Lee, M. C., and Ivy, J. L.,** Muscle glycogen storage postexercise: effect of mode of carbohydrate administration, *J. Appl. Physiol.,* 66, 720, 1989.

Chapter 14

NUTRITIONAL ERGOGENIC AIDS

_____ Luke R. Bucci

CONTENTS

0-8493-7911-3/94/$0.00+$.50
© 1994 by CRC Press, Inc.

I. INTRODUCTION

Since the ancient Greeks advocated a diet rich in animal flesh instead of the usual lacto-ovo vegetarian diet for elite athletes in the 6th century B.C.,[1-3] humans have endeavored to improve exercise and sports performance by dietary alterations. Knowledge of human physiology and nutrition has increased greatly this century, and so has application of dietary alterations and supplementation with specific nutrients. Modulation of dietary composition and/or supplementation with specific nutrients with the intent of improving human physical performance is a working definition of nutritional ergogenic aids.

This chapter will consider nutrients currently hypothesized or applied as ergogenic aids, and examine experimental evidence for the central questions: What are the effects of nutrient X on human performance? Are other physiological changes of interest to exercise performance observed?

The tone of this chapter is an overview, with a plethora of data distilled into conclusions of effectiveness (or lack thereof) for performance enhancement, rather than lengthy discussions of mechanisms of action. Where possible, guidelines for practical usage, including applicable conditions and dosages, will be presented. For further information on nutritional ergogenic aids, the reader is referred to several excellent reviews.[4-15]

Nutritional ergogenic aids can be classified as macronutrients (water, electrolytes, carbohydrates, proteins, and fats) and micronutrients. Macronutrients are normally consumed in gram quantities per day, while micronutrients are consumed in milligram or microgram quantities per day. Micronutrients can be further subdivided into two categories: indispensable (essential vitamins and minerals), and dispensable (nonessential dietary components or metabolic intermediates like caffeine or carnitine).

II. ALTERATION OF DIETARY MACRONUTRIENTS

A. Water and Electrolytes

Body fluids are composed primarily of water and salt (sodium chloride),[16] and will be considered simultaneously. Minor amounts of potassium, calcium, magnesium, and phos-

TABLE 1 Conditions for Ergogenic Properties of Water and Electrolytes

Condition	Parameters
Prior dehydration	
High ambient temperature	>30°C (>80°F)
High body temperature	>39°C (>104°F)
High relative humidity	>80%
High solar radiation	Sunshine, reflective surfaces (sand, snow, water, concrete)
Lack of air movement	No wind or light rear wind
High rate of sweating	>2 l/h
Lack of heat acclimatization	
Untrained subjects	
Exercise intensity	>75% $\dot{V}O_2$ max
Exercise duration	>1 h
Exercise intensity-duration product	
High body fat percentage	>25% body fat by weight
Heat-trapping or excessive clothing	
Underwater exercise	Scuba-diving, snorkeling, swimming, water polo
Altitude	>1500 km (>1 mile)
Voluntary fluid restriction	Making weight practices for wrestlers, boxers, bodybuilders, weightlifers
Diuretic drugs	Caffeine overdoses, thiazides, furosemide, bumetanide, spironolactone, etc.
Certain diseases	Diabetes, renal diseases

phates are also present in body fluids and considered to be electrolytes. Water and electrolytes in body fluids are important to exercise performance by: (1) maintaining blood volume and osmolality in order to transport and transfer oxygen, fuels, cellular waste products, and regulatory molecules; (2) thermoregulation to prevent dangerous overheating; (3) shock-absorbing and lubricating properties; and (4) homeostasis of enzymic and neuromuscular functions.[16-25]

Loss of body fluids containing water and electrolytes during exercise is mostly by sweating. Table 1 lists the major causes of dehydration. Increasing loss of body fluids is associated with progressive decreases in ability to control body temperature, muscular endurance, muscular strength, and physical performance.[16-25] Losses of body fluids equivalent to 5% of body weight are associated with overt symptoms of muscle cramps and obvious decreases in physical performance. Further losses of water and electrolytes (>6% of body weight lost) may lead to heat exhaustion, heat stroke (mental confusion, headache, disorientation), coma, and death. Since several deaths per year among exercising individuals, including healthy athletes, are attributed to dehydration and/or heat stroke, attention to proper hydration is vital to life.

When compared to limited or no fluid intake during exercise, ingestion of water and/or electrolytes often improves performance.[16-25] Thus, it appears that water administration during exercise can maintain optimal performance or prevent fatigue until other factors initiate fatigue. Can supranormal amounts of water (hyperhydration, superhydration, or overhydration) offer further increases in performance? Several studies compared normal hydration states to forced hyperhydration (ingesting 1.5 to 2 l of water before exercise, infusing saline solutions, and/or antidiuretic hormone administration). Hyperhydration did not change performance or physiological parameters for 30 min of cycling at 55% $\dot{V}O_2$ max at 35°C.[26] However, other studies that utilized higher temperatures, longer durations or higher intensities of exercise in the heat (48.8°C, 120°F) found significant improvements in performance,[27]

**TABLE 2 Guidelines for Prevention of Thermal Injury During
Endurance Exercise in the Heat (>80°F, >30°C)**

1. Drink 500 ml (1 pint) of cold water (or dilute electrolyte drink) 20–30 min
    before exercise.
2. During exercise, every 15–20 min (or 2–3 km) drink 100–200 ml (6–7 fl oz) of
    cold water (or dilute electrolyte drink).
3. A total of 1.4–4.2 l of water should be consumed every hour (amounts >2
    l/h are difficult to consume in practice).

Notes: 1. Thirst is not an adequate indicator of dehydration. Liquids must be
consumed *before* thirst is noticed.
2. Choose water or dilute electrolyte solutions that are good-tasting in
order to encourage liquid consumption.

From The American College of Sports Medicine, *Med. Sci. Sports Exercise*, 16, IX,
1984. With permission.

decreased heart rate,[26,28-32] and decreased body temperature.[26,28-32] These changes should prevent or delay adverse effects of dehydration.

Other results demonstrated that hyperhydration is not universally applicable. Consumption of 1 to 1.5 l of water immediately before a 200-yard swimming medley actually slowed race times significantly.[33] Several individuals consuming large amounts of water (without electrolytes) during an ultramarathon experienced hyponatremia (loss of sodium), with a serious detriment to both performance and health.[34] Short-term (20 min), intense (84% $\dot{V}O_2$ max) exercise performance was not influenced by saline infusion.[35]

The American College of Sports Medicine has published a position statement for prevention of thermal injury (heat stroke) during distance running (or other sports activities such as football practice) in the heat.[36] Guidelines are listed in Table 2.

Electrolyte depletion is only a problem when high rates of sweating occur, usually over several days of vigorous exercise in the heat, after several events in one day (tennis tournaments), or after daily training.[16,17,22] Exercise under other conditions may actually lead to higher electrolyte concentrations in the blood, since sweat is hypotonic. Thus, the total amount of sweat in a given time period is a key parameter to measure. Losses of 5 to 6 lbs (>2 kg) of body weight may indicate electrolyte depletion and a need for increased dietary intake of sodium, potassium, and chloride.[22,29] Individuals may vary widely in their sweating rates (over fourfold),[37,38] and close attention must be given to those who seem to sweat more than others.

At one time, salt tablets were freely administered and consumed by subjects exercising and sweating in the heat. However, a consensus of limited research has agreed that adding small amounts of salt to meals from a salt shaker on the table or during cooking is sufficient to prevent losses of sodium chloride detrimental to performance during exercise or training.[22] Alternatively, conservative use of salt tablets (three to six 500-mg tablets daily with meals) will accomplish the same intake levels of salt for individuals who consume low amounts of dietary salt. Excessive use of salt tablets or salt (>10 g/d) is to be discouraged in average settings, since excess sodium may induce potassium excretion and loss.[22,39-41]

Potassium supplements have helped to prevent muscle cramping and heat stroke in susceptible individuals.[42-45] Daily doses of supplemental potassium ranged from 0.75 to 3 g/d. Again, similar to sodium, high intakes of potassium (>10 g/d) are known to be hazardous to health. Fresh fruits and vegetables are rich in potassium, and their consumption is to be encouraged before resorting to potassium supplements. Daily dietary intake of ≥3 g of potassium appears to be adequate to replace potassium losses from exercise in the heat.[44,45] Table 3 lists conditions for which potassium may be an ergogenic aid.

TABLE 3 Conditions for Potassium as an Ergogenic Aid

1. Low dietary potassium intake (few fruits or vegetables)
2. Individuals susceptible to muscle cramps or heat exhaustion
3. Excessive (>10 g/d) salt intake
4. Excessive sweating (>2 kg of body loss per day)

In summary, water is an important and essential ergogenic aid for the conditions listed in Table 1. Hyperhydration is recommended for exercise of long duration in the heat. Electrolyte replenishment (sodium, potassium, and chloride) is important for large, repetitive losses of sweat, especially when subjects are not acclimatized. Other conditions may not exhibit improved performance after consumption of water and/or electrolytes, but at least a decrease in performance is unlikely.

B. Carbohydrates

Availability of carbohydrate to muscles is a limiting factor in exercise performance.[46-53] Since carbohydrates supply about 50% of energy sources during submaximal exercise (<70% $\dot{V}O_2$ max) and the majority of energy at intensities >70% $\dot{V}O_2$ max,[49] fatigue is closely related to carbohydrate availability. Depletion of carbohydrate sources (tissue glycogen and blood glucose) has been repeatedly documented to cause fatigue and reduce exercise performance.[13,46,50,51,54] Furthermore, carbohydrate storage is directly dependent on recent dietary history, since relatively little (approximately 2000 kcal) is stored in the body.

Glucose is the carbohydrate currency of human metabolism, and can be stored in branched-chain polymers called glycogen, primarily in muscle and liver. Blood glucose levels are carefully regulated by an elegant hormonal system including insulin, glucagon, catecholamines, glucocorticoids, somatotropin, and eicosanoids. Muscle glycogen stores are utilized preferentially during exercise.[46-48,50-52] If exercise is of sufficient duration and/or intensity (usually >2 h), muscle glycogen becomes depleted, and muscles become reliant upon blood glucose for carbohydrate supply.[46-48,50,51] Liver glycogen, gluconeogenesis (formation of glucose by breakdown of amino acids) and exogenous dietary sources of carbohydrate then maintain blood glucose levels as long as possible.[46-48,50,51] When blood glucose levels decrease below normal physiological levels (70 mg/dl or 5.0 mmol/l), performance deteriorates rapidly. Thus, maintenance of glucose supply to working muscles should prolong performance and delay fatigue, resulting in ergogenic effects when compared to lack of maintenance for glucose levels.

Studies on the role of carbohydrates as ergogenic aids are numerous, and detailed descriptions would demand more space than is necessary for an overview. At this time, there is no doubt that exogenous carbohydrate ingestion and/or supplementation benefits exercise performance under the proper conditions.[46-48,50-53] Thus, a focus on what exercise conditions have shown benefit from carbohydrate supplementation, and how to apply the findings, will be presented.

1. Glycogen Supercompensation (Carbohydrate Loading)

Two basic types of carbohydrate manipulation are used to enhance exercise performance: (1) increasing glycogen stores, and (2) consuming carbohydrate during exercise. The practice of glycogen supercompensation, popularly known as carbohydrate loading, can produce supranormal levels of muscle glycogen, which can lead to improved performance, compared to a typical diet.[13,24,46-48,51-53,55] Glycogen supercompensation is designed for optimal performance during a single endurance event, such as a triathlon, marathon, ultramarathon, long cycling road races, or competitive sports events. Any event lasting over 90 min and

TABLE 4 Exercise Activities With Ergogenic Benefits from Glycogen Supercompensation (Carbohydrate Loading)

More Benefits	Less Benefits
Soccer	Runs <10 km
Marathon	Sprinting
Triathlon	Weightlifting
Ultramarathon	Hockey games
Ultra-endurance events	Football games
Cross-country skiing	Baseball games
Cycling time trials	Basketball games
Long-distance swimming	Most rowing events
Long-distance canoe or kayak	Most track and field events
Rock climbing	Walking and hiking
Mountain climbing	Downhill ski runs

leading to exhaustion signals a need for glycogen supercompensation.[46-48,51] However, glycogen supercompensation should not be performed more than two or three times per month.

The preferred method of glycogen supercompensation starts 7 d before an event. During the next week, one should consume a large amount (70% of total calories) of foods rich in complex carbohydrates (starches). Up to 600 g of carbohydrates daily is considered to be a high-carbohydrate diet. In practical terms, 600 g of carbohydrates is equivalent to 2 loaves of bread, 3 cups of sugar, 15 medium baked potatoes, or 12 cups of rice. Every second day, exercise amount is cut in half, until no exercise is performed the day before the event. Carbohydrate consumption is continued throughout the pre-event period, culminating in a preexercise meal. A high-carbohydrate (>300 g), preexercise meal should be consumed 3 to 4 h before the event. Preexercise carbohydrates should be low-fiber, low-fat, complex carbohydrates (starches) instead of sugars, to avoid an insulin response with resulting hypoglycemia during exercise.

Glycogen supercompensation (carbohydrate loading) is recommended for the conditions listed in Table 4. In general, long-term endurance events lasting more than 90 min, or repetitive events occurring in a single or multiple days (such as cycling road races) are primary conditions for maintaining a high-carbohydrate diet.

2. Carbohydrate Supplementation During Exercise

Similar to the prodigious amount of information on glycogen supercompensation, a voluminous body of literature (over 100 original articles) exploring the effects of exogenous carbohydrate supplementation ingested *during* exercise is available.[4,13,24,25,46,50,51,55-58] A consensus of research has shown that carbohydrate ingestion during exercise can improve long-term endurance performance (lasting 90 min or more) and delay fatigue 30 to 60 min. Many reports have isolated one or more of the conditions listed in Table 5, leading to exercise conditions which may be benefitted by carbohydrate supplementation during exercise. Endurance events lasting longer than 90 min (listed in Table 4) showed the most benefits from carbohydrate supplementation during exercise.

During the 1980s, as research showed that water, electrolytes, and carbohydrates could be combined into an "electrolyte/energy replacement drink", commercial interest resulted in a sport-drink market that reached $700 million in annual sales in the U.S. in 1991.[59] Many commercial products have been examined in peer-reviewed literature publications, and shown to possess ergogenic benefits, lending credibility to practical usage. Since drinks containing carbohydrates were found to extend performance better than water (flavored or

**TABLE 5   Variables Affecting Ergogenic Effects of
Carbohydrate Supplementation During Exercise**

Muscle and liver glycogen levels (prior diet)
Gastric emptying rate of ingested food/fluid
Rate of glucose oxidation in muscle
Identity of supplemental carbohydrate
Concentration of supplemental carbohydrate
Volume (amount of supplemental carbohydrate)
Exercise intensity
Exercise duration
Exercise intensity-duration product
Feeding schedule
Electrolyte content
Individual variations in $\dot{V}O_2$ max, sweating rate, stomach disten-
   tion, and other physiological considerations

unflavored) in studies of endurance exercise, the use of electrolyte/carbohydrate drinks is perceived as more ergogenic than plain water. Also, most sports drinks taste better than plain water, encouraging adequate water intake.

The most recent guidelines on carbohydrate supplementation during exercise gave the following recommendations:

1. Immediately before exercise, consume 200 to 400 ml of a moderately concentrated (5 to 7%) carbohydrate drink, preferably as glucose polymers.
2. Continue consuming 100 to 150 ml of the same drink at 10- to 15-min intervals for the first 2 h of exercise.
3. After 2 h, switch to a more concentrated drink (15 to 20% carbohydrate). Consume 100 to 150 ml every 15 min. For exhaustive events lasting less than 2 h, consume the more concentrated drink during the last quarter of exercise. At least 200 to 300 ml total of the more concentrated drink should be consumed. Mild gastric discomfort is acceptable; however, nausea indicates an excess has been consumed.

Table 6 lists some commercially available carbohydrate/electrolyte drinks listed in order of their carbohydrate concentration (%). It is highly recommended that each individual choose a drink that tastes palatable, a matter of individual preference. At this time, it is not certain if additional ingredients (vitamins, minerals, lactic acid buffers) offer further benefits.

One alternative to purchasing sports drinks is to dilute any fruit juice 1:1 with water, and add a teaspoon of salt per liter (quart). This should approximate carbohydrate, electrolyte, and osmolality values of commercial sports drinks.

3. Carbohydrates and Recovery From Exercise

For those engaging in highly strenuous activities on successive days (such as cycling road races), rapid replenishment of carbohydrate stores is advisable, since insufficient time for carbohydrate loading is available. Again, a burst of recent research has suggested the following guidelines to maximize glycogen stores to support exhausting, repetitive tasks.[46,60]

1. Initiate carbohydrate feeding immediately (within 2 h) after exhausting exercise.
2. Consume simple sugars (0.7 g glucose or sucrose/kg body weight or 50 g carbohydrate) rather than complex carbohydrates every 2 h for the first 4 to 6 h after exercise.
3. After 6 h, complex carbohydrates may be consumed. In the 20 to 24 h after exercise, a total of 500 to 700 g of carbohydrates should be consumed, preferably from low-fat, low-fiber foods (much like a preexercise meal).

TABLE 6 Commercial Carbohydrate/Electrolyte Drinks and Carbohydrate Concentration

Drink (8 fl oz or 237 ml)	CHO Conc. (%)[a]	Carbohydrate Type
Gatorade Light	3	Glucose
Workout Light	3	Maltodextrin, glucose polymer
Rehydrate	5	Fructose
Body Cooler	6	Fructose, maltodextrin
Gatorade	6	Glucose, sucrose
Glucolyte	6	Fructose, maltodextrin
Power-Ade	6	Fructose, sucrose
Power Burst	6	Fructose
Body Fuel 750	7	Fructose, maltodextrin
Exceed Fluid Replacement	7	Fructose, glucose polymer
Hydra-Fuel	7	Glucose, fructose, maltodextrin
Hypo-Cell FX	7	Glucose polymer
Cyto Max	8	Fructose, maltodextrin[b]
Workout	8	Fructose, maltodextrin, glucose polymer
Max	10	Fructose, maltodextrin
Mountain Dew Sport	10	Fructose, sucrose
Performance	11	Fructose, maltodextrin
10-K	15	Sucrose, fructose

[a] CHO Conc. = carbohydrate concentration.
[b] Also contains polylactate.

Rapid replenishment with carbohydrates after exercise hastens recuperation, allowing a quicker return to training and maintenance of performance during strenuous daily events.

C. Protein and Amino Acids

Until this century, protein was thought to be the most important nutrient for exercise performance.[1] However, the myriad of studies comparing endurance performance of low- and high-carbohydrate diets clearly showed that diets high in protein do not improve long-term endurance performance (see previous section on carbohydrates). Although protein catabolism and resulting gluconeogenesis by the liver can account for 5 to 10% of energy production during long-term endurance exercise,[61-64] this amount is apparently insufficient to delay fatigue or improve performance after high-protein diets. Instead of providing energy during exercise, the potential ergogenic effects of protein (and their constituents — amino acids) are related to muscle mass formation.

While most published exercise physiology research has concentrated on endurance exercise such as running or cycling, much public interest has focused on building larger muscles and strength (football, bodybuilding, weightlifting, wrestling, sprinting, and cross-training). Muscular hypertrophy has not enjoyed the same research attention that endurance performance has enjoyed. This makes the large number of persons trying to increase muscle mass more open to speculation about the role of nutrients in muscle hypertrophy.

Because of the obvious association between protein and muscle, and many anecdotal claims from obviously well-muscled individuals about the virtues of high-protein diets,[1] and near-epidemic use of anabolic steroids (with emphasis on dietary protein to better utilize drug effects), protein and their components, amino acids, have great market appeal. Modern food technology has provided affordable and ample amounts of protein derivatives, including singular amino acids, providing the opportunity to utilize protein in a pharmacological manner.

TABLE 7 Sophisticated Selection of Protein Supplements Available to Athletes

Protein-rich dietary foodstuffs
    Meat (beef, pork, sheep, poultry, fish, seafood, wild game, muscle flesh, organ meats)
    Eggs
    Milk and dairy products (cheese, yogurt)
    Soybeans and derivatives (tofu)
    Legumes (lentils, beans, peas)
    Algae (*Spirulina, Chlorella*)
Purified protein powders
    Whole milk protein
    Caseinates
    Whey (lactalbumin)
    Soy
    Rice
    Bovine muscle
Protein hydrolysates (same sources as protein powders)
Amino acid mixtures
Purified protein powders fortified with individual amino acids
Protein hydrolysate/amino acid mixtures

1. Dietary Protein and Muscle Mass

The U.S. Recommended Dietary Allowance (RDA) has set an adequate protein intake at 0.8 g/kg/d.[1,64] Protein status can be assessed by measurement of nitrogen intake and excretion (nitrogen balance), as well as muscle mass (approximated by fat-free body mass and strength). Of great interest is the question: Can additional dietary protein enhance exercise-induced muscular hypertrophy?

Early studies by Kraut and co-workers on four total subjects suggested that high protein intakes (2.0 g/kg/d) aided strength and muscle mass increases induced by heavy training.[65,66] Other studies did not find an effect of protein supplements (25 g/d or 0.69 g/kg/d) on strength or power.[67,68] Subsequent studies found that increased dietary protein intakes ($\geq$300% RDA), compared to lower intakes (100 to 275% RDA), improved nitrogen retention, lean body mass, strength, thigh muscle sizes, and urine creatine excretion (a crude measure of muscle mass).[69-74] Taken together, these studies suggest that high protein intakes (>168 g/d or >2.4 g/kg/d or >300% RDA) may facilitate muscular hypertrophy during initiation of strength-promoting exercise.

Another potential need for manipulation of protein intake is to prevent muscle mass loss during periods of strenuous endurance training. Several studies have found that protein needs are elevated 50 to 100% during the first month of initiated or increased workloads, as determined by nitrogen balance.[61,75] Afterwards, a slightly increased protein intake (1.2 to 1.4 g/kg/d or 85 to 98 g/d) was adequate to provide a favorable nitrogen balance.[61,75] It is still unclear whether protein intake manipulation would affect endurance performance.

An additional issue of commercial significance is the validation of perceived advantages of sophisticated protein supplements compared to protein-rich foodstuffs. Table 7 lists some of the bewildering number of options facing an athlete who wishes to augment dietary protein intake. At this time, there is no direct evidence in exercising individuals of any differences in effect among the various types of protein supplements and protein-rich foodstuffs.

2. Single Amino Acids

Components of proteins, the individual amino acids, are available in large quantities. Each amino acid has unique metabolic uses and properties in human physiology, and many of these have been exploited in an effort to enhance or improve human exercise performance.

a. Arginine and Ornithine

Arginine and its metabolic relative, ornithine, are involved in several physiological areas of interest to athletes:

1. Protein synthesis, as a component of polypeptide chains (arginine only)
2. Release of somatotropin (theoretical benefits for muscular hypertrophy and fat loss)
3. Release of insulin (theoretical benefits for muscular energy and protein synthesis)
4. Creatine synthesis (theoretical benefits for muscular strength and energy)
5. Removal of ammonia (a fatigue-causing byproduct of muscular exhaustion[76-78])
6. Polyamine synthesis (regulation of cellular and muscular growth[79])

Both arginine and ornithine have been used to elicit a large release of somatotropin after intravenous administration of 15 to 30 g.[80-86] Somatotropin release after oral administration of arginine or arginine salts has been observed.[87-90] Arginine pyroglutamate (L-arginine-2-pyrrolidone-5-carboxylate) combined with L-lysine hydrochloride (1200 mg each) was administered to 15 healthy male volunteers.[90] Plasma somatotropin levels increased two to eight times, insulin levels doubled, and somatomedin A levels tripled. Similarly, oral ornithine hydrochloride (170 mg/kg) led to fourfold increases in serum somatotropin in 12 bodybuilders.[91] However, insulin levels were not affected,[92] and osmotic diarrhea was encountered at the dose of 170 mg/kg.[91] Lower doses of ornithine (70, 100 mg/kg) did not significantly affect somatotropin levels. The practical aspects of somatotropin release on demand are not clear at this time, although strength athletes remain convinced that higher somatotropin levels accelerate muscular hypertrophy and loss of body fat.[93]

Ten subjects received 1 g each of arginine and ornithine, in two daily losses, and eight other subjects received a placebo.[94] All subjects (untrained middle-aged adult males) initiated a 5-week resistance training program. After 5 weeks, body fat decreased significantly more in the supplemented group (-0.85 vs. -0.20%) and body mass decreased significantly more in the supplemented group (-1.3 vs. -0.81 kg), but composite muscle girth changes were not different.

These results suggest that a moderate dose of arginine and ornithine may have enhanced body fat loss associated with resistance training, an attribute partially modulated by somatotropin. Thus, there is some evidence to suggest that arginine/ornithine may have ergogenic effects for resistance training.

b. Aspartates

Like arginine and ornithine, aspartic acid is a dispensable amino acid with many metabolic uses: (1) transport of minerals to subcellular sites,[95] (2) participant in tricarboxylic acid cycle (cellular energy), and (3) part of urea cycle (removal of ammonia). Early reports implicated a medical use for potassium and magnesium L-aspartate salts as antifatigue agents,[96,97] but this use was refuted since fatigue estimation was subjective.[98]

Administration of 2 g/d of potassium and magnesium-L-aspartate to 38 subjects measured by weightlifting performance, grip strength, and submaximal and maximal treadmill exercises showed no convincing effects.[99,100] However, three reports measured increased times to exhaustion (23 to 50%) for cycle ergometry after administration of 7 or 13 g/d of potassium and magnesium-DL-aspartate.[101-103] Another report found a significant improvement in treadmill performance for untrained subjects, but not trained subjects after 2 weeks of 2 g/d of potassium and magnesium-L-aspartate.[104] Acute administration of 10 g of potassium–magnesium aspartate to seven trained athletes in a double-blind crossover study found a significant increase (14%) in time to exhaustion for treadmill runs at 75% $\dot{V}O_2$ max.[105] The two studies that measured blood ammonia levels both found a trend towards decreased ammonia levels after aspartate administration, consistent with aspartate metabolic roles.

However, three double-blind studies with trained athletes found no effects on short-term exercise, treadmill walking performance, or cycle ergometry to exhaustion after administration of up to 8.4 g/d of potassium–magnesium aspartates.[106-108]

Aspartate salts appear to possess some ergogenic benefits when given in high doses (>7 g) before endurance exercise. However, benefits appeared in untrained subjects rather than trained subjects. Also differences between DL- and L-aspartates need further clarification. Conflicting results from studies will require further research to determine what conditions are necessary to reproduce ergogenic effects of aspartates.

c. Glutamate

Glutamate is used by muscle cells to remove ammonia, forming glutamine.[76-78] Thus, enhanced glutamate levels are hypothesized to prevent fatigue by reduction of exercise-induced ammonia levels. Monosodium glutamate (MSG) was administered intravenously (9 g at 200 mg/min) to six healthy, untrained men before exercise to exhaustion on a cycle ergometer.[109] Compared to saline infusion, MSG infusion decreased postexercise blood ammonia levels by half, although lactate, pyruvate, urate, glucose, and urea values were unchanged. Unfortunately, MSG infusion produced nausea in most subjects, making further studies of MSG as an ergogenic aid questionable. Also, incidence of toxicity from MSG (but not glutamic acid or glutamate dipeptides), known as the "Chinese Restaurant Syndrome", means that future research should explore other chemical forms of glutamate.

d. Glycine

Another single amino acid that has been explored as an erogenic aid is glycine, the simplest amino acid. Early interest in glycine was stimulated by its role as a precursor for creatine, and clinical use in muscular dystrophy and myasthenia gravis (both exhibiting muscular weakness and creatine loss).[110] Like aspartate, glycine was tried as an antifatigue agent in clinical situations, and discounted for lack of objective measurements.[110-113] During the 1940s, several reports on the ergogenic effects of glycine administration (5 to 12 g/d) found enhancement of exercise[114,115] or not.[116-119] However, results are suspect because of lack of experimental controls. At least large oral doses of glycine were well tolerated.

Similar to arginine and ornithine, glycine has been shown to elicit increases in serum somatotropin after intravenous[120] and oral (6.75 and 30 g)[121,122] administration to normal subjects. However, these effects have not been examined in association with exercise or in athletes. Thus, research on glycine as an ergogenic aid is still incomplete, but it does not appear to have dramatic effects.

e. Lysine

No differences in the physical performance test scores of "sub-par" college males were noted after consumption of placebo or 790 mg of L-lysine per day with a multiple vitamin.[123] Serum somatotropin levels were not affected by 1200 mg L-lysine, but were increased when lysine was co-administered with 1200 mg of arginine pyroglutamate.[90] However, a rationale for continued study of lysine as an ergogenic aid is lacking.

f. Tryptophan

Although several reports have found increased levels of serum somatotropin after oral tryptophan administration, side effects of drowsiness and mellow feelings were noted.[124-128] Total exercise time and total work load performed were greatly increased (49%) after supplementation with 1200 mg of L-tryptophan 24 h before a treadmill test, compared to a placebo.[129] Ratings of perceived exertion were lowered, suggesting a possible effect on endogenous levels of endorphin/enkephalins, increasing pain tolerance and work performance.

Unfortunately, in the U.S., tryptophan sales and distribution have been banned since 1989 by the Food and Drug Administration (except for parenteral feeding solutions and protein fortification) after outbreaks of eosinophilia myalgia syndrome (EMS) were related to tryptophan supplement consumption.[130-133] EMS cases were ultimately connected to ingestion of products manufactured from one of three batches of L-tryptophan produced by one Japanese manufacturer. Abnormal tryptophan dimer formation occurred after procedural changes during purification of tryptophan.[130-133] Research and use of tryptophan as an ergogenic aid is not feasible at this time.

g. Summary

Single amino acids may have effects on levels of endogenous hormones involved in exercise physiology. Whether these effects are sufficient to enhance performance or muscular hypertrophy has not been tested adequately.

D. Fat

Body fat stores (adipose tissue) represent an enormous amount of potential fuel for muscular exertion.[49] However, in order to be metabolized on a cellular level, fat must be converted from triglycerides into its components: glycerol and free fatty acids. Fatty acids are then taken up into mitochondria with the assistance of carnitine, and metabolized to produce energy.

One important difference between trained and untrained subjects is the ability of exercise training to enable athletes to metabolize less carbohydrate and more fat for muscular energy.[49,134] It seems logical that increased blood levels of fats (as fatty acids and glycerol) would result in improved aerobic performance. However, research has consistently shown that increased dietary fat and/or blood levels of fats do not improve exercise performance, and can actually impair performance.

"Fat-loading", akin to carbohydrate loading, has involved consuming a high-fat diet (60 to 80% of caloric intake) for 3 to 7 d before exercise trials. The numerous studies of carbohydrate loading compared high-fat diets to high-carbohydrate diets, with almost every one finding more benefits from carbohydrate loading.[13,24,46-48,51-53,55] These studies suggest indirectly that fat loading is not ergogenic. Specific studies on fat loading for 3 to 7 d before exercise have found significant impairment of both endurance and anaerobic exercise performance, compared to mixed or high-carbohydrate diets.[135-138] Longer periods of high dietary fat intake (3 to 4 weeks) either noted no changes in time to exhaustion for cycling exercise,[139] or decreases in leg power and parameters of aerobic performance.[140] Likewise, preexercise meals high in fat (50 to 60 g)[141-143] did not improve exercise performance times, and led to gastric distress due to the slow gastric emptying rate of fatty meals.

The other component of fat, glycerol, was given to athletes at a dose of 1 g/kg.[144] Glycerol delayed the decline in blood glucose after timed cycle ergometer or treadmill runs, suggesting that glycerol can be converted into glucose during exercise (a potentially beneficial situation). Performance was not measured.

On a different note, supplementation of 16 males with menhaden fish oil capsules plus salmon steaks for 10 weeks led to improvements in aerobic metabolism, although benefits were quantitatively less than aerobic exercise programs.[145] This study offers some evidence that postulated mechanisms of omega-3 fatty acids[146] are applicable to exercise performance.[147] In a series of studies not published in peer-reviewed journals, omega-3 fatty acid supplementation was associated with increased muscular strength and improved aerobic performance for collegiate and professional football teams.[147] Postulated mechanisms of omega-3 fatty acids include enhancement of somatotropin release, vasodilatory properties, erythrocyte flexibility, and antiplatelet aggregatory effects, mediated by changes in eicosanoid production.[145-147]

E. Alcohol (Ethanol)

Although ethanol is not an essential macronutrient, its inclusion in this section stems from structural similarity to glycerol and carbohydrates, as well as widespread consumption in common foodstuffs. From a legal perspective, ethanol is considered to be a drug or substance of abuse, and its presence in body fluids may cause disqualification in some athletic competitions.

Ethanol has important and conflicting impacts on exercise performance. Small amounts can reduce psychological tension and insecurity, leading to increased self-confidence and improved physical performance via strictly psycological, not physiological means.[148-150] Larger doses of alcohol, corresponding to blood levels of 0.040 to 0.075%, compromise motor performance, coordination, reaction times, and judgment, even though physiological parameters such as $\dot{V}O_2$ max, heart rate, or peak lactate levels generally show little or no changes. However, higher blood levels of ethanol ($>0.10\%$) are considered legally intoxicating and possess detrimental physiological properties that definitely deteriorate physical performance. Furthermore, ethanol can increase dehydration and hypothermia in cold temperatures. Chronic excess ethanol consumption can lead to excess caloric intake with associated body fat increase, or displacement of nutrient-rich foods.

Individual variations in response to ethanol ingestion are large. However, in general, one alcoholic drink per day is not associated with physical harm or performance deficits. One drink is defined as 12 oz of beer, 4 oz (one small glass) of wine, or 1 oz of hard liquor (100 proof).

III. MICRONUTRIENTS AS ERGOGENIC AIDS

Micronutrients include essential and nonessential dietary components with normal intakes less than 1 g/d, and usually in the milli- or microgram ranges. Food and pharmaceutical technology has provided abundant supplies of micronutrients. It seems that if a role in exercise metabolism exists for a particular micronutrient, then a rationale for use, followed by commercial products, also exists. Proliferation of available micronutrient products has far outstripped the scientific ability to test for ergogenic effects of such products. This section will thus be concerned with reported ergogenic studies on micronutrients, with brief mention of micronutrients as yet untested (but commercially available).

A. Antioxidants

The generation of free radicals (chemically unstable species with an unpaired electron) is a normal byproduct of life. Because of their nonspecific and potent chemical reactivity, free radicals alter and damage biological structures and molecules.[151,152] Intense scientific effort is focused on antioxidants as protectors against aging and degenerative diseases.[151,152] Exercise increases oxidative processes of muscles, leading to increased generation of free radicals and their byproducts in humans.[153-159] There appears to be an association of increased free radical production with increasing exercise intensity.[159] Intense exercise also decreased antioxidant status in humans.[160] Free radicals have been observed to be intimately associated with fatigue during exercise.[153-155] Therefore, a rationale for antioxidant supplementation to prevent free radical damage and delay fatigue during exercise is hypothesized.

Antioxidants in human tissues and diets are listed in Table 8. The administration of combined (rather than single) antioxidants to humans in ergogenic studies is a new approach. When 23 runners were given a daily supplement of 10 mg beta-carotene, 800 IU vitamin E, and 1000 mg vitamin C for 3 to 4 weeks, postexercise measurements of antioxidant status showed less muscle damage (lower creatine phosphokinase [CPK] and lactose dehydrogenase [LDH] enzyme levels in blood), fewer decreases in antioxidant status (less oxidized and more reduced plasma glutathione), and quicker recovery of antioxidant status after downhill treadmill running at 65% $\dot{V}O_2$ max.[161]

TABLE 8 Antioxidants in Human Tissues

Endogenous Production	Dietary Source
Bilirubin	Anthocyanidins
Catalase	Ascorbic acid (vitamin C)[a]
Coenzyme Q_{10} (ubiquinone)	Beta-carotene (pro-vitamin A)[a] and other carotenoids
Cysteine	
Glutathione	Bioflavonoids
Glutathione peroxidase	Curcumin (turmeric)
Histidine	Mannitol
Protein sulfhydryl groups	Methionine[a]
Superoxide dismutase	Plant phenolic acids (gallates, ferulates, ellagates, etc.)
Taurine	Polyphenols (tannins)
	Synthetic antioxidants (BHA, BHT, TBHQ, ethoxyquin)
	Synthetic spin trappers (DMPO, PBN, POBN)
	Tocopherols (vitamin E)[a]
	Zinc[a]

[a] Essential (indispensible) nutrients.

BHA, butylated hydroxyanisole; BHT, butylated hydroxytoluene; TBHQ, *tert*-butyl hydroquinone; DMPO, 5,5-dimethyl-1-pirrolyn-*N*-oxide; PBN, *N*-*tert*-butyl-α-phenylnitrone; POBN, α-4-pyridyil-1-oxide-*N*-*tert*-butyl-nitrone.

A personal communication from Kantner, Noble, and Holloszy reported by Singh found that daily supplementation with 28 mg of beta-carotene, 727 mg of *dl*-α-tocopherol, and 1000 mg of ascorbic acid significantly reduced serum lipid peroxide levels and breath pentane after exhaustive treadmill exercise.[155]

Another study administered 10 mg of beta-carotene, 533 mg of *d*-α-tocopherol, and 1000 mg of ascorbic acid daily for 28 d.[162] Compared to a presupplementation exercise bout (90 min of cycle ergometry at 65% $\dot{V}O_2$ max), antioxidant supplementation did not affect urinary output of 8-hydroxyguanosine, a measure of free radical damage to RNA. Blood levels of antioxidants were significantly increased.

Supplementation with 400 IU of vitamin E and 500 mg of vitamin C daily for 6 months led to stimulation of T-cell mitogenesis and enhanced prostaglandin E synthesis by stimulated lymphocytes in both fit and sedentary subjects.[163] The authors concluded that physical conditioning and antioxidant vitamin supplementation can stimulate cellular immune function in adults.

Unfortunately, none of these studies explored whether antioxidant supplementation affected exercise performance. They did illustrate that antioxidant supplementation can beneficially alter fatigue parameters during endurance exercise, indicating that ergogenic properties are possible.

In addition to combined antioxidants, supplementation with single antioxidant nutrients has generated a considerable body of ergogenic-related literature.

1. Ascorbic Acid (Vitamin C)

Few nutrients have attracted as much scientific and popular attention as vitamin C. Widespread availability, popularity, use, and low cost has prompted numerous studies on human physical performance, with mostly contradictory results. Vitamin C is primarily involved in antioxidant functions in the body,[164] and a proposed mechanism of protection and/or facilitation of oxidative reactions has been proposed.[165] Interestingly, about 36 studies on ergogenic effects of vitamin C can be discounted due to lack of suitable controls, substandard measurements of performance, failure to provide experimental data, or relatively low doses of vitamin C.[6] No adequately controlled study administered less than 500 mg/d of vitamin C and revealed ergogenic effects, suggesting a dose threshold.[4] Eleven studies which did administer $\geq$500 mg/d of vitamin C have yielded conflicting conclusions.

Four hours after ingestion of 600 mg of vitamin C, 15 young males did not exhibit any differences in maximum grip strength or muscular endurance measured by a hand dyna-mometer in a double-blind crossover study.[166] Track athletes given doses of vitamin C ranging from 0 to 1 g/d for several weeks showed no observable effects on field tests of sprinting, long-distance running, or the Harvard step test.[167] Two hours after ingestion of 0.5 to 2.0 g of vitamin C, maximal cycle ergometer workloads were not affected.[168] Twenty-one days of 1 g/d vitamin C supplementation to 16 out of 33 total subjects had no effect on $\dot{V}O_2$ max or anaerobic capacities measured by cycle ergometry in a double-blind study.[169] Two weeks of 1 g/d of vitamin C supplementation to 13 athletes did not find changes in total work performed.[170] Twelve weeks of 1 g/d of vitamin C supplementation to 112 U.S. Air Force officers did not affect performance of a 12-min walk–run test, compared to 100 officers given a placebo.[171] Five days of supplementation with 2 g/d of vitamin C given to both smokers and nonsmokers did not affect respiratory adjustment or oxygen utilization before, during, or after exercise.[172] Seven days of 3 g/d of vitamin C supplementation to 10 athletes did not affect ventilation, heart rate, or respiratory quotient during cycle ergometry at 60% $\dot{V}O_2$ max.[173]

Finally, a recent study administered both 0.5- and 2.0-g doses of vitamin C in acute (4 h before testing) or chronic (for 7 d) modes of administration to 24 subjects in a double-blind, placebo-controlled fashion.[174] Acute dosing with 0.5 g of vitamin C did not affect quadriceps endurance or pectoral strength and endurance. Acute dosing with 2.0 g of vitamin C did not change $\dot{V}O_2$ max or muscular strength and endurance. Chronic supplementation with 0.5 g/d vitamin C significantly reduced $\dot{V}O_2$ max and muscular endurance (quadriceps and pectoral muscles). Chronic supplementation with 2.0 g/d of vitamin C resulted in significantly reduced $\dot{V}O_2$ max.

On the positive side, after 5 d of 1 g/d of vitamin C supplementation, efficiency of submaximal work at a constant load of 120 W for 20 min was significantly increased.[175] A similar study protocol showed a 25% increase in efficiency for a 5-min step test, along with significant reductions in total energy cost, oxygen debt, oxygen consumption, pulmonary ventilation, and heart rate.[176] Two weeks of 1 g/d of vitamin C supplementation to 13 athletes (in the study which did not find changes in total work performed) did find significant increases in peak work capacity at 170 W, with a lower heart rate.[170] In addition, blood glucose levels were slightly but significantly decreased, plasma free fatty acid levels were significantly increased, and urinary vanillylmandelic acid excretion was significantly in-creased (indicating a higher turnover rate of catecholamines) during the vitamin C period compared to the placebo period.[170] Seven days of 3 g/d of vitamin C supplementation to 10 athletes produced a significantly lower blood lactate level after cycle ergometry at 60% $\dot{V}O_2$ max, although other physiological parameters were unchanged.[173] Finally, returning to the recent study that examined acute and chronic administration of 0.5 or 2.0 g of vitamin C to 24 subjects, the following conditions exhibited ergogenic benefits. Acute dosing with 0.5 g of vitamin C led to significantly improved quadriceps strength. Acute dosing with 2.0 g of vitamin C showed no significant changes in strength or endurance. Chronic dosing with 0.5 g/d of vitamin C resulted in significantly increased muscular strength, and chronic dosing with 2.0 g/d of vitamin C did not affect strength.

In summary, there are no clear-cut or reproducible ergogenic benefits from vitamin C supplementation of doses ranging from 0.5 to 3.0 g/d. These doses appear safe, with no side effects noted. Indices of free radical activity or antioxidant status have not been measured in any study. Thus, it has not been shown if ergogenic effects from doses of vitamin C sufficient to influence antioxidant status are possible or not.

2. Tocopherols (Vitamin E)

Biological functions of vitamin E are almost entirely due to its function as the major fat-soluble antioxidant.[154] Initial ergogenic studies on vitamin E utilized wheat germ oil as the supplemental source.[177] However, factors other than vitamin E in wheat germ oil accounted for observed ergogenic effects.[177] Similar to vitamin C, many early reports on vitamin E supplementation as an ergogenic aid were made suspect by lack of controls, reliance on anecdotal data, or unreliable measurements of performance.[6]

Several studies have shown no enhancement of exercise performance after vitamin E supplementation, especially for swimming times.[156,178-186] Swim and run racing times, $\dot{V}O_2$ max, pulmonary function, muscular strength, electrocardiograph (ECG) readings, postexercise blood lactate, postexercise serum CPK levels, and other physical factors were measured. Doses of vitamin E ranged from 400 to 1600 IU/d, which are generally regarded as levels sufficient to benefit antioxidant status in humans. However, other than postexercise serum CPK levels (an indicator of muscle trauma), measures of antioxidant status were not performed in these studies. Thus, correlation of failure of vitamin E to exhibit ergogenic effects could not be directly compared to its primary biological function.

Other studies have found significant effects of vitamin E supplementation on physiological exercise parameters. Vitamin E supplementation was associated with lower postexercise blood lactate levels compared to controls.[187] Decreased elevations in breath pentane,[156,188] blood lipid peroxides,[158,189] and leakage of muscle enzymes (including CPK)[158,190,191] were observed after exercise when daily doses of vitamin E greater than 400 IU/d were given for longer than 7 d. At high altitudes, evidence of free radical damage (blood rheological changes, elevated breath pentane) was completely reversed by 400 IU/d of vitamin E supplementation, along with improvements in physical performance.[156,188,192] Likewise, at altitudes of 5,000 and 15,000 ft, vitamin E supplementation significantly improved $\dot{V}O_2$ max, submaximal oxygen uptake, and oxygen debt in 12 subjects.[193]

Inhaled ozone is another source of free radical exposure during exercise, especially in urban areas, that can adversely affect antioxidant status and exercise performance.[151,156] Vitamin E supplementation, followed by exercise with ozone exposure, did not affect respiratory parameters,[156,194] but did significantly reduce free radical indices of damage.[156] Vitamin E supplementation was recommended for athletes participating in the 1984 Summer Olympic Games at Los Angeles to protect against smog-related free radical exposure.[195]

In summary, vitamin E administration has reproducibly decreased free radical damage induced by intense exercise, or by other conditions causing free radical production during exercise in humans (high altitude, ozone exposure). At high altitudes, vitamin E prevents degradation of physical performance, while at sea level, vitamin E supplements do not appear to enhance performance. Effective doses of vitamin E appear to be 400 to 800 IU/d of either *d*-α-tocopherol (nature-identical form) or *dl*-α-tocopheryl esters (less expensive, synthetic forms). Vitamin E can be considered an ergogenic aid at high altitudes. Otherwise, vitamin E is an ergogenic aid in the sense that recovery and long-term protection from possible adverse effects of overtraining or exposure to free radicals have been exhibited following intense exercise. Vitamin E supplementation cannot be expected to improve aerobic performance under usual conditions.

3. Other Antioxidants

Other antioxidant compounds have been applied to human exercise physiology studies. Similar to vitamin E findings, when 15 untrained subjects were given BHT (20 mg/kg every

48 h for 15 d), breath pentane was greatly decreased after exhaustive cycling.[154] Performance was not studied.

The ultratrace, essential mineral selenium is an antioxidant because it is a component of the intracellular enzyme glutathione peroxidase (GPx), perhaps the most important intracellular antioxidant.[151,152] Deficiencies of selenium decrease GPx activity, which is the major system for removal of peroxides,[151,152] and can lead to cardiomyopathies (Keshan disease) and muscle weakness.[196] At the Sports Polyclinic in Romania, 33 elite swimmers in a crossover study were supplemented with 150 μg of selenium (as selenite) for 2 weeks.[197] Postexercise levels of serum lipid peroxides (a measure of free radical damage) were significantly reduced, and improvements in antioxidant status were measured.[197] The selenium status of subjects was not assessed, so results could be due to correcting marginal status, or to a true ergogenic effect. Nevertheless, the modest dose of selenium employed (150 μg) is well within the Estimated Safe and Adequate Daily Dietary Intake of 50 to 200 μg.[196] Increased attention for selenium as a possible ergogenic acid seems warranted.

Beta-carotene and other carotenoids have received much recent publicity about their protective roles against cancer and heart disease.[151,152] However, although beta-carotene is a potent quencher of singlet oxygen,[198] no studies in humans or animals have examined the effects of beta-carotene alone on exercise performance. Beta-carotene is a precursor for vitamin A (retinol) with excellent safety and tolerability,[199] making it ideal for supplementation studies. As presented earlier in this section, beta-carotene was a component of antioxidant mixtures that showed protection from free radical effects during exercise.[155,161,162]

In conclusion, antioxidants have shown definite ability to reduce indices of free radical damage associated with intense exercise or other conditions producing free radicals. However, except at high altitudes, exercise performance has not been improved in studies to date examining single antioxidants. A comprehensive mixture of antioxidants has not been specifically examined for effects on physical performance. Speculative doses of a comprehensive antioxidant mixture might include 400 to 800 IU/d of vitamin E (*d*-α-tocopherol, 25,000 to 100,000 IU/d of beta-carotene, 0.5 to 2.0 g/d of vitamin C (ascorbate), 100 to 250 μg of selenium (sodium selenite), and perhaps 2 to 5 g of *N*-acetyl-cysteine (to provide precursors for glutathione synthesis). Regardless of effects on exercise performance, antioxidant supplements show great promise to protect against adverse effects of free radicals, with long-term health benefits, in both sedentary and trained subjects.[151,152]

B. B Complex Vitamins

Table 9 lists the compounds included in the B complex family of vitamins and their roles related to exercise. Most B vitamins are involved with the metabolism of foodstuffs into energy and, thus, have attracted research interest as ergogenic aids. B vitamins have been studied for ergogenic effects since the 1920s.[4,6] Early studies usually suffered from lack of controls, lack of statistical analysis, and/or low doses of B vitamins, and so their results will not be considered further in this section. Results from more recent studies are presented. Other excellent reviews on B vitamins and exercise have been published.[4,6,7,173,200-202]

1. Individual B Complex Vitamins

Thiamin (vitamin B_1) supplementation (900 mg/d for 3 d) to 15 trained cyclists led to consistent and significant improvements in anaerobic thresholds, heart rates, blood lactate levels, and blood glucose levels during maximal cycle ergometry.[203]

Riboflavin (vitamin B_2) supplementation (10 mg before exercise) led to lowering of neuromuscular irritability after electrical stimulation, suggesting that improvement of muscular hyperexcitability and glycolytic capability is possible.[204] Theoretically, performance can be benefitted by these changes. Supplementation with 60 mg/d of riboflavin for 16 to

TABLE 9 B Vitamin Complex: Functions Related to Exercise

Vitamin B₁ (Thiamin)

Role: Energy production from foodstuffs, especially carbohydrates.
Function: Coenzyme for transketolase (pentose phosphate pathway); pyruvate dehydrogenase and α-ketoglutarate dehydrogenases (entry of acetyl groups and α-ketoglutarate into tricarboxylic acid cycle).
Needs: 0.5 mg per 1000 kcal

Vitamin B₂ (Riboflavin)

Role: Energy production and cellular respiration.
Function: As coenzymes flavin adenine dinucleotide (FAD) and flavin mononucleotide (FMN), vital for large number of redox reactions, releasing energy from carbohydrates, fats and proteins.
Needs: 0.6 mg per 1000 kcal

Niacin, Niacinamide (Nicotinic Acid, Nicotinamide, Vitamin B₃)

Roles: Energy production, cellular respiration, fat synthesis.
Function: As coenzymes nicotinamide adenine dinucleotide (NAD) and nicotinamide adenine dinucleotide phosphate (NADP), vital for many redox reactions, releasing energy from breakdown of carbohydrates, fats, and proteins; glycogen synthesis.
Needs: 6.6 niacin equivalents per 1000 kcal (1 niacin equivalent = 1 mg niacin)

Vitamin B₆ (Pyridoxine, Pyridoxal, Pyridoxamine)

Roles: Amino acid metabolism and energy production.
Function: As coenzyme pyridoxal phosphate (PLP), vital for numerous reactions involving transamination (transfer of amino groups), deamination (removal of amino groups), desulfuration (transfer of sulfhydryl groups), decarboxylation (removal of organic acid group), heme formation, conversion of tryptophan to niacin, glycogen breakdown, eicosanoid synthesis.
Needs: 2.0–2.2 mg per day

Vitamin B₁₂ (Cobalamins)

Roles: Prevention of anemia, sustains growth of rapidly dividing tissues.
Function: Vital for transfer of methyl groups and folate metabolism, breakdown of odd-chain fatty acids and branched-chain amino acids.
Needs: 3.0 µg per day

Folic Acid (Folacin, Folinic Acid, Pteroylglutamates)

Roles: Formation of blood cells and rapidly growing cells.
Function: Primary carrier of one-carbon units used for myriad biosynthetic reactions.
Needs: 0.4 mg per day

Pantothenic Acid

Roles: Energy production from carbohydrates, fats, and proteins.
Function: As coenzyme A, vital for entry of carbohydrates, fats, and proteins into tricarboxylic acid cycle, and for many biosynthetic pathways.
Needs: 4–7 mg per day (estimate)

Biotin

Roles: Energy production and fat metabolism.
Function: Biosynthesis of fatty acids, replenishment of tricarboxylic acid cycle, gluconeogenesis.
Needs: 100–300 µg per day

Sources

Brown, M. L., Ed., *Present Knowledge in Nutrition*, International Life Sciences Institute — Nutrition Foundation, Washington, D.C., 1990.

Devlin, T. M., Ed., Principles of nutrition II: Micronutrients, in *Textbook of Biochemistry*, 3rd ed., Wiley-Liss, New York, 1992, 1115.

Krause, M. V. and Mahan, L. K., Eds., Vitamins, in *Food, Nutrition, and Diet Therapy*, 7th ed., W. B. Saunders, Philadelphia, 1984, 99.

Machlin, L. J., Ed., *Handbook of Vitamins*, 2nd ed., Marcel Dekker, New York, 1991.

Williams, M. H., The role of vitamins in physical activity, in *Nutritional Aspects of Human Physical Performance*, 2nd ed., Williams, M. H., Ed., Charles C Thomas, Springfield, 1985, 147.

20 d to elite swimmers did not find any changes compared to a placebo group for swimming performance, $\dot{V}O_2$ max, or anaerobic threshold. Presupplementation riboflavin status was assessed and found to be normal.[205]

Niacin (nicotinic acid, vitamin B_3) supplementation (300 go 2000 mg before exercise) was found to prevent the normal rise in plasma free fatty acid levels seen during exercise.[206-211] Although five of these reports did not find changes in endurance performance after acute niacin administration, niacin caused greater perceived fatigue[210] and decreased endurance in glycogen-depleted subjects compared to unsupplemented, glycogen-depleted subjects.[211] Therefore, excessive amounts of niacin (>300 mg) are not ergogenic and may actually be anti-ergogenic in settings of exhaustion or low dietary carbohydrate intake. The effects of niacinamide (the usual form of vitamin B_3 in supplements) on exercise performance has not been specifically studied. Since niacinamide does not share pharmacological properties of niacin at high doses, it is possible that the amounts of niacinamide in multiple vitamin/mineral products is insufficient to affect free fatty acid levels in most persons.

Pyridoxine (vitamin B_6) supplementation (51 to 985 mg/d for 30 to 180 d) did not affect endurance performance of trained swimmers,[179] exercise workload after carbohydrate-rich diets,[201] or $\dot{V}O_2$ max and peak lactate levels after supramaximal treadmill runs.[212] Supplementation with 8 mg/d of pyridoxine to four subjects caused a more rapid emptying of muscle glycogen stores during cycling,[213] while an intake of 10.4 mg/d of pyridoxine found increased glycogen utilization and decreased serum free fatty acid levels, compared to an intake of 2.4 mg/d of pyridoxine.[214] Pyridoxine augmented the normal increase in serum somatotropin levels induced by intense cycling exercise.[215] Taken together, these results suggest that pyridoxine supplementation is not beneficial for endurance performance, but may have a positive effect on short-term anaerobic exercises (such as weightlifting), which rely chiefly on rapid glycogenolysis.

Cyanocobalamin (vitamin B_{12}) supplementation (10, 50, or 1000 μg/d for 42 to 49 d) had no effect on half-mile run time,[216] grip strength,[217,218] heart rate recovery, maximal cycling times,[218] $\dot{V}O_2$ max, or other standard strength tests.[219] Since 1986, commercial availability of one coenzymatic form of vitamin B_{12} (Dibencozide, cobamamide, 5,6-dimethyl-benzimidazolyl cobamide coenzyme) from European pharmaceutical companies has turned into a fad for weightlifters and bodybuilders, promoted as an anabolic steroid replacement.[220,221] An oft-cited study of malnourished Polish children (who were very likely deficient in vitamin B_{12} and other nutrients) seemed to show better growth responses and lean body mass accretion after supplementation with cobamamide compared to anabolic steroid administration.[222] No studies exist to support benefits of vitamin B_{12} for weightlifters, despite common usage and belief in efficacy by users.[216-219] However, since deficiency symptoms of vitamin B_{12} include psychological disturbances and neurological symptoms (including fatigue) that are difficult to diagnose by the usual clinical laboratory tests, a possible placebo-like effect for high doses of vitamin B_{12} cannot be excluded at this time.

Folate supplementation (5 mg/d for 11 weeks) to 10 nonanemic, folate-deficient female marathon runners raised serum folate levels three- to fourfold, but did not change $\dot{V}O_2$ max, maximal treadmill performance, heart rates, and blood lactate levels compared to placebo subjects.[223] There has been no obvious research into possible deleterious effects of megaloblastic anemia (caused by deficiencies of vitamin B_{12} and/or folate) on exercise performance in athletes. Folate deficiencies in women are not uncommon, making this topic an overlooked facet of nutrition and exercise interactions.

Pantothenate supplementation (1 g/d for 2 weeks) to 18 trained runners did not affect treadmill run times to exhaustion or blood glucose, CPK, or bicarbonate levels compared to a placebo period.[224] Pantothenate supplementation (2 g/d for 2 weeks) to trained distance runners led to decreased blood lactate levels and oxygen consumption during prolonged, strenuous cycling.[225] Pantothenate may exhibit ergogenic effects for endurance performance if previous findings are confirmed.

Biotin, inositol, and *p*-**aminobenzoic acid (PABA)** are untested for effects on human exercise performance. These compounds are present in some mixtures considered later in this chapter, although at rather small doses.

In general, administration of individual B vitamins showed no ergogenic effects unless very large doses were given (thiamin and pantothenate). However, since B vitamins work in concert with each other and other metabolic processes, it is much more logical to administer supplemental B vitamins as a mixture.

2. Mixtures of B Complex Vitamins

Before 1950, all of the B complex vitamins were not yet characterized, and thus, mixtures did not contain what is considered to be a complete B complex. This fact, coupled with doses known to be insufficient to affect body levels, rendered results of most early studies on effects of B complex vitamins suspect.[4,6,7,173,201]

Table 10 exhibits doses and conclusions from studies on B vitamins as ergogenic aids. Read and McGuffin found no change in treadmill endurance after 6 weeks of supplementation with a relatively low-dose B vitamin complex supplement.[226] However, a positive correlation between thiamin intake and treadmill running times to exhaustion was seen in some trials. Van der Beek et al.[227] measured functional performance of 23 subjects fed a diet deficient in thiamin, riboflavin, pyridoxine, and ascorbate for 8 weeks. All subjects were given a supplement containing twice the RDA for other vitamins (A, D, E, B_{12}, folate, biotin, niacinamide, pantothenate) and adequate minerals. Eleven subjects were also given a supplement supplying twice the RDA for thiamin, riboflavin, pyridoxine, and ascorbate. Fully supplemented subjects exhibited no changes in $\dot{V}O_2$ max, maximal workload, and blood lactate levels, while the deficient group exhibited decreases in each parameter. Compared to the deficient group, the supplemented group showed no differences in submaximal exercise performance, although mental performance (reaction time) deteriorated in the deficient group. Biochemical markers of vitamin status for the deficient group demonstrated a vitamin-deficient state, while the supplemented group showed no changes from normal status. This study is important because it illustrated that doses of B vitamins at twice the RDA level did not affect vitamin status, and also did not affect exercise performance. Thus, evidence for a dose-response effect of B vitamins and ergogenic effects can be seen (Table 10). Results emphasize the importance of correlating measurements of nutrient status with exercise performance results before a conclusion on effectiveness of nutrients as ergogenic aids is stated.

This concept is dramatized by the results of Buzina et al.,[228] who found a small but significant increase in $\dot{V}O_2$ max in 80 school children (12 to 15 years old) after 3 months of supplementation with RDA amounts of riboflavin, pyridoxine, and ascorbate. Measurement of biochemical deficiencies for one or more of the supplemented vitamins was found in 34% of subjects, indicating observed ergogenic effects may have been due to repletion of B vitamin deficiencies, which are known to cause decreased exercise performance,[173,200-202] rather than a true ergogenic effect.

Boncke and Nickel administered high doses of thiamin, pyridoxine, and vitamin B_{12} (at two dose levels) for 8 weeks to trained marksman (pentathletes) in a double-blind study.[229] Better control of fine muscles, less muscle tremor, and significantly improved marksmanship were attributed to both supplemented groups (the higher-dose group showed more significant results). Another double-blind study administered relatively higher doses of B vitamins to high school runners in a hot environment.[230] Compared to a placebo group, supplemented subjects reported decreased fatigue after running successive 50-yard dashes.

Finally, a novel B vitamin complex, pyridoxine α-ketoglutarate (PAK) was supplemented (30 mg/kg/d for 30 d) to 20 trained runners.[212] A significant increase in $\dot{V}O_2$ max and

TABLE 10 Correlation of Dose and Ergogenic Effects of Recent Controlled Human Studies on B Vitamin Supplements

Investigators (year)	B₁ (mg)	B₂ (mg)	Niacin (mg)	B₆ (mg)	B₁₂ (μg)	Panto. (mg)	Folate (mg)	Length of Admin.	Ergogenic Results[a]	Ref.
Knippel et al. (1986)	900	—	—	—	—	—	—	3 d	+	203
Haralambie (1976)	—	10	—	—	—	—	—	Acute [b]	+	204
Tremblay et al. (1984)	—	60	—	—	—	—	—	16–20	+	205
Jenkins (1965)	—	—	300	—	—	—	—	Acute	—	207
Carlson et al. (1963)	—	—	500	—	—	—	—	Acute	—	206
Bergstrom et al. (1969)	—	—	1,600	—	—	—	—	Acute	—[c]	210
Pernow and Saltin (1971)	—	—	1,200	—	—	—	—	Acute	—[c]	211
Norris et al. (1978)	—	—	2,000	—	—	—	—	Acute	—	208
Gilman and Lemon (1982)	—	—	?	—	—	—	—	6 months	—	209
Lawrence et al. (1974)	—	—	—	51	—	—	—	30 d	—	179
Marconi et al. (1982)	—	—	—	985[d]	—	—	—	—	—	212
Wetzel et al. (1952)	—	—	—	—	10	—	—	7 weeks	—	217
Montoye et al. (1955)	—	—	—	—	50	—	—	6 weeks	—	216,218
Tin-May-Than et al. (1978)	—	—	—	—	1,000	—	—	11 weeks	—	219
Matter et al. (1987)	—	—	—	—	—	—	5	14 d	—	223
Nice et al. (1984)	—	—	—	—	—	1,000	—	14 d	—	224
Litoff et al. (1985)	—	—	—	—	—	2,000	—	14 d	+	225
Buzina[e] et al. (1982)	—	2	—	2	—	—	—	3 months	+	228
Boncke and Nickel (1989)	90	—	—	60	120	—	—	8 weeks	+	229
Boncke and Nickel (1989)	300	—	—	600	600	—	—	8 weeks	+	229
van der Beek et al.[f] (1988)	2.5	4	—	4	—	—	—	8 weeks	—	227
Read and McGuffin (1983)	5	5	25	2	0.5	12.5	—	Acute	—	226
Early and Carlson (1969)	100	8	100	5	25,000	30	—	Acute	+	230

[a] + indicates improved physiological change or enhanced exercise performance; − indicates no effect on performance or physiological variables.

[b] Acute signifies administration 0–2 h before exercise.

[c] Performance and/or physiological measurements showed detrimental changes.

[d] Actual administration was 16 mg/kg with a mean body weight of 61.6 ± 1.6 (S.E.M.) kg, for an average dose of 985 mg/d.

[e] Up to one third of subjects showed clinical or biochemical symptoms of deficiencies for supplemented vitamins. This fact may mean observed benefits were due to repletion of deficiencies, which are known to decrease performance. Vitamin C (70 mg/d) was included in the supplement.

[f] Supplement included 2× RDA amounts of vitamins A, D, E, B₁₂, folate, biotin, niacinamide, and pantothenate plus 100 mg vitamin C to both the control and experimental groups.

TABLE 11 Potential Guidelines for Supplementation with B Complex Vitamins for Ergogenic Effects

Vitamin	Daily Dose	% RDA[a]
Thiamin (Vitamin B_1)	100–1,000 mg	6,667–66,667
Riboflavin (Vitamin B_2)	10–100 mg	5,556–55,556
Niacinamide (Vitamin B_3)	22 mg	100
Pantothenate	50–2,000 mg	714–28,571[b]
Pyridoxine (Vitamin B_6)	2–10 mg	100–500
Cyanocobalamin (Vitamin B_{12})	2–100 μg	100–5,000
Folate	400–800 μg	100[c]

[a]   % RDA = % Recommended Daily Allowances for adult males (1985).
[b]   % RDA value for pantothenate is actually calculated from the upper limit of the Estimated Safe and Adequate Daily Dietary Intake of 4–7 mg/d.
[c]   Levels of folate in nutritional supplements are restrained by the FDA to 400 μg/d for adults or 800 μg/d for pregnant women per unit of delivery (tablet, capsule, pill). Higher doses require a prescription from a licensed physician.

significant decrease in blood lactate accumulation after a supramaximal treadmill run was measured for the supplemented group, but not for the control period or a placebo group. Neither pyridoxine or α-ketoglutarate alone was effective.

It is clear that rather large doses of mixtures of B complex vitamins are needed before ergogenic benefits are possible. When sufficiently large doses of one or more B vitamins have been given, some type of ergogenic effects have been measured. Thus, sufficiently large doses of some, but not all, B complex vitamins may offer ergogenic properties for a wide range of exercising individuals, and perhaps, result in a small improvement in performance, in the order of 5 to 10%.

Table 11 lists potential guidelines for B vitamin complex supplementation. Thiamin and pantothenate are associated with large safety margins and most pertinent metabolic mechanisms. Pyridoxine and niacin have a real potential for toxicity, and also have few documented ergogenic effects. Riboflavin, vitamin B_{12}, and folate appear to have little or no ergogenic effects, but are safe in very large oral doses, and are included in order to prevent possible imbalances in metabolism among other B vitamins. Nevertheless, further research on B complex vitamins is recommended to confirm dose–response effects in mixtures and to determine the practicality of ergogenic benefits.

C. Bicarbonate (Alkalinizers)

Acidosis (decrease in pH or increase in hydrogen ion concentration) in muscle tissue is one major factor causing fatigue during exercise.[231] Acidosis is produced by exercise that accumulates lactic acid (especially anaerobic exercise).[231] Bicarbonate ions are the chief buffering system of the body.[231] Thus, research efforts have focused on increasing bodily bicarbonate reserve to neutralize acidity produced by anaerobic exercise, delay fatigue, and improve exercise performance.

Induced metabolic acidosis before exercise (usually from ammonium chloride administration) has been able to decrease exercise performance reproducibly.[232-242] Conversely, induced metabolic alkalosis from bicarbonate administration before exercise has been able to improve exercise performance in many studies.[236,237,243-272] In general, sodium bicarbonate (0.2 to 0.3 g/kg) was given, dissolved in water or flavored drinks, 1 to 3 h before exercise (an acute mode of administration). Most studies exhibiting improved performance after bicarbonate loading also reported reduced perception of fatigue, lowered serum levels of enzymes released after muscular damage (CPK, LDH, glutamate oxalacetate transaminase [GOT], glutamate pyruvate transaminase [GPT], ornithine transcarbamylase [OCT], aldolase), increased blood lactate levels, increased blood pH, increased base excess, and increased blood bicarbonate levels.[236,237,243-272]

However, not all studies have discovered ergogenic benefits from bicarbonate loading.[240,241,254,272-289] Comparing these studies to ones showing an ergogenic effect of bicarbonate found insufficient exercise time, aerobic submaximal work, variability in subject training, insufficient dose, few experimental details reported, methodological difficulties, or no changes in blood pH or lactate for some studies, but not all.

The types of exercise that appear to be benefitted from bicarbonate loading are any *exhaustive* exercise lasting 1 to 7 min; maximal races (200 to 800 m), and repeated short-term, maximal, anaerobic exercise bouts. Cycling, running, swimming, and weightlifting are examples of exercises studied in reports showing ergogenic benefits. For example, subjects ran an 800-m race an average of 2.9 s faster than the control period, and 2.2 s faster than a placebo period, which works out to a distance of up to 19 m, a large and dramatic difference![258]

In summary, a wealth of data from a large number of well-conducted and well-controlled studies supports the use of acute bicarbonate loading 1 to 3 h before exhausting exercise lasting 1 to 7 min. A dose of 0.2 to 0.3 g/kg is necessary, which equates to 14 to 21 g of sodium bicarbonate (baking soda) for one 70-kg person.

Two caveats must be observed: (1) large volumes of water (*ad libitum* drinking) must be consumed to prevent possible osmotic diarrhea, cramping, and abdominal pain;[272] and (2) a large sodium load (up to 5.5 g of sodium for a 70-kg person) is ingested, meaning those on sodium-restricted diets should consult their physician before attempting bicarbonate loading. Accurate weighing of bicarbonate is essential to prevent over- or under-dosing. Bicarbonate loading is useless for endurance events and is not recommended for events lasting longer than 7 to 10 min. Bicarbonate loading is a well-supported ergogenic aid, when used under the appropriate circumstances.

D. Caffeine

Caffeine is a methylxanthine occurring naturally in coffee beans, tea leaves, chocolate, cocoa beans, cola nuts, Guarana herb, and added to carbonated beverages and pharmaceuticals.[290,291] Almost every social culture on earth reveres caffeinated foodstuffs for their socially acceptable, readily available, and inexpensive stimulant properties. Caffeine is able to stimulate the central nervous system, neurons, cardiac muscles, epinephrine release, gastric acid secretion, diuresis, relaxation of smooth muscles, lipolysis of adipose tissue triglycerides, with resulting increased serum free fatty acid levels (and corresponding reduction in carbohydrate oxidation).[290,292] Oxygen uptake ($\dot{V}O_2$)[293-296] and respiratory exchange ratios (R)[294,296-299] were improved in some, but not all, studies on caffeine given to exercising subjects. Therefore, one mechanism of action for caffeine is increased oxidation of fat by muscles, with sparing of glycogen stores, enabling performance to continue longer before glucose availability is compromised to fatigue.

Almost every study administered 200 to 350 mg of caffeine (3 to 5 mg/kg) per subject 1 h before exercise (an acute mode of administration), which reflected the well-known pharmacokinetics of caffeine in humans.[290,292]

A large number of reports has found significant increases in exercise performance after ingestion of caffeine.[293,297,300-306] Increased times to exhaustion, total work performed, and decreased race times for cycling, cross-country skiing, and treadmill runs were observed. For example, nine competitive cyclists given 330 mg of caffeine increased their time to exhaustion for a maximal cycle ergometry test from 76 to 90 min.[297]

However, an equally large number of reports did not find significant effects on exercise performance.[298,306-312] Caffeine doses and exercise parameters were similar between studies that succeeded or failed to measure ergogenic effects of caffeine. However, two important variables were usually not controlled in most studies: (1) caffeine habituation to tolerance, and (2) composition of muscle fiber types (slow vs. fast twitch).

Caffeine habituation, which is caused by chronic drinking of 1 to 2 cups of coffee (or the equivalent amount of 100 mg/d of caffeine from any source),[313,314] has been shown to blunt metabolic responses to the usual effects of caffeine during exercise.[295,306,307] In fact, caffeine-habituated subjects that were fully withdrawn from caffeine exhibited significant changes in metabolism and performance that were not seen when habituated to caffeine.[306]

Muscle fiber types from mouse soleus (slow twitch) and gastrocnemius (fast twitch) muscles showed large differences in metabolism when exposed to caffeine *in vitro*.[315] Differences in proportion of muscle fiber types in humans may account for individual variations seen in almost every caffeine study (and many other studies as well), and could account for lack of significance of result from some studies.

Two drawbacks to caffeine use exist. First, excessive amounts of caffeine (over five cups of coffee at a time) can produce urinary caffeine levels deemed unacceptable by sports governing agencies.[316] Urine caffeine levels >15 µg/ml are considered doping and grounds for disqualification from sporting events. Second, caffeine is not without toxicity.[290-292,317] Of foremost concern is the diuretic action of caffeine, which may be deleterious in hot, humid conditions. Large excesses of caffeine can produce delirium, hallucinations, anxiety, memory impairment, insomnia, cardiac arrhythmias, and gastric upset.[290,317]

In summary, caffeine is an inexpensive, convenient, and generally safe means to attempt to enhance endurance performance if one is not accustomed to regular intake of caffeine. Not everyone will derive ergogenic benefits from caffeine, but those who do (maybe 40 to 70% of a general population) will experience significant improvements in endurance performance. Caffeine loading can be accomplished by drinking two to three cups of strong, fresh-brewed coffee 1 h before exercise. Caffeine loading is indicated for endurance events lasting more than 1 h, such as running, cycling, cross-country skiing, and other aerobic endurance activities.

E. Calcium

Few reports on the effects of calcium supplementation on exercise preformance are available. However, acute administration of small, single doses of calcium (as controls or placebos for bicarbonate or pangamate studies) has been performed many times, but no obvious ergogenic effects were noted.[4,6]

Calcium status is important for maintenance of bone mass in cases where bone mass is already reduced, or in thin, amenorrheic women.[318] Adequate calcium can be ingested from increased intake of dairy products, tofu, and green leafy vegetables. Calcium supplements, in the form of calcium citrate/malate, calcium citrate, calcium gluconate, or calcium lactate, at doses of 500 to 1000 mg/d are in common use. However, at this time, there appears to be no evidence for considering calcium as an ergogenic aid.

F. Carnitine

L-Carnitine is an alpha-hydroxy acid primarily located in muscle, where it is required for entry of long-chain fatty acids into mitochondria.[319] Thus, carnitine influences energy production from fats. Much recent research has shed further light on the importance of carnitine for exercise performance.[320] Exercise of sufficient intensity and duration (60 to 90% $\dot{V}O_2$ max or work loads between lactate threshold and maximal work capacity) results in a negative carnitine balance from muscles.[6,319,320]

A very recent review on carnitine supplementation and physical performance found that 1 to 6 g/d for periods up to 6 months consistently improved carnitine status with no adverse side effects or toxicity in exercising individuals.[320] Using these dosage amounts, several studies have found significant improvements in $\dot{V}O_2$ max,[321-323] lipid utilization during exercise,[321,322,324-327] carnitine metabolism,[321,323,325,328-330] and enhancement of exercise performance.[320,321,323-325,331,332] Increases in treadmill run times,[321] evoked muscular potential,[324,325] peak anaerobic power,[320] power output from maximal treadmill exercise,[323] and improved submaximal exercise performance (lower heart rate for a given work output)[331] were the observed enhancements of exercise performance. Supplementation with carnitine or propionyl-L-carnitine decreased serum markers of free radical damage after exercise.[333]

Studies which did not show physiological or ergogenic benefits from L-carnitine supplementation either used low doses (0.5 g/d) of carnitine, a shorter duration of supplementation (<14 d), or utilized submaximal exercise now known to be insufficient to elicit a demand on carnitine metabolism.[320,331,332,334-336] Trained subjects seemed to exhibit better responses to carnitine supplementation than untrained subjects.

Another use for carnitine that also has considerable research documentation is in medical conditions of muscular hypoxia (chronic respiratory insufficiency,[337-338] cardiovascular conditions (angina pectoris, peripheral vascular disease, or congestive heart failure),[338-349] and hemodialysis patients.[350] For each condition, exercise performance was significantly enhanced, along with improvement in cardiac performance, total work output, time to exertional pain, and reduction in blood lipid levels. Doses and administration schedules were similar to studies in healthy subjects. The implications for amelioration of symptoms and ability of exercise tolerance to be increased by carnitine is of major medical importance.

In summary, supplementation with L-carnitine for extended periods (>28 d) with large doses (1 to 6 g/d) has shown the ability to improve utilization of lipids as energy sources during strenuous aerobic exercise (>60% $\dot{V}O_2$ max) for trained subjects. Carnitine represents a recent addition to compounds with documented erogogenic abilities.

G. Chromium

Chromium is involved with efficient use of insulin, and is known as the glucose tolerance factor (GTF).[351] Efficient metabolism of carbohydrates, fats, and proteins is the essential function of chromium. Exercising individuals are at risk for developing chromium deficiencies, since low dietary intakes are common and exercise of sufficient intensity increases excretion of chromium.[351-353] Therefore, chromium supplementation is hypothesized to enhance metabolic processes, allowing for greater effects of exercise training. In two studies on collegiate weightlifers, supplementation with 200 μg of chromium (as chromium picolinate) for 40 d to 41 subjects was associated with significant increases in lean body mass and decreased body fat, compared to a placebo group.[354] A similar study of 59 men and women in a 12-week weightlifting program found increased lean body mass in females, but not males.[355]

Research into chromium as an ergonenic acid is still seminal, but preliminary results suggest that attention be paid to the role of chromium in exercising persons. At this time, it is still unclear whether a true ergogenic effect of chromium was observed, or if repletion of marginally deficient states occurred. Nevertheless, chromium has been widely touted as an anabolic agent worthy of anabolic steroid replacement. While any guidelines for use of chromium as an ergonenic aid are premature at this time, doses of 200 μg/d are safe, and almost every athlete is a candidate for chromium depletion and, thus, supplementation.

H. Coenzyme Q_{10} (Ubiquinone)

Coenzyme Q_{10} is similar to carnitine in that endogenous synthesis has prevented both from being defined as essential vitamins. Like carnitine, coenzyme Q_{10} fills a vital role in cellular energy production, as a gateway for progression of electrons from the tricarboxylic acid cycle and other sources to the electron transport chain in mitochondria.[356] Coenzyme Q_{10} is thus vital for aerobic energy production. In addition, coenzyme Q_{10} is lipid-soluble, inhabits membranes, and is a potent antioxidant.[356,357] The scope and breadth of research on coenzyme Q_{10} worldwide is prodigious, as evidenced by several reviews.[356,358,359]

Like other metabolic intermediates, intense or exhaustive exercise leads to loss of coenzyme Q_{10} from plasma of athletes.[360-362] However, training leads to increased levels of coenzyme Q_{10} in muscles, correlating with increased mitochondrial content.[360,361] Since normal coenzyme Q_{10} levels do not saturate associated energy-producing enzymes,[363] there is a valid rationale for provision of additional coenzyme Q_{10} to increase energy production and, thus, exercise performance.

Several studies have found increased exercise performance after supplementation with coenzyme Q_{10} (60 to 100 mg/d for 4 to 8 weeks).[364-367] Submaximal and maximal exercise capacities,[364] cardiac function,[364,368] lipid utilization improvements,[367,369-371] treadmill exercise times,[365] total work capacity,[366,367] and $\dot{V}O_2$ max[365-368] were significantly improved. Overall, every study reported either an improvement in a physiological parameter related to exercise performance and/or an actual improvement in exercise performance. Thus, coenzyme Q_{10} has reproducibly and consistently shown ergogenic effects for aerobic exercise tasks for a variety of submaximal and maximal exercises. These findings indicate that prolonged administration of 100 mg/d of coenzyme Q_{10} may be suitable as an ergogenic aid for all types of exercise tasks, both aerobic and anaerobic. Few compounds have shown the consistency and success of coenzyme Q_{10} in tests of exercise enhancement. With its well-studied safety and pharmacokinetics, coenzyme Q_{10} deserves much attention as an ergogenic aid.

Similar to carnitine, coenzyme Q_{10} supplementation (100 mg/d for at least 4 weeks) has repeatedly been associated with improvements in exercise tolerance, exercise performance, peak work capacity, and cardiac function in patients with angina or cardiac ischemia.[372-380] Coenzyme Q_{10} supplementation should be strongly considered for cardiac disease patients wishing to use exercise as a therapeutic modality.

I. Ferulates (Gamma Oryzanol)

A little-known, but almost ubiquitous, plant phenolic compound (ferulic acid) has shown properties of possible benefit to weightlifters.[381] Ferulic acid is a potent antioxidant, with properties similar to tocopherol and ascorbate.[381-383] The molecular structure of ferulic acid closely resembles the structure of normetanephrine, the primary metabolite of norepinephrine.[381] Administration of ferulate to animals has shown increased somatotropin levels in serum.[381,384] Interactions with catecholamine receptors are also possible.[381] These mechanisms suggested that ferulate supplementation may be useful for recovery from the stress of intense exercise, possibly aiding results of exercise training programs.

Gamma oryzanol is a lipophilic ferulate ester of phytosterols found in rice bran.[381] Both it and ferulic acid have been supplemented to athletes undertaking a variety of resistance-training programs.[381,385,386] Body weight and one-repetition maximum strength were significantly increased for supplemented groups (30 mg of ferulate per day for 8 weeks) compared to placebo groups. In another type of study, ferulate supplementation augmented postexercise serum beta-endorphin levels, but not levels of cortisol or testosterone, indicating a possible norepinephrine-like effect on the hypothalamus to peripheral tissues.[387]

Ferulates are promoted as safe alternatives to anabolic steroids to weightlifters and bodybuilders. Potentially useful research results indicate that confirmation of observed effects to date is needed.

TABLE 12 Topics Concerning Iron and Exercise Performance

Dietary/Nutritional Factors
    Intake surveys (prevalence of deficient intake)
    Interfering dietary components (fiber, oxalates)
    Augmentation of iron absorption (heme, vitamin C)
    Iron salts supplementation characteristics
Iron Status
    Clinical laboratory tests and interpretations for determination of iron status
    Clinical signs of iron deficiency
    Iron excretion/loss pathways
    Iron metabolism
    Iron metalloproteins: biochemistry and physiology
    Prevalence of deficient status (pre-anemia, anemia)
Exercise and Iron
    Effects of exercise on iron loss
    Effects of exercise on iron metabolism
    Iron requirements: alterations by exercise
    Iron repletion
    Iron supplementation during normal iron status
    "Sports anemia"

Note: Details on these topics are presented in many reviews.[394-405]

J. Ginseng

The root of the ginseng plant (*Panax ginseng* or *P. quinquefolium*) has been revered as an overall tonic for centuries by Oriental cultures, and is still a popular herbal supplement, with a worldwide market of $1 billion.[388] Human studies on exercise performance after ginseng supplementation have shown mixed results. On one hand, several studies have shown no changes in physiological parameters (lactate, glucose, insulin, glycerol, free fatty acids, somatotropin, $\dot{V}O_2$ max, heart rate) or exercise performance after doses of 200 to 2000 mg/d of ginseng root for 4 to 9 weeks.[389-391] However, even the highest doses only contained a dose of 0.4 mg/kg of ginsenosides (the putative active components of ginseng based on animal studies), compared to doses of 200 mg/kg of ginsenosides given to animals in studies showing ergogenic effects.[6]

One study did find increased muscle strength and $\dot{V}O_2$ max after 1 g/d of *P. ginseng* root administration, compared to a placebo period.[392] Another study found improvements in work capacity and muscular oxygenation after supplementation of 50 sports teachers with either a placebo or a supplement containing ginseng extract, dimethylaminoethanol bitartrate (DMAE), vitamins, and minerals for 6 weeks.[393]

The variability in choosing a ginseng preparation for study presents obstacles to further research of ginseng as an ergogenic aid for humans. Dose–response issues and ginsenoside amounts have not been resolved. Further investigations of ginseng as an ergogenic aid are necessary before firm conclusions about effectiveness can be drawn.

K. Iron

The importance of iron for exercise performance relates to its role as an integral component of hemoglobin, myoglobin, dehydrogenases, cytochromes, and other mitochondrial iron–sulfur proteins.[394-405] These proteins are essential for oxygen transport and generation of cellular energy in aerobic metabolism, both major determinants of fatigue and exercise capacity.[394-405] Due to the common nature of iron deficiency in the world, and especially in female endurance athletes, dozens of reports have appeared which present much detailed information on the interactions of iron and exercise.[394-405] Table 12 lists some of the topics on iron and exercise that have been extensively studied. This section will only review effects of iron supplementation on exercise performance under different conditions of iron status.

Given the vital importance of iron for exercise and widespread prevalence of deficient iron states, it is understandable that anemia of iron deficiency definitely decreased exercise performance for almost every type of exercise task.[394-399] Repletion of deficient iron status and resolution of anemia will improve exercise performance.[394-399] Thus iron supplementation (and increased intake of dietary sources rich in iron) will definitely improve exercise performance in iron-deficient, anemic subjects.

During the progression of iron deficiency, before the end-stage of anemia, is a period of progressive loss of iron status (nonanemic iron deficiency). Recent attention has focused on whether iron supplementation/repletion will improve exercise performance during nonanemic iron-deficient status. Results have been mixed, with some studies reporting improvement of exercise performance, and others showing no effects (usually because performance was not yet compromised).[394-399] Nevertheless, iron supplementation is recommended to replete iron stores and prevent progression to anemia.

Effect of iron supplementation on exercise performance in iron-replete, nonanemic individuals has also shown mixed results.[394] However, further studies are needed before any conclusions can be inferred.

Iron status is a common cause of decreased physical performance in humans, especially in women. Laboratory testing can easily determine functional iron status, so anyone concerned with their exercise performance is recommended to periodically consult a physician knowledgeable in iron metabolism to initiate testing and interpretation of results. Table 13 lists the usual clinical laboratory tests used to determine iron status.

If subnormal iron status is discovered, dietary modification is recommended. Pertinent dietary changes to improve iron intake and uptake are listed in Table 13. Iron supplements may also be used to replenish iron stores (doses of 18 mg/d), or prevent depletion (10 to 25 mg/d for extended periods). Organic chelates of iron are the preferred type of supplementation because of enhanced bioavailability and better tolerance (see Table 13). Excessive doses of iron can be toxic and even life-threatening. Do not exceed recommended intakes.

In summary, iron status greatly affects exercise performance. It is strongly recommended for serious athletes, those whose performance has reached a plateau, and female endurance athletes to seek medical consultation for determination of iron status. If deficient in any way, iron repletion by dietary manipulation and/or iron supplementation is wise. Seeking the services of a professional to analyze dietary intake and learn more about iron-rich foodstuffs is also recommended. These practices should prevent ergogenic deficits from iron deficiency from occurring.

L. Magnesium and Boron

Magnesium and boron are considered together since very recent research has linked the two minerals. Magnesium plays so many vital roles in metabolism (glycolysis, contractility, membrane permeability, membrane transport, any enzyme using ATP, osmoregulation, phosphorylations, hexose monophosphate shunt) that its essentiality is well documented. Magnesium losses during exercise and subnormal magnesium status have been detected in athletes.[394,404,406-411] In one case report, hypomagnesemia caused muscle cramps, which were alleviated by magnesium gluconate supplements (500 mg/d).[406] Magnesium supplementation has enhanced physical capacity of endurance athletes[412] and also increased quadriceps torque measurements following resistance training.[413] Doses of magnesium ranged up to 8 mg/kg/d, corresponding to 600 mg/d for a 70-kg person. These doses are well tolerated in normal persons.[404]

In addition, studies examining ergogenic effects of potassium–magnesium aspartate have been reviewed earlier in this chapter.[96-108] Magnesium amounts were not trivial, and ranged from 40 to 400 mg/d. Although potassium and aspartate were ingested, these studies suggest that magnesium supplementation may have ergogenic effects under certain conditions.

TABLE 13 Determinants of Iron Status and Dietary Practices to Replete Iron Stores

Clinical Laboratory Tests for Iron Status
CBC (Complete Blood Count) includes:
Hemoglobin (Hb or Hgb in g/dl)
Hematocrit (Hct in %)
Erythrocyte count (RBC in 10^6 cells/mm^3)
Leukocyte count (WBC in 10^3 cells/mm^3)
Leukocyte differential (cell %)
Mean corpuscular volume (MCV in fl)
Mean corpuscular hemoglobin (MCH in μg)
Mean corpuscular hemoglobin concentration (MCHC in %)
Platelet count (10^3/mm^3)
Serum ferritin
Serum iron (Fe)
Total iron-binding capacity (TIBC)
Transferrin saturation (calculated from Fe and TIBC)
Free erythrocyte protoporphyrin
Additional Laboratory Tests to Rule Out Non-Iron Deficiency Anemias
Serum and erythrocyte folate
Serum vitamin B$_{12}$
Erythropoietin
Microbial assays for vitamin B$_6$ levels
Functional vitamin B$_6$ assays (erythrocyte transaminase saturation indices)
Serum copper
NOTE: Reference ranges for each test may differ between laboratories.
Dietary Changes to Improve Iron Intake and Uptake
1. Increase ingestion of heme iron by increasing intake of cooked muscle meats or blood, preferably lean red meats
2. Increase consumption of vitamin C at same time as iron-rich foods or iron supplements by increasing *fresh* citrus fruits and green leafy vegetable intakes; Vitamin C supplements (100–1000 mg/d) are also appropriate
3. Iron supplements (optional 10–25 mg/d to replete nonanemic iron deficiency; or higher doses for shorter periods — determined by a health care professional — in iron deficiency anemia) should be considered, especially for strict or lacto-ovo vegetarians
4. Better iron supplements: ferritin, ferrous glycinate, ferrous lactate, ferrous gluconate, ferrous fumarate, iron dextran; less ideal iron supplements: ferrous sulfate, reduced iron, carbonyl iron, ferric orthophosphate

Further studies, including dietary histories and determinations of magnesium status, are needed to confirm the reported ergogenic effects of magnesium supplementation. At issue is whether deficient states are being repleted, resulting in normalization of performance, or whether a true ergogenic effect is possible.

Boron is an obscure ultratrace mineral that, until recently, has attracted little research attention. A possible beneficial effect on bone metabolism via interactions with calcium and magnesium metabolism has been reported.[414] Boron supplementation improved magnesium status in sedentary and athletic females, with positive implications for bone mass.[415]

Boron has attracted recent attention as an anabolic steroid alternative because of a report finding a tripling of serum testosterone levels in elderly women after boron supplementation (3 mg/d as borate for 42 d).[414] These results have stimulated a fad of boron supplement consumption by bodybuilders and weightlifters wanting an anabolic steroid effect. This commerical interest stimulated a study by Ferrando and Green, who administered a boron supplement (2.5 mg/d) to ten bodybuilders, and a placebo to nine bodybuilders for 7 weeks.[416] Although serum boron levels increased in the supplemented group, no effects of boron could be found for plasma total and free testosterone, lean body mass, or strength (one repetition maximum squat and bench press values).[416] Large individual variations suggest that group trends could be obscured by small number of subjects, but the results strongly suggest that

2.5 mg of boron is insufficient to be an anabolic steroid alternative in humans. An animal report found a "physiological role for boron in energy metabolism regulation possible at the site of lactate formation and/or utilization" after 36 d of exercise training and feeding a diet containing 2.0 mg/kg of boron.[459] Thus, potential ergogenic effects of boron are not obvious, and may relate to interactions with magnesium status. Boron does form unusual bridge bonds that augment hydroxylation of steroid rings (vitamin D, androgens, estrogens, progestins, corticosteroids). Further research on boron using higher doses should consider hormonal effects before confirmation or denial of boron as an ergogenic acid.

M. Methyl Donors (DMG, Pangamate, Lecithin, Choline)

Methyl donors are a group of compounds found in intermediary metabolism. Functionally, vitamin B_{12}, folate, and methionine are also methyl donors, and their ergogenic possibilities have already been discussed earlier in this chapter. Betaine (trimethylglycine or TMG), sarcosine, and S-adenosylmethionine (SAM), are also components of methyl group metabolism.

Ergogenic effects of methyl donors on athletes have focused on two compounds: lecithin and dimethylglycine (DMG). Lecithin (soybean oil phospholipids containing 17 to 35% phosphatidyl choline) was the first inexpensive commerical source of methyl donors. Putative mechanisms of enhanced creatine synthesis and improved function of neural and muscular membranes have been proposed. However, no recent studies have examined ergogenic effects of lecithin or choline supplementation, even though plasma choline levels in runners after a marathon race were severely depleted.[417]

Ergogenic research on methyl donors has focused on DMG and its related compound, pangamic acid. Russian research reported enhanced performance following supplementation with 100 to 300 mg/d of pangamate.[418] Rumored use of pangamate by successful Russian Olympic athletes in the 1960s initiated a cult status for pangamate use by athletes in the U.S. The use of pangamate gave way to its active principle, DMG. Interestingly, no other food supplement has attracted the regulatory attention that pangamate and DMG have enjoyed, making researcher bias in studies on these compounds a major variable.[419]

Only three studies found any sort of ergogenic effect from pangamate or DMG supplementation.[419-421] One study showed very large increases of treadmill time to exhaustion and $\dot{V}O_2$ max after a small dose of 5 mg/d of pangamic acid.[420] The other studies found increased work tolerance and decreased blood lactate levels after exercise.[419,421]

However, five well-controlled studies found no beneficial ergogenic effects from DMG in maximal or submaximal exercises after daily doses of 100 to 200 mg/d.[422-427] Thus, ergogenic capabilities of DMG (and pangamate) are unproven at the doses studied.

N. Nucleotides (Inosine)

Like pangamic acid, a fad of inosine supplementation is still sweeping the U.S. after rumors of use by Russian and Eastern Bloc athletes (especially weightlifters). Inosine has been touted as a precursor for ATP that also possesses inotropic effects which have been thought to improve oxygen utilization, and thus, anaerobic performance.[4,6,428]

Inosine supplementation (3 g/d) to four trained weightlifters in a double-blind, matched-pairs crossover study appeared to increase one-repetition maximum strength, but no statistical analysis was presented.[428] The investigator commented that prolonged use of inosine tended to exhaust athletes.[428] Another recent report actually found decreased time to exhaustion during treadmill running after inosine supplementation (6 g/d for 2 d) to nine trained endurance runners.[429]

Inosine supplementation is theoretically an antiergogenic aid because: (1) inosine metabolism increases free radical production during exercise; (2) inosine metabolism increases serum urate levels, contributing to gout in susceptible individuals; (3) inosine metabolism is associated with increased formation of fatigue-producing ammonia; and (4) inosine is also a degradation product of ATP metabolism during exercise.[430]

Inosine supplementation may be more detrimental than ineffective for changing performance, and is not recommended under any circumstances (unless one wants to sabotage exercise performance). Hopefully, the low doses found in most nutritional supplements sold to athletes are insufficient to alter tissue levels of inosine, but this concept is untested.

O. Octacosanol and Wheat Germ Oil

A long-chain (C_{28}) waxy alcohol, octacosanol is a common plant compound, and is found in many edible plants (especially wheat germ oil). A series of experiments by Cureton on wheat germ oil eventually identified octacosanol as the active ingredient.[177] Improvements in endurance times and reaction times were reported,[177] but since no obvious mechanism of action was convincingly demonstrated, and other early reports did not reproduce Cureton's findings, use of wheat germ oil and octacosanol has fallen out of favor as an ergogenic aid.[431]

One report did not find effects of octacosanol supplementation (1000 μg/d for 8 weeks) to 16 subjects on aerobic metabolism, but did find improved reaction times to visual and auditory stimuli, along with increased grip strength.[432] Thus, octacosanol may act by neuromuscular membrane stabilization. This interesting study, if replicated, would indicate that octacosanol may affect performance in skill sports requiring hand–eye coordination and split-second timing, such as tennis, racquetball, squash, baseball, jai-alai, race car driving, equestrian events, soccer, basketball, hockey, lacrosse, and football.

P. Phosphates

Phosphates were initially studied as ergogenic aids because of the early observations of phosphate compounds (ATP) as being crucial for cellular energy production and muscular function. Use of phosphate salts dates back to World War I.[173] Many early reports suffered from lack of data, lack of statistical analysis, lack of experimental controls, or subjective measurements of fatigue and performance.[173] At least the safety of large oral doses (1 to 10 g/d) of phosphate salts was proven.

Phosphate supplementation (4 g/d of neutral-buffered phosphates for 3 d) or placebo supplementation (0.4 g/d of sodium citrate) consisting of two trials with each type of supplement found increased $\dot{V}O_2$ max, increased serum phosphate levels, increased 2,3-diphosphoglycerate (2,3-DPG) levels in erythrocytes, and decreased midexercise blood lactate levels during exhaustive treadmill runs after phosphate loading.[433] Subjects ran from one to three increments higher during phosphate periods than during placebo periods, indicating improved maximal exercise performance. Another study did not find any changes in leg power, $\dot{V}O_2$, or exhaustive treadmill run times following phosphate loading (1.24 g sodium–potassium phosphate 1 h before exercise or 3.73 g/d for 6 d).[434] Biochemical measurements were not performed.

The conflicting results of these two studies show a need for further testing of phosphate loading to assess potential ergogenic effects.

Q. Pollen

Bee pollen (flower pollen) has attracted considerable popular use as an ergogenic aid and tonic food.[431] Several European studies reported increased work capacity,[435] and improved lactate levels, ECG readings, and respiratory performance[436] for weightlifters. However, five other studies did not find ergogenic effects from bee pollen.[431,436-439] Doses of bee pollen ranged from unspecified to 2700 mg/d. Thus, bee pollen has not been proven consistently as an ergogenic aid, and the bulk of evidence does not favor ergogenic properties.

A new type of pollen product has recently appeared (Polbax), made from fertilized pollen tubes harvested at a specific growth stage to provide measurable levels of superoxide dismutase (SOD) activity.[440] Supplementation with unspecified amounts of Polbax or placebo for 4 weeks found significant reductions in postexercise indices of free radical damage and higher muscle glycogen contents after Polbax administration.[440] Thus, a possible antioxidant effect was apparent, even though previous research has not found evidence of absorption of purified SOD into circulation after oral administration.[441,442] At present, use of pollen as an ergogenic aid is not supported.

R. Vitamins A, D, and K

The fat-soluble vitamins A, D, and K have not shown any ergogenic effects after supplementation to humans, and also have no clear mechanism or rationale for enhancement of performance.[4,6,199-201] The only vitamin studied for ergogenic effects was vitamin D (calciferols), and two reports failed to find any effects on cycle ergometer performance after high doses of vitamin D supplementation (1500 IU/d).[443,444]

The fat-soluble vitamins are associated with significant toxicity when ingested in large amounts for long time periods. Vitamin A (retinol), but *not* beta-carotene, has caused toxicity in a soccer player[445] and many others.[199,446] Doses of 50,000 IU/d or more of retinol equivalents can eventually be toxic to adults. In addition, high doses of retinol may be teratogenic, causing fetal malformations.[199]

Symptoms of vitamin A toxicity include headaches, dry skin, hair loss, fatigue, muscle pain, bone pain, joint pain, diarrhea, anorexia, edema, bulging fontanelles (foreheads), liver and spleen enlargement, insomnia, irritability, nausea, vomiting, and weight loss.[199]

Similarly, very high doses of vitamin D (>50,000 IU/d for adults) can be toxic, causing hypercalcemia, hypercalciuria, anorexia, nausea, vomiting, thirst, polyuria, muscle weakness, joint pains, bone demineralizations, disorientation, and soft tissue calcifications (including arteries).[447]

No hazards from natural food sources of vitamin K have been reported, but pharmacological doses may antagonize coumarin function (an anticoagulant drug given to some patients).[448] Loading with fat-soluble vitamins A, D, or K is not recommended because of toxicity and lack of ergogenic effects.

S. Vitamin–Mineral Combinations

Although an almost limitless number of products containing only vitamins and minerals are possible (and it seems, available), most products are actually very similar and frequently the only real differences are doses of B vitamins and the presence/absence of trace minerals. Addition of other nutrients discussed in this chapter to vitamins and minerals is also quite common, leading to literally hundreds of such products available commercially. Only a very few commercial mixture products have been studied for ergogenic effects.

Of the studies listed in Table 14,[123,201,431,449-454] only three showed any evidence of improved performance,[449-451] but each suffered from a lack of experimental control, leaving results suspect. Thus, in general, studies of comprehensive nutrient combinations have not shown ergogenic effects, possibly due to low doses of each particular nutrient.

T. Other Untested Compounds with Theoretical Benefits

Table 15 lists the nutrient compounds that have been advocated as ergogenic aids for either anaerobic exercise (weightlifting) or endurance exercises. An example is gamma-hydroxybutyrate (GHB), or sodium oxybate, which enjoyed a brief life as a nutritional supplement from 1989 to 1991 (Bucci, unpublished data). On paper, GHB appeared to be an ideal candidate for a nutritional ergogenic aid. Promotional literature from companies

TABLE 14 Contents and Ergogenic Effects of Nutrient Combinations, Including Multiple Vitamin–Mineral Formulations

Investigator (Year) (Exercise type studied)	Supplement Contents	Ergogenic Effects	Ref.
Cockerill and Bucci (1987)	B complex vitamins Vitamin C Amino acids Arginine and ornithine Gamma oryzanol Octacosanol Chlorophyll Coenzyme Q_{10} Glandulars	↓ Body fat ↑ Muscle girth	449
Ushakov (1978) (submaximal step test)	B complex vitamins Vitamins A, C Calcium Magnesium Phosphates Amino acids Nucleic acid Rutin	↓ Heart rate	450
Keul and Haralambie (1974) (submaximal cycle ergometry)	B complex vitamins Vitamins C, E Calcium Magnesium Potassium Phosphates Complex carbohydrates	↓ Heart rate ↑ Work efficiency	451
McCollum (1960) (variety of exercise tests)	B complex vitamins Vitamins A, C, D ± Lysine	Physical performance, NS	123
Williams (1985) (cycle ergometry, vertical jump, sprint times)	Multiple vitamin–mineral	Endurance power, NS	201
Williams (1985) (arm ergometry, cable tensiometry)	Caffeine Glucose Citrate (sodium) Phosphate Vitamins B_1, C	Endurance, recovery, strength, NS	431
Barnett and Conlee (1984) (65–70% $\dot{V}O_2$ max treadmill runs)	Multiple vitamin–mineral	$\dot{V}O_2$ max, lactate, glucose, free fatty acids, glycogen depletion, NS	452
Weight et al. (1988) (running performance)	Multiple vitamin–mineral (composition not listed)	All measures of running performance, NS	453
Anderson et al. (1990) (swim times, treadmill test)	Vitamin E succinate Inosine Coenzyme Q_{10} Magnesium glycerol phosphate Cytochrome c	Swim times, $\dot{V}O_2$ max, NS	454

TABLE 15 Putative Nutritional Ergogenic Aids with Commercial Availability

Alpha ketoacids	Glutathione
Ascorbyl palmitate	Herbs (numerous)
Adenosine phosphates	Lactate, polylactates
Amino acids not previously tested	Lipoic acid (thioctic acid)
Avena sativa (wild oats)	NADH, NADPH
Betaine (trimethylglycine, TMG)	Pantethine, pantetheine
Carnosine	Phytosterols (beta sitosterol, etc.)
Chlorophyll	Pyruvate
Cytochrome c	Sarcosine
Citrulline malate	Sarsaparilla
Colloidal silicates	*Smilax* extracts
Dessicated liver	Somatomedins
Dihydroepiandrostenedione (DHEA)	Succinates
Ecdysterone	Tricarboxylic acid cycle intermediates
Gamma hydroxybutyrate (GHB)	Vanadium salts
Glandulars (dried raw animal organs)	Yohimbine bark

selling GHB distributed pamphlets with explanations of peer-reviewed research articles on physiological effects of GHB administration to humans, complete with bar charts and tables of data. Some excerpts from this literature are listed as follows:

> GHB is the most powerful GH (growth hormone) releaser yet discovered: Independent studies show GH (growth hormone) levels increase 9–16 times higher than resting levels, after administration of GHB.

> GHB is proven to reduce body fat and increase muscle mass:

> ... long-term administration of large doses (4–9 grams per day) for long periods of time (up to nine years) have shown no negative side effects whatsoever.

Included with promotional literature were copies of several research articles on GHB, none of which studied athletes or effects on exercise performance.[455-458] Thus, while the documented effects of GHB ingestion on serum somatotropin levels were strongly promoted, other properties of GHB were ignored or stated to be insignificant in promotional literature, which is a far different conclusion from that which a biochemist or physician would deduce.

Although promotional literature recommended taking GHB only before bedtime or naptime, the potent anesthetic, hypnotic, and neurobehavioral effects were not explained. It turns out that GHB, as sodium oxybate, is classified as a drug, and utilized to induce anesthesia in Japan and Europe. Side effects of muscle movements, nausea, vomiting, respiratory depression, hypokalemia, bradycardia, and occasional emergence delirium were found during a computer search of the Martindale Drug Information Database.

Although GHB did possess a property desirable to bodybuilders, there were enough other, potent effects to argue against indiscriminate use without medical supervision. In 1990, GHB was advocated as a legal hallucinogen (Bucci, unpublished data). Soon, reports from Florida of persons ingesting 10 to 30 g of GHB for recreational drug purposes listed nausea, vomiting, respiratory depression, dyskinesia, seizures, and coma. The Food and Drug Administration (FDA) banned and confiscated all known nutritional supplies of GHB as an unapproved drug.

Of course, the unique and potent properties of GHB turned the usual practices of promoting intermediary metabolites into a potentially dangerous business. This story illustrates the point

TABLE 16 Guidelines for Rational Use of Nutritional Ergogenic Aids with Documented Efficacy

Aerobic Exercise: running, cycling, swimming, skiing, sports events or training lasting longer than 60 min

1. Carbohydrate/Electrolyte Drinks — 400–600 ml before event, and 100–200 ml every 15 min during event
2. Glycogen Supercompensation (Carbohydrate Loading) — single events: 60–70% carbohydrate diet started one week before event; taper exercise down by half every 2nd day until event; consume >300 g carbohydrates (low fat, low fiber, complex) 3–4 h before event; consume 500–700 mg carbohydrates (sugars) immediately after exercise
3. Protein Intake — maintain 1.8–2 g protein/kg/d intake during strenuous training
4. Iron — if anemic or iron-depleted, add 15–50 mg of supplemental iron from organic chelates; increase dietary heme iron (lean meats) and vitamin C (fresh fruits and vegetables)
5. Caffeine — 200–300 mg (2–3 fresh brewed cups of coffee) 1 h before event
6. B Complex Vitamins — high doses of thiamin and pantothenate (100–2000 mg/d each)
7. L-carnitine — 1.0–3.0 g/d
8. Coenzyme Q_{10} — 60–100 mg/d
9. Antioxidant Mixture — vitamin E, 400–800 IU/d; vitamin C, 500–2,000 mg/d; beta-carotene, 25,000–100,000 IU/d; selenium, 100–250 µg/d

Anaerobic Exercise: weightlifting, bodybuilding, track and field, maximal intensity events (short-term or <60 min exhaustive exercise)

1. Protein Intake — 100–200 g/d (2.0–2.5 g protein/kg/d)
2. Sodium Bicarbonate (baking soda) — 0.2–0.3 g/kg 1–3 h before exercise; consume water *ad libitum*
3. Antioxidant Mixture — (same as for aerobic exercise)

that any perceived benefit from previously unmarketed nutrients will be avidly sought after and exploited, regardless of scientific research findings. Research on ergogenic effects of nutrients listed in Table 15 will assist in determining whether a given nutrient has ergogenic potential.

IV. SUMMARY AND CONCLUSIONS

A bottom line for efficacy of nutritional ergogenic aids is that manipulation of diet or addition of specific compounds at adequate doses for adequate length of time has the ability to improve exercise performance compared to a nonmanipulated or nonsupplemented state. Magnitude of performance improvement can range from slightly better than normal (not apparent in real-life situations) to finishing otherwise impossible tasks. Certainly, psychological and training contributions to exercise performance are usually of greater magnitude than nutritional modulations. In other words, there is still no pill or diet that will transform a sedentary, middle-aged clerk into a world-class Olympic track and field athlete. However, when training, motivation, and talent are already optimal, nutritional ergogenic aids offer a viable option to provide a small but significant improvement in performance. In addition, the practice of nutritional modulation offers a placebo response itself.

Research on nutritional ergogenic aids is adequate to deduce general guidelines for water, electrolytes, and carbohydrates. Other nutrients need further work before definite guidelines can be regarded as dogma. However, enough evidence has accumulated to make convincing cases for supplementation with protein, iron, caffeine, B complex vitamins, L-carnitine, coenzyme Q_{10}, bicarbonate, and antioxidants in specific conditions, as listed in Table 16.

Experimental variables that need more attention in future studies are (1) effects of muscle fiber type composition, (2) dosage level, dose response, and dose threshold effects, (3) training status of subjects, (4) nutritional status and dietary intakes of subjects before, during, and after study periods, and (5) exercise type, intensity, and duration effects.

A final conclusion from the brief overview of research on nutritional ergogenic aids is that there is no question that dietary manipulation or supplements can improve human exercise performance in certain settings. A prevailing opinion that supplementation of athletes with nutrients is useless, harmful, or quackery is rapidly melting under the heat of scientific findings. Table 16 lists nutritional ergogenic aids with documentation of efficacy.

ACKNOWLEDGMENTS

The author would like to thank Rose Kelly and Naniece Bucci for excellent handling of the manuscript.

REFERENCES

1. **Hickson, J. F., Jr. and Wolinsky, I.,** Human protein intake and metabolism in exercise and sport, in *Nutrition in Exercise and Sport,* Vol. 1, Hickson, J. F., Jr. and Wolinsky, I., Eds., CRC Press, Boca Raton, FL, 1989, 5.
2. **Simopoulos, A. P.,** Opening address. Nutrition and fitness from the first Olympiad in 776 BC to 393 AD and the concept of positive health, *Am. J. Clin. Nutr.,* 49 (Suppl.), 921, 1989.
3. **Finley, M. I. and Pleket, H. W., Eds.,** *The Olympic Games: The First Thousand Years,* Chatto & Windus, London, 1976, 93.
4. **Bucci, L. R.,** *Nutrients as Ergogenic Aids in Exercise and Sport,* CRC Press, Boca Raton, 1993.
5. **Lamb, D. R. and Williams, M. H.,** *Perspectives in Exercise Science and Sports Medicine,* Vol. 4, *Ergogenics: The Enhancement of Sports Performance,* Benchmark Press, Indianapolis, 1991.
6. **Bucci, L. R.,** Nutritional ergogenic aids, in *Nutrition in Exercise and Sport,* Hickson, J. F., Jr. and Wolinsky, I., Eds., CRC Press, Boca Raton, FL, 1989, 107.
7. **Williams, M. H.,** Vitamin supplementation and athletic performance, *Int. J. Vit. Nutr. Res. Suppl.,* 30, 163, 1989.
8. **Horton, E. S. and Terjung, R. L., Eds.,** *Exercise, Nutrition and Metabolism,* Macmillan, New York, 1988.
9. **Garrett, W. E. and Malone, T. E., Eds.,** *Muscle Development: Nutritional Alternatives to Anabolic Steroids,* Ross Laboratories, Columbus, 1988.
10. **Winick, M., Ed.,** *Nutrition and Exercise,* John Wiley & Sons, New York, 1986.
11. **Williams, M. H., Ed.,** *Nutritional Aspects of Human Physical and Athletic Performance,* 2nd ed., Charles C Thomas, Springfield, 1985.
12. **Williams, M. H., Ed.,** *Ergogenic Aids in Sports,* Human Kinetics Publishers, Champaign, 1983.
13. **Fox, E. L., Ed.,** *Ross Symposium on Nutrient Utilization During Exercise,* Ross Laboratories, Columbus, 1983.
14. **Haskell, W., Scala, J., and Whittam, J., Eds.,** *Nutrition and Athletic Performance,* Bull Publishing, Palo Alto, 1982.
15. **Morgan, W. P., Ed.,** *Ergogenic Aids and Muscular Performance,* Academic Press, New York, 1972.
16. **Pivarnik, J. M.,** Water and electrolytes during exercise, in *Nutrition in Exercise and Sport,* Hickson, J. F., Jr. and Wolinsky, I., Eds., CRC Press, Boca Raton, FL, 1989, 185.
17. **Greenleaf, J. E.,** The body's need for fluids, in *Nutrition and Athletic Performance,* Haskell, W., Scala, J., and Whittam, J., Eds., Bull Publishing, Palo Alto, 1982.
18. **Fink, W. J.,** Fluid intake for maximizing athletic performance, in *Nutrition and Athletic Performance,* Haskell, W., Scala, J., and Whittam, J., Eds., Bull Publishing, Palo Alto, 1982, 52.
19. **Herbert, W. G.,** Water and electrolytes, in *Ergogenic Aids in Sports,* Williams, M. H., Ed., Human Kinetics Publishers, Champaign, 1983, 56.
20. **Gisolfi, C. V.,** Water and electrolyte metabolism in exercise, in *Ross Symposium on Nutrient Utilization During Exercise,* Fox, E. L., Ed., Ross Laboratories, Columbus, 1983, 21.
21. **Sawka, M. N., Francesconi, R. P., Young, A. J., and Pandolf, K. B.,** Influence of hydration level and body fluids on exercise in the heat, *JAMA,* 252, 1165, 1984.
22. **Williams, M. H.,** The role of water and electrolytes in physical activity, in *Nutritional Aspects of Human Physical and Athletic Performance,* 2nd ed., Williams, M. H., Ed., Charles C Thomas, Springfield, 1985, 219.
23. **Saltin, B. and Costill, D. L.,** Fluid and electrolyte balance during prolonged exercise, in *Exercise, Nutrition and Metabolism,* Horton, E. S. and Terjung, R. L., Eds., Macmillan, New York, 1988, 150.

24. **Buskirk, E. R. and Puhl, S.,** Nutritional beverages: Exercise and sport, in *Nutrition in Exercise and Sport,* Hickson, J. F., Jr. and Wolinsky, I., Eds., CRC Press, Boca Raton, FL, 1989, 201.

25. **Maughan, R. J. and Noakes, T. D.,** Fluid replacement and exercise stress. A brief review of studies on fluid replacement and some guidelines for the athlete, *Sports Med.,* 12(1), 16, 1991.

26. **Nadel, E. R., Fortney, S. M., and Wenger, C. B.,** Effect of hydration state on circulatory and thermal regulations, *J. Appl. Physiol.,* 49, 715, 1980.

27. **Blythe, C. and Burt, J.,** Effect of water balance on ability to perform in high ambient temperatures, *Res. Q. Am. Assoc. Health Phys. Educ.,* 32, 301, 1961.

28. **Moroff, S. V. and Bass, D. E.,** Effects of overhydration on man's physiological responses to work in the heat, *J. Appl. Physiol.,* 20, 267, 1965.

29. **Greenleaf, J.,** Exercise and water electrolyte balance, in *Nutrition and Physical Activity,* Blix, G., Ed., Almqvist & Wiksells, Uppsala, Sweden, 1967, 54.

30. **Greenleaf, J. and Castle, B.,** Exercise temperature regulation in man during hypohydration and hyperhydration, *J. Appl. Physiol.,* 30, 847, 1971.

31. **Nielsen, B.,** Thermoregulation in exercising man during dehydration and hyperhydration with water and saline, *Int. J. Biometeorol.,* 15, 195, 1971.

32. **Gisolfi, C. and Copping, J.,** Thermal effects of prolonged treadmill exercise in the heat, *Med. Sci. Sports,* 6, 108, 1974.

33. **Foley, P.,** Effect of ingesting water in swimming, *Swimming Technique,* 8, 34, 1971.

34. **Noakes, T. D., Goodwin, N., Rayner, B. L., Branken, T., and Taylor, R. K. N.,** Water intoxication: a possible complication during endurance exercise, *Med. Sci. Sports Exercise,* 17, 370, 1985.

35. **Deschamps, A., Levy, R. D., Cosio, M. G., Marliss, E. B., and Magder, S.,** Effect of saline infusion on body temperature and endurance during heavy exercise, *J. Appl. Physiol.,* 66, 2799, 1989.

36. American College of Sports Medicine, Position stand on prevention of thermal injuries during distance running, *Med. Sci. Sports Exercise,* 16, ix, 1984.

37. **Greenhaff, P. L. and Clough, P. J.,** Predictors of sweat loss in man during prolonged exercise, *Eur. J. Appl. Physiol.,* 58, 348, 1989.

38. **Maughan, R. J.,** Thermoregulation and fluid balance in marathon competition at low ambient temperature, *Int. J. Sports Med.,* 6, 15, 1985.

39. **Schamadam, J. and Snively, W.,** The role of potassium in diseases due to heat stress, *Ind. Med. Surg.,* 36, 785, 1967.

40. **Knochel, J. P. and Vertel, R. M.,** Salt loading as a possible factor in the production of potassium depletion, rhabdomyolysis, and heat injury, *Lancet,* 1, 659, 1967.

41. **Costill, D.,** Water and electrolytes, in *Ergogenic Aids and Muscular Performance,* Morgan, W., Ed., Academic Press, New York, 1972.

42. **Schamadam, J. and Snively, W.,** Evaluation of potassium-rich electrolytes solutions as oral prophylaxis for heat stress, *Ind. Med. Surg.,* 37, 677, 1968.

43. **Settineri, L. and Allgayer, C.,** Utilization of potassium chloride "per os" for the prevention of muscle cramps in athletes, in *Nutrition and Sport,* Litvinova, V., Ed., Leningrad Institute of Physical Culture, Leningrad, 1976.

44. **Lane, H. W. and Cerda, J.,** Potassium requirements and exercise, *J. Am. Diet. Assoc.,* 73, 64, 1978.

45. **Lane, H. W. and Cerda, J.,** Potassium requirements and exercise, *Am. Correct. Ther. J.,* 33, 67, 1979.

46. **Costill, D. L. and Hargreaves, M.,** Carbohydrate nutrition and fatigue, *Sports Med.,* 13(2), 86, 1992.

47. **Miller, G. D. and Massaro, E. J.,** Carbohydrate in ultra-endurance performance, in *Nutrition in Exercise and Sport,* Hickson, J. F., Jr. and Wolinsky, I., Eds., CRC Press, Boca Raton, FL, 1989, 51.

48. **Pate, T. D. and Brunn, J. C.,** Fundamentals of carbohydrate metabolism, in *Nutrition in Exercise and Sport,* Hickson, J. F., Jr. and Wolinsky, I., Eds., CRC Press, Boca Raton, FL, 1989, 37.

49. **Nagle, F. J. and Bassett, D. R.,** Energy metabolism, in *Nutrition in Exercise and Sport,* Hickson, J. F., Jr. and Wolinsky, I., Eds., CRC Press, Boca Raton, FL, 1989, 87.

50. **Valeriani, A.,** The need for carbohydrate intake during endurance exercise, *Sports Med.,* 12(6), 349, 1991.

51. **Williams, M. H.,** The role of carbohydrates in physical activity, in *Nutritional Aspects of Human Physical and Athletic Performance,* 2nd ed., Williams, M. H., Ed., Charles C Thomas, Springfield, 1985, 58.

52. **Wilmore, J. H. and Freund, B. J.,** Nutritional enhancement of athletic performance, in *Nutrition and Exercise,* Winick, M., Ed., John Wiley & Sons, New York, 1986, 67.

53. **Sherman, W. H.,** Carbohydrates, muscle glycogen and muscle glycogen supercompensation, in *Ergogenic Aids in Sports,* Williams, M. H., Ed., Human Kinetics Publishers, Champaign, 1983, 3.

54. **Bergstrom, J., Hermansen, L., Hultman, E., and Saltin, B.,** Diet, muscle glycogen, and physican performance, *Acta Physiol. Scand.,* 71, 140, 1967.

55. **Costill, D. L.,** Carbohydrates for exercise: dietary demands for optimal performance, *Int. J. Sports Med.,* 9, 1, 1988.

56. **Coyle, E. F.,** Carbohydrate supplementation during exercise, *J. Nutr.,* 122, 788, 1992.

57. **Hawley, J. A., Dennis, S. C., and Noakes, T. D.,** Oxidation of carbohydrate ingested during prolonged endurance exercise, *Sports Med.,* 14, 27, 1992.

58. **Maughan, R.,** Carbohydrate-electrolyte solutions during prolonged exercise, in *Perspectives in Exercise Science and Sports Medicine,* Vol. 4, *Ergogenics, Enhancement of Performance in Exercise and Sport,* Lamb, D. R. and Williams, M. H., Eds., Benchmark Press, Indianapolis, 1991, 35.

59. **Applegate, L.,** Drinks to your health, *Runner's World,* 26, 24, 1991.

60. **Friedman, J. E., Neufer, P. D., and Dohm, G. L.,** Regulation of glycogen resynthesis following exercise. Dietary considerations, *Sports Med.,* 11(4), 232, 1991.

61. **Lemon, P. W. R.,** Protein and exercise: update 1987, *Med. Sci. Sports Exercise,* 19, S179, 1987.

62. **Lemon, P. W. R. and Proctor, D. N.,** Protein intake and athletic performance, *Sports Med.,* 12(5), 313, 1991.

63. **Kaufmann, D. A,.** Protein as an energy substrate during intense exercise, *Ann. Sports Med.,* 5, 142, 1990.

64. **Williams, M. H.,** The role of protein in physical exercise, in *Nutritional Aspects of Human Physical and Athletic Performance,* 2nd ed., Williams, M. H., Ed., Charles C Thomas, Springfield, 1985, 120.

65. **Kraut, H. and Müller, E. A.,** Muselkrafte und Eiweissration, *Biochem. Z.,* 320, 302, 1950.

66. **Kraut, H., Müller, E. A., and Müller-Wecker, H.,** Der Einfluss zu Zusammensetzung des Nahrungseiweisses auf Stickstoffbilanz und Muskeltraining, *Int. Z. Angew. Physiol.,* 17, 378, 1958.

67. **Rasch, P. and Pierson, W.,** The effect of a protein dietary supplement on muscular strength and hypertrophy, *Am. J. Clin. Nutr.,* 11, 530, 1962.

68. **Rasch, P., Hamby, J. W., and Burns, H. J.,** Protein dietary supplementation and physical performance, *Med. Sci. Sports,* 1, 195, 1969.

69. **Consolazio, C. F., Johnson, H. L., Nelson, R. A., Dramise, J. G., and Skala, J. H.,** Protein metabolism during intensive physical training in the young adult, *Am. J. Clin. Nutr.,* 28, 29, 1975.

70. **Oddoye, E. B. and Margen, S.,** Nitrogen balance studies in humans: long-term effect of high nitrogen intake on nitrogen accretion, *J. Nutr.,* 109, 363, 1979.

71. **Marable, N. L., Hickson, J. F., Korslund, M. K., Herbert, W. G., and Desjardins, R. F.,** Urinary nitrogen excretion as influenced by a muscle-building exercise program and protein intake variation, *Nutr. Rep. Int.,* 19, 795, 1979.

72. **Dragan, G. I., Vasiliu, A., and Georgescu, E.,** Effects of increased supply of protein on elite weight lifters, in *Milk Proteins '84,* Galesloot, T. E. and Timbergen, B. J., Eds., Pudoc, Waningen, Netherlands, 1985, 176.

73. **Hecker, A. L. and Wheeler, K. B.,** Protein: a misunderstood nutrient for the athlete, *NSCA J.,* 7(6), 28, 1985.

74. **Frontera, W. R., Meredith, C. N., O'Reilly, K. P., Knuttgen, G., and Evans, W. J.,** Strength conditioning in older men: skeletal muscle hypertrophy and improved function, *J. Appl. Physiol.,* 64, 1038, 1988.

75. **Dohm, G. L.,** Protein nutrition for the athlete, *Clin. Sports Med.,* 3, 595, 1985.

76. **Banister, E. W. and Cameron, B. J. C.,** Exercise-induced hyperammonemia: peripheral and central effects, *Int. J. Sports Med.,* 11, S129, 1990.

77. **Mutch, B. J. C. and Banister, E. W.,** Ammonia metabolism in exercise and fatigue: a review, *Med. Sci. Sports Exercise,* 15, 41, 1983.

78. **Banister, E. W., Rajendra, W., and Mutch, B. J. C.,** Ammonia as an indicator of exercise stress: implications of recent findings to sports medicine, *Sports Med.,* 2, 34, 1985.

79. **Maudsley, D. V.,** Regulations of polyamine biosynthesis, *Biochem. Pharmacol.,* 38, 153, 1979.

80. **Knopf, R. F., Conn, J. W., Falans, S. S., Floyd, J. C., Guntsche, E. M., and Rull, J. A.,** Plasma growth hormone responses to intravenous administration of amino acids, *Clin. Endocrinol.,* 25, 1140, 1965.

81. **Merimee, T. J., Rabinowitz, D., Riggs, L., Burgess, J. A., Rimoin, D. L., and McKusick, V. A.,** Plasma growth hormone after arginine infusion. Clinical experiences, *N. Engl. J. Med.,* 276, 434, 1967.

82. **Bratusch-Marrain, P. and Waldhausl, W.,** The influence of amino acids and somatostatin on prolactin and growth hormone release in man, *Acta Endocrinol.,* 90, 403, 1979.

83. **Onishi, T., Itoh, K. F., Miyai, K., Izumi, K., Shima, K., and Kumahara, Y.,** Prolactin response to arginine in normal subjects and in patients with hyperthyroidism, *J. Clin. Endocrinol.,* 42, 148, 1976.

84. **Gourmelen, M., Donnadieu, M., Schimpff, R. M., Lestradet, H., and Girard, F.,** Effect of ornithine monochloride on plasma HGH levels, *Ann. Endocrinol.,* 33, 526, 1972.

85. **Donnadieu, M., Combourieu, M., and Schimpff, R. M.,** Comparison de différentes épreuves de stimulation utilisées pour l'etude de la fonction somatotrope chez l'infant, *Pathol. Biol.,* 19, 293, 1971.

86. **Evian-Brion, D., Donnadieu, M., Roger, M., and Job, J. C.,** Simultaneous study of somatotrophic and corticotrophic pituitary secretions during ornithine infusion test, *Clin. Endocrinol.,* 17, 119, 1982.

87. **Mathieni, G.,** Growth hormone secretion by arginine stimulus: the effect of both low doses and oral arginine, *Boll. Soc. It. Sper. Biol.,* 56, 2254, 1980.

88. **Besset, L.,** Increase in sleep related growth hormone and prolactin secretion after chronic arginine aspartate administration, *Acta Endocrinol.,* 99, 18, 1982.

89. **Elsair, C.,** Effets de l'arginine, administrie par voie orale, *C. R. Soc. Biol.,* 179, 608, 1985.
90. **Isidori, A., Lo Monaco, A., and Cappa, M.,** A study of growth hormone release in man after oral administration of amino acids, *Curr. Med. Res. Opinion,* 7, 475, 1981.
91. **Bucci, L. R., Hickson, J. F., Pivarnik, J. M., Wolinsky, I., McMahon, J. C., and Turner, S. D.,** Ornithine ingestion and growth hormone release in bodybuilders, *Nutr. Res.,* 10, 239, 1990.
92. **Bucci, L. R., Hickson, J. F., Wolinsky, I., and Pivarnik, J. M.,** Ornithine supplementation and insulin release in bodybuilders, *Int. J. Sports Nutr.,* 2, 287, 1992.
93. **Macintyre, J. G.,** Growth hormone and athletes, *Sports Med.,* 4, 129, 1987.
94. **Elam, R. P.,** Morphological changes in adult males from resistance exercise and amino acid supplementation, *J. Sports Med.,* 28, 35, 1988.
95. **Nieper, H. A. and Blumberger, K.,** Electrolyte transport therapy of cardiovascular diseases, in *Electrolytes and Cardiovascular Diseases,* Vol. 2, Bajusz, E., Ed., S. Karger, Basel, 1966, 141.
96. **Kruse, C. A.,** Treatment of fatigue with aspartic acid salts, *Northwest Med.,* 60, 597, 1961.
97. **Shaw, D. L., Chesney, M. A., Tullis, I. F., and Agersborg, M. P. K.,** Management of fatigue: a physiological approach, *Am. J. Med. Sci.,* 243, 758, 1962.
98. Council on Drugs, American Medical Association, Potassium and magnesium aspartate (Spartase), *JAMA,* 183, 362, 1963.
99. **Fallis, N., Wilson, W. R., Tetreault, L. L., and Lasagna, L.,** Effect of potassium and magnesium aspartate on athletic performance, *JAMA,* 185, 129, 1963.
100. **Consolazio, C. F., Nelson, R. A., Matoush, L. O., and Isaac, G. J.,** Effects of aspartic acid salts (Mg and K) on physical performance of men, *J. Appl. Physiol.,* 19, 257, 1964.
101. **Ahlborg, B., Ekelund, L. G., and Nilsson, C. G.,** Effect of potassium-magnesium aspartate on the capacity for prolonged exercise in man, *Acta Physiol. Scand.,* 74, 238, 1968.
102. **Gupta, J. S. and Srivastava, K. K.,** Effect of potassium-magnesium aspartate on endurance work in man, *Ind. J. Exp. Biol.,* 11, 392, 1973.
103. **Von Franz, I. W. and Chintanaseri, C.,** Über die Wirkung des Kalium-Magnesium-Aspartates auf die Ausdauerleistung unter besonderer Berücksichtigung des Aspartates, *Sportarzt. Sportmed.,* 28, 37, 1977.
104. **Nagle, F. J., Balke, B., Ganslen, R. V., and Davis, A. W.,** The mitigation of physical fatigue with "Spartase", *U.S. Civil Aeromed. Res. Inst.,* 1, 1, 1963.
105. **Wesson, M., McNaughton, L., Davies, P., and Tristram, S.,** Effects of oral administration of aspartic acid salts on the endurance capacity of trained athletes, *Res. Q. Exercise Sport,* 59, 234, 1988.
106. **de Hann, A., van Doom, J. E., and Westra, H. G.,** Effects of potassium and magnesium aspartate on muscle metabolism and force development during intensive static exercise, *Int. J. Sports Med.,* 6, 44, 1985.
107. **Hagen, R. D., Upton, S. J., Duncan, J. J., Cummings, J. M., and Gettman, L. R.,** Absence of effect of potassium-magnesium aspartate on physiologic response to prolonged work in aerobically trained man, *Int. J. Sports Med.,* 3, 177, 1982.
108. **Maughan, R. J. and Sadler, D. J. M.,** The effects of oral administration of salts of aspartic acid on the metabolism response to prolonged exhausting exercise in man, *Int. J. Sports Med.,* 4, 119, 1983.
109. **Brodan, V., Kuhn, E., Pechar, J., Placer, Z., and Slabochova, Z.,** Effects of sodium glutamate infusion on ammonia formation during intense physical exercise in man, *Nutr. Rep. Int.,* 9, 223, 1974.
110. **Boothby, W. M.,** The clinical effect of glycine in progressive muscular dystrophy, in simple fatigability and on normal controls, *Proc. Staff Meet. Mayo Clin.,* 9, 600, 1934.
111. **Hench, P. S.,** A consideration of muscular pain and fatigue with a note on glycine: preliminary comment, *Proc. Staff Meet. Mayo Clin.,* 9, 603, 1934.
112. **McGuire, S.,** Glycine in the treatment of chronic fatigability, *Int. J. Med. Surg.,* 47, 459, 1934.
113. **Wilder, R. M.,** Discussion of reports by Drs. Boothby and Hench, *Proc. Staff Meet. Mayo Clin.,* 9, 606, 1934.
114. **Beard, H. H., Ed.,** *Creatine and Creatinine Metabolism,* Brooklyn Chemical Publishers, Brooklyn, NY, 1943.
115. **Chaikelis, A. S.,** The effect of glycocoll (glycine) ingestion upon the growth, strength and creatinine-creatine excretion in man, *Am. J. Physiol.,* 132, 578, 1941.
116. **Maison, G. L.,** Failure of gelatin or aminoacetic acid to increase the work ability, *JAMA,* 115, 1439, 1940.
117. **Horvath, S. M., Knehr, C. A., and Dill, D. B.,** The influence of glycine of muscular strength, *Am. J. Physiol.,* 134, 469, 1941.
118. **King, E. Q., McCaleb, L. B., Kennedy, H. F., and Klumpp, T. G.,** Failure of aminoacetic acid to increase the work capacity of human subjects, *JAMA,* 118, 594, 1942.
119. **Hilsendager, D. and Karpovich, P. V.,** Ergogenic effect of glycine and niacin separately and in combination, *Res. Q. Exerc. Sport,* 35, 389, 1964.
120. **Kasai, K., Suzuki, H., Nakamura, T., Shiina, H., and Shimoda, S.,** Glycine stimulates growth hormone in man, *Acta Endocrinol.,* 93, 283, 1980.

121. **Braverman, E. R. and Pfeiffer, C. C.,** Glycine, in *The Healing Nutrients Within. Facts, Findings and New Research on Amino Acids,* Braverman, E. R., and Pfeiffer, C. C., Eds., Keats Publishing, New Canaan, CT, 1986, 237.

122. **Kasai, K., Kobayashi, M., and Shimoda, S.,** Stimulatory effect of glycine on human growth hormone secretion, *Metabolism,* 27, 201, 1978.

123. **McCollum, R. H.,** The Effect of L-Lysine and a Vitamin Compound upon the Physical Performance of Subpar College Men, Ed.D. thesis, University of Oregon, Eugene, 1960.

124. **Muller, E. E., Brambilla, F., Cavagnini, F., Peracchi, M., and Panerai, A.,** Slight effect of L-tryptophan on growth hormone release in normal human subjects, *J. Clin. Endocrinol. Metab.,* 39, 1, 1974.

125. **Woolf, P. D. and Lee, L.,** Effect of the serotonin precursor, tryptophan, on pituitary hormone secretion, *J. Clin. Endocrinol. Metab.,* 45, 123, 1977.

126. **Fraser, W. M., Tucker, H. S., Grubb, S. R., Wigand, J. P., and Blackard, W. G.,** Effect of L-tryptophan on growth hormone and prolactin release in normal volunteers and patients with secretory pituitary tumors, *Horm. Metab. Res.,* 11, 149, 1979.

127. **Glass, A. R., Schaaf, M., and Dimond, R. C.,** Absent growth hormone response to L-tryptophan in acromegaly, *J. Clin. Endocrinol. Metab.,* 48, 664, 1979.

128. **Koulu, M. and Lammintausta, R.,** Effect of methionine on L-tryptophan and apomorphine-stimulated growth hormone secretion in man, *J. Clin. Endocrinol. Metab.,* 49, 70, 1979.

129. **Segura, R. and Ventura, J. L.,** Effect of L-tryptophan supplementation on exercise performance, *Int. J. Sports Med.,* 9, 301, 1988.

130. **Slutsker, L.,** Eosinophilia-myalgia syndrome associated with exposure to tryptophan from a single manufacturer, *JAMA,* 264(2), 213, 1990.

131. **Belongia, R.,** An investigation of the cause of the eosinophilia-myalgia syndrome associated with tryptophan use, *N. Engl. J. Med.,* 323(6), 357, 1990.

132. **Jaffe, R.,** Eosinophilia myalgia syndrome secondary to contaminated trypotophan — clinical experience, *J. Nutr. Med.,* 2, 195, 1991.

133. **Aldhous, P.,** Yellow light on L-tryptophan, *Nature,* 353, 490, 1991.

134. **Williams, M. H.,** The role of fat in physical activity, in *Nutritional Aspects of Human Physical and Athletic Performance,* 2nd ed., Williams, M. H., Ed., Charles C Thomas, Springfield, 1985, 106.

135. **Maughan, R. and Poole, D.,** The effects of a glycogen-loading regimen on the capacity to perform anaerobic exercise, *Eur. J. Appl. Physiol.,* 46, 211, 1981.

136. **Jansson, E. and Kaijser, L.,** Effect of diet on the utilization of blood-borne and intramuscular substrates during exercise in man, *Acta Physiol. Scand.,* 115, 19, 1982.

137. **Jansson, E. and Kaijser, L.,** Effect of diet on muscle glycogen and blood glucose utilization during short-term exercise in man, *Acta Physiol. Scand.,* 115, 341, 1982.

138. **Jansson, E., Hjemdahl, P., and Kaijser, L.,** Diet induced changes in sympatho-adrenal activity during submaximal exercise in relation to substrate utilization in man, *Acta Physiol. Scand.,* 114, 171, 1982.

139. **Phinney, S., Bistrian, B. R., Evans, W. J., Gervino, E., and Blackburn, G. L.,** The human metabolic response to chronic ketosis without caloric restriction: preservation of submaximal exercise capability with reduced carbohydrate oxidation, *Metabolism,* 32, 769, 1983.

140. **Cooney, M. M., Haymes, E. M., and Lucariello, G.,** The effects of a low carbohydrate-ketogenic diet in trained females, *Med. Sci. Sports Exercise,* 15, 129, 1983.

141. **Costill, D. L., Coyle, E., Dalsky, G., Evans, W., Fink, W., and Hoopes, D.,** Effects of elevated plasma FFA and insulin on muscle glycogen usage during exercise, *J. Appl. Physiol.,* 43, 695, 1977.

142. **Ivy, J., Costill, D. L., Fink, W. J., and Maglischo, E.,** Contribution of medium and long chain triglyceride intake to energy metabolism during prolonged exercise, *Int. J. Sports Med.,* 1, 15, 1980.

143. **Ivy, J., Costill, D. L., Van Handel, P. J., Essig, D. A., and Lower, R. W.,** Alteration in the lactate threshold with changes in substrate availability, *Int. J. Sports Med.,* 2, 139, 1981.

144. **Miller, J., Coyle, E. F., Sherman, W. M., Hagberg, J. M., Costill, D. L., Fink, W. J., Terblanche, S. E., and Holloszy, J. O.,** Effect of glycerol feeding on endurance and metabolism during prolonged exercise in man, *Med. Sci. Sports Exercise,* 15, 237, 1983.

145. **Brilla, L. R. and Landerholm, T. E.,** Effect of fish oil supplementation and exercise on serum lipids and aerobic fitness, *J. Sports Med.,* 30(2), 173, 1990.

146. **Simopoulos, A. P.,** Omega-3 fatty acids in health and disease and in growth and development, *Am. J. Clin. Nutr.,* 54, 438, 1991.

147. **Sears, B.,** BIOSYN Training Manual, Marblehead, 1990.

148. **Williams, M. H.,** Drug foods — alcohol and caffeine, in *Nutritional Aspects of Human Physical and Athletic Performance,* 2nd ed., Williams, M. H., Ed., Charles C Thomas, Springfield, 1985, 272.

149. **Williams, M. H., Ed.,** *Drugs and Athletic Performance,* Charles C Thomas, Springfield, 1974.

150. **McArdle, W. D., Katch, E. L., and Katch, V. L.,** Special aids to performance and conditioning, in *Exercise Physiology, Energy, Nutrition, and Human Performance,* 2nd ed., McArdle, W. D. et al., Eds., Lea & Febiger, Philadelphia, 1986, 401.

151. **Halliwell, B. and Gutteridge, J. M. C.,** *Free Radicals in Biology and Medicine,* 2nd ed., Clarendon Press, Oxford, 1989.

152. **Simic, M. G., Taylor, K. A., Ward, J. F., and von Sonntag, C., Eds.,** *Oxygen Radicals in Biology and Medicine,* Plenum Press, New York, 1988.

153. **Sjodin, B., Westing, Y. H., and Apple, F. S.,** Biochemical mechanisms for oxygen free radical formation during exercise, *Sports Med.,* 10, 236, 1990.

154. **Kagan, V. E., Spirichev, V. B., and Erin, A. N.,** Vitamin E in physical exercise and sport, in *Nutrition in Exercise and Sport,* Vol. 1, Hickson, J. F., Jr. and Wolinsky, I., Eds., CRC Press, Boca Raton, FL, 1989, 255.

155. **Singh, V. N.,** A current perspective on nutrition and exercise, *J. Nutr.,* 122, 760, 1992.

156. **Dillard, C. J., Litov, R. E., Savin, W. M., Dumelin, E. E., and Tappel, A. L.,** Effects of exercise, vitamin E and ozone on pulmonary function and lipid peroxidation, *J. Appl. Physiol.,* 45, 927, 1978.

157. **Kantner, M. M., Lesmes, G. R., Kaminsky, L. A., La Ham-Saeger, J., and Nequin, N. D.,** Serum creatine kinase and lactate dehydrogenase changes following an eighty kilometer race. Relationship to lipid peroxidation, *Eur. J. Appl. Physiol.,* 57, 60, 1988.

158. **Sumida, S., Tanaka, K., Kitao, H., and Nakadamo, F.,** Exercise-induced lipid peroxidation and leakage of enzymes before and after vitamin E supplementation, *Int. J. Biochem.,* 21, 835, 1989.

159. **Lovlin, R., Cottle, W., Pyke, I., Kavanagh, M., and Belcastro, A. N.,** Are indices of free radical damage related to exercise intensity, *Eur. J. Appl. Physiol.,* 56, 313, 1987.

160. **Corbucci, G. G., Montanari, G., Cooper, M. B., Jones, D. A., and Edwards, R. H. T.,** The effect of exertion on mitochondrial oxidative capacity and on some antioxidant mechanisms in muscle from marathon runners, *Int. J. Sports Med.,* 5 (Suppl.), 135, 1984.

161. **Viguie, C. A., Packer, L., and Brooks, G. A.,** Antioxidant supplementation affects indices of muscle trauma and oxidant stress in human blood during exercise, *Med. Sci. Sports Exercise,* 21(2), S16, 1989.

162. **Witt, E. H., Reznick, A. Z., Viguie, C. A., Starke-Reed, P., and Packer, L,** Exercise, oxidative damage and effects of antioxidant manipulation, *J. Nutr.,* 122, 766, 1992.

163. **Ismail, A. H., Petro, T. M., and Watson, R. R.,** Dietary supplementation with vitamin E and C in fit and nonfit adults: biochemical and immunological changes, *Fed. Proc.,* 42, 335, 1983.

164. **Moser, U. and Bendich, A.,** Vitamin C, in *Handbook of Vitamins,* 2nd ed., Machlin, L. J., Ed., Marcel Dekker, New York, 1991, 195.

165. **Williams, M. H.,** Vitamin, iron and calcium supplementation: effect on human physical performance, in *Nutrition and Athletic Performance,* Haskell, W., Scala, J., and Whittam, J., Eds., Bull Publishing, Palo Alto, 1982, 106.

166. **Keith, R. E. and Merrill, E.,** The effects of vitamin C on maximum grip strength and muscular endurance, *J. Sports Med.,* 23, 253, 1983.

167. **Bender, A. and Nash, A.,** Vitamin C and physical performance, *Plant Foods for Men,* 1, 217, 1975.

168. **Inukai, M.,** The effect of vitamin C on anaerobic activities. Committee report on vitamin C, *Jpn. Phys. Educ. Assoc.,* No. 5, 1977.

169. **Keren, G. and Epstein, Y.,** The effect of high dosage vitamin C intake on aerobic and anaerobic capacity, *J. Sports Med.,* 20, 145, 1980.

170. **Howald, H., Segesser, B., and Korner, W. F.,** Ascorbic acid and athletic performance, *Ann. N.Y. Acad. Sci.,* 258, 458, 1975.

171. **Gey, G. O., Cooper, K. H., and Bottenberg, R. A.,** Effect of ascorbic acid on endurance performance and athletic injury, *JAMA,* 211, 105, 1970.

172. **Bailey, D. A., Carron, A. V., Teece, R. G., and Wehner, H. J.,** Vitamin C supplementation related to physiological response to exercise in smoking and nonsmoking subjects, *Am. J. Clin. Nutr.,* 23, 905, 1970.

173. **Keys, A.,** Physical performance in relation to diet, *Fed. Proc.,* 2, 164, 1943.

174. **Bramich, K. and McNaughton, L.,** The effects of two levels of ascorbic acid on muscular endurance, muscular strength and on VO_2 max, *Int. Clin. Nutr. Rev.,* 7, 5, 1987.

175. **Hoogerweif, A. and Hoitink, A.,** The influence of vitamin C administration on the mechanical efficiency of the human organism, *Int. Z. Angew. Physiol.,* 20, 164, 1963.

176. **Spioch, F., Kobza, R., and Mazur, B.,** Influence of vitamin C upon certain functional changes and the coefficient of mechanical efficiency in humans during physical effort, *Acta Physiol. Pol.,* 17, 204, 1966.

177. **Cureton, T. K., Ed.,** *The Physiological Effects of Wheat Germ Oil on Humans in Exercise,* Charles C Thomas, Springfield, 1972.

178. **Sharman, I. M., Down, M. G., and Sen, R. N.,** The effects of vitamin E and training on physiological function and athletic performance in adolescent swimmers, *Br. J. Nutr.,* 26, 265, 1971.

179. **Lawrence, J., Smith, J., Bower, R., and Riehl, W.,** The effect of alpha-tocopherol (vitamin E) and pyridoxine HCl (vitamin B6) on the swimming endurance of trained swimmers, *J. Am. Coll. Health Assoc.,* 23, 219, 1974.

180. **Lawrence, J., Bower, R., Riehl, W., and Smith, J.,** Effects of alpha-tocopherol acetate on the swimming endurance of trained swimmers, *Am. J. Clin. Nutr.,* 28, 205, 1974.

181. **Shephard, R. J., Campbell, R., Pimm, P., Stuart, D., and Wright, G.,** Vitamin E, exercise and the recovery from physical activity, *Eur. J. Appl. Physiol.,* 33, 119, 1974.

182. **Shephard, R. J., Stuart, R., Campbell, R., Wright, G., and Pimm, P.,** Do athletes need vitamin E?, *Phys. Sportsmed.,* 2, 57, 1974.

183. **Watt, T., Romet, T. T., McFarlane, I., McGuey, D., Allen, C., and Goode, R. C.,** Vitamin E and oxygen consumption, *Lancet,* 2, 354, 1974.

184. **Sharman, I. M., Down, M. G., and Morgan, N. G.,** The effects of vitamin E on physiological function and athletic performance of trained swimmers, *J. Sports Med.,* 16, 215, 1976.

185. **Talbot, D. and Jamieson, J.,** An examination of the effect of vitamin E on the performance of highly trained swimmers, *Can. J. Appl. Sci.,* 2, 67, 1977.

186. **Helgheim, I., Hetland, O., Nilsson, S., Ingjer, F., and Stromme, S. B.,** The effects of vitamin E on serum enzyme levels following heavy exercise, *Eur. J. Appl. Physiol.,* 40, 283, 1979.

187. **Shephard, R. J.,** Vitamin E and athletic performance, *J. Sports Med.,* 23, 461, 1983.

188. **Simon-Schnass, I. and Pabst, H.,** Influence of vitamin E on physical performance, *Int. J. Vitam. Nutr. Res.,* 58, 49, 1988.

189. **Goldfarb, A. H., Todd, M. K., Boyer, B. T., Alessio, H. M., and Cutler, R. G.,** Effect of vitamin E on lipid peroxidation at 80% VO_2 max, *Med. Sci. Sports Exercise,* 21(2), S16, 1989.

190. **Cannon, J. C., Orencole, S. F., Fielding, R. A., Meydani, M., Meydani, S. N., Fiatarone, M. A., Blumberg, J. B., and Evans, W. J.,** Acute phase response in exercise: interaction of age and vitamin E on neutrophils and muscle enzyme release, *Am. J. Physiol.,* 259, R1214, 1990.

191. **Cannon, J. G., Meydani, S. N., Fielding, R. A., Fiatarone, M. A., Meydani, M., Farhangmehr, M., Orencole, S. F., Blumberg, J. B., and Evans, W. J.,** Acute phase response in exercise. II. Associations between vitamin E, cytokines, and muscle proteolysis, *Am. J. Physiol.,* 260, R1235, 1991.

192. **Simon-Schnass, I. M.,** Nutrition at high altitude, *J. Nutr.,* 122, 778, 1992.

193. **Kobayashi, Y.,** Effect of Vitamin E on Aerobic Work Performance in Man During Acute Exposure to Hypoxic Hypoxia, Ph.D. dissertation, University of New Mexico, Albuquerque, 1974.

194. **Hackney, J. D., Linn, W. S., Buckley, R. D., Jones, M. P., Wightman, L. H., Karuza, S. K., Blessey, R. L., and Hislop, H. J.,** Vitamin E supplementation and respiratory effects of ozone in humans, *J. Toxicol. Environ. Health,* 7, 383, 1981.

195. **Shephard, R. J.,** Athletic performance and urban air pollution, *Can. Med. Assoc. J.,* 131, 105, 1984.

196. **Levander, O. A. and Burk, R. F.,** Selenium, in *Present Knowledge in Nutrition,* Brown, M. L., Ed., International Life Sciences Institute — Nutrition Foundation, Washington, D.C., 1990, 268.

197. **Dragan, I., Dinu, V., Mohora, M., and Cristea, E.,** Studies regarding the antioxidant effects of selenium on top swimmers, *Rev. Rhoum. Physiol.,* 27(1), 15, 1990.

198. **Krinsky, N. I. and Denke, S. M.,** The interaction of oxygen and oxyradicals with carotenoids, *J. Natl. Cancer Inst.,* 69, 205, 1982.

199. **Olson, J. A.,** Vitamin A, in *Handbook of Vitamins,* 2nd ed., Machlin, L. J., Ed., Marcel Dekker, New York, 1991, 1.

200. **Keith, R. E.,** Vitamins in sport and exercise, in *Nutrition in Exercise and Sport,* Hickson, J. F., Jr. and Wolinsky, I., Eds., CRC Press, Boca Raton, FL, 1989, 233.

201. **Williams, W. H.,** The role of vitamins in physical activity, in *Nutritional Aspects of Human Physical and Athletic Performance,* 2nd ed., Williams, M. H., Ed., Charles C Thomas, Springfield, 1985, 147.

202. **Cormier, M.,** Regulatory mechanisms of energy needs: vitamins in energy utilization, *Prog. Food Nutr. Sci.,* 2, 347, 1977.

203. **Knippel, M., Mauri, L., Belluschi, R., Bana, G., Galli, C., Pusterla, G. L., Spreafico, M., and Troina, E.,** The action of thiamin on the production of lactic acid in cyclists, *Med. Sport,* 39(1), 11, 1986.

204. **Haralambie, G.,** Vitamin B2 status in athletes and the influence of riboflavin administration on neuromuscular irritability, *Nutr. Metab.,* 20, 1, 1976.

205. **Tremblay, A., Boiland, F., Breton, M., Bessette, H., and Roberge, A. G.,** The effects of a riboflavin supplementation on the nutritional status and performance of elite swimmers, *Nutr. Res.,* 4, 201, 1984.

206. **Carlson, L., Havel, R., Ekelund, L., and Holmgren, A.,** Effect of nicotinic acid on the turnover rate and oxidation of the free fatty acids of plasma during exercise, *Metabolism,* 12, 837, 1963.

207. **Jenkins, D. J. A.,** Effects of nicotinic acid on carbohydrate and fat metabolism during exercise, *Lancet,* 1, 1307, 1965.

208. **Norris, B., Schade, D. S., and Eaton, R. P.,** Effects of altered free fatty acid mobilization on the metabolic response to exercise, *J. Clin. Endocrinol. Metab.,* 46, 254, 1978.

209. **Gilman, W. D. and Lemon, P. W. R.,** Effects of altered free fatty acid levels and environmental temperature on lactate threshold, *Med. Sci. Sports Exercise,* 14, 113, 1982.

210. **Bergstrom, J., Hultman, E., Jorfeldt, L., Pernow, B., and Wahren, J.,** Effect of nicotinic acid on physical working capacity and on metabolism of muscle glycogen in man, *J. Appl. Physiol.,* 26, 170, 1969.

211. **Pernow, B. and Saltin, B.,** Availability of substrates and capacity for prolonged heavy exercise in man, *J. Appl. Physiol.,* 31, 416, 1971.

212. **Marconi, C., Sassi, G., and Cerretalli, P.,** The effect of an alphaketoglutarate-pyroxidine complex on human maximal aerobic performance, *Eur. J. Appl. Physiol.,* 49, 307, 1982.

213. **deVos, A. M., Leklem, J. E., and Campbell, D. E.,** Carbohydrate loading, vitamin B6 supplementation, and fuel metabolism during exercise in man, *Med. Sci. Sports Exercise,* 14, 137, 1982.

214. **Manore, M. M. and Leklem, J. E.,** Effect of carbohydrate and vitamin B6 on fuel substrates during exercise in women, *Med. Sci. Sports Exercise,* 20, 233, 1988.

215. **Moretti, C., Fabri, A., Gnessi, L., Bonifacio, V., Fraioli, F., and Isidori, A.,** Pyridoxine (B6) suppresses the rise in prolactin and increases the rise in growth hormone induced by exercise, *N. Engl. J. Med.,* 307(7), 444, 1982.

216. **Montoye, H., Spata, P., Pinckney, V., and Barron, L.,** Effects of vitamin B12 supplementation on physical fitness and growth of young boys, *J. Appl. Physiol.,* 7, 589, 1955.

217. **Wetzel, N. C., Hopwood, H. H., Kuechle, M. E., and Grueninger, R. M.,** Growth failure in school children: further studies of vitamin B_{12} dietary supplements, *J. Clin. Nutr.,* 1, 17, 1952.

218. **Montoye, H.,** Vitamin B12: a review, *Res. Q. Am. Assoc. Health Phys. Educ.,* 26, 308, 1955.

219. **Tin-May-Than, Ma-Win-May, Khin-Sann-Aung, and Mya-Tu, M.,** The effect of vitamin B12 on physical performance capacity, *Br. J. Nutr.,* 40, 269, 1978.

220. **Roundtable,** Popularized ergogenic aids, *NSCA J.,* 11(1), 10, 1989.

221. **Wagner, J. C.,** Use of chromium and cobamamide by athletes, *Clin. Pharm.,* 8, 832, 1989.

222. **Stpopzyk, K.,** Kobalin — a new anabolic drug from the coenzyme group, *Przaglad Lekarski,* 25, 723, 1969.

223. **Matter, M., Stittfall, R., Graves, J., Myburgh, K., Adams, B., Jacobs, P., and Noakes, T. D.,** The effect of iron and folate therapy on maximal exercise performance in female marathon runners with iron and folate deficiency, *Clin. Sci.,* 72, 415, 1987.

224. **Nice, C., Reeves, A. G., Brinck-Johnsen, T., and Noll, W.,** The effects of pantothenic acid on human exercise capacity, *J. Sports Med.,* 24, 26, 1984.

225. **Litoff, D., Scherzer, H., and Harrison, J.,** Effects of pantothenic acid supplementation on human exercise, *Med. Sci. Sports Exercise,* 17, 287, 1985.

226. **Read, M. H. and McGuffin, S. L.,** The effect of B-complex supplementation on endurance performance, *J. Sports Med.,* 23, 178, 1983.

227. **van der Beek, E. J., van Dokkum, W., Schrijver, J., Wedel, M., Gaillard, A. W. K., Wesstra, A., van de Weerd, H., and Hermus, R. J. J.,** Thiamin, riboflavin, and vitamins B-6 and C: impact of combined restricted intake on functional performance in man, *Am. J. Clin. Nutr.,* 48, 1451, 1988.

228. **Buzina, R., Grgic, A., Jusic, M., Sapunar, J., Milanovic, N., and Brubacher, G.,** Nutritional status and physical working capacity, *Hum. Nutr. Clin. Nutr.,* 36C, 429, 1982.

229. **Bonke, D. and Nickel, B.,** Improvement of fine motoric movement control by elevated dosages of vitamin B_1, B_6, and B_{12} in target shooting, *Int. J. Vitam. Nutr. Res.,* 30 (Suppl.), 198, 1989.

230. **Early, R. G. and Carlson, R. B.,** Water-soluble vitamin therapy in the delay of fatigue from physical activity in hot climatic conditions, *Int. Z. Angew Physiol.,* 27, 43, 1969.

231. **Hultman, E. and Sahlin, K.,** Acid-base balance during exercise, *Exercise Sport Sci. Rev.,* 8, 41, 1980.

232. **Dennig, H., Peters, K., and Schneikert, O.,** Die Beeinflussung köperlicher Arbeit durch Azidose und Alkalose, *Arch. Exp. Pathol. Pharmakol.,* 165, 161, 1932.

233. **Hewitt, J. and Callaway, E.,** Alkali reserve of the blood in relation to swimming performance, *Res. Q. Am. Assoc. Health Phys. Educ.,* 7, 83, 1936.

234. **Jones, N. L., Sutton, J. R., Lin, J., Ward, G., Richardson, W., and Toews, C. J.,** Effects of acidosis on exercise performance and muscle glycolysis in man, *Clin. Res.,* 23, 636A, 1976.

235. **Sutton, J. R., Jones, N. L., and Toews, C. J.,** Growth hormone secretion in acid-base alterations at rest and during exercise, *Clin. Sci. Mol. Med.,* 50, 241, 1976.

236. **Jones, N. L., Sutton, J. R., Taylor, R., and Toews, C. J.,** Effect of pH on cardiorespiratory and metabolic responses to exercise, *J. Appl. Physiol.,* 43, 959, 1977.

237. **Kostka, C. E. and Cafarelli, E.,** Effect of pH on sensation during cycling exercise, *Med. Sci. Sports Exercise,* 13, 85, 1981.

238. **Ehrsam, R. E., Heigenhauser, G. J. F., and Jones, N. L.,** The effect of respiratory acidosis on metabolism in exercise, *Med. Sci. Sports Exercise,* 12, 112, 1980.

239. **Sutton, J. R., Jones, N. L., and Toews, C. J.,** Effect of pH on muscle glycolysis during exercise, *Clin. Sci.,* 61, 331, 1981.

240. **Kowalchuk, J. M., Heigenhauser, G. J. F., and Jones, N. L.,** The effect of acid-base disturbances on ventilatory and metabolic reponsese to progressive exercise, *Med. Sci. Sports Exercise,* 15, 111, 1983.

241. **McCartney, N., Heigenhauser, G. J. F., and Jones, N. L.,** Effects of pH on maximal power output and fatigue during short-term dynamic exercise, *J. Appl. Physiol.,* 55, 225, 1983.

242. **Bulbulian, R., Girandola, R. N., Wiswell, R. A., and Koyal, S. N.,** The effect of NH₄Cl induced chronic metabolic acidosis on work capacity in man, *Med. Sci. Sports Exercise,* 13, 85, 1981.

243. **Maughan, R. J., Leiper, J. B., and Litchfield, P. E.,** The effects of induced acidosis and alkalosis on isometric endurance capacity in man, in *Exercise Physiology. Current Selected Research,* Vol. 2, Dotson, C. O. and Humphrey, J. H., Eds., AMS Press, New York, 1986, 73.

244. **Denning, H., Talbott, J. H., Edwards, H. T., and Dill, D. B.,** Effect of acidosis and alkalosis upon capacity for work, *J. Clin. Invest.,* 9, 601, 1931.

245. **Dill, D. B., Edwards, H. T., and Talbott, J. H.,** Alkalosis and the capacity for work, *J. Biol. Chem.,* 97, lviii, 1932.

246. **Margaria, R., Edwards, H. T., and Dill, D. B.,** The possible mechanisms of contracting and paying the oxygen debt and the role of lactic acid in muscular contraction, *Am. J. Physiol.,* 106, 689, 1933.

247. **Dennig, H.,** Über Steigerung der körperlichen Leistungsfähigkeit durch Eingriffe in den Säurebasenhaushalt, *Dtsche. Med. Wochenschr.,* 63, 733, 1937.

248. **Dennig, H., Becker-Fregseng, H., Rendenbach, R., and Schostak, G.,** Leistungssteigerung in künstlicher Alkalose bei wiederholter Arbeit, *Naunyn-Schmiedebergs Arch.,* 195, 261, 1940.

249. **Dorow, H., Galuba, B., Hellwig, H., and Becker-Freyseng, H.,** Der Einfluss künstlicher Alkalose auf die sportliche Leistung von Laufern und Schwimmern, *Naunyn-Schmiedebergs Arch.,* 195, 264, 1940.

250. **Margaria, R., Aghemo, P., and Sassi, G.,** Effect of alkalosis on performance and lactate formation in supramaximal exercise, *Int. Z. Angew. Physiol.,* 29, 215, 1971.

251. **Simmons, R. and Hardt, A.,** The effect of alkali ingestion on the performance of trained swimmers, *J. Sports Med.,* 13, 159, 1973.

252. **Inbar, O., Rotstein, A., Jacobs, I., Kaiser, P., Dlin, R., and Dotan, R.,** Effect of induced alkalosis on short maximal exercise performance, *Med. Sci. Sports Exercise,* 13, 128, 1981.

253. **Grassi, M., Messuna, B., Fraiolo, A., Schietroma, M., Giacomo, M. L. D., and Grossi, F.,** Effects of bicarbonate-alkaline earth water (Sangemini) on some parameters of blood chemistry in wrestlers after exertion, *J. Sports Med.,* 23, 102, 1983.

254. **Wilkes, D., Gledhill, N., Smyth, R., and Tomlinson, J.,** The effect of acute induced metabolic alkalosis on anaerobic performance, *Med. Sci. Sports Exercise,* 13, 85, 1981.

255. **Robertson, R., Falkel, J., Drash, A., Spungen, S., Metz, K., Swank, A., and LeBoeuf, J.,** Effect of induced alkalosis on differentiated perceptions of exertion during arm and leg movement, *Med. Sci. Sports Exercise,* 14, 158, 1982.

256. **Costill, D. L., Verstappen, F., Kuipers, H., Jansson, E., and Funk, W.,** Acid-base balance during repeated bouts of exercise: influence of HCO₃⁻, *Med. Sci. Sports Exercise,* 15, 115, 1983.

257. **Rupp, J. C., Bartels, R. L., Zuelzer, W., Fox, E. L., and Clark, R. N.,** Effect of sodium bicarbonate ingestion on blood and muscle pH and exercise performance, *Med. Sci. Sports Exercise,* 15, 115, 1983.

258. **Wilkes, D., Gledhill, N., and Smyth, R.,** Effect of acute induced metabolic alkalosis on 800-m racing time, *Med. Sci. Sports Exercise,* 15, 277, 1983.

259. **Costill, D. L., Verstappen, F., Kuipers, H., Janssen, E., and Fink, W.,** Acid-base balance during repeated bouts of exercise: influence of HCO₃, *Int. J. Sports Med.,* 5, 228, 1984.

260. **Horewill, C. A., Gao, J., and Costill, D. L.,** Oral NaHCO₃ improves performance in interval swimming, *Med. Sci. Sports Exercise,* 20, S3, 1988.

261. **Pfefferle, K. P. and Wilkinson, J. G.,** Induced alkalosis and supramaximal cycling in trained and untrained men, *Med. Sci. Sports Exercise,* 20, 525, 1988.

262. **Bouissou, P., Defer, G., Guezennec, C. Y., Estrade, P. Y., and Serrurier, B.,** Metabolic and blood catecholamine responses to exercise in alkalosis, *Med. Sci. Sports Exercise,* 20, 228, 1988.

263. **Messina, B., Cairella, M., Trasatti, M., and Vecchi, L.,** Azione della terapia con un'acqua bicarbonato-alcalino-terrosa (Sangemini) su alcuni aspetti della sindrome da affaticamento negli sportivi, *Clin. Term.,* 17, 227, 1964.

264. **Messina, B., Cairella, M., Simonotti, P. L., and Vecchi, L.,** Comportamento di alcune costanti ematochimiche in corso di prova da sforzo negli sportivi, *Clin. Term.,* 17, 399, 1964.

265. **Messina, B., Cairella, M., Nasta, G., Simonotti, P. L., and Vecchi, L.,** Osservazioni sul trattamento con acqua bicarbonato-alcalino-terrosa (Sangemini) in atleti in allenamento, *Med. Sport,* 20, 690, 1966.

266. **Messina, B., Grassi, M., Fraioli, A., Pellegrino, M. R., Di Giacomo, M. L., and Grossi, F.,** Variazioni enzimatische sieriche in nuotatori dopo sforzo (influenza di un trattamento con acqua bicarbonato-alcalino-terrosa), *Med. Sport,* 35, 121, 1982.

267. **Miscia, G.,** Modificazioni del dolore muscolare da sforzo indotte dalla somministrazione di un'acqua bicarbonato-calcica, *Med. Sport,* 37, 4, 1984.

268. **Inbar, O., Rotstein, A., Jacobs, I., Kaiser, P., and Dlin, R.,** The effects of alkaline treatment on short-term maximal exercise, *J. Sport Sci.,* 1, 95, 1983.

269. **McKenzie, D. C., Coutts, K. D., Stirling, D. R., Hoeben, H. H., and Kazara, G.,** Maximal work production following two levels of induced metabolic alkalosis, *J. Sports Sci.,* 4, 35, 1986.

270. **Parry-Billings, M. and MacLaren, D. P. M.,** The effect of sodium bicarbonate and sodium citrate ingestion on anaerobic power during intermittent exercise, *Eur. J. Appl. Physiol.,* 55, 524, 1986.

271. **Grassi, M., Fraioli, A., Messina, B., Mammucari, S., and Mennuni, G.,** Mineral waters in treatment of metabolic changes from fatigue in sportsmen, *J. Sports Med.,* 30(4), 441, 1990.

272. **Linderman, J. and Fahey, T. D.,** Sodium bicarbonate ingestion and exercise performance. An update, *Sports Med.,* 11(2), 71, 1991.

273. **Parade, G. W. and Otto, H.,** Alkali-Reserve und Leistung, *Z. Klin. Med.,* 137, 7, 1939.

274. **Karpovich, P.,** Ergogenic aids in work and sports, *Res. Q. Suppl.,* 12, 432, 1941.

275. **Johnson, W. R. and Black, D. H.,** Comparison of effects of certain blood alkalinizers and glucose upon competitive endurance performance, *J. Appl. Physiol.,* 5, 577, 1953.

276. **Karpovich, P. and Sinning, W., Eds.,** *Physiology of Muscular Activity,* W. B. Saunders, Philadelphia, 1971, 264.

277. **Poulus, A. J., Docter, H. J., and Westra, H. G.,** Acid-base balance and subjective feelings of fatigue during physical exercise, *Eur. J. Appl. Physiol.,* 33, 207, 1974.

278. **Kinderman, W., Keul, J., and Huber, G.,** Physical exercise after induced alkalosis (bicarbonate or Tris buffer), *Eur. J. Appl. Physiol.,* 37, 197, 1977.

279. **Hunter, C., Van Huss, W., Boosharga, K., Smoak, B., Ho, K., and Heusner, W.,** The effects of sodium bicarbonate and diet upon acid-base balance in exhaustive work of short duration, *Med. Sci. Sports Exercise,* 12, 127, 1980.

280. **Balberman, S. E. and Roby, F. B.,** The effects of induced alkalosis and acidosis on the work capacity of the quadriceps and hamstrings muscle groups, *Int. J. Sports Med.,* 4, 143, 1983.

281. **Katz, A., Costill, D. L., King, D. S., Hargreaves, M., and Fink, W. J.,** Effect of oral alkalizer on maximal exercise tolerance, *Med. Sci. Sports Exercise,* 15, 126, 1983.

282. **Katz, A., Costill, D. L., King, D. S., Hargreaves, M., and Fink, W. J.,** Maximal exercise tolerance after induced alkalosis, *Int. J. Sports Med.,* 5, 107, 1984.

283. **Wignen, S., Verstappen, F., and Kuipers, H.,** The influence of intravenous $NaHCO_3$-administration on interval exercise: acid-base balance and endurance, *Int. J. Sports Med.,* 5(Suppl.), 130, 1984.

284. **Robins, K. and Verity, L. S.,** Effect of induced alkalosis on rowing ergometer performance (REP) during repeated 1-mile workouts, *Med. Sci. Sports Exercise,* 19, S68, 1987.

285. **Klein, L.,** The effect of bicarbonate ingestion on upper body power in trained athletes, *Med. Sci. Sports Exercise,* 19, S67, 1987.

286. **Hooker, S., Morgan, C., and Wells, C.,** Effect of sodium bicarbonate ingestion on time to exhaustion and blood lactate of 10K runners, *Med. Sci. Sports Exercise,* 19, S67, 1987.

287. **Horswill, C. A., Costill, D. L., Fink, W. J., Flynn, M. G., Kirwan, J. P., Mitchell, J. B., and Houmard, J. A.,** Influence of sodium bicarboante on sprint performance: relationship to dosage, *Med. Sci. Sports Exercise,* 20, 566, 1988.

288. **George, K. P. and MacLaren, D. P. M.,** The effect of induced alkalosis and acidosis on endurance running at an intensity corresponding to 4mM blood lactate, *Ergonomics,* 31(11), 1639, 1988.

289. **Verity, L. S. and Robinson, K.,** Effect of induced alkalosis on rowing ergometer performance during repeated 1-mile workouts, in *Exercise Physiology. Current Selected Research,* Vol. 4, Dotson, C. O. and Humphrey, J. H., Ed., AMS Press, New York, 1990, 111.

290. **Williams, M. H.,** Drug foods — alcohol and caffeine, in *Nutritional Aspects of Human Physical and Athletic Performance,* 2nd ed., Williams M. H., Ed., Charles C. Thomas, Springfield, 1985, 272.

291. **Graham, D. M.,** Caffeine — its identity, dietary sources, intake and biological effects, *Nutr. Rev.,* 36, 97, 1978.

292. **Slavin, J. L. and Joensen, D. J.,** Caffeine and sports performance, *Phys. Sportsmed.,* 13, 191, 1985.

293. **Temples, T. and Haymes, E.,** The effects of caffeine on substrate metabolic and body temperature responses during exercise in a cold and neutral environment, *Med. Sci. Sports Exercise,* 15, 157, 1983.

294. **Temples, T. and Haymes, E.,** The effects of caffeine on substrates in a cold and neutral environment, *Med. Sci. Sports Exercise,* 14, 176, 1982.

295. **Toner, M. M., Kirkendall, D. T., Delio, D. J., Chase, J. M., Clearly, P. A., and Fox, E. L.,** Metabolic and cardiovascular responses to exercise with caffeine, *Ergonomics,* 25, 1175, 1982.

296. **Axelrod, J. and Reichenthal, J.,** The fate of caffeine in man and a method for its estimation in biological material, *J. Pharmacol. Exp. Ther.,* 107, 519, 1953.

297. **Costill, D. L., Dalsky, G. P., and Fink, W. J.,** Effects of caffeine ingestion on metabolism and exercise performance, *Med. Sci. Sports Exercise,* 10, 155, 1978.

298. **Essig, D., Costill, D. L., and Van Handel, P. J.,** Effects of caffeine ingestion on utilization of muscle glycogen and lipid during leg ergometer cycling, *Int. J. Sports Med.,* 1, 86, 1980.

299. **Knapik, J. J., Jones, B. J., Toner, M. M., Daniels, W. L., and Evans, W. J.,** Influence of caffeine on serum substrate changes during running in trained and untrained individuals, in *Biochemistry of Exercise,* Knuttgen, H. G., Vogel, J. A., and Poortmans, J., Eds., Human Kinetics Publishers, Champaign, 1983, 514.

300. **Berglund, B. and Hemmingson, P.,** Effects of caffeine ingestion on exercise performance at low and high altitudes in cross-country skiers, *Int. J. Sports Med.,* 3, 234, 1982.

301. **Giles, D. and Maclaren, D.,** Effects of caffeine and glucose ingestion on metabolic and respiratory functions during prolonged exercise, *J. Sports Sci.,* 2, 35, 1984.

302. **Jacobson, B. H. and Edwards, S. W.,** Caffeine and neuromuscular performance, *Med. Sci. Sports Exercise,* 19, S44, 1987.

303. **Mamimori, G. H., Hetzler, R. K., Somani, S. M., Knowlton, R. G., and Perkins, R. M.,** The interactive effects of obesity and route of administration on caffeine metabolism during prolonged submaximal exercise, *Med. Sci. Sports Exercise,* 19, S44, 1987.

304. **Ivy, J. L., Costill, D. L., Fink, W. J., and Lower, R. W.,** Influence of caffeine and carbohydrate feedings on endurance performance, *Med. Sci. Sports Exercise,* 11, 6, 1979.

305. **Sasaki, H., Maeda, J., Usui, S., and Ishiko, T.,** Effect of sucrose and caffeine ingestion on performance of prolonged strenuous exercise, *Int. J. Sports Med.,* 8, 261, 1987.

306. **Fisher, S. M., McMurray, R. G., Berry, M., Mar, M. H., and Forsythe, W. A.,** Influence of caffeine on exercise performance in habitual caffeine users, *Int. J. Sports Med.,* 7, 276, 1986.

307. **Perkins, R. and Williams, M. H.,** Effect of caffeine upon maximal muscular endurance of females, *Med. Sci. Sports,* 7, 221, 1975.

308. **Ben-Ezra, V. and Vaccaro, P.,** The influence of caffeine on the anaerobic threshold of competitively trained cylists, *Med. Sci. Sports Exercise,* 14, 176, 1982.

309. **Powers, S., Byrd, R., Tulley, R., and Callender, T.,** Effects of caffeine ingestion on metabolism and performance during graded exercise, *Eur. J. Appl. Physiol.,* 40, 301, 1983.

310. **Butts, N. K. and Crowell, D.,** Effect of caffeine ingestion on cardiorespiratory endurance in men and women, *Res. Q., Exercise Sport,* 56, 301, 1985.

311. **Gaessner, G. A. and Rich, R. G.,** Influence of caffeine on blood lactate response during incremental exercise, *Int. J. Sports Med.,* 6, 207, 1985.

312. **Titlow, L. W., Ishee, J. H., and Riggs, C. E.,** Failure of caffeine to affect exercise metabolism, *Med. Sci. Sports Exercise,* 19, S44, 1987.

313. **Colton, T., Gosswlin, R. E., and Smith, R. P.,** The tolerance of coffee drinkers to caffeine, *Clin. Pharmacol. Ther.,* 9, 31, 1968.

314. **Robertson, D., Wade, D., Workman, R., Woosley, R. L., and Oats, J. A.,** Tolerance to the humoral and hemodynamic effects of caffeine in man, *J. Clin. Invest.,* 67, 1111, 1981.

315. **Brust, M.,** Fatigue and caffeine effects in fast-twich and slow-twich muscles of the mouse, *Pflugers Arch.,* 367, 189, 1976.

316. **Delbeke, F. T. and Debackere, M.,** Caffeine: use and abuse in sports, *Int. J. Sports Med.,* 5, 179, 1984.

317. **Stillner, V., Popkin, M. K., and Pierce, C. M.,** Caffeine induced delirium during prolonged competitive stress, *Am. J. Psychiatr.,* 135, 855, 1978.

318. **Wolinsky, I. and Hickson, J. F., Jr.,** Calcium and bone in physical activity and sport, in *Nutrition in Exercise and Sport,* Hickson, J. F., Jr. and Wolinsky, I., Eds., CRC Press, Boca Raton, FL, 1989, 279.

319. **Siliprandi, N.,** Carnitine and physical exercise, in *Biochemical Aspects of Physical Exercise,* Benzi, G., Packer, L., and Siliprandi, N., Eds., Elsevier, Amsterdam, 1986, 197.

320. **Cerretelli, P. and Marconi, C.,** L-Carnitine supplementation in humans. The effects on physical performance, *Int. J. Sports Med.,* 11(1), 1, 1990.

321. **Marconi, C., Sassi, G., Carpinelli, A., and Cerretelli, P.,** Effects of L-carnitine loading on the aerobic and anaerobic performance of endurance athletes, *Eur. J. Appl. Physiol.,* 54, 131, 1985.

322. **Dragan, G. J., Vasiliu, A., Georgescu, E., and Dumas, I.,** Studies concerning chronic and acute effects of L-carnitine on some biological parameters in elite athletes, *Physiologie,* 24, 23, 1987.

323. **Vecchiet, L., Di Lisa, F., Pieralisi, G., Ripari, P., Menabo, R., Giamberardino, M. A., and Siliprandi, N.,** Influence of L-carnitine administration on maximal physical performance, *Eur. J. Appl. Physiol.,* 61, 486, 1990.

324. **Dragan, A. M., Vasiliu, A., Eremia, N. M., and Georgescu, E.,** Studies concerning some acute biological changes after endovenous administration of 1 g L-carnitine in elite athletes, *Physiologie,* 24, 231, 1987.

325. **Dragan, I. G., Vasiliu, A., Georgescu, E., and Eremia, N.,** Studies concerning chronic and acute effects of L-carnitine in elite athletes, *Physiologie,* 26, 111, 1989.

326. **Wyss, V., Ganzit, G. P., and Rienzi, A.,** Effect of L-carnitine administration on VO_2 max and the aerobic-anaerobic threshold in normoxia and hypoxia, *Eur. J. Appl. Physiol.,* 60, 1, 1990.

327. **Gorostiaga, E. M., Maurer, C. A., and Eclache, J. P.,** Decrease in respiratory quotient during exercise following L-carnitine supplementation, *Int. J. Sports Med.,* 10, 1989, 169.

328. **Angelini, C., Vergani, L., Costa, L., Martinuzzi, A., Dunner, E., Marescotti, C., and Nosadini, R.,** Use of carnitine in exercise physiology, *Adv. Clin. Enzymol.,* 4, 103, 1986.

329. **Arenas, J., Ricoy, J. R., Encinas, A. R., Pola, P., Diddio, S., Zeviani, M., Didonato, S., and Corsi, M.,** Carnitine in muscle, serum and the urine of nonprofessional athletes: effects of physical exercise, training and L-carnitine administration, *Muscle Nerve,* 14, 598, 1991.

330. **Soop, M., Bjorkamn, O., Cederblad, G., Hagenfeldt, H., and Wahren, J.,** Influence of carnitine supplementation on muscle substrate and carnitine metabolism during exercise, *Eur. J. Appl. Physiol.,* 64, 2394, 1988.

331. **Greig, C., Finch, K. M., Jones, D. A., Cooper, M., Sargeant, A. J., and Forte, C. A.,** The effect of oral supplementation with L-carnitine on maximum and submaximum exercise capacity, *Eur. J. Appl. Physiol.,* 56, 457, 1987.

332. **Cereda, G. and Scolari, M.,** Effect of an energy stimulator on the performance of a group of young people: evaluation of a videogame test, *Acta Vitaminol. Enzymol.,* 6, 63, 1984.

333. **Corbucci, G. G., Montanari, G., Mancinelli, G., and Diddio, S.,** Metabolic effects induced by L-carnitine and propionyl-L-carnitine in human hypoxic muscle tissue during exercise, *Int. J. Clin. Pharmacol. Res.,* 10, 197, 1990.

334. **Dal Negro, R., Pomari, G., Zoccatelli, O., and Turco, P.,** Changes in physical performance of untrained volunteers: effects of L-carnitine, *Clin. Trials J.,* 23, 242, 1986.

335. **Otto, R. M., Shores, K. V. M., and Perez, H. R.,** The effect of L-carnitine supplementation on endurance exercise, *Med. Sci. Sports Exercise,* 19, S68, 1987.

336. **Shores, K. V., Otto, R. M., Wygand, J. W., Perez, H. R.,** Effect of L-carnitine supplementation on maximal oxygen consumption and free fatty acid serum levels, *Med. Sci. Sports Exercise,* 19, S68, 1987.

337. **Dal Negro, R., Pomari, G., Zoccatelli, O., and Turco, P.,** L-Carnitine and rehabilitative physiokinesitherapy: metabolic and ventilatory response in chronic respiratory insufficiency, *Int. J. Clin. Pharmacol. Ther. Toxicol.,* 24, 453, 1986.

338. **Dal Negro, R., Turco, P., Pomari, C., and De Conti, F.,** Effects of L-carnitine on physical performance in chronic respiratory insufficiency, *Int. J. Clin. Pharmacol. Ther. Toxicol.,* 26, 269, 1988.

339. **Kosolcharoen, P., Nappi, J., Peducci, P., Shug, A., Patel, A., Filipek, T., and Thomsen, J. H.,** Improved exercise tolerance after administration of L-carnitine, *Curr. Ther. Res.,* 30, 753, 1981.

340. **Kamikawa, T., Suzuki, Y., Kobayashi, A., Hayashi, H., Masumura, Y., Nishihara, K., Abe, M., and Yamazaki, N.,** Effects of L-carnitine on exercise tolerance in patients with stable angina pectoris, *Jpn. Heart J.,* 25, 587, 1984.

341. **Cherchi, A., Lai, C., Angelino, F., Trucco, G., Caponnetto, S., Mereto, P. E., Rosolen, G., Manzoli, U., Schiavoni G., Reale, J. A., Romeo, F., Rizzon, P., Sorgente, L., Strano, A., Novo, S., and Immordino, R.,** Effects of L-carnitine on exercise tolerance in chronic stable angina: a multicenter, double-blind, randomized placebo controlled crossover study, *Int. J. Clin. Pharmacol. Ther. Toxicol.,* 23, 569, 1985.

342. **Goa, K. L. and Brogden, R. N.,** L-Carnitine. A preliminary review of its pharmacokinetics, and its therapeutic use in ischaemic heart disease and primary and secondary carnitine deficiencies in relationship to its role in fatty acid metabolism, *Drugs,* 34, 1, 1987.

343. **Brevetti, G., Chairiello, M., Ferulano, G., Policicchio, A., Nevola, E., Rossinin, A., Attisano, R., Ambrosio, G., Siliprandi, M., and Angelini, C.,** Increases in walking distance in patients with peripheral vascular disease treated with L-carnitine: a double-blind, cross-over study, *Circulation,* 77, 767, 1988.

344. **Canale, C., Terrachini, V., Biagini, A., Vallebons, A., Masperone, M. A., Valice, S., and Castellano, A.,** Bicycle ergometer and echocardiographic study in healthy subjects and patients with angina pectoris after administration of L-carnitine: semiautomatic computerized analysis of M-mode tracing, *Int. J. Clin. Pharmacol. Ther. Toxicol.,* 26, 221, 1988.

345. **Cherchi, A., Lai, C., Onnis, E., Orani, E., Pirisi, R., Pisano, M. R., Soro, A., and Corsi, M.,** Propionyl carinitine in stable effort angina, *Cardiovasc. Drugs Ther.,* 4(2), 481, 1990.

346. **Cacciatore, L., Cerio, R., Ciarimboli, M., Cocozza, M., Coto, V., DAlessandro, A., DAlessandro, L., Grattarola, G., Imparato, L., and Lingetti, M.,** The therapeutic effect of L-carnitine in patients with exercise-induced stable angina: a controlled study, *Drugs Exp. Clin. Res.,* 17, 225, 1991.

347. **Brevetti, G., Perna, S., Sabba, C., Rossini, A., Scotto di Uccio, V., Berardi, E., and Godi, L.,** Superiority of L-propionylcarnitine vs L-carnitine in improving walking capacity in patients with peripheral vascular disease: an acute, intravenous, double-blind, cross-over study, *Eur. Heart J.,* 13, 251, 1992.

348. **Kobayashi, A., Masumura, Y., and Yamazaki, N.,** L-Carnitine treatment for congestive heart failure — experimental and clinical study, *Jpn. Circ. J.,* 56, 86, 1992.

349. **Lagioia, R., Scrutinio, D., Mangini, S. G., Ricci, A., Mastropasqua, F., Valentini, G., Ramunni, G., Totaro-Fila, G., and Rizzon, P.,** Propionyl-L-carnitine: a new compound in the metabolic approach to treatment of effort angina, *Int. J. Cardiol.,* 34, 167, 1992.

350. **Ahmad, S., Robertson, H. T., Golper, T. A., Wolfson, M., Kurtin, P., Katz, L. A., Hirschberg, R., Nicora, R., Ashbrook, D. W., and Kopple, J. D.,** Multicenter trial of L-carnitine in maintenance hemodialysis patients. II. Clinical and biochemical effects, *Kidney Int.,* 38, 912, 1990.

351. **Stoecker, B. J.**, Chromium, in *Present Knowledge in Nutrition*, Brown, M. L., Ed., International Life Sciences Institute — Nutrition Foundation, Washington, D.C., 1990, 287.

352. **Anderson, R. A., Polansky, M. M., and Bryden, N. A.**, Strenuous running: acute effects on chromium, copper, zinc, and selected clinical variables in urine and serum of male runners, *Biol. Trace Element Res.*, 6, 327, 1984.

353. **Anderson, R. A., Bryden, N. A., Polansky, M. M., and Deuster, P. A.**, Exercise effects on chromium excretion of trained and untrained men consuming a constant diet, *J. Appl. Physiol.*, 64, 249, 1988.

354. **Evans, G. W.**, The effect of chromium picolinate on insulin controlled parameters in humans, *Int. J. Biosc. Med. Res.*, 11, 163, 1989.

355. **Clarkson, P. M.**, Nutritional ergogenic aids: chromium, exercise, and muscle mass, *Int. J. Sports Nutr.*, 1, 289, 1991.

356. **Lenaz, G., Ed.**, Coenzyme Q. Biochemistry, Bioenergetics and Clinical Applications of Ubiquinone, John Wiley & Sons, Chichester, 1985.

357. **Ernster, L. and Beyer, R. E.**, Antioxidant functions of coenzyme Q: some biochemical and pathophysiological implications, in *Biomedical and Clinical Aspects of Coenzyme Q*, Vol. 6, Folkers, K., Yamagami, T., and Littarru, G. P., Eds., Elsevier/North-Holland, Amsterdam, 1991, 45.

358. **Lenaz, G., Barnabei, O., Rabbi, A., and Battino, M., Eds.**, *Highlights in Ubiquinone Research*, Taylor & Francis, London, 1990.

359. **Folkers, K., Yamagami, T., and Littarru, G. P., Eds.**, *Biomedical and Clinical Aspects of Coenzyme Q*, Vol. 6, Elsevier/North Holland, Amsterdam, 1991.

360. **Karlsson, J., Diamant, B., Theorell, H., and Folkers, K.**, Skeletal muscle coenzyme Q_{10} in healthy man and selected patient groups, in *Biomedical and Clinical Aspects of Coenzyme Q*, Vol. 6, Folkers, K., Yamagami, T., and Littarru, G. P., Eds., Elsevier/North-Holland, Amsterdam, 1991, 191.

361. **Karlsson, J., Diamant, B., Folkers, K., Edlung, P.-O., Lund, B., and Theorell, H.**, Skeletal muscle and blood CoQ_{10} in health and disease, in *Highlights in Ubiquinone Research*, Lenaz, G., Barnabei, O., Rabbi, A., and Battino, M., Eds., Taylor & Francis, London, 1990, 288.

362. **Guerra, G. P., Ballardini, E., Lippa, S., Oradei, A., and Littarru, G. P.**, Effetto della somministrazione di Ubidecarenone nel consume massimo di ossigeno e sulla performance in un gruppo di giovani ciclisti, *Med. Sport*, 40, 359, 1987.

363. **Lenaz, G., Fato, R., Castelluccio, C., Batino, M., Cavazzoni, M., Rauchova, H., and Castelli, G. P.**, Coenzyme Q saturation kinetics of mitochondrial enzymes: theory, experimental aspects and biomedical implications, in *Biomedical and Clinical Aspects of Coenzyme Q*, Vol. 6, Folkers, K., Yamagami, T., and Littarru, G. P., Eds., Elsevier/North-Holland, Amsterdam, 1991, 11.

364. **Vanfraechem, J. and Folkers, K.**, Coenzyme Q_{10} and physical performance, in *Biomedical and Clinical Aspects of Coenzyme Q*, Vol. 3, Folkers, K. and Yamamura, Y., Eds., Elsevier/North-Holland, Amsterdam, 1981, 325.

365. **Yamabe, H. and Fukuzaki, H.**, The beneficial effect of coenzyme Q_{10} on the impaired aerobic function in middle aged women without organic disease, in *Biomedical and Clinical Aspects of Coenzyme Q*, Vol. 6, Folkers, K., Yamagami, T., and Littarru, G. P., Eds., Elsevier/North-Holland, Amsterdam, 1991, 535.

366. **Zeppilli, P., Merlino, B., de Luca, A., Palmieri, V., Santini, C., Vannicelli, R., la Rosa Gangi, M., Caccese, R., Cameli, S., Servidei, S., Ricci, E., Silvestri, G., Lippa, S., Oradei, A., and Littarru, G. P.**, Influence of coenzyme Q_{10} on physical work capacity in athletes, sedentary people and patients with mitochondrial disease, in *Biomedical and Clinical Aspects of Coenzyme Q*, Vol. 6, Folkers, K., Yamagami, T., and Littarru, G. P., Eds., Elsevier/North-Holland, Amsterdam, 1991, 541.

367. **Wyss, V., Lubich, T., Ganzit, G. P., Cesaretti, D., Fiorella, P. L., Dei Rocini, C., Bargossi, A. M., Battistoni, R., Lippi, A., Grossi, G., Sprovieri, G., and Battino, M.**, Remarks on prolonged ubiquinone administration in physical exercise, in *Highlights in Ubiquinone Research*, Lenaz, G., Barnabei, O., Rabbi, A., and Battino, M., Eds., Taylor & Francis, London, 1990, 303.

368. **Amadio, E., Palermo, R., Peloni, G., and Littarru, G. P.**, Effect of CoQ_{10} administration on VO_2max and diastolic function in athletes, in *Biomedical and Clinical Aspects of Coenzyme Q*, Vol. 6, Folkers, K., Yamagami, T., and Littarru, G. P., Eds., Elsevier/North-Holland, Amsterdam, 1991, 525.

369. **Zuliani, U., Bonetti, A., Campana, M., and Cerioli, G.**, The influence of ubiquinone (CoQ_{10}) on the metabolic response to work, *J. Sports Med.*, 29(1), 57, 1989.

370. **Cerioli, G., Tirelli, G., and Musiani, L.**, Effect of CoQ_{10} on the metabolic response to work, in *Biomedical and Clinical Aspects of Coenzyme Q*, Vol. 6, Folkers, K., Yamagami, T., and Littarru, G. P., Eds., Elsevier/North-Holland, Amsterdam, 1991, 521.

371. **Fiorella, P. L., Bargossi, A. M., Grossi, G., Motta, R., Senaldi, R., Battino, M., Sassi, S., Sprovieri, G., and Lubich, T.**, Metabolic effects of coenzyme Q_{10} treatment in high level athletes, in *Biomedical and Clinical Aspects of Coenzyme Q*, Vol. 6, Folkers, K., Yamagami, T., and Littarru, G. P., Eds., Elsevier/North-Holland, Amsterdam, 1991, 513.

372. **Awata, N., Ishiyama, T., Harada, H., Sawamura, A., Ogura, K., Tanimoto, T., Azuma, J., Hasegawa, H., Morita, Y., and Yamamura, Y.,** The effect of coenzyme Q_{10} on ischemic heart disease evaluated by dynamic exercise test, in *Biomedical and Clinical Aspects of Coenzyme Q*, Vol. 2, Yamamura, Y., Folkers, K., and Ito, Y., Eds., Elsevier/North-Holland, Amsterdam, 1980, 247.

373. **Hiasa, Y., Ishida, T., Maeda, T., Iwano, K., Aihara, T., and Mori, H.,** Effects of coenzyme Q_{10} on exercise tolerance in patients with stable angina pectoris, in *Biomedical and Clinical Aspects of Coenzyme Q*, Vol. 4, Folkers, K. and Yamamura, Y., Eds., Elsevier/North-Holland, Amsterdam, 1984, 291.

374. **Vanfraechem, J. H. P., Picalusa, C., and Folkers, K.,** Effects of CoQ$_{10}$ on physical performance and recovery in myocardial failure, in *Biomedical and Clinical Aspects of Coenzyme Q*, Vol. 5, Folkers, K. and Yamamura, Y., Eds., Elsevier, Amsterdam, 1986, 371.

375. **Motomiya, T., Iyeki, K., Watanabe, K., Tokuyasu, Y., Sakurada, H., Ejiri, N., and Nanba, K.,** Elevated beta thromboglobulin in peripheral venous blood of patients with exercise-induced myocardial ischemia and its prevention with coenzyme Q_{10}, in *Biomedical and Clinical Aspects of Coenzyme Q*, Vol. 5, Folkers, K. and Yamamura, Y., Eds., Elsevier, Amsterdam, 1986, 379.

376. **Schardt, F., Welzel, D., Schiess, W., and Toda, K.,** Effect of coenzyme Q_{10} on ischaemia-induced ST-segment depression: a double-blind, placebo-controlled crossover study, in *Biomedical and Clinical Aspects of Coenzyme Q*, Vol. 5, Folkers, K. and Yamamura, Y., Eds., Elsevier, Amsterdam, 1986, 385.

377. **Yamazaki, M., Kamikawa, T., Kobayashi, A., and Yamashita, T.,** Effects of coenzyme Q_{10} on exercise tolerance in stable angina: a double-blind, randomized, placebo-controlled crossover trial, in *Biomedical and Clinical Aspects of Coenzyme Q*, Vol. 5, Folkers, K. and Yamamura, Y., Eds., Elsevier, Amsterdam, 1986, 395.

378. **Rossi, E., Lombardo, A., Testa, M., Lippa, S., Oradei, A., Littarru, G. P., Lucente, M., Coppola, E., and Manzoli, U.,** Coenzyme Q_{10} in ischaemic cardiopathy, in *Biomedical and Clinical Aspects of Coenzyme Q*, Vol. 6, Folkers, K., Yamagami, T., and Littarru, G. P., Eds., Elsevier/North-Holland, Amsterdam, 1991, 321.

379. **Wilson, M. F., Frishman, W. H., Giles, T., Sethi, G., Greenberg, S. M., and Brackett, D. J.,** Coenzyme Q_{10} therapy and exercise duration in stable angina, in *Biomedical and Clinical Aspects of Coenzyme Q*, Vol. 6, Folkers, K., Yamagami, T., and Littarru, G. P., Eds., Elsevier/North-Holland, Amsterdam, 1991, 339.

380. **Greenberg, S. M. and Frishman, W. H.,** Coenzyme Q_{10}: a new drug for myocardial ischemia, *Med. Clin. North Am.*, 72, 243, 1988.

381. **Bruni, O. J.,** *Gamma Oryzanol — The Facts*, Claudell Publishing, Houston, 1989.

382. **Yagi, K. and Ohishi, N.,** Action of ferulic acid and its derivatives as antioxidants, *J. Nutr. Sci. Vitaminol.*, 25, 127, 1979.

383. **Ishihara, M.,** Effect of gamma oryzanol on serum lipid peroxide level and clinical symptoms of patients with climacteric disturbances, *Asia-Oceania J. Obstet. Gynaecol.*, 10(3), 317, 1984.

384. **Gorewit, R. C.,** Pituitary and thyroid hormone responses of heifers after ferulic acid administration, *J. Dairy Sci.*, 66, 624, 1983.

385. **Bucci, L. R.,** A natural magic bullet?, *Flex*, April, 1989, p. 25.

386. **Bucci, L. R., Blackman, G., Defoyd, W., Kaufmann, R., Mandel-Tayes, C., Sparks, W. S., Stiles, J. C., and Hickson, J. F.,** Effect of ferulate on strength and body composition of weightlifters, *J. Appl. Sport Sci. Res.*, 4(3), 104, 1990.

387. **Bonner, B., Warren, B., and Bucci, L.,** Influence of ferulate supplementation on postexercise stress hormone levels after repeated exercise stress, *J. Appl. Sport Sci. Res.*, 4(3), 110, 1990.

388. **Anon.,** Ginseng: western myth or eastern promise?, *IPU Rev.*, 9, 69, 1984.

389. **Forgo, I. and Kirchdorfer, A.,** Ginseng steigert die Körperliche Leistung, *Arztlich. Praxis*, 33, 1784, 1981.

390. **Knapik, J. J., Wright, J. E., Welch, M. J., Patton, J. F., Suek, L. L., Mello, R. P., Rock, P. B., and Teves, M. A.,** The influence of Panax ginseng on indices of substrate utilization during repeated, exhaustive exercise in man, *Fed. Proc.*, 42, 336, 1983.

391. **Teves, M. A., Wright, J. E., Welch, M. J., Patton, J. F., Mello, R. P., Rock, P. B., Knapik, J. J., Vogel, J. A., and der Marderosian, A.,** Effects of ginseng on repeated bouts of exhaustic exercise, *Med. Sci. Sports Exercise*, 15, 162, 1983.

392. **McNaughton, L., Egan, G., and Caelli, G.,** A comparison of Chinese and Russian ginseng as ergogenic aids to improve various facets of physical fitness, *Int. Clin. Nutr. Rev.*, 9(1), 32, 1989.

393. **Pieralisi, G.,** Effects of a standardized ginseng extract combined with dimethylaminoethanol bitartrate, vitamins, minerals, and trace elements on physical performance during exercise, *Clin. Ther.*, 13(3), 373, 1991.

394. **Williams, M. H.,** The role of minerals in physical activity, in *Nutritional Aspects of Human Physical Performance*, 2nd ed., Williams, M. H., Ed., Charles C Thomas, Springfield, 1985, 186.

395. **Sherman, A. E. and Kramer, B.,** Iron nutrition and exercise, in *Nutrition in Exercise and Sport,* Hickson, J. F., Jr. and Wolinsky, I., Eds., CRC Press. Boca Raton, FL, 1989, 291.

396. **McDonald, R., Strause, L., Hegenaure, J., Saltman, P., and Sucec, A. A.,** Limitations to maximum exercise performance: implications of iron deficiency, in *Exercise Physiology. Current Selected Research,* Vol. 1, Dotson, C. O. and Humphrey, J. H., Eds., AMS Press, New York, 1985, 99.

397. **Weaver, C. M. and Rajaram, S.,** Exercise and iron status, *J. Nutr.,* 122, 782, 1992.

398. **Klingsshirn, L. A., Pate, R. A., Bourque, S. P., Davis, J. M., and Sargent, R. G.,** Effect of iron supplementation on endurance capacity in iron-depleted female runners, *Med. Sci. Sports Exercise,* 24, 819, 1992.

399. **Clement, D. B. and Sawchuck, L. L.,** Iron status and sports performance, *Sports Med.,* 1, 65, 1984.

400. **Haymes, E. M.,** Nutritional concerns: need for iron, *Med. Sci. Sports Exercise,* 19, S197, 1987.

401. **Pate, R. R.,** Sports anemia: a review of the current research literature, *Phys. Sportsmed.,* 11, 115, 1983.

402. **Newhouse, I. and Clement, D. B.,** Iron status in athletes. An update, *Sports Med.,* 5, 337, 1988.

403. **Yoshimura, H.,** Anemia during physical training (sports anemia), *Nutr. Rev.,* 28, 251, 1970.

404. **McDonald, R. and Keen, C. L.,** Iron, zinc and magnesium nutrition and athletic performance, *Sports Med.,* 14, 152, 1986.

405. **Eichner, E. R.,** The anemias of athletes, *Phys. Sportsmed.,* 14, 122, 1986.

406. **Liu, L., Borowski, G., and Rose, L. I.,** Hypomagnesemia in a tennis player, *Phys. Sportsmed.,* 11, 79, 1983.

407. **Casoni, I., Guglielmini, C., Graziano, L., Reali, M. G., Mazzotta, D., and Abbasciano, V.,** Changes of magnesium concentrations in endurance athletes, *Int. J. Sports Med.,* 11(3), 234, 1990.

408. **Deuster, P. A.,** Magnesium in sports medicine, *J. Am. Coll. Nutr.,* 8, 462, 1989.

409. **Stendig-Lindberg, G. and Wacker, W. E. C.,** The magnesium deficiency of strenuous effort, *J. Am. Coll. Nutr.,* 8, 463, 1989.

410. **Franz, K. B.,** Serum and erythrocyte magnesium changes during aerobic endurance events, *J. Am. Coll. Nutr.,* 8, 463, 1989.

411. **Dolev, E., Burstein, R., Wishnitzer, R., and Deuster, P. A.,** Longitudinal study of magnesium status of Israeli military recruits, *J. Am. Coll. Nutr.,* 8, 463, 1989.

412. **Steinacker, J. M., Grünert-Fuchs, M., Steininger, K., and Wodick, R. E.,** Effects of long-time administration of magnesium on physical capacity, *Int. J. Sports Med.,* 8, 151, 1987.

413. **Brilla, L. and Haley, T.,** Effect of magnesium supplementation on strength training in humans, *J. Am. Coll. Nutr.,* 11, 326, 1992.

414. **Nielsen, F. H., Hunt, C. D., Mullen, L. M., and Hunt, J. R.,** Effect of dietary boron on mineral, estrogen, and testosterone metabolism in postmenopausal women, *FASEB J.,* 1, 394, 1987.

415. **Darnton, S., Taper, J., and Volpe-Snyder, S.,** The effects of boron supplementation on bone mineral density, blood and urinary calcium, magnesium, phosphorus and urinary boron in female athletes, *FASEB J.,* 6, A1945, 1992.

416. **Ferrando, A. and Green, N. R.,** The effect of boron supplementation on lean body mass, plasma testosterone levels and strength in male weightlifers, *FASEB J.,* 6, A1946, 1992.

417. **Conaly, L. A., Wurtman, R. J., Blusztaijn, K., Coviella, I. L. G., Maher, T. J., and Evoniuk, G. E.,** Decreased plasma choline concentrations in marathon runners, *N. Engl. J. Med.,* 315, 892, 1986.

418. **Yakovlev, N. N., Leshkevich, L. G., and Kolomeitseva, B. I.,** The effect of pangamic acid (vitamin B15) on metabolism during physical exercise of varying duration, in *Vitamin B15 (Pangamic Acid). Properties, Functions and Uses,* Michlin, V. N., Ed., Science Publishing House (Nauka), Moscow, 1965, 182.

419. **Gray, M. E. and Titlow, L. W.,** B$_{15}$: myth or miracle?, *Phys. Sportsmed.,* 10, 107, 1982.

420. **Pipes, T. V.,** The effect of pangamic acid on performance in trained athletes, *Med. Sci. Sports Exercise,* 12, 98, 1980.

421. **Kemp, G. L.,** A clinical study and evaluation of pangamic acid, *J. Am. Osteopath. Assoc.,* 58, 714, 1959.

422. **Girandola, R. N., Wiswell, R. A., and Bulbulian, R.,** Effects of pangamic acid (B-15) ingestion on metabolic response to exercise, *Med. Sci. Sports Exercise,* 12, 98, 1980.

423. **Girondola, R. N., Wiswell, R. A., and Bulbulian, R.,** Effects of pangamic acid (B-15) ingestion on metabolic response to exercise, *Biochem. Med.,* 24, 218, 1980.

424. **Black, D. G. and Suec, A. A.,** Effects of calcium pangamate on aerobic endurance parameters. A double-blind study, *Med. Sci. Sports Exercise,* 13, 93, 1981.

425. **Gray, M. E. and Titlow, L. W.,** The effect of pangamic acid on maximal treadmill performance, *Med. Sci. Sports Exercise,* 14, 424, 1982.

426. **Harpaz, M., Otto, R. M., and Smith, T. K.,** The effect of $N'N'$-dimethylglycine ingestion upon aerobic performance, *Med. Sci. Sports Exercise,* 17, 287, 1985.

427. **Bishop, P. A., Smith, J. F., and Young, B.,** Effects of N,N-dimethylglycine on physiological response and performance in trained runners, *J. Sports Med. Phys. Fitness,* 27, 53, 1987.

428. **Colgan, M.,** Inosine, *Muscle Fitness,* 49, 94, 1988.

429. **Williams, M. H., Krieder, R. B., Hunter, D. W., Somma, C. T., Shall, L. M., Woodhouse, M. L., and Rokitski, L.,** Effect of inosine supplementation on 3-mile treadmill run performance and VO_2 peak, *Med. Sci. Sports Exercise,* 22, 517, 1990.

430. **Lowenstein, J. M.,** The purine nucleotide cycle revisited, *Int. J. Sports Med.,* 11(Suppl. 2), S37, 1990.

431. **Williams, M. H.,** Ergogenic foods, in *Nutritional Aspects of Human Physical Performance,* 2nd ed., Williams, M. H., Ed., Charles C Thomas, Springfield, 1985, 312.

432. **Saint-John, M. and McNaughton, L.,** Octacosanol ingestion and its effects on metabolic responses to submaximal cycle ergometry, reaction time and chest and grip strength, *Int. Clin. Nutr. Rev.,* 6, 81, 1986.

433. **Cade, R., Conte, M., Zauner, C., Mars, D., Peterson, J., Lunne, D., Hommen, N., and Packer, D.,** Effects of phosphate loading on 2,3-diphosphoglycerate and maximal oxygen uptake, *Med. Sci. Sports Exercise,* 16, 263, 1984.

434. **Duffy, D. J. and Conlee, R. K.,** Effects of phosphate loading on leg power and high intensity treadmill exercise, *Med. Sci. Sports Exercise,* 18, 674, 1986.

435. **Jethon, Z., Szczurek, A. L., and Put, A.,** Effects of additional supply of minerals and vitamins on physical work capacity in strength sports, in *Symposium for Sportsmen,* Cernelle, A. B., Ed., Cernitin, Helsingborg, Sweden, 1972, 173.

436. **Steven, R. E., Wells, J. C., and Harless, I. L.,** The effect of bee pollen tablets on the improvement of certain blood factors and performance of male collegiate swimmers, *J. Natl. Athletic Trainers Assoc.,* 11, 124, 1976.

437. **Steben, R. E. and Boudreaux, P.,** The effects of pollen and protein extracts on selected factors and performance of athletes, *J. Sports Med.,* 18, 221, 1978.

438. **Maughan, R. J. and Evans, S. P.,** Effects of pollen extract upon adolescent swimmers, *Br. J. Sports Med.,* 16, 142, 1982.

439. **Chandler, J. V. and Hawkins, J. D.,** The effect of bee pollen on physiological performance, *Med. Sci. Sports Exercise,* 17, 287, 1985.

440. Polbax — Nature's Own Antioxidant, Holomed Int., Malmo, Sweden, 1991.

441. **Giri, S. N. and Misra, H. P.,** Fate of superoxide dismutase in mice following oral route of administration, *Med. Biol.,* 62, 285, 1984.

442. **Zidenburg-Cherr, S., Keen, C. L., Lonnerdal, B., and Hurley, L. S.,** Dietary superoxide dismutase does not affect tissue levels, *Am. J. Clin. Nutr.,* 37, 5, 1983.

443. **Seidl, E. and Hettinger, T.,** Der Einfluss von Vitamin D3 auf Kraft und Leistungfähgkeit des gesunden Erwachsenen, *Int. Z. Angew. Physiol.,* 16, 365, 1957.

444. **Berven, H.,** The physical working capacity of healthy children. Seasonal variation and effect of ultraviolet radiation and vitamin D supply, *Acta Pediatr.,* 148 (Suppl.), 1, 1963.

445. **Fumich, R. and Essig, G.,** Hypervitaminosis. A case report in an adolescent soccer player, *Am. J. Sports Med.,* 11, 37, 1983.

446. **Korner, W. F. and Vollm, J.,** New aspects of the tolerance of retinol in humans, *Int. J. Vitam. Nutr. Res.,* 45, 363, 1975.

447. **Collins, E. D. and Norman, A. W.,** Vitamin D, in *Handbook of Vitamins,* 2nd ed. Machlin, L. J., Ed., Marcel Dekker, New York, 1991, 59.

448. **Suttie, J. W.,** Vitamin K, in *Handbook of Vitamins,* 2nd ed., Machlin, L. J., Ed., Marcel Dekker, New York, 1991, 59.

449. **Cockerill, D. L. and Bucci, L. R.,** Increases in muscle girth and decreases in body fat associated with a nutritional supplement program, *Chir. Sports Med.,* 1, 73, 1987.

450. **Ushakov, A.,** Effect of vitamin and amino acid supplements on human physical performance during heavy mental and physical work, *Aviat. Space Environ. Med.,* 49, 1184, 1978.

451. **Keul, J. and Haralambie, G.,** Effect of a multivitamin-electrolyte-granulate on blood circulation and metabolism in protracted effort, *Schweiz Z. Sportmed.,* 22, 164, 1974.

452. **Barnett, D. W. and Conlee, R. K.,** The effects of a commercial dietary supplement on human performance, *Am. J. Clin. Nutr.,* 40, 586, 1984.

453. **Weight, L. M., Myburgh, K. H., and Noakes, T. D.,** Vitamin and mineral supplementation: effect on the running performance of trained athletes, *Am. J. Clin. Nutr.,* 47, 192, 1988.

454. **Anderson, T., Moffit, J., Fahrenbach, B., and Dunford, M.,** The ergogenic effect of Enerzymes, *J. Appl. Sport Sci. Res.,* 4(3), 111, 1990.

455. **Oyama, T. and Takiguchi, M.,** Effects of gamma-hydroxybutyrate and surgery on plasma human growth hormone and insulin levels, *Agressologie,* 11, 289, 1970.

456. **Takahara, J., Yunoki, S., Yakushiji, W., Yamauchi, J., Yamane, Y., and Ofuji, T.,** Stimulatory effects of gamma-hydroxybutyric acid on growth hormone and prolactin release in humans, *J. Clin. Endocrinol. Metab.,* 44, 1014, 1977.

457. **Mamelak, M., Scharf, M. B., and Woods, M.,** Treatment of narcolepsy with γ-hydroxybutyrate. A review of clinical and sleep laboratory findings, *Sleep,* 9, 285, 1986.

458. **Mamelak, M.,** Gammahydroxybutyrate: an endogenous regulator of energy metabolism, *Neurosci. Biobehav. Rev.,* 13, 187, 1989.

459. **Hunt, C. D. and Herbel, J. L.,** Dietary boron modifies the effects of exercise training on energy metabolism in the rat, *FASEB J.,* 6, A1946, 1992.

Chapter 15

NUTRITIONAL CONCERNS OF FEMALE ATHLETES

Jaime S. Ruud
Ann C. Grandjean

CONTENTS

0-8493-7911-3/94/$0.00+$.50
© 1994 by CRC Press, Inc.

I. INTRODUCTION

Title IX legislation has had a tremendous impact on women's athletics. Millions of women now take part regularly in both competitive and recreational sports. Accompanying these changes has been a greater interest in the special needs of the female athlete. While men and women athletes should observe the same basic dietary principles, there are nutritional concerns unique to active women, such as low energy intakes, eating disorders, iron deficiency, amenorrhea, and premenstrual syndrome. This chapter will provide a nutritional review of these issues.

II. ENERGY REQUIREMENTS

The energy requirement of an athlete depends on several factors, including age, sex, body composition, type of sport, and the intensity and duration of the sport. Ideally, energy intake should balance energy expended. If intake is consistently above or below an athlete's requirement, weight gain or weight loss can be expected. An energy imbalance can have a negative impact on health and performance.

Results of several studies which measured energy intake of female athletes are shown in Table 1. It is difficult to make comparisons, due to differences in research design, sample size, body size, level of competition, and manner in which the data are reported. Additionally, athletes' energy intakes vary due to the stage of training, intensity of effort, and weight control practices. Data by Gong and associates[1] and Tarasuk and Beaton[2] reported higher energy intakes during the luteal phase than the follicular phase, suggesting that studies assessing food intake of females should consider the different stages of the menstrual cycle. Few studies have done so. Considering these limitations, the studies cited herein should be viewed with caution.

As can be seen, a wide range of energy intakes exists between sport groups (Table 1). Female triathletes studied by Green et al.[3] had the highest mean absolute energy intake (4149 kcal/d). Swimmers examined by Berning et al.[4] and cyclists surveyed by Grandjean[5] also reported high energy intakes, 3572 and 3029 kcal/d, respectively. The lowest energy intakes were found in female gymnasts (1552 kcal/d),[6] distance runners (1603 kcal/d),[7] and dancers (1358 kcal/d).[8]

There is also a wide range of energy intakes within sport groups. For example, mean intakes of female runners ranged from 1603 kcal/d (27.5 kcal/kg body weight) to 2489 kcal/d (48.3 kcal/kg body weight). The differences in energy intakes may be explained in part by training abilities. The runners studied by Nieman et al.[9] and Pate et al.[7] were not highly trained. Mean energy intakes of elite female cyclists (3029 kcal/d) studied by Grandjean[5] were also higher than intakes of cyclists reported by Keith et al.[10] (1781 kcal/d).

The methods used to assess dietary intake may underestimate actual energy values.[11] Nevertheless, the energy intakes of female gymnasts and dancers are consistently low, especially when considered as total daily intake. In these sports, body shape is important and many young athletes feel constant pressure to lose weight. As total energy intake decreases, so does nutrient intake, particularly calcium and iron.[12] Low energy intakes also place women at greater risk for other problems, namely, amenorrhea, decreased bone density, and eating disorders. Severely restricting energy intake can result in failure to grow, impaired maturation, glycogen depletion, and fatigue.[13,14]

There are reported discrepancies between energy intake and energy expenditure in female athletes. Deuster et al.[15] found a mean daily energy intake of 2397 kcal for 51 highly trained female runners, while energy expenditure was estimated at 2600 kcal/d. Similarly, the energy intake of Swedish dancers was 1989 kcal/d (34 kcal/kg body weight), while energy requirement was estimated to be 2457 kcal/d (42 kcal/kg body weight).[11]

Researchers[11,16] have raised the question as to why some athletes are not consistently losing weight if reported energy intakes really reflect day-to-day eating habits. One explanation

TABLE 1 Summary of Energy Intakes of Female Athletes

N	Age	kcal	kcal/kg	Ref.
		Runners		
8	27	2489	48.3	121
51	29	2397	46.3	15
27	—	2386	42.0	143
18	31	—	40.2	144
56	38	1868	34.3	9
17	21	2026	—	51
10	34	2272	—	71
14	32	2331	—	145
11	20	1823	—	54
9	31	1922[a]	—	86
103	30	1603	27.5	7
7	29	1973	37.0	20
		Swimmers		
6	22	2472	39.6	21
10	16	2064	35.0	16
19	19	2493	—	84
7	—	2248	—	146
9	—	2468	—	147
16	—	2193	—	62
21	15	3572	61.4	4
		Cyclists		
12	26[b]	3029	51.0[b]	5
21	23	—	39.2	144
8	22	1781	—	10
		Triathletes		
34	—	4149	—	3
10	39	2474	—	148
19	36	2557	—	47
		Gymnasts		
10	16[b]	1935	43.5[b]	5
26	12	1552	42.8	6
11	15	—	37.8	144
97	13	1838	—	80
9	19	1827	32.0	149
13	15	1923	—	39
6[c]	8	1637	74.0	150
5[d]	18	2298	51.0	150
22	11-14	1706	—	81
29	7-10	1651	—	81
		Dancers		
14	24	1989	34.0	11
34	22	1358	—	8
92	14.6	1890	—	83
9	—	1909	—	146
12	24	1673	—	36

[a] Original data presented as kilojules.
[b] Unpublished data.
[c] Amateur gymnasts.
[d] Elite gymnasts.

may be the decrease in resting metabolic rate (RMR) that reportedly occurs in response to energy restriction.[17] Other possible factors include (1) errors in methods available for calculating energy expenditure and/or intake,[11] (2) under-reporting of energy intakes by subjects,[18,19] and (3) a high incidence of unreported binge eating.[8] Inaccuracies in the nutrient data base are also possible. In the case of highly trained women, energy efficiency may also be a factor.[20,21]

III. EATING DISORDERS

Weight and/or body fat restrictions are imposed in a number of competitive sports. Female gymnasts, dancers, and runners typically maintain a very lean body for esthetic and/or athletic reasons. While athletics alone is not a direct cause of eating disorders, a single event or comments from the coach, trainer, or teammate can trigger a problem. An off-handed remark can become deeply ingrained in the mind of a potential anorexic or bulimic. Rosen and Hough[22] found 75% of the gymnasts who were told by their coaches that they were too heavy resorted to dangerous weight measures to lose weight. In another study, Zucker et al.[23] concluded that one or two suggestions about reducing body fat can lead to destructive eating behaviors which may adversely affect the athlete's health and performance. In a survey of 182 female collegiate athletes,[24] 32% reported practicing at least one pathogenic weight control behavior, which included self-induced vomiting, weekly binges, laxative abuse, diet pills, and/or diuretics. Borgen and Corben[25] analyzed the responses to a questionaire completed by 101 nonathletes, 35 athletes whose sports emphasize leanness and 32 whose sports do not. They found 6% of the nonathletes, 20% of the athletes whose sports emphasize leanness, and 10% of all the athletes were either exceptionally preoccupied with weight or had tendencies toward eating disorders.

Extreme methods of weight control are health-threatening and can, in susceptible people, lead to anorexia nervosa and bulimia nervosa. Anorexia nervosa is self-imposed starvation in an obsessive effort to lose weight. It occurs most often in adolescent and young women who have an intense fear of being fat.[26] Bulimia nervosa is defined as recurring episodes of uncontrolled binge-eating, usually followed by purging. Vomiting, laxative abuse, and intense exercise are purging methods often used in an effort to relieve guilt and avoid weight gain.

It is estimated that anorexia nervosa occurs as often as one in a hundred persons in a vulnerable population, such as female high school or college students.[27] Bulimia nervosa, now the most common eating disorder, is thought to occur in as many as 4 to 5% of female college freshmen.[28] Estimates of the prevalence of eating disorders vary widely, however, depending on the diagnostic criteria used.[29] Although eating disorders are more common in young women and girls, 5 to 10% of cases occur in men and boys.[30]

Reports of the prevalence of eating disorders in female athletes vary depending upon the sport and the diagnostic tool used to measure eating disorders. In studies of female ballet dancers, 6 to 33% were reportedly at risk for anorexia nervosa.[31-33] Data by Kurtzman et al.[34] demonstrated, overall, dancers reported the highest prevalence of anorexia nervosa symptoms (27%) when compared to other groups of university female students. Similarly, Brooks-Gunn et al.[35] concluded ballet dancers showed more restraint when eating than did skaters or swimmers.

Amenorrhea is one of the diagnostic criteria for anorexia (Table 2). In ballet dancers, a high incidence of amenorrhea and irregular menstrual cycles has been demonstrated.[8,36] Thirty-three percent of the university and professional dancers studied by Benson et al.[37] experienced abnormal or absent cycles. In another study of 89 young professional ballet dancers, 15% reported secondary amenorrhea and 30% reported irregular cycles.[38]

A few studies have attempted to assess the incidence of eating problems in gymnasts, swimmers, and distance runners. In gymnastics, there is a constant desire to be thin and

TABLE 2 Diagnostic Criteria for Anorexia Nervosa and Bulimia

Anorexia Nervosa

1. Refusal to maintain body weight over a minimal normal weight for age and height. For example, the athlete works at keeping weight 15% below the target weight. Or, doesn't grow as should during childhood or teen years and results in a body weight 15% below expected.
2. Intense fear of becoming obese, even when underweight.
3. Not accurately seeing one's body weight, size, or shape. In other words, claiming to "feel fat" even when emaciated. Believing that one area of the body is "too fat" even when obviously underweight.
4. In females, absence of at least three menstrual cycles in a row.

Bulimia

1. Binge eating is hurried eating of large amounts of food in usually less than 2 h.
2. During the eating binges, there is a fear of not being able to stop eating.
3. Regularly engaging in either self-induced vomiting, use of laxatives, or rigorous dieting or fasting in order to get rid of the food or the calories from the food eaten during binge eating.
4. At least two binge-eating sessions per week for at least 2 months.

From the American Psychiatric Association, *Diagnostic and Statistical Manual of Mental Disorders*, 3rd ed. rev., American Psychiatric Association, Washington, D.C., 1987.

esthetically appealing.[22,39] A number of weight control practices such as diet pills, self-induced vomiting, or fasting are used by female gymnasts.[22] When compared to female swimmers, however, the gynmasts studied by Benson et al.[40] exhibited fewer tendencies towards eating disorders, 11 vs. 1%. Elite-level gymnasts reportedly are less likely to be dissatisfied with their bodies and less concerned about their weight than nonelite gymnasts.[41] However, according to Weight and Noakes,[42] elite distance runners are more likely than nonelite distance runners to exhibit physical and psychological features of anorexia nervosa.

The prevalence of eating disorder-related symptoms may be greater than the prevalence of eating disorders. Schotte and Stunkard[29] conducted a survey of 1965 university students and found that although binge-eating and self-induced vomiting were common among college women, clinically significant bulimia, as described in the Diagnostic Statistical Manual of Mental Disorders (DSM-III), is not. While a female athlete may have abnormal eating habits or amenorrhea, these symptoms alone are not sufficient for diagnosis of an eating disorder. Key clues that an eating disorder is present include emotional liability and withdrawal from social relationships.[43] Mallick et al.[43] examined three groups of young females (eating disordered, athletes, and students) to determine menstrual, dieting, and exercise patterns, as well as self-images. Eating-disordered subjects had the poorest self-images and scored lower on emotional tone and social relationships compared to the other groups.

IV. IRON DEFICIENCY

Iron is present in all cells of the body and plays a key role in numerous biochemical reactions. It performs a vital role in the transport of oxygen, synthesis of hemoglobin and myoglobin, and the activation of oxygen, and is present in a number of enzymes responsible for electron transport. Thus, a deficiency of iron can affect several metabolic functions related to the production of energy.

One of the difficulties in drawing conclusions from the literature on iron status of athletes is the inconsistencies in the terminology and the lack of a standardized definition of those terms, e.g., "iron deficiency," "iron depletion," and "prelatent iron deficiency." Secondly, there is lack of agreement as to what serum values are "normal" for athletes or which tests or levels define iron deficiency in athletes.

Furthermore, the point in the menstrual cycle, degree of menstrual blood loss, and past pregnancy can influence measures of iron status.[44] Rarely are these factors accounted for in studies on women athletes.

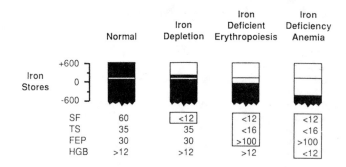

FIGURE 1. Parameters of iron status in relationship to body iron stores (milligrams). Negative iron stores indicate the amount of iron that must be replaced in circulating red cells before iron reserves can reaccumulate. (Adapted from Cook, J. D. and Finch, C. A., *Am. J. Clin. Nutr.*, 32, 2115, 1979.)

A. Measuring Iron Status

Several blood parameters have been used to measure iron status, including: serum ferritin (SF), transferrin saturation (TS), hemoglobin (Hgb), hematocrit (Hct), total iron-binding capacity (TIBC), and serum iron (Fe). As shown in Figure 1, a deficiency of iron develops gradually, progressing through several stages before anemia is evident.[45] In the first stage, when iron stores are adequate, all measurements are normal. In the second stage, iron stores become depleted, as reflected by a decrease in serum ferritin, while transferrin saturation, free erythrocyte protoporphyrin (FEP), and hemoglobin levels are normal. With continued iron loss, lower iron stores are reflected by low transferrin saturation levels ($<16\%$) and an increase in free erythrocyte protoporphyrin (>100 µg/dl), indicating the production of red blood cells with insufficient iron. In the final stage, iron deficiency anemia can be identified by a significant fall in circulating hemoglobin (<12 g in adult women) in addition to the other abnormal measures.

Typically, serum ferritin levels provide a useful guide to detecting early stages of iron depletion, which is a reduction in the size of iron stores. According to Balaban et al.,[46] normal serum ferritin levels for female athletes range from 20 to 140 ng/ml. However, there is a lack of agreement as to what values represent "depletion." Some researchers use serum ferritin levels <12 ng/ml as a cut-off; others use <20 ng/ml. Some investigators classify subjects as iron-depleted based on serum ferritin measurements alone, where others use several parameters. These issues should be considered when reviewing the literature.

In a study by O'Toole et al.,[47] eight triathletes (five men, three women) ($n = 50$) reportedly had serum ferritin concentrations within normal limits (21 to 81 ng/ml), but abnormally low serum iron (<50 µg/dl) and transferrin saturation levels ($<16\%$), demonstrating the importance of using more than one criterion to assess iron status in well-trained athletes. More than one blood sample should also be collected due to day-to-day variation in iron status indicators. Borel et al.[48] evaluated the day-to-day variation of hemoglobin, hematocrit, serum ferritin, and serum iron in 20 healthy men and women. The variation in the iron-status measures was similar between men and women except for serum ferritin, for which the day-to-day variation was greater in women. They found that three to ten independent measures were required to accurately determine serum ferritin and serum iron, whereas one was adequate for hemoglobin and hematocrit.

A recent study by Telford and Cunningham[49] suggests hematological values of highly trained athletes vary according to sex, sport, and body size. The shorter, mesomorphic athlete is predicted to have hematological concentrations at the high end of the range while the tall, ectomorphic athlete will be at the lower end of the range. However, it is not clear what values represent "the normal range." Highly trained athletes are likely to be at variance genetically from the nonathletic population,[44] and thus textbook reference values may not be useful for analyzing and comparing data.

When comparing studies of athletes, the number of subjects, type and intensity of sport, and criteria used to measure iron status should be considered. Furthermore, diagnosis of iron deficiency based solely on serum ferritin or hemoglobin values can be inaccurate. For a complete assessment of iron status, a battery of tests is indicated.

B. Prevalence of Iron Deficiency Among Female Athletes

The prevalence of iron deficiency in female athletes has been investigated.[46,50] Risser[50] studied 100 female intercollegiate athletes in a variety of sports and reported a high prevalence of iron deficiency (31%) as determined by serum ferritin (<12 ng/ml) and transferrin saturation levels (<16%). Iron deficiency without anemia was more common than anemia; only 7% of the athletes had hemoglobin levels <12 g/dl. Likewise, Balaban et al.[46] concluded iron deficiency in elite athletes is no more frequent when compared with nonathletes, about 25%. Therefore, athletics does not appear to be a contributing factor of iron deficiency. However, as in the general population, the incidence of iron deficiency is higher in female than male athletes[46,51,52] and in those consuming vegetarian diets.[12,53]

1. Runners

Distance runners have been identified as a group that is at particularly high risk for iron deficiency. Nickerson et al.[52] studied female cross-country runners and reported 34% were iron-deficient during the running season, which the authors attributed to gastrointestinal bleeding and previously low iron stores. Another study of 52 elite women runners stated more than 35% had diminished iron stores (serum ferritin levels <12 ng/ml).[15] Clement and Asmundson[51] reported a higher incidence (82%) of iron deficiency in Canadian female endurance runners. However, they used a serum ferritin value of <25 ng/100 ml and a transferrin saturation level of <21% to classify their subjects. Haymes and Spillman[54] compared the iron status of competitive female runners and sprinters with a control group and concluded low serum ferritin levels are more common in women who engage in distance running than sprinting events. The authors believe this difference may be due to differences in bioavailability of food iron intake, which was significantly greater ($P < .05$) for the sprinters' diets than that of the runners and control group, 1.41, 0.97, and 0.96 mg/d, respectively.

The most widely accepted explanations for reduced iron levels in athletes during endurance-type training, such as distance running and swimming, are hemodilution[55] and physiological adaptation.[56,57] Studies have shown that endurance athletes have a relatively large total blood volume compared to nonathletes.[55,58,59] Brotherhood and co-workers[58] measured blood volume and hematological status of middle- and long-distance runners whose training mileage was between 100 and 250 km a week. Blood volumes were 20% higher in the runners than in the controls. Based on numerous studies with similar results, it has been speculated that in some athletes a decrease in hemoglobin levels may result from an increase in plasma volume.

2. Other Sports

While numerous studies have been conducted on runners, the iron status of female triathletes, ballet dancers, field hockey players, and swimmers has also been evaluated.[36,47,60-62]

Selby and Eichner[61] measured iron status in collegiate swimmers during the competitive season and reported 57% of the female swimmers had low serum ferritin levels (<15 ng/ml). They believe the cause may have been dilutional, as shown by an increase in plasma volume.

C. Factors Contributing to Iron Deficiency

There are a number of factors which may contribute to iron deficiency in athletes, including red blood cell hemolysis,[63-65] increased iron losses through sweating,[64,66] and gastrointestinal (GI) blood loss.[52,67-69]

In female athletes, the cause of iron deficiency is most likely nutrition-related, due to a low intake of dietary iron.[36,50,51,70-72] Women also face a potentially greater loss of iron as a result of menstruation, pregnancy, and lactation. The average menstrual blood loss is estimated at about 0.6 mg/d with excesses of 1.5 mg/d being reported.[73]

1. Decreased Iron Absorption

Unlike other minerals, there is no physiological regulation of iron metabolism through increased or decreased excretion. The primary control for maintaining adequate levels of iron is the intestinal absorption system, which is influenced in part by the iron status of the individual. Persons who are iron-deficient generally absorb a higher percentage of dietary iron than those who are iron-replete.[74]

While dietary iron intake is positively related to total calorie intake, iron absorption is dependent on the bioavailability of iron.[75] Iron is absorbed as heme and nonheme, and its availability from food sources varies greatly. Heme iron (meat, poultry, fish) is well absorbed (15 to 35%) by the body regardless of the dietary composition of a meal.[76] Nonheme iron, found primarily in plant foods, is not well absorbed (2 to 20%). Also, the rate of absorption is highly dependent upon enhancing and blocking substances in the diet and the amount of iron stores.[75] Meat, poultry, and fish (MPF) and ascorbic acid increase nonheme iron availability,[77] while tea, coffee, and wheat bran act as inhibitors.[75]

Female athletes consuming vegetarian diets may be at risk for iron deficiency due to poor absorption of nonheme iron. In female runners consuming a modified vegetarian diet (<100 g red meat/week), Snyder et al.[53] reported the bioavailability of iron was significantly lower ($P < .05$) than in female runners who consumed red meat. There were no differences in total calorie intake, and both groups consumed approximately 14 mg of dietary iron. However, the athletes who ate red meat consumed greater amounts of heme iron (1.2 vs. 0.2 mg/d, respectively) and had higher serum ferritin levels than athletes consuming a modified vegetarian diet (19.8 vs. 7.4 ng/100 ml, respectively). van Erp-Baart et al.[12] also report a negative influence on iron absorption in endurance athletes with vegetarian food habits.

2. Inadequate Dietary Iron Intake

Inadequate dietary iron intake appears to be a major contributing factor to the prevalence of iron deficiency.[78] Some groups of female athletes, particularly young gymnasts, reportedly consume less than the 1989 Recommended Dietary Allowance (RDA) of 15 mg/d of iron.[79] Reggiani et al.[6] evaluated the diets of 26 gymnasts (average age of 12 years) and reported a mean iron intake of 6.2 mg/d with a range of 2.7 to 12.6. Low mean iron intakes were also noted in gymnasts studied by Moffatt,[39] Loosli et al.,[80] and Benardot et al.[81] Whether these athletes were iron deficient could not be determined because hematological data were not assessed. In adolescent female gymnasts surveyed by van Erp-Baart et al.,[12] the mean iron intake was 9.9 mg/d with nonheme iron contributing three times as much as heme iron to total iron intake, 7.6 vs. 2.3 mg.

Adolescents are often at risk of iron deficiency, not only because of their increased physiological needs, but because of low energy intakes. Many young females consume less than 1800 kcal/d and, as a result, limit their intake of dietary iron. According to survey data from the Second National Health and Nutrition Examination Survey (NHANES II), females aged 18 to 24 years averaged 1687 kcal/d and 10 mg of iron.[82] Surveys of female adolescent athletes show mean energy intakes ranging from 1706 to 3572 kcal/d, with an average of 13 mg of iron/d.[4,39,81,83,84]

The 1989 RDA concludes that a daily intake of 15 mg of iron from a typical U.S. diet should be sufficient to replace iron losses of most women. Others believe the present RDA for females is too low. Based on calculations by Hallberg and Rossander-Hulten,[85] the amount of iron needed to be absorbed to cover the iron requirements of adult menstruating women is 2.84 mg/d. For this amount to be absorbed from typical Western-type meals, it appears the diet should contain 18.9 mg of iron daily. This would be 9.4 mg of iron/1000 kcal for a woman consuming approximately 2000 kcals per day. In one of the few studies on female athletes which determined iron intake per 1000 kcal, Manore et al.[71] reported a group of runners averaged 6 mg of iron/1000 kcal with a range of 4.3 to 8.8 mg/1000 kcal. If this is representative, female athletes will have difficulty meeting iron needs if energy intake is low.

3. Training

The question of whether or not training alters iron status in female athletes has been examined.[60,62,70-72,86,87] Diehl et al.[60] determined the effects of training and competition on serum ferritin levels of collegiate female field hockey players during consecutive seasons over a 3-year period. Serum ferritin levels decreased significantly ($P < .05$) following successive seasons of competition. Although the athletes' daily intake of iron averaged only 10 mg/d, it was the authors' feeling that psychological stress from competition, rather than factors such as diet, menstruation, or hemodilution, may have been the primary factor producing the greater decrease in serum ferritin in the second and third season.

Cooter and Mowbray[87] reported that a 4-month training program did not significantly alter serum iron, total iron-binding capacity, hemoglobin, and percent saturation levels in female basketball athletes. Serum ferritin levels, however, were not reported in this study. More recently, Manore et al.[71] studied 10 long-distance runners for a 9-week period. Over 50% of the runners reportedly had latent iron deficiency, which the authors attributed to increased iron losses, low iron intakes, and low iron absorption. The women averaged <3 oz of meat, fish, or poultry a day; only 11 to 14% of dietary iron was from animal sources (4 to 6% heme iron). The authors indicated that the individuals with the most miles run each week had the lowest ferritin levels, regardless of dietary iron intake. It must be noted, however, that Manore defined low ferritin as <20 ng/ml.

D. Effects of Iron Deficiency on Performance

It is well known that iron deficiency anemia limits the physical work capacity of experimental animals[88] and man.[89,90] Iron deficiency without anemia, however, does not appear to have a significant impact on performance. Newhouse et al.[78] studied the effects of prelatent/latent iron deficiency in 40 female endurance runners before and after 8 weeks of oral iron supplementation (320 mg ferrous sulfate). Iron supplementation did not significantly enhance work capacity, although it did increase serum ferritin levels. The authors concluded the presence of a serum ferritin <20 ng/ml does not significantly affect performance. Similar results were found by Matter et al.[91]

Another study[50] examined the impact of iron deficiency on female intercollegiate athletes and also reported that iron deficiency without anemia has little effect on performance. The only notable difference between iron-deficient and nondeficient athletes was that the iron-deficient athletes were less satisfied with their performance at the beginning of the season than their teammates.

E. Iron Supplementation

Surveys have shown that many athletes, particularly female endurance runners, are taking iron supplements.[15,92] Whether iron supplements are of value for athletes remains to be determined. Deuster et al.[15] surveyed elite female runners and reported 27 out of 51 women took nutritional supplements. Iron was the most common supplement taken and the one taken in the greatest amounts. Supplemental iron contributed more to total intake than did food iron. Thirty-one percent (31%) of varsity athletes studied by Barr[92] also reported using iron supplements.

Because women potentially face a greater chance of being iron deficient due to increased iron loss through menses and poor dietary iron intake, it has been suggested that female athletes consider routine use of iron supplements,[93] particularly during periods of heavy training.[94] The effects of iron supplements on nonanemic female athletes have been studied and no significant improvement in performance was found.[87,95] In women athletes with iron deficiency without anemia, no change in performance was noted with iron supplementation.[78,91,96]

V. ATHLETIC AMENORRHEA

Amenorrhea is the absence of menstrual cycles, characterized by low levels of circulating estrogen.[97] Many factors have been associated with athletic amenorrhea. Frequently cited are low calorie intake, training intensity, delayed menarche, eating disorders, stress, low body weight, and low percent body fat.[98-102]

A. Prevalence

The prevalence of amenorrhea varies among sport groups. In a study of 226 elite athletes, gymnasts had the highest incidence of amenorrhea (71%), followed by lightweight rowers (46%) and runners (45%).[99] Amenorrhea was defined as no more than one period in the 6 months prior to the study.

In ballet dancers, the reported incidence of amenorrhea is approximately 27 to 50%.[8,37,99] Part of the variance may be explained by the fact that different definitions of amenorrhea were used in all three studies.

B. Factors Associated with Amenorrhea

1. Low Body Fat

Athletic amenorrhea has been linked to low body fat, but the results of studies are difficult to compare due to differences in methods used to measure percent body fat. More recent data have criticized the "fat hypothesis" theory. Sanborn et al.[103] measured percent body fat in regularly menstruating and amenorrheic long-distance runners of the same somatotype using underwater weighing and found percent body fat for both groups was the same: 17.4 ± 2.1% and 17.7 ± 2.17%, respectively. Kaiserauer et al.[100] and Marcus et al.[102] also found no difference in percent body fat between amenorrheic and eumenorrheic distance runners. Furthermore, many female runners with low percentage body fat levels (<17%) have regular menstrual cycles.[102,104] Brownell and colleagues[105] suggest that amenorrhea may be mediated in part by regional fat distribution rather than total body fat.

2. Nutrition and Stress

Nutrition and stress may play a role in the etiology of amenorrhea.[38,98] Adolescent athletes who train vigorously and consume a low-energy diet exhibit secondary amenorrhea and reduced estradiol levels.[101] In a study by Baer and Taper,[101] amenorrheic runners averaged 40 miles per week and had been training for approximately 4 years, while the eumenorrheic athletes ran 20 miles per week and had been training for only 2 years.

Studies comparing the diets of regularly menstruating athletes to amenorrheic athletes indicate that amenorrheic athletes tend to eat fewer calories[97,100,102,106] and have lower fat intakes.[15,97,107,108] Investigators have also found a significantly lower resting metabolic rate (RMR) in amenorrheic runners and a tendency toward a bulimic pattern of binging and purging.[106]

3. Vegetarian Habits

A vegetarian diet can contribute to changes in hormone status. Vegetarians, because of a high fiber intake, have a large fecal output and lose two to three times more estrogen in feces than women on omnivorous diets.[109] Additionally, low fat intake, low body fat, low dietary protein, low tryptophan intake, and high fiber intake, which are more common among vegetarian women, have been associated with reduced prolactin levels and may alter the menstrual cycle.[110]

Endocrine status is more severely affected in women who consume a low-calorie, vegetarian diet. There is a higher prevalence of anovulatory cycles and lower levels of reproductive hormones in the luteal phase.[111-113] Pedersen et al.[112] reported the incidence of menstrual irregularities was 4.9% among nonvegetarian women compared to 26.5% in vegetarian women.

Researchers have tried to determine whether a lack of red meat in the diet contributed to amenorrhea.[15,97,100,106] In a survey of the dietary habits of elite runners, 61% of the amenorrheic subjects did not eat red meat compared with 43% of the menstruating group.[114] Kaiserauer et al.[100] reported 44% of the regularly menstruating distance runners ate no red meat compared to 100% of the amenorrheic subjects.

C. Amenorrhea and Bone Health

Amenorrhea is not a harmless alteration of endocrine status. It is associated with decreased bone mineral content of the lumbar spine,[97,107] a greater incidence of scoliosis among adolescents,[115] and a greater incidence of stress fractures.[102,104,116] Although the long-term consequences of amenorrhea are unknown, one of the major concerns is osteoporosis. Extended periods of amenorrhea, if left untreated, can lead to irreversible bone loss.[117]

It is important for regular menstrual cycles to be maintained and adequate calcium intake to be achieved in order to ensure that adult bone is well mineralized.[118] According to Lloyd et al.,[119] young women who have missed 50% of their expected menstrual periods are likely to reach the age of 20 with reduced peak bone mass, putting them at greater risk for the development of osteoporosis. Consuming inadequate dietary calcium during adolescence may also cause a reduction in peak bone mass and density and risk for osteoporosis later in life.

Many female athletes, particularly those who strive for thinness, have less than optimal calcium intakes.[36,39,120] One hundred and ten female athletes studied by Grandjean et al.[121] had an average calcium intake of 981 mg $\pm$ 379, which for all subjects combined represents 92% of the RDA. However, of the 54 female athletes 19 years and older, 26% had a calcium intake under 70% of the RDA, while 55% of the female athletes 18 years and under consumed less than 70% of the RDA. Young female athletes should be aware of dietary sources of calcium and consume at least 100% of the RDA, which is 1200 mg/d.

Although the efficacy of calcium supplements in the prevention or treatment of osteoporosis has not been proven, calcium supplements are being used by an increasing number of adult women to reduce the risk of osteoporosis. Calcium carbonate is the most widely used supplement because it is inexpensive and contains the highest percentage of calcium. The women who are most likely to benefit from calcium supplements are those whose usual dietary intake of calcium is less than 400 mg/d, and calcium citrate malate may be more effective than supplementation with calcium carbonate.[122] However, when taken with food, calcium carbonate as well as calcium citrate and calcium phosphate reduce iron absorption, making it difficult for women to meet their daily iron requirement.[123,124]

VI. PREMENSTRUAL SYNDROME

Premenstrual syndrome (PMS) is of particular interest to athletes and coaches because of possible effects on athletic performance. Dalton[125] described PMS as "the recurrence of symptoms in the premenstruum with absence in the postmenstruum." The manifestations are varied and range in severity from mild to incapacitating.[126] The symptoms, which usually occur 7 to 10 d prior to the onset of menses, can be divided into two categories: those of a physical nature and those of a psychological nature. Among a group of adolescents studied by Fisher et al.,[127] general discomfort and water retention were the mostly commonly reported physical symptoms, while impaired social function and depression were the most commonly reported categories of change in mood and behavior.

A. Prevalence

The reported prevalence of PMS among menstruating women in the U.S. ranges from 60 to 95%.[127,128] The etiology of PMS has been associated with excessive levels of estrogen[129] and a deficiency of progesterone in the luteal phase of the menstrual cycle.[130] However, there is a lack of data to support either theory. Fisher and colleagues[127] found that female adolescents having greater premenstrual physical changes were more likely to be white, have heard of PMS, have dysmenorrhea during their periods, and were not currently using an oral contraceptive.

B. Effects on Performance

Of greater concern to the female athlete is the effect of PMS on performance. Brooks-Gunn et al.[131] investigated the effect of the cycle phase on the performance of postmenarcheal adolescent swimmers. Results showed the fastest times for the 100-yard freestyle and 100-yard best event occurred during the menstrual phase and the slowest times during the premenstrual phase. One possible explanation for these findings is premenstrual fluid retention and menstrual fluid reduction.

It has been suggested that women who are physically active tend to suffer less from PMS, although there is little data to support this theory. Prior and colleagues[132] conducted a 3-month controlled study involving eight women who began an exercise training program and six sedentary control women. The exercising women reported significant decreases in overall molimina, breast tenderness, and fluid retention after 3 months of gradual training.

C. Treatment

A variety of therapeutic approaches have been recommended for PMS, but none have been fully accepted. Progesterone is the most widely prescribed treatment even though there are few well-controlled studies demonstrating its efficacy. Freeman et al.[133] recently conducted a randomized, placebo-controlled, double-blind crossover study of 168 women receiving progesterone suppositories in doses of 400 and 800 mg or a placebo. Premenstrual symptoms were not significantly improved by progesterone compared with placebo in any measure used in the study.

A number of dietary interventions have been used to treat PMS. Dietary recommendations include restricting sodium and caffeine, decreasing intake of refined sugar, and increasing intake of complex carbohydrate.[134] Rossignol and Bonnlander[135] found that consumption of caffeine-containing beverages was related to the prevalence of PMS. In women with more severe symptoms, the effect was higher, per amount of exposure, for consumers of tea and coffee than for soft-drink consumers over the range of consumption studied (0 to 8 cups of soft drink, and 0 to 3 cups of tea or coffee).

Supplementation with vitamin B_6 has been a popular approach to treating PMS. Arguments for the use of vitamin B_6 are based on the role of this vitamin as a cofactor for several enzymes[136] and the relationship between low levels of the neurotransmitter serotonin and depression.[137] Williams et al.[138] reported a significant improvement in women receiving 100 to 200 mg of vitamin B_6 daily compared to those receiving a placebo. More recently, Berman et al.[139] observed favorable trends in symptom improvements with dietary modification and 250 mg/d of vitamin B_6 in an experimental group compared to a control group of women. However, differences in these two groups were not significant. While the RDA for vitamin B_6 is 1.6 mg/d for women ages 19 to 50,[79] some women have been known to take 50 to 300 mg/d supplemented by a variety of multivitamin preparations.[140] In view of the fact that excessive amounts of vitamin B_6 can produce neurological disorders,[141] caution is indicated and indiscriminate use is not advised.

Magnesium supplementation reportedly has been successful in relieving premenstrual mood fluctuations in PMS sufferers. Facchinetti et al.[142] conducted a double-blind randomized study involving 28 women with confirmed PMS. For 2 months, magnesium carboxylic acid (360 mg of Mg) or placebo was administered three times a day from the 15th day of the menstrual cycle to the onset of menstrual flow. Magnesium supplementation was shown to be more effective than placebo in improvement of PMS mood, providing preliminary evidence that this nutrient may have pharmacological benefits.

VII. CONCLUSIONS AND RECOMMENDATIONS

Female athletes, their coaches, and support staff need to be aware of the nutritional problems associated with low energy intakes. Indiscriminate reduction in total food intake, or exclusion of major food categories, and extreme methods of weight control can have adverse effects on health and performance. Iron and calcium are two key nutrients that may be compromised. Female athletes are at risk for iron deficiency because of low iron intake and increased iron losses. Routine screening tests should be performed on prospective female athletes to detect early stages of iron depletion. More than one indicator should be used, i.e., serum ferritin, hemoglobin, hematocrit, serum iron, or transferrin saturation. Those athletes found to be deficient should receive dietary counseling. Supplemental iron may be indicated in individual cases; however, routine use of iron supplements by all athletes is not warranted and requires further investigation.

Female athletes who train vigorously and consume a low-energy diet are at risk for amenorrhea. These are typically gymnasts, dancers, and runners who maintain a very lean body for esthetic and/or athletic reasons. Amenorrhea is associated with decreased bone density and reduced levels of estrogen, both of which are considered risk factors for osteoporosis. It is important that regular menstrual cycles be maintained and adequate calcium intake achieved. If the athlete has a history of stress fractures and/or menstrual dysfunction, training should be reduced so as not to compromise bone health.

REFERENCES

1. **Gong, E. J., Garrel, D., and Calloway, D. H.,** Menstrual cycle and voluntary food intake, *Am. J. Clin. Nutr.,* 49, 252, 1989.
2. **Tarasuk, V. and Beaton, G. H.,** Menstrual-cycle patterns in energy and macronutrient intake, *Am. J. Clin. Nutr.,* 53, 442, 1991.

3. **Green, D. R., Gibbons, C., O'Toole, M., and Hiller, W. B. O.,** An evaluation of dietary intakes of triathletes: are RDAs being met?, *J. Am. Diet. Assoc.,* 89, 1653, 1989.

4. **Berning, J. R., Troup, J. P., Van Handel, P. J., Daniels, J., and Daniels, N.,** The nutritional habits of young adolescent swimmers, *Int. J. Sports Nutr.,* 1, 240, 1991.

5. **Grandjean, A. C.,** Macronutrient intake of US athletes compared with the general population and recommendations made for athletes, *Am. J. Clin. Nutr.,* 49, 1070, 1989.

6. **Reggiani, E., Arras, G. B., Trabacca, S., Senarega, D., and Chiodini, G.,** Nutritional status and body composition of adolescent female gymnasts, *J. Sports Med.,* 29, 285, 1989.

7. **Pate, R. R., Sargent, R. G., Baldwin, C., and Burgess, M. L.,** Dietary intake of women runners, *Int. J. Sports Med.,* 11, 461, 1990.

8. **Calabrese, L. H., Kirkendall, D. T., Floyd, M., Rapoport, S., Williams, G. W., Weiker, G. G., and Bergfeld, J. A.,** Menstrual abnormalities, nutritional patterns, and body composition in female classical ballet dancers, *Phys. Sportsmed.,* 11, 86, 1983.

9. **Nieman, D. C., Butler, J. V., Pollett, L. M., Dietrich, S. J., and Lutz, R. D.,** Nutrient intake of marathon runners, *J. Am. Diet. Assoc.,* 89, 1273, 1989.

10. **Keith, R. E., O'Keeffe, K. A., Alt, L. A., and Young, K. L.,** Dietary status of trained female cyclists, *J. Am. Diet. Assoc.,* 89, 1620, 1989.

11. **Dahlstrom, M., Jansson, E., Nordevang, E., and Kaijser, L.,** Discrepancy between estimated energy intake and requirement in female dancers, *Clin. Physiol.,* 10, 11, 1990.

12. **van Erp-Baart, A. M. J., Saris, W. H. M., Binkhorst, R. A., Vos, J. A., and Elvers, J. W. H.,** Nationwide survey on nutritional habits in elite athletes. II. Mineral and vitamin intake, *Int. J. Sports Med.,* 10, S11, 1989.

13. **Hermansen, L., Hultman, E., and Saltin, B.,** Muscle glycogen during prolonged severe exercise, *Acta Physiol. Scand.,* 71, 129, 1967.

14. **Pugliese, M. T., Lifshitz, F., Grad, G., Fort, P., and Marks-Katz, M.,** Fear of obesity: a cause of short stature and delayed puberty, *N. Engl. J. Med.,* 309, 513, 1983.

15. **Deuster, P. A., Kyle, S. B., Moser, P. B., Vigersky, R. A., Singh, A., and Schoomaker, E. B.,** Nutritional survey of highly trained women runners, *Am. J. Clin. Nutr.,* 44, 954, 1986.

16. **Barr, S. I.,** Women, nutrition and exercise: a review of athletes' intakes and a discussion of energy balance in active women, *Prog. Food Nutr. Sci.,* 11, 307, 1987.

17. **Bray, G. A.,** Effect of caloric restriction on energy expenditure in obese patients, *Lancet,* II, 397, 1969.

18. **Rosenberg, I. H., Ed.,** Errors in reporting habitual energy intake, *Nutr. Rev.,* 49, 215, 1991.

19. **Mertz, W., Tsui, J. C., Judd, J. T., Reiser, S., Hallfrisch, J., Morris, E. R., Steele, P. D., and Lashley, E.,** What are people really eating? The relationship between energy intake derived from estimated diet records and intake determined to maintain body weight, *Am. J. Clin. Nutr.,* 54, 291, 1991.

20. **Mulligan, K. and Butterfield, G. E.,** Discrepancies between energy intake and expenditure in physically active women, *Br. J. Nutr.,* 64, 23, 1990.

21. **Vallieres, F., Tremblay, A., and St.-Jean, L.,** Study of the energy balance and the nutritional status of highly trained female swimmers, *Nutr. Res.,* 9, 699, 1989.

22. **Rosen, L. W. and Hough, D. O.,** Pathogenic weight-control behaviors of female college gymnasts, *Phys. Sportsmed.,* 16, 141, 1988.

23. **Zucker, P., Avener, J., Bayder, S., Brotman, A., Moore, K., and Zimmerman, J.,** Eating disorders in young athletes, *Phys. Sportsmed.,* 13, 88, 1985.

24. **Rosen, L. W., McKeag, D. B., Hough, D. O., and Curley, V.,** Pathogenic weight-control behavior in female athletes, *Phys. Sportsmed.,* 14, 79, 1986.

25. **Borgen, J. S. and Corben, C. B.,** Eating disorders among female athletes, *Phys. Sportsmed.,* 15, 89, 1987.

26. American Psychiatric Association, *Diagnostic and Statistical Manual of Mental Disorders* (DSM-III), 3rd ed., American Psychiatric Association, Washington, D.C., 1980.

27. **Krey, S. H., Palmer, K., and Porcelli, K. A.,** Eating disorders: the clinical dietitian's changing role, *J. Am. Diet. Assoc.,* 89, 41, 1989.

28. American Psychiatric Association, *Diagnostic and Statistical Manual of Mental Disorders* (DSM-III), 3rd ed. rev., American Psychiatric Association, Washington, D.C., 1987.

29. **Schotte, D. E. and Stunkard, A. J.,** Bulimia vs. bulimic behaviors on a college campus, *JAMA,* 258, 1213, 1987.

30. **Barry, A. and Lippmann, S. B.,** Anorexia nervosa in males, *Postgrad. Med.,* 87, 161, 1990.

31. **Garner, D. M. and Garfinkel, P. E.,** Socio-cultural factors in the development of anorexia nervosa, *Psychol. Med.,* 10, 647, 1980.

32. **Brooks-Gunn, J., Warren, M. P., and Hamilton, L. H.,** The relation of eating problems and amenorrhea in ballet dancers, *Med. Sci. Sports Exercise,* 19, 41, 1987.

33. **Evers, C. L.,** Dietary intake and symptoms of anorexia nervosa in female university dancers, *J. Am. Diet. Assoc.,* 87, 66, 1987.

34. **Kurtzman, F. D., Yager, J., Landsverk, J., Wiesmeier, E., and Bodurka, D. C.,** Eating disorders among selected female student populations at UCLA, *J. Am. Diet. Assoc.,* 89, 45, 1989.

35. **Brooks-Gunn, J., Burrow, C., and Warren, M. P.,** Attitudes toward eating and body weight in different groups of female adolescent athletes, *Int. J. Eating Disorders,* 7, 749, 1988.

36. **Cohen, J. L., Potosnak, L., Frank, O., and Baker, H.,** A nutritional and hematologic assessment of elite ballet dancers, *Phys. Sportsmed.,* 13, 43, 1985.

37. **Benson, J. E., Geiger, C. J., Eiserman, P. A., and Wardlaw, G. M.,** Relationship between nutrient intake, body mass index, menstrual function, and ballet injury, *J. Am. Diet. Assoc.,* 89, 58, 1989.

38. **Frisch, R. E., Wyshak, G., and Vincent, L.,** Delayed menarche and amenorrhea in ballet dancers, *N. Engl. J. Med.,* 303, 17, 1980.

39. **Moffatt, R. J.,** Dietary status of elite female high school gymnasts: inadequacy of vitamin and mineral intake, *J. Am. Diet. Assoc.,* 84, 1361, 1984.

40. **Benson, J. E., Allemann, Y., Theintz, G. E., and Howald, H.,** Eating problems and calorie intake levels in Swiss adolescent athletes, *Int. J. Sports Med.,* 11, 249, 1990.

41. **Harris, M. B. and Greco, D.,** Weight control and weight concern in competitive female gymnasts, *J. Sports Exercise Psychol.,* 12, 427, 1990.

42. **Weight, L. M. and Noakes, T. D.,** Is running an analog of anorexia?: a survey of the incidence of eating disorders in female distance runners, *Med. Sci. Sports Exercise,* 19, 213, 1987.

43. **Mallick, M. J., Whipple, T. W., and Huerta, E.,** Behavioral and psychological traits of weight-conscious teenagers: a comparison of eating-disordered patients and high- and low-risk groups, *Adolescence,* 23, 157, 1987.

44. **Sherman, A. R. and Kramer, B.,** Iron nutrition and exercise, in *Nutrition in Exercise and Sport,* Hickson, J. F. and Wolinsky, I., Eds., CRC Press, Boca Raton, FL, 1989, 291-300.

45. **Cook, J. D. and Finch, C. A.,** Assessing iron status of a population, *Am. J. Clin. Nutr.,* 32, 2115, 1979.

46. **Balaban, E. P., Cox, J. V., Snell, P., Vaughan, R. H., and Frenkel, E. P.,** The frequency of anemia and iron deficiency in the runner, *Med. Sci. Sports Exercise,* 21, 643, 1989.

47. **O'Toole, M. L., Iwane, H., Douglas, P. S., Applegate, E. A., and Hiller, D. B.,** Iron status in ultraendurance triathletes, *Phys. Sportsmed.,* 17, 90, 1989.

48. **Borel, M. J., Smith, S. M., Derr, J., and Beard, J. L.,** Day-to-day variation in iron-status indices in healthy men and women, *Am. J. Clin. Nutr.,* 54, 729, 1991.

49. **Telford, R. D. and Cunningham, R. B.,** Sex, sport, and body-size dependency of hematology in highly trained athletes, *Med. Sci. Sports Exercise,* 23, 788, 1991.

50. **Risser, W. L., Lee, E. J., Poindexter, H. B. W., West, M. S., Pivarnik, J. M., Risser, J. M. H., and Hickson, J. F.,** Iron deficiency in female athletes: its prevalence and impact on performance, *Med. Sci. Sports Exercise,* 20, 116, 1988.

51. **Clement, D. B. and Asmundson, R. C.,** Nutritional intake and hematological parameters in endurance runners, *Phys. Sportsmed.,* 10, 37, 1982.

52. **Nickerson, H. J., Holubets, M. C., Weiler, B. R., Haas, R. G., Schwartz, S., and Ellefson, M. E.,** Causes of iron deficiency in adolescent athletes, *J. Pediatr.,* 114, 657, 1989.

53. **Snyder, A. C., Dvorak, L. L., and Roepke, J. B.,** Influence of dietary iron source on measures of iron status among female runners, *Med. Sci. Sports Exercise,* 21, 7, 1989.

54. **Haymes, E. M. and Spillman, D. M.,** Iron status of women distance runners, sprinters, and control women, *Int. J. Sports Med.,* 10, 430, 1989.

55. **Oscai, L. B., Williams, B. T., and Hertig, B. A.,** Effect of exercise on blood volume, *J. Appl. Physiol.,* 24, 622, 1968.

56. **Dressendorfer, R. H., Wade, C. E., and Amsterdam, E. A.,** Development of pseudoanemia in marathon runners during a 20-day road race, *JAMA,* 246, 1215, 1981.

57. **Steenkamp, I., Fuller, C., Graves, J., Noakes, T. D., and Jacobs, P.,** Marathon running fails to influence RBC survival rates in iron-replete women, *Phys. Sportsmed.,* 14, 89, 1986.

58. **Brotherhood, J., Brozovic, B., and Pugh, L. G. C.,** Haematological status of middle and long-distance runners, *Clin. Sci. Mol. Med.,* 48, 139, 1975.

59. **Dill, D. B., Braithwaite, K., Adams, W. C., and Bernauer, E. M.,** Blood volume of middle-distance runners: effect of 2,300 m altitude and comparison with non-athletes, *Med. Sci. Sports Exercise,* 6, 1, 1974.

60. **Diehl, D. M., Lohman, T. G., Smith, S. C., and Kertzer, R.,** Effects of physical training and competition on the iron status of female field hockey players, *Int. J. Sports Med.,* 7, 264, 1986.

61. **Selby, G. B. and Eichner, E. R.,** Endurance swimming, intravascular hemolysis, anemia, and iron depletion, *Am. J. Med.,* 81, 791, 1986.

62. **Lukaski, H. C., Hoverson, B. S., Gallagher, S. K., and Bolonchuk, W. W.,** Physical training and copper, iron, and zinc status of swimmers, *Am. J. Clin. Nutr.,* 51, 1093, 1990.
63. **Miller, B. J., Pate, R. R., and Burgess, W.,** Foot impact force and intravascular hemolysis during distance running, *Int. J. Sports Med.,* 9, 56, 1988.
64. **Colt, E. and Heyman, B.,** Low ferritin levels in runners, *J. Sports Med.,* 24, 13, 1984.
65. **Eichner, E. R.,** Runner's macrocytosis: a clue to footstrike hemolysis, *Am. J. Med.,* 78, 321, 1985.
66. **Lamanca, J. J., Haymes, E. M., Daly, J. A., Moffatt, R. J., and Waller, M. F.,** Sweat iron loss of male and female runners during exercise, *Int. J. Sports Med.,* 9, 52, 1988.
67. **Lampe, J. W., Slavin, J. L., and Apple, F. S.,** Iron status of active women and the effect of running a marathon on bowel function and gastrointestinal blood loss, *Int. J. Sports Med.,* 12, 173, 1991.
68. **Stewart, J. G., Ahlquist, D. A., McGill, D. B., Ilstrup, D. M., Schwartz, S., and Owen, R. A.,** Gastrointestinal blood loss and anemia in runners, *Ann. Intern. Med.,* 100, 843, 1984.
69. **McMahon, L. F., Ryan, M. J., Larson, D., and Fisher, R. L.,** Occult gastrointestinal blood loss in marathon runners, *Ann. Intern. Med.,* 100, 846, 1984.
70. **Ehn, L., Carlmark, B., and Hoglund, S.,** Iron status in athletes involved in intense physical activity, *Med. Sci. Sports Exercise,* 12, 61, 1980.
71. **Manore, M. M., Besenfelder, P. D., Wells, C. L., Carroll, S. S., and Hooker, S. P.,** Nutrient intakes and iron status in female long-distance runners during training, *J. Am. Diet. Assoc.,* 89, 257, 1989.
72. **Strand, S. M., Clarke, B. A., Slavin, J. L., and Kelly, J. M.,** Effects of physical training and iron supplementation on iron status of female athletes, *Med. Sci. Sports Exercise,* 16, 161, 1984.
73. **Hallberg, L., Hogdahl, A. M., Nilsson, L., and Rybo, G.,** Menstrual blood loss — a population study, *Acta Obstet. Gynecol. Scand.,* 45, 320, 1966.
74. **Raper, N. R., Rosenthal, J. C., and Woteki, C. E.,** Estimates of available iron in diets of individuals 1 year old and older in the Nationwide Food Consumption Survey, *J. Am. Diet. Assoc.,* 84, 783, 1984.
75. **Monsen, E. R., Hallberg, L., Layrisse, M., Hegsted, D. M., Cook, J. D., Mertz, W., and Finch, C. A.,** Estimation of available dietary iron, *Am. J. Clin. Nutr.,* 31, 134, 1978.
76. **Monsen, E. R. and Balintfy, J. L.,** Calculating dietary iron bioavailability: refinement and computerization, *J. Am. Diet. Assoc.,* 80, 307, 1982.
77. **Layrisse, M., Martinez-Torres, C., and Roche, M.,** Effect of interaction of various food on iron absorption, *Am. J. Clin. Nutr.,* 21, 1175, 1968.
78. **Newhouse, I. J., Clement, D. B., Taunton, J. E., and McKenzie, D. C.,** The effects of prelatent/latent iron deficiency on physical work capacity, *Med. Sci. Sports Exercise,* 21, 263, 1989.
79. Food and Nutrition Board, *Recommended Dietary Allowances,* 10th rev. ed., National Academy of Sciences, Washington, D.C., 1989.
80. **Loosli, A. R., Benson, J., Gillien, D. M., and Bourdet, K.,** Nutrition habits and knowledge in competitive adolescent female gymnasts, *Phys. Sportsmed.,* 14, 118, 1986.
81. **Benardot, D., Schwarz, M., and Heller, D. W.,** Nutrient intake in young, highly competitive gymnasts, *J. Am. Diet. Assoc.,* 89, 401, 1989.
82. **Murphy, S. P. and Calloway, D. H.,** Nutrient intakes of women in NHANES II, emphasizing trace minerals, fiber, and phytate, *J. Am. Diet. Assoc.,* 86, 1366, 1986.
83. **Benson, J., Gillien, D. M., Bourdet, K., and Loosli, A. R.,** Inadequate nutrition and chronic calorie restriction in adolescent ballerinas, *Phys. Sportsmed.,* 13, 79, 1985.
84. **Tilgner, S. A. and Schiller, M. R.,** Dietary intakes of female college athletes: the need for nutrition education, *J. Am. Diet. Assoc.,* 89, 967, 1989.
85. **Hallberg, L. and Rossander-Hulten, L.,** Iron requirements in menstruating women, *Am. J. Clin. Nutr.,* 54, 1047, 1991.
86. **Lampe, J. W., Slavin, J. L., and Apple, F. S.,** Poor iron status of women runners training for a marathon, *Int. J. Sports Med.,* 7, 111, 1986.
87. **Cooter, G. R. and Mowbray, K. W.,** Effects of iron supplementation and activity on serum iron depletion and hemoglobin levels in female athletes, *Res. Q.,* 49, 114, 1978.
88. **Edgerton, V. R., Bryant, S. L., Gillespie, C. A., and Gardner, G. W.,** Iron deficiency anemia and physical performance and activity of rats, *J. Nutr.,* 102, 381, 1972.
89. **Andersen, H. T. and Barkve, H.,** Iron deficiency and muscular work performance, *Scand. J. Clin. Lab. Invest.,* 114S, 9, 1970.
90. **Viteri, F. E. and Torun, B.,** Anaemia and physical work capacity, *Clin. Haematol.,* 3, 609, 1974.
91. **Matter, M., Stittfall, T., Graves, J., Myburgh, K., Adams, B., Jacobs, P., and Noakes, T. D.,** The effect of iron and folate therapy on maximal exercise performance in female marathon runners with iron and folate deficiency, *Clin. Sci.,* 72, 415, 1987.
92. **Barr, S. I.,** Nutrition knowledge of female varsity athletes and university students, *J. Am. Diet. Assoc.,* 87, 1660, 1987.

93. **Haymes, E. M.,** Iron supplementation, in *Encyclopedia of Physical Education, Fitness, and Sports,* Stull, G. A. and Cureton, T. K., Eds., Brighton Publications, Salt Lake City, 1980, 335.

94. **de Wijn, J. F., de Jongste, J. L., Mosterd, W., and Willebrand, D.,** Haemoglobin, packed cell volume, serum iron and iron binding capacity of selected athletes during training, *J. Sports Med.,* 11, 42, 1971.

95. **Pate, R. R., Maguire, M., and Van Wyk, J.,** Dietary iron supplementation in women athletes, *Phys. Sportsmed.,* 7, 81, 1979.

96. **Schoene, R. B., Escourrou, R., Robertson, H. T., Nilson, K. L., Parsons, J. R., and Smith, N. J.,** Iron repletion decreases maximal exercise lactate concentrations in female athletes with minimal iron-deficiency anemia, *J. Lab. Clin. Med.,* 102, 306, 1983.

97. **Nelson, M. E., Fisher, E. C., Catsos, P. D., Meredith, C. N., Turksoy, R. N., and Evans, W. J.,** Diet and bone status in amenorrheic runners, *Am. J. Clin. Nutr.,* 43, 910, 1986.

98. **Schweiger, U., Laessle, R., Schweiger, M., Herrmann, F., Riedel, W., and Pirke, K.,** Calorie intake, stress, and menstrual function in athletes, *Fertil. Steril.,* 49, 447, 1988.

99. **Wolman, R. L. and Harries, M. G.,** Menstrual abnormalities in elite athletes, *Clin. Sports Med.,* 1, 95, 1989.

100. **Kaiserauer, S., Snyder, A. C., Sleeper, M., and Zierath, J.,** Nutritional, physiological, and menstrual status of distance runners, *Med. Sci. Sports Exercise,* 21, 120, 1989.

101. **Baer, J. T. and Taper, L. J.,** Amenorrheic and eumenorrheic adolescent runners: dietary intake and exercise training status, *J. Am. Diet. Assoc.,* 92, 89, 1992.

102. **Marcus, R., Cann, C., Madvig, P., Minkoff, J., Goddard, M., Bayer, M., Martin, M., Gaudiani, L., Haskell, W., and Genant, H.,** Menstrual function and bone mass in elite women distance runners, *Ann. Intern. Med.,* 102, 158, 1985.

103. **Sanborn, C. F., Albrecht, B. H., and Wagner, W. W.,** Athletic amenorrhea: lack of association with body fat, *Med. Sci. Sports Exercise,* 19, 207, 1987.

104. **Howat, P. M., Carbo, M. L., Mills, G. Q., and Wozniak, P.,** The influence of diet, body fat, menstrual cycling, and activity upon the bone density of females, *J. Am. Diet. Assoc.,* 89, 1305, 1989.

105. **Brownell, K. D., Nelson Steen, S., and Wilmore, J. H.,** Weight regulation practices in athletes: analysis of metabolic and health effects, *Med. Sci. Sports Exercise,* 19, 546, 1987.

106. **Myerson, M., Gutin, B., Warren, M. P., May, M. T., Contento, I., Lee, M., Pi-Sunyer, F. X., Pierson, R. N., and Brooks-Gunn, J.,** Resting metabolic rate and energy balance in amenorrheic and eumenorrheic runners, *Med. Sci. Sports Exercise,* 23, 15, 1991.

107. **Drinkwater, B. L., Nilson, K., Chestnut, C. H., Bremner, W. J., Shainholtz, S., and Southworth, M. B.,** Bone mineral content of amenorrheic and eumenorrheic athletes, *N. Engl. J. Med.,* 311, 277, 1984.

108. **Frusztajer, N. T., Dhuper, S., Warren, M. P., Brooks-Gunn, J., and Fox, R. P.,** Nutrition and the incidence of stress fractures in ballet dancers, *Am. J. Clin. Nutr.,* 51, 779, 1990.

109. **Goldin, B. R., Adlercreutz, H., Gorbach, S. L., Warram, J. H., Dwyer, J. T., Swenson, L., and Woods, M. N.,** Estrogen excretion patterns and plasma levels in vegetarian and omnivorous women, *N. Engl. J. Med.,* 307, 1542, 1982.

110. **Shultz, T. D., Wilcox, R. B., Spuehler, J. M., and Howie, B. J.,** Dietary and hormonal interrelationships in premenopausal women: evidence for a relationship between dietary nutrients and plasma prolactin levels, *Am. J. Clin. Nutr.,* 46, 905, 1987.

111. **Pirke, K. M., Schweiger, U., Laessle, R., Dickhaut, B., Schweiger, M., and Waechtler, M.,** Dieting influences the menstrual cycle: vegetarian versus nonvegetarian diet, *Fertil. Steril.,* 46, 1083, 1986.

112. **Pedersen, A. B., Bartholomew, M. J., Dolence, L. A., Aljadir, L. P., Netteburg, K. L., and Lloyd, T.,** Menstrual differences due to vegetarian and nonvegetarian diets, *Am. J. Clin. Nutr.,* 53, 879, 1991.

113. **Schweiger, U., Laessle, R., Pfister, H., Hoehl, C., Schwingenschloegel, M., Schweiger, M., and Pirke, K. M.,** Diet-induced menstrual irregularities: effects of age and weight loss, *Fertil. Steril.,* 48, 746, 1987.

114. **Clark, N., Nelson, M., and Evans, W.,** Nutrition education for elite female runners, *Phys. Sportsmed.,* 16, 124, 1988.

115. **Warren, M. P., Brooks-Gunn, J., Hamilton, L. H., Warren, L. F., and Hamilton, W. G.,** Scoliosis and fractures in young ballet dancers, *N. Engl. J. Med.,* 314, 1348, 1986.

116. **Cann, C. E., Martin, M. C., Genant, H. K., and Jaffe, R. B.,** Decreased spinal mineral content in amenorrheic women, *JAMA,* 251, 626, 1984.

117. **Drinkwater, B. L., Bruemner, B., and Chesnut, C. H.,** Menstrual history as a determinant of current bone density in young athletes, *JAMA,* 263, 545, 1990.

118. **Grimston, S. K., Engsberg, J. R., Kloiber, R., and Hanley, D. A.,** Menstrual, calcium, and training history: relationship to bone health in female runners, *Clin. Sports Med.,* 2, 119, 1990.

119. **Lloyd, T., Myers, C., Buchanan, J. R., and Demers, L. M.,** Collegiate women athletes with irregular menses during adolescence have decreased bone density, *Obstet. Gynecol.,* 72, 639, 1988.

120. **Perron, M. and Endres, J.,** Knowledge, attitudes, and dietary practices of female athletes, *J. Am. Diet. Assoc.,* 85, 573, 1985.

121. **Grandjean, A. C. et al.,** unpublished data, 1991.

122. **Dawson-Hughes, B., Dallal, G. E., Krall, E. A., Sadowski, L., Sahyoun, N., and Tannenbaum, S.,** A controlled trial of the effect of calcium supplementation on bone density in postmenopausal women, *N. Engl. J. Med.,* 323, 878, 1990.

123. **Cook, J. D., Dassenko, S. A., and Whittaker, P.,** Calcium supplementation: effect of iron absorption, *Am. J. Clin. Nutr.,* 53, 106, 1991.

124. **Hallberg, L., Brune, M., Erlandsson, M., Sandberg, A. S., and Rossander-Hulten, L.,** Calcium: effect of different amounts on nonheme- and heme-iron absorption in humans, *Am. J. Clin. Nutr.,* 53, 112, 1991.

125. **Dalton, K.,** *Premenstrual Syndrome and Progesterone Therapy,* 2nd ed., Yearbook Medical, Chicago, 1985, 39.

126. **Sharma, V.,** Premenstrual syndrome, *Practitioner,* 226, 1091, 1982.

127. **Fisher, M., Trieller, K., and Napolitano, B.,** Premenstrual symptoms in adolescents, *J. Adolescent Health Care,* 10, 369, 1989.

128. **Woods, N. F., Most, A., and Dery, G. K.,** Prevalence of perimenstrual symptoms, *Am. J. Public Health,* 72, 1257, 1982.

129. **Frank, R. T.,** The hormonal causes of premenstrual tension, *Arch. Neurol. Psychiatry,* 26, 1053, 1931.

130. **Reid, R. L. and Yen, S. S. C.,** Premenstrual syndrome, *Am. J. Obstet. Gynecol.,* 139, 85, 1981.

131. **Brooks-Gunn, J., Gargiulo, J. M., and Warren, M. P.,** The effect of cycle phase on the performance of adolescent swimmers, *Phys. Sportsmed.,* 14, 182, 1986.

132. **Prior, J. C., Vigna, Y., and Alojada, N.,** Conditioning exercise decreases premenstrual symptoms, *Eur. J. Appl. Physiol.,* 55, 349, 1986.

133. **Freeman, E., Rickels, K., Sondheimer, S. J., and Polansky, M.,** Ineffectiveness of progesterone suppository treatment for premenstrual syndrome, *JAMA,* 264, 349, 1990.

134. **Abraham, G. E.,** Nutritional factors in the etiology of the premenstrual tension syndromes, *J. Reprod. Med.,* 28, 446, 1983.

135. **Rossignol, A. M. and Bonnlander, H.,** Caffeine-containing beverages, total fluid consumption, and premenstrual syndrome, *Am. J. Public Health,* 80, 1106, 1990.

136. **Adams, P. W., Wynn, V., Seed, M., and Folkard, J.,** Vitamin B6 depression, and oral contraception, *Lancet,* 2, 516, 1974.

137. **Rose, D. P.,** The interactions between vitamin B6 and hormones, *Vitam. Horm.,* 36, 53, 1978.

138. **Williams, M. J., Harris, R. I., and Dean, B. C.,** Controlled trial of pyridoxine in the premenstrual syndrome, *J. Int. Med. Res.,* 13, 174, 1985.

139. **Berman, M. K., Taylor, M. L., and Freeman, E.,** Vitamin B-6 in premenstrual syndrome, *J. Am. Diet. Assoc.,* 90, 859, 1990.

140. **Dalton, K.,** Pyridoxine overdose in premenstrual syndrome, *Lancet,* 1, 1168, 1985.

141. **Schaumburg, H., Kaplan, J., Windebank, A., Vick, N., Rasmus, S., Pleasure, D., and Brown, M. J.,** Sensory neuropathy from pyridoxine abuse, *N. Engl. J. Med.,* 309, 445, 1983.

142. **Facchinetti, F., Borella, P., Sances, G., Fioroni, L., Nappi, R. E., and Genazzani, A. R.,** Oral magnesium successfully relieves premenstrual mood changes, *Obstet. Gynecol.,* 78, 177, 1991.

143. **Blair, S. N., Ellsworth, N. M., Haskell, W. L., Stern, M. P., Farquhar, J. W., and Wood, P. D.,** Comparison of nutrient intake in middle-aged men and women runners and controls, *Med. Sci. Sports Exercise,* 13, 310, 1981.

144. **van Erp-Baart, A. M. J., Saris, W. H. M., Binkhorst, R. A., Vos, J. A., and Elvers, J. W. H.,** Nationwide survey on nutritional habits in elite athletes. I. Energy, carbohydrate, protein, and fat intake, *Int. J. Sports Med.,* 10, S11, 1989.

145. **Singh, A., Deuster, P. A., Day, B. A., and Moser-Veillon, P. B.,** Dietary intakes and biochemical markers of selected minerals: comparison of highly trained runners and untrained women, *J. Am. Coll. Nutr.,* 9, 65, 1990.

146. **Short, S. H. and Short, W. R.,** Four-year study of university athletes' dietary intake, *J. Am. Diet. Assoc.,* 82, 632, 1983.

147. **Smith, M. P., Mendez, J., Druckenmiller, M., and Kris-Etherton, P. M.,** Exercise intensity, dietary intake, and high-density lipoprotein cholesterol in young female competitive swimmers, *Am. J. Clin. Nutr.,* 36, 251, 1982.

148. **Khoo, C. S., Rawson, N. E., Robinson, M. L., and Stevenson, R. J.,** Nutrient intake and eating habits of triathletes, *Ann. Sports Med.,* 3, 144, 1987.

149. **Hickson, J. F., Schrader, J., and Trischler, L. C.,** Dietary intakes of female basketball and gymnastics athletes, *J. Am. Diet. Assoc.,* 86, 251, 1986.

150. **Chen, J. D., Wang, J. F., Li, K. J., Zhao, Y. W., Wang, S. W., Jiao, Y., and Hou, X. Y.,** Nutritional problems and measures in elite and amateur athletes, *Am. J. Clin. Nutr.,* 49, 1084, 1989.

Chapter 16

SURVEYS OF DIETARY INTAKE AND NUTRITION KNOWLEDGE OF ATHLETES AND THEIR COACHES

Sarah H. Short

CONTENTS

0-8493-7911-3/94/$0.00+$.50
© 1994 by CRC Press, Inc.

I. INTRODUCTION

The goals of this chapter are to:

*   Investigate the nutritional knowledge of those involved in physical activity and athletic performance
*   Investigate the nutritional knowledge of coaches and those who supervise the training of athletes
*   Discuss nutritional surveys
*   Consider dietary intake of athletes

Peak performance and good health involve proper nutrition and physical fitness. There are no magic diets that will make an athlete win. Good genes, good conditioning, *and* a proper diet are needed to build a fit body or an elite athlete. There is too much misinformation in the field of sports nutrition and too many sales of super wonder pills. Why is this? Athletes want the "edge", a fast way to become a winner. There are also at least four problems with communicating scientific nutrition information in the U.S.

Under the First Amendment, anyone can write a book that contains nutrition inaccuracies or outright falsehoods. This means that many of the nutrition books published for the public should be listed under "books of fiction". Readers should investigate the author's qualifications before they follow the recommendations in the book.

Second, if the product is not labeled a food or a drug, it falls between the cracks of the Federal Food, Drug, and Cosmetic Act (FDCA). This act is the laws that protects consumers against harmful and misleading food, drugs, devices, and cosmetics.[1] However, the Proxmire Amendment[2] modified the law so that the Food and Drug Administration (FDA) cannot set limits on the potency of vitamin and mineral supplements except for reasons of safety and cannot declare them drugs only because they exceed the level of potency determined to be nutritionally rational or useful. According to FDA Deputy Associate Commissioner Dykstra " . . . it is no secret that in terms of safety of dietary supplements, FDA is not doing much today. It is really buyer beware! . . . The framework simply is not in place today to give consumers the type of assurance that they demanded."[3] Recently, the FDA Dietary Supplement Task Force has been investigating vitamin and minerals, amino acids, and a "catch-all" category (including such products as coenzyme Q_{10}, garlic oil, and herbs) for safety and nutritive value, among other concerns. It is hoped that athletes, as well as the general public, soon will be better protected when they buy dietary supplements.

The third problem associated with nutrition education for athletes and the public is that anyone can call themselves a nutritionist. A nutritionist may be someone who purchases a degree from a nonaccredited institution, someone who has a Ph.D. in nutrition, a physician who specializes in nutrition, a dietitian, or others. A registered dietition (R.D.) has graduated from an accredited university, an internship, or similar experience, passed an examination by the American Dietetic Association, and has continuing education credits.[4] Dietitians may also be licensed by some states and use L.D. after their names. Athletes should ask for credentials before they follow nutritional advice.

An added problem is that research scientists go public with their conclusions before their study or experiments have been duplicated. One research study or one epidemiological survey does not test a scientific theory. Since athletics are big business in the U.S., all of these problems are intensified when it comes to sports nutrition information and products. Misinformation spreads through electronic and print media to the players, their coaches, and trainers.

Nutrition has been one of the most neglected areas in sports medicine.[5] Too few involved in sports and fitness know that there are qualified sports nutritionists/dietitians in the practice of sports and cardiovascular nutrition. These dietitians are organized to promote the integration of nutrition, exercise, and respiratory fitness to achieve and maintain optimal health. A registered dietitian is an essential part of the sports medicine team.

"There is still no sphere of nutrition in which faddism and ignorance are more obvious than in athletics." Athletes need and want correct nutrition information. "There is a growing need for sports nutrition counseling and education to help athletes improve their eating habits."[7]

Even general nutrition textbooks are not blameless. In many cases, advice for athletes is presented as if all athletes had the same needs. Nutrition advice must be *individualized*. When providing nutritional information, it is necessary to know if the athlete is involved in an endurance or short-term event, body composition (if possible), age, time spent practicing and training, and whether the athlete is training for a meet/match/tournament lasting one day or held on successive days. Nutrition advice that is provided for "athletes in general" makes little sense.

"Although coaches, trainers and athletes usually well understand the principles of physical training, they often neglect the equally well-developed principles of nutrition."[8] It is important for coaches to know enough about nutrition concepts to have a sports nutritionist help with the team, since many sports have weight constraints. This leads to tension between the coaches and their athletes, especially women athletes.[9]

In order to best serve elite athletes, it is necessary to know something about what the coaches are telling the players, what the athletes know about nutrition, and what the athletes are actually eating. Surveys of nutrition knowledge provides a starting point for nutrition education of athletes, their coaches, and those professionals caring for athletes. Surveys of dietary intake provide information on nutrient intake which should be translated into changes in dietary habits. This should serve as a basis for sports nutrition education over a lifetime. Before using survey results, it should be noted that sampling and data processing survey activities "are more scientifically based than the questionnaire design, which remains essentially an art".[10]

II. NUTRITION KNOWLEDGE
A. What Do Athletic Coaches and Others Know About Nutrition?

It is important to investigate the nutrition knowledge of coaches, trainers, and others who influence the athletes, since coaches, especially, can greatly influence all aspects of the athlete's life, including their eating habits. Coaches, however, may have learned from their coaches, thereby promulgating nutrition myths.

Over 100 college coaches in North Carolina were surveyed to measure nutrition knowledge, identify recommendations for dietary practices, and to discover sources of the coaches' nutrition information.[11] A short true–false nutrition test was answered correctly by 70% of the coaches, but only one third of the coaches were certain their answers were correct. Most (82%) of the coaches never took a college nutrition course, but 48% planned the pregame meals. These coaches (80%) knew little about the amount of carbohydrate, fat, and protein appropriate for an athlete's diet. The majority of the coaches reported that eating ''junk food'' was the worst dietary problem. Three of the coaches did urge their athletes to enroll in a college nutrition course. Recommendations of vitamin/mineral supplements (60%), carbohydrate loading (40% of male coaches), protein supplements (20%), fluid restriction (12% of the male coaches), and milk restriction (24% of male coaches) all indicated that more nutrition education was needed. These coaches indicated that their nutrition information came from ''books'', physician's advice, ''professional journals'', and ''popular literature''. Dietitians or nutritionists were consulted by only 2% of the coaches. The authors recommended special nutrition workshops to increase the coaches' nutrition information.

A survey of 303 North Carolina high school coaches and trainers found that trainers knew more about 15 nutrition questions than coaches, and that trainers more frequently recommended better nutrition procedures for their athletes.[12] The trainers probably are more knowledgeable because those certified by the National Athletic Trainers Association must have passed a nutrition course or the equivalent and the state of North Carolina requires an additional nutrition course. It was interesting to note that coaches considered that they should provide nutrition information to the athletes, while the trainers believed the responsibility should be shared between coaches and trainers. Nutrition information was gained from professional publications, meetings, workshops, and textbooks. The professional most consulted for nutrition information was a physician. However, trainers usually consulted with other trainers, while coaches asked other coaches or trainers for advice.

A nutrition knowledge survey of 342 high school coaches from Alabama found that 69% could not recommend a correct diet for athletes, 32% recommended protein supplements, 20% recommended salt tablets, 62% told their athletes to take vitamin and mineral supplements.[13]

The Iowa Dairy Council, the Iowa High School Athletic Association, and an area hospital held a conference for high school coaches to learn about sports nutrition.[14] Coaches indicated that they would use the nutrition information for their athletes, but no follow-up was reported.

Texas high school coaches were studied using a questionnaire.[15] More than half of the coaches suggested that athletes supplement with vitamins or multivitamins with minerals. Water was recommended to hydrate by the majority of coaches, but set times were not scheduled for drinking the water. Some (12%) of the coaches recommended salt tablets for their athletes.

A nutrition knowledge survey of 348 coaches, 179 athletic trainers, and 2977 athletes in high school and college settings throughout the U.S. reported that over 70% of the athletic trainers (ATC) certified by the National Athletic Trainers Association had taken nutrition courses and felt that they should provide the athletes with nutrition information.[16] Despite the fact that only 27% of the coaches had taken a formal nutrition course, half of them stated that they should provide the nutrition education. Athletic trainers not certified (81%) believed they should counsel the athletes on diet, although over 25% had little nutrition education. The coaches and both groups of trainers reported fluids as the prime nutritional concern for the athletes. This was ranked third by the athletes, themselves, after concerns about weight and vitamins. Sources of nutrition information reported by athletes were parents (ranked first or second by 77%) followed by print or electronic media. Athletes were asked about their familiarity with, and daily use of, three nutritional guides. Most (68%) of the athletes were very familiar with the daily food guides and 71% of them used this guide daily. Since the athletes were not asked to define these nutritional guides, it would be difficult to judge if these guidelines were actually being used. Additionally, these guidelines were not formulated for athletes. Athletes were not identified by their event except to state that wrestlers and swimmers relied more on coaches for nutrition information, while football and baseball players relied on their trainers.

The Daily "Four" Food guide is mentioned in several surveys. The Daily Food Guide was divided into six food groups by the United States Department of Agriculture.[17] The groups consisted of bread/cereal, milk/cheese, meat/poultry/fish/beans, fruit, vegetable, and the "other group" of fats/sweets/alcohol. The Eating Right Pyramid, A Guide to Daily Food Choices was released as an official United States Department of Agriculture publication in 1992. In this scheme, the bread/cereal group is at the bottom of the pyramid with 6 to 11 servings suggested per day. Next on the pyramid are the vegetable group (3 to 5 servings) and the fruit group with 2 to 4 servings. The meat/poultry/fish/beans group has 2 to 3 servings and the milk group suggests 2 to 3 servings, while the top of the pyramid suggests that fats, oils, and sweets be used sparingly.

High school football, basketball, and track coaches in Texas were surveyed to determine their nutrition knowledge.[18] Only 11% had taken a separate college course in nutrition but 86% provided nutrition information on a monthly basis to the athletes. A majority (73%) indicated that their preparation for advising athletes was sufficient, but almost all of them stated that a nutrition course or workshop would be beneficial. The coaches indicated that their source of nutrition information came mainly from professional journals and popular magazines. They believed that the coach is responsible for nutrition in relation to athletic performance.

Nutritional practices surveys were answered by 137 coaches in the Big Ten conference.[19] Of these college coaches, representing 153 men's and women's varsity teams, only two used dietary surveys to measure the nutritional health of their athletes. However, some were dispensing vitamins (17% of the coaches), protein supplements (8%), and minerals (8%). The coaches reported that they relied on popular magazines, trainers, physicians, players, and other coaches for nutrition information. Many (69%) stated that they rarely read about nutrition, but 78% did feel the need for more knowledge about sports nutrition.

Many of the physical education majors in college will become the coaches and teachers working with athletes in schools. When these students were questioned about their source of nutrition information, those who ranked college nutrition courses as their first source of nutrition knowledge had higher mean test scores than those who listed college course as third or not at all.[20] Students who ranked coaches low on their list of information sources scored higher on the test. There was no difference in scores for those who participated in athletics as compared with those who did not.

Information was collected from 75 coaches and trainers (mostly involved with football programs) concerning their nutrition knowledge.[21] Over half (51%) believed that a desirable diet should be 45% protein, 45% carbohydrate, and 10% fat. All of the group indicated they did not possess current nutrition information, but only 56% felt they needed more information. The authors concluded that trainers should take a college nutrition course, coaches should become more knowledgeable about nutrition, and that a nutrition expert should discuss sports nutrition information with high school athletes.

The nutrition knowledge of aerobic dance instructors was surveyed nationwide using a mailed questionnaire.[22] The 544 instructors averaged 59% on the nutrition test covering weight control, nutrient requirements, and nutrient sources. Most of those responding suggested that nutrition education be part of their program.

B. What do Athletes Know About Nutrition? What Are Their Sources?

What do athletes know about general or sports nutrition, and from what source is this information gained? It is difficult to sort out sources when the public is being bombarded by the media, and athletes are surrounded by older players with their ideas of nutrition "facts". Some studies have been reported which attempt to discover nutrition knowledge of athletes. More studies are needed to describe methods of providing correct information and persuading athletes to change their diets in a suitable direction.

A study of nutrition knowledge and food practices of college athletes (115) compared to nonathletes (55) found that nonathletes and females had significantly higher nutrition knowledge scores and lower nutrient intakes (from a 24-h recall) than athletes and male subjects.[23] Nutrition knowledge was not related to better dietary intakes.

Adolescents may know more about nutrition than they apply to their own diets. While investigating conceptual relationships between training and eating in high school distance runners, it was concluded that nutrition knowledge was poor (52% on test scores) and that educators should make the nutrition message more meaningful to the individual adolescent.[24]

While looking at bone densities of 13 female college track team members, 14 college dancers, 14 nonathletic college women, and 18 postmenopausal women, subjects were given nutrition knowledge and attitude tests.[25] Nutrition knowledge and attitude scores were not significantly correlated with each other. All of the nonathletic group had taken a college nutrition course and earned higher scores on the nutrition test. The knowledge scores of the dancers were the lowest. Nutrition knowledge was positively correlated with age and milk drinking and negatively correlated with the use of carbonated beverages. Sources of nutrition education for the dancers were parents and friends and then the media. The track team gained their nutrition information from the media and then parents and friends. Only one dancer and two track team members had consulted a registered dietition.

Unfortunately, too little research has been published on wheelchair athletes. One survey, completed by 157 athletes who had competed in the National Veterans Wheelchair games, found the mean of correctly answered sports nutrition questions was 54%.[26] Most of the incorrect answers concerned information about protein, vitamins, and energy needs. Magazines, television, and books provided most of the nutrition information. The athletes listed dietitians, followed by physicians and trainers, as the best source of nutrition knowledge.

Division I football and basketball players at the University of Southern Mississippi were given a nutrition test resulting in a mean score of 57%.[27] The conclusion from the test and dietary assessment was that these athletes should be provided with information about increasing complex carbohydrates in the diet and decreasing simple sugar, total fat, and saturated fat.

Nutrition knowledge and weight control practices of 317 high school wrestlers and 81 National Junior Olympic boxing competitors were compared.[28] These adolescent athletes had similar nutrition knowledge and agreed that fasting was dangerous and that weight should be lost by proper dieting and exercise. However, over 90% of both groups were losing weight and many were using techniques such as saunas, rubber suits, and vomiting. Both groups considered that their coaches were the most important source of nutrition information about weight control, with their fellow team members rated second for information.

To determine if exercising adult members of a university wellness center have greater nutrition knowledge and better eating habits, 240 subjects were interviewed by a mail survey.[29] It was found that exercisers were significantly better informed and had better eating patterns than nonexercisers.

Self- and group instruction for teaching sports nutrition to college athletes were developed covering athletes' basic diet, pregame meal, fluids, and ergogenic aids.[30] The mean gain in post-test scores was 23 for the self-instruction and 17 for the group instruction, which may have been due to the fact that the self-instruction group received review questions while the other group had no review. This is certainly a step in the right direction, since the athletes knew only about half the information before they started.

Others have found that nutrition education in an extracurricular setting over a 2-month period was an effective method of providing nutrition information to Little League cheerleaders.[31]

Trent[32] studied the nutrition knowledge of active-duty United States Navy personnel using a questionnaire based on the Navy Nutrition and Weight Control Guide.[33] The mean score from 2938 participants was 65%. Knowledge was low in the area of calories/food intake and carbohydrates and strongest in vitamin/minerals and fiber. It was concluded that efforts should be intensified to reach low-scoring subgroups and to develop point-of-choice nutrition education programs for military dining facilities.

The United States Miliary Academy at West Point provided their 1040 cadets with 2-h lessons on sports nutrition, which included worksheets on energy expenditure and fluid replacement during exercise.[34] Students also receive 3 h of nutrition education, but it was not stated if this was three credit hours or three clock hours of study.

Since the relationship between nutrition and sports has become of "increasing interest in college athletics", a study done at Florida International University found that nutrition education during six weekly small group lectures improved nutrition knowledge for the female athletes, but little difference was noted for the male athletes.[35]

A family health history as well as physical and blood measurements were taken for 49 male athletes at the University of Nevada–Reno.[36] The nutrition exam testing knowledge of dietary sodium and fat found 43% of the sample scored below 70%.

A study of the nutrition knowledge of female varsity athletes (70) and university students (129), found test scores averaging 34% for both groups.[37] Sources of nutrition information for both groups came mainly from magazines, followed by books, and teammates or friends. The "most useful" sources were listed as magazines or books, followed by school courses. The coach was listed at the bottom of the "most useful" list, but listed as a source used by 30% of the varsity athletes.

Primary sources of nutrition information used by 106 dancers (age 8 to 66) were investigated.[38] Over half of the group enrolled in ballet (many were professional dancers) received their nutrition information from magazines or books, while 37% found their information from other dancers or friends. The total group of dancers reported their source of nutrition knowledge from magazines (39%), books (24%), friends (24%), other dancers (23%), doctors (20%), nutritionists (15%), dance instructors (12%), health food stores (12%), parents and family (8%), and college/school (8%). It is not very encouraging to learn that only slightly more dancers choose nutritionists over health food stores as a source of information.

Nutrition knowledge, attitudes, and dietary practices were compared among female college athletes (dancers and track team), nonathletic college women, and postmenopausal women.[39] The nonathletic group earned a higher score on the knowledge test than did the dancers or track team, and their score was slightly higer than the postmenopausal women. It should be noted that the nonathletes had all taken a college nutrition course. The four groups showed no significant difference in attitude scores. The source of nutrition information reported by most of the track team was the media. Dancers relied on parents, nonathletes learned most from their college nutrition course, while the postmenopausal women most frequently listed friends, physicians, and the media.

As part of a study to investigate dietary patterns and gastrointestinal complaints of recreational triathletes, researchers at the Uniformed Services University of the Health Sciences administered a nutrition knowledge test.[40] There was no significant difference in scores between the triathletes (21 women and 50 men) and the control group, but women athletes scored higher on the test than men athletes. Their nutrition information was mostly derived from newspapers and sports magazines. There seemed to be widespread misinformation since they believed that spinach is a good source of iron, that peanut butter is high in cholesterol, and many of the athletes used nutritional supplements and had atypical eating patterns.

A study of 75 male members of college track, basketball, and football teams questioned about their nutrition knowledge and the sources of this information found that less than half could define glycogen loading, list good food sources of carbohydrates, recommend a healthy pregame meal, or knew major functions of vitamins.[41] More than half, however, knew about fluid intake for athletes, food sources of fat, functions of carbohydrates, and how muscle mass is increased. The major sources of nutrition information for these men were parents first and then high school physical education/health courses. Only about 10% cited nutritionists/dietitions as sources of their nutrition information. Most of the athletes on all three teams believed that nutrition can influence performance. Few thought they had current nutrition information, but up to 70% of the team members believed they had adequate knowledge.

The majority of 104 female marathon runners and 105 fitness club members studied found their nutrition information in magazines and books.[42] Runners found books most useful, while fitness club members found books and their fitness class most useful. The mean for the general nutrition knowledge and sports nutrition tests were slightly higher for runners than for the fitness class. Dietetic interns, completing the same test, scored well on the general nutrition knowledge, but low on sports nutrition. Dietetic programs need to include more information on sports nutrition in their coursework.

Walsh[43] studied the health beliefs and practices of 77 runners and 66 nonrunners using a mailed questionnaire, one section of which covered nutrition. Results of the nutrition test were not presented, but it was stated that because of the runner's emphasis on leanness and strict weight control, "nutrition counseling often is indicated".

Competitive adolescent female gymnasts (age 11 to 17) practicing at least 9 h a week did poorly on nutrition questions about fuel for energy and food sources of carbohydrate.[44] Half of the girls could not describe a complex carbohydrate, and they knew little about the role of carbohydrates as a fuel during exercise.

National male and female elite adolescent swimmers, who train between 10,000 and 16,000 m a day at 85 to 90% of $\dot{V}O_2$ max, given a nutrition test did well on basic knowledge but poorly on choosing foods high in specific nutrients such as carbohydrates or proteins.[45] If they were unable to answer questions on food sources, it seems improbable that they would be able to choose the correct diet.

Less than half of 31 female volleyball team members age 13 to 17 correctly answered general nutrition or sports nutrition questions.[46] These volleyball players knew little about protein in the diet, carbohydrate loading, sodium levels, or energy needed during exercise. The subjects were knowledgeable about reducing diets, vitamin supplements, plant oils vs. animal fats, and the value of eating a variety of food. Less than one third believed that nutrition was a coach's responsibility, but they did not state who should have that responsibility. The scores on nutrition knowledge and attitude did not correlate with dietary intakes, indicating other forces shaped their dietary habits. These forces might be a desire to be thin, or easily accessible high caloric foods.

Most of the 171 college athletes, questioned about their nutritional beliefs, indicated that a high-protein diet would improve athletic performance and increase muscle mass.[47] Over 75% felt that athletes need a larger quantity of vitamins as compared with nonathletes and that natural vitamin supplements are better than synthetic. Half of the athletes thought that water is the best fluid for athletes, but only 13% strongly agreed that athletes need more water than thirst dictates. Almost half thought that athletes should use salt tablets in hot weather.[48]

Investigators looking at the nutrition knowledge of two college wrestling teams concluded that "the wrestlers lacked a good understanding of basic nutrition and were prone to common food fallacies''.[49] It was found that 32% of the wrestlers avoided breads, pasta, and potatoes, preferred high-protein foods, and believed that protein was nonfattening. Only 8% of these men thought that fluids were essential for training or performance.

Wisconsin was the first state to have a mandatory body composition testing for wrestlers in the high schools.[50] Dietitians dispensed sports nutrition education in 158 high schools in 1990, providing hope that sports nutrition education will be viewed as important.

A test of nutritional knowledge and food practices of 943 male and female high school athletes showed a mean of 55% on nutrition questions.[51] Of the 18 different sports teams in this study, members of the cross-country team and track-and-field participants scored higher on nutrition knowledge than the high school athletes in other sports. Athletes who had participated in their sport for a longer period of time had higher nutrition knowledge scores. When asked to rate their sources of nutrition information from outside the school, most ranked parents first, then popular books and magazines. Only 10% ranked medical personnel first. From within the school, science courses and home economics courses were ranked first as sources of nutrition information by half the students. Only 15% of the students ranked their coaches as a major source of information about sports nutrition.

A survey was conducted among 94 college women participating in 10 different competitive sports to ascertain their nutrition knowledge and attitudes.[52] The athletes scored higher on the sports nutrition section than on general nutrition and were least knowledgeable about common food misconceptions. They expressed favorable attitudes toward nutrition with very positive attitudes toward the relationship of good eating habits to good health, nutrition counseling for weight control, and the importance of coaches having favorable attitudes toward nutrition. Athletes who had nutrition education in high school or college had higher knowledge and attitude scores. Nutrition knowledge and attitude did not correlate with the frequency of food consumption.

A survey of the nutrition knowledge of 101 competitive swimmers (age 13 to 20) in the areas of general and sports nutrition found a low level of nutrition knowledge.[53] The majority believed that a well-balanced meal was necessary at all times, that a balanced diet without supplements was adequate for top performance, that eating steak did not provide extra strength before competition, and 41% felt that not everyone should take iron supplements. Almost half, however, stated that everyone should take supplements, extra energy is derived from taking vitamin B supplements, vitamin E supplements improve performance, drinking milk the day of the event decreases performance, and that protein supplements improved performance.

A nutrition knowledge survey of 120 males and females, who participated in either private or commercial, corporate, community, or a cardiac rehabilitation facility, found higher scores on health and fitness than on nutrient functions.[54] Those exercising for 20 to 45 min had higher mean scores than those exercising for only 20 min.

Although millions of adolescents take part in school sports in the U.S., less than 45% of 179 secondary schools surveyed in one state had health intervention nutrition programs for the athletes.[55] Over 60% of the respondents (health teachers, nurses, and coaches) stated that the coaches were qualified to supervise the intervention programs, although no nutritional qualifications were given.

Young athletes in community sports programs are often entrusted to inexperienced and untrained coaches.[56] Several organizations in the U.S. and Canada are attempting to remedy this situation. Nutrition information is included in some of the guides published by such organizations as Little League.[57] However, too many supervisors of young athletic teams leave the children to pick up sports nutrition information from their families or the media.

Learning nutrition information from their families may not be the best direction to take. When investigating over 2300 members of the public, health care workers, university graduate students, and health club attenders, it was found that 90% did not know the recommendations for calcium, salt, vitamin A, and fiber.[58] The majority of these subjects with college degrees or higher were ignorant of the nutrition information needed to use the dietary guidelines.

III. DIETARY SURVEYS AND THEIR PROBLEMS
A. Overall Problems

Surveys cannot document cause-and-effect relationships, even if subjected to statistical analysis, but they can point the way for further research. It has been pointed out that researchers "carrying out statistical analyses, often of an elaborate nature, have a tendency to find the answers they set out in search of and they are quick to ignore problematic aspects of and sources of uncertainty in the data they analyze."[59]

"With mounting interest in health and fitness, has come an increase in research relating diet and nutrition to physical performance."[60] Should we assume "that the athlete is a normal human whose needs can be ascertained by a standard population study? Or is the competitive athlete able to excel because he or she is metabolically unique as a result of a genetic chance or training?"[61] There are many problems associated with trying to assess the nutritional status of the athlete.

Reports of survey methods for populations and for individuals are numerous. Methods for individuals will be emphasized in this section. Gibson[62] has written an excellent book on various methods of nutritional assessment, including body composition and assessment of specific nutrients.

When judging the usefulness of dietary surveys, several problem areas should be examined: (1) the method of collecting the dietary intake of the athlete, (2) the nutrient comparison standard, (3) the data base of nutrients and food composition, and (4) how to provide athletes with feedback from the dietary assessment.

B. Methods of Obtaining Dietary Intake

Individual food intake information may be obtained from a variety of methods, including a 24-h recall, records of various lengths (commonly 1, 3, or 7 d), diet history, food frequency list, weighed food intake, electronic monitoring, or a combination of methods. There are advantages and disadvantages connected with the use of all these methods. Guidelines for the use of dietary intake data have been published.[63]

A comprehensive article by Medlin and Skinner[65] presents a 50-year history of methods used to collect individual dietary intakes.

No matter which method is used, the number of days the diet is monitored is important, since usual intake varies for an individual.[64] For more accurate results in both individuals and groups, caloric intake would need to be recorded for the fewest days (31 d for individuals and 3 for this reported group of 29), and the most days would be required to predict the intake of vitamin A (433 d for individuals and 41 for the group).[65] From 2 to 3 weeks would be needed for dietary cholesterol or the ratio of polyunsaturated fatty acids to saturated fatty acids.[66] Food habits change over a lifetime, and food intake changes from season to season. Some foods are eaten every day while others are eaten rarely. Therefore, the time necessary for a dietary survey is unknown. It depends on the precision required and varies for the nutrients under study. It may be impractical to try for more than 80% correctly classified in top and bottom thirds of a needed nutrient.

One of the more difficult aspects of collecting dietary information is the estimation of food portion sizes. Using food models or household measures increased the accuracy of estimating the amount of food eaten.[67]

Diets should be assessed for both weekends and weekdays, since significant differences were found in the number of meals and snacks eaten, energy intake throughout the day, type of food eaten, and nutrient intake when comparing weekdays to Saturday and Sunday intakes.[68]

1. Weighed Intake of All Food

A weighed food intake report is costly and time consuming, and it is difficult to achieve the desired accuracy. This method may interfere with a subject's eating patterns, which should be taken into account. An article written in the early 1970s compared weighing the subject's food intake with a diet history and concluded that there is always a bias when trying to study dietary intake.[69]

The method of duplicate food collection involves collecting duplicate amounts of all food and beverages consumed for analysis. One study concluded that the intakes of subjects during these collection periods did not represent their habitual levels of intake at other times throughout the year.[70]

A technique for quantitating individual dietary intake was described which enables individuals to self-weigh and identify all foods ingested.[71] The computer program instructs and guides the subject to ensure complete food records.

Energy intake was measured by a 7-d weighed dietary record at the same time doubled labeled water from daily urine samples were recorded. The average recorded energy intakes were found to be significantly lower than the measured expenditure in subjects whose weight was stable. This indicated a bias in reported caloric intake.[72]

Repeatability of intakes does not necessarily signify validity. Even the so-called "gold standard" for diet records (7-d weighed-food records) energy intakes were still only about 80% of outputs as assessed over a 2-week period with doubly labeled water.[73] The errors in energy intakes reported exceed 20% in more than half of the subjects studied.

2. A 24-h Recall of Food Eaten Within a Day

A 24-h recall requires an accurate memory, a 1-d diet may not be representative of usual intake, and the subject may change the intake information in an effort to please the interviewer. An advantage of this method is that the interviewer may ask for more details about the intake and its logistical simplicity.[74] Increasing to three recalls at 6-week intervals improves the reliability of the estimate for all nutrients.

A report from the National Center for Health Statistics stated that the 24-h recall method has provided accurate and reproducible estimates of the mean intakes of population groups, but information from multiple days is necessary for characterizing an individual's usual nutrient intake.[75] Others agree that the validity of the 24-h dietary recall is unsatisfactory on the individual level.[76] Some call 1-d data meaningless[77] and valueless for individual dietary intakes.[78]

Foods reported as most often omitted in men's recalls were auxiliary foods such as accompaniments, salad dressings, crackers, salty snacks, gravies and sauces, desserts such as fruits, and items such as cheese, breads, and vegetables.[79]

3. Written Personal Diet Records

Diet records need the subject's cooperation. The validity decreases with the time the record is being kept, and may depend on the time of the week or the season.[80]

Some researchers state that there is a greater stability of mean nutrient intakes from 3-d that from 1-d dietary records,[81] while others prefer a 4-d record (Friday through Monday) over a 3-d record, since weekend intakes are the most variable for individuals.[82] A 7-d dietary record was deemed sufficiently precise to describe dietary intake and show relationships of dietary intake to serum nutritional indicators.[83] However, another study indicated that classifying 106 females into quintiles even with a 7-d record was less than 55% for calories, calcium, vitamin A, and vitamin C.[84]

Mertz et al.[85] compared the estimated 7-d diet records of 263 free-living volunteers with the intake determined to maintain weight and found an under-reporting of 18%. The authors suggest caution in the interpretation of food consumption data.

A random sample of 3 d of dietary records provided closer estimates of energy and nutrients intake than did consecutive-day samples when compared with a 16-d average taken over a year-long study.[86]

Using 7-d, or even 4-d, estimated records based on detailed food descriptions with portion sizes estimated using household measures and standardized photographs were almost as reliable as weighed records and were more convenient, which perhaps increased compliance.[87]

Nutrient intake is more variable in children (age 5 to 14 years) than in adults.[88] The minimum of days of food records needed to estimate energy intake was 7 for boys and 8 for girls, with more than 20 d required for an estimate of vitamin intake. Validation of mother's reports of dietary intake by 4- to 7-year-old children was reported to be useful for classifying children by intake of calories, macronutrients, and micronutrients, but is a less accurate measure of actual food eaten, portion sizes, and nutrient levels consumed.[89]

Nationwide food consumption and dietary surveys have been conducted every 10 years by the United States Department of Agriculture since the mid-1930s. Since 1977, 3 d of intake data have been collected using 1-d recall and 2-d records.[90]

4. Dietary History

A dietary history is an interview by a trained dietition that may take an hour or longer and may include a 24-h recall, a 3-day record, and a questionnaire. The interviewer collects information about the subject's eating habits and patterns, food likes and dislikes, frequency and size of intake portions, and other diet- and health-related questions.[91] This method takes time and expertise.

A self-administered diet history questionnaire was validated using three 4-d diet records collected over a year. Correlations in the range of 0.65 were found between the questionnaire and the diet records.[92] It was pointed out that these correlations are in the same range as physiologic measures such as repeated measures of cholesterol, adult blood pressure, and uric acid.

A dietary history was developed and used with 5116 young adults.[93] This included a short questionnaire about general dietary practices, a comprehensive food frequency questionnaire for selected foods using the previous month as a reference for recall, follow-up questions concerning serving size, frequency of consumption, and common additions to these foods. This interview took 45 min.

5. Food Frequency Questionnaires

Food frequency questionnaires provide information about the quality of the diet but require a good memory since the subject is required to remember both frequency and amount of various food categories eaten over a period of time. Dietary changes during time between questionnaires contributes to poor reproducibility and validity.[94]

Questionnaires are useful in categorizing individuals and groups by food intake characteristics.[75] Food frequency questionnaire validity is limited by the adequacy of the food list and the ability of respondents to report usual intake patterns. It can only place individuals into broad categories.[95]

Food frequency reports for 1184 subjects were compared to reports from the previous 15 years.[96] Those whose diets changed least over the 15-year period had the greatest diet reproducibility. Greater reproducibility was found among men with higher education and among women of less than 110% of desirable weight.

A study of college students sought to develop a time-efficient method of assessing short-term intake by comparing a 7-d food frequency questionnaire with 24-h recalls taken three times during the week.[97] Moderately high reliability was shown. A revised food frequency questionnaire was later published.[98]

One problem with using a food frequency questionnaire is the need to know portion size eaten. The use of a standard portion size would reduce interview time for both the interviewer and the respondent. However, results of a comparison using reported and standard portion sizes indicated that this leads to different results.[99] People do not always eat standard portions.

A food-use checklist was developed as a simplification of the 24-h recall consisting of 19 yes–no questions about foods consumed during the previous day.[100] For most items agreement was good, but for items requiring knowledge of food (high-fiber cereal), it was poor.

Questionnaires can be adapted for computer use. A data collection and nutrient analysis flexible computer program was designed to permit modification of the questionnaires.[101] The program checks for unusual or omitted answers. A computer-assisted method to assess food intakes used a portion of a composite recipe stored in the computer and concluded that the time of investigation should not be shorter than 2 weeks.[102]

A food behavior checklist consisting of yes–no questions about food consumed the previous 24 h was developed and tested against a 24-h recall where the agreement was good to excellent. There was a trend to over-report general food categories (luncheon meats) but not specific foods (ice cream).[95] The authors state that this is a simple dietary assessment tool when group-level data on dietary behavior are needed to evaluate intervention programs or monitor dietary change.

A 32-item eating behavior questionnaire was developed for use in a 5-year dietary intervention project in which 287 adults were encouraged to gradually change eating habits to reduce risk factors for coronary heart disease.[103] It was concluded that the questionnaire is an inexpensive, reliable, and valid instrument for rapid assessment of eating habits and diet composition. The changes in survey scores correlated with changes in plasma cholesterol levels taken at the beginning and end of the 5-year period.

In 1992, there was a flurry of articles discussing the advantages and disadvantages of the food frequency questionnaire method of assessing dietary intake.[104-110] Monsen,[111] editor of the *Journal of the American Dietetic Association*, states that "there is a pressing need for objective methods that accurately assess food intake". Comparing dietary assessment methods to a standard is difficult when there are apprehensions about the standards.

6. Other Methods

Direct observation of children's consumption of bag lunches brought from home and eaten in school was reported to be a reliable method for assessing energy and nutrient intake of children.[112] This seems very time consuming, since one observer could only watch two children and must have many hours of training.

The study investigating if current diet reflects long-term intake concluded that in long-term studies, continuous monitoring is needed and that current intake is not a good estimator of past intake for most nutrients, especially for calcium.[113]

The selection of an appropriate dietary method depends on the level of measurement required. The dietary assessment method should be validated to ensure it is measuring what it claims to measure.[114] Validity can be measured by comparing method in use against a reference method chosen for its accuracy or against biochemical markers. Examples of biochemical markers are 24-h urinary nitrogen excretion to measure protein, urinary excretion of sodium and potassium as measures of intakes, and fatty acid composition of subcutaneous adipose tissue as a measure of fatty acid composition of the diet.

Objective verification of dietary intake by measurement of urine osmolality has been described.[115] The urinary osmol load consists primarily of compounds derived from consumed foods, specifically nitrogen-containing compounds and sodium and potassium salts. A measured osmol load lower than the predicted value indicates a lower food intake than that recorded in a food record.

Overweight women (BMI* 24 to 30) reported a smaller intake of energy and protein than lean women. Significant under-reporting of dietary intake by overweight women was revealed by the urine nitrogen test, indicating the necessity of using an independent validation test in surveys.[116] Comparisons of self-reported energy intake with energy expenditure measured by doubly labeled water have shown that errors in energy intake are much larger than previously suspected,[117] creating a dilemma for the interpretation of intake data. Double-labeled water is a method of measuring carbon dioxide, which is the end product of macronutrient oxidation. Intake must be assessed, but should be viewed as only a cautious estimate of habitual intake and interpretations based on such data.

An automated food-selection system with two vending machines containing a large variety of foods was used to measure food intake in 10 male volunteers on a metabolic ward.[118] *Ad libitum* intake resulted in a 7-d overfeeding of 6468 kJ (1546 kcal) per day above weight maintenance requirements, leading to a 2.3-kg gain. However, many of the foods in the vending machine were high-calorie, high-fat foods, and there was no skim milk available. This automated system allowed entrees, snacks, and beverages to be freely accessible to the subjects with continuous monitoring by the computer.

A photographic procedure for the measurement of individual food consumption was used to record the lunches of 13 subjects eating together.[119] The food was weighed at the same time and a 24-h recall was taken the next day. Results showed that the mean recalled estimate was lower than the mean actual weight of food items. The photographic procedure could predict the actual weight of a food item better than the recall.

Ten subjects weighed and photographed their own total food intake for 1 d.[120] Analysis of the photographic record was done by computer program as well as a nutrient analysis. Results indicated that the daily nutrient intakes estimated from photographs compared well with those obtained from a weighed record.

In order to increase the accuracy of estimating serving sizes, computer graphics were used.[121] When subjects were satisfied that the computer graphics (size could be changed on the screen) were the same as the food item, it was recorded. The results confirmed that using computer graphics increased the accuracy of serving size estimates.

7. Conclusions

One might conclude (as many have done), that there is no accurate method of determining what an athlete regularly eats. This may be true, but the more information collected, the nearer the goal of providing the best nutrition for each athlete.

Bingham[122] wrote an outstanding review of dietary assessment techniques making many important points. Asking people to estimate the weight of food as opposed to actually weighing the food may produce a variation of about 50% for foods and 20% for nutrients. Differences in nutrient intake from a 24-h recall compared with direct observation may range from 4 to 400%. Evidence suggests that estimations of food eaten in the past are impossible to obtain. Energy intakes of groups found to be less than 1.4 times the basal metabolic rate are underestimates. A 3-d record is recommended for groups. In clinical work, a 14-d record is best, depending on which nutrient is being considered. In research, records with weights of food are recommended. Sources of error include food tables used, coding errors, wrong

---

* The Body Mass Index (BMI) is defined as W/H^2, where W is weight in kilograms and H is height in centimeters.

weights of food, reporting error, variation with time, wrong frequency of consumption, change in diet, response bias, and sampling bias. All results from dietary surveys are dependent on the quality of the food tables unless food is analyzed in the laboratory. If the subject is going to weigh the food, use electronic balances. Errors in estimating portion weights of food can reach 90%. The 24-h recall is especially prone to reporting error. Overall average energy intake may be underestimated by 21%. It was concluded that the daily recall method can be associated with unacceptably large errors, no matter whether the foods alone or nutrients are considered. A diet history may include errors in the amount and frequency of food eaten. Diet histories obtained by interview only, even through carefully done, have little quantitative value. When subjects are asked to keep a record of everything they eat, there is the risk they will change their normal dietary habits. It is easier to make incorrect statements during an interview than when writing a record. The perceived importance of survey is critical and affects response rates and attitudes. There is a lack of agreement between measured dietary intake and that estimated from questionnaires. A search for a shortened method of dietary assessment of individuals seems hopeless. A diet history is thought to be highly repeatable, but this is not supported for individuals. The results of biological markers, such as a 24-h urine nitrogen for protein intake, are reported as scientifically accurate, but there are daily variations in nitrogen excretion. "Categorically, a single 24 hour record or recall should never be used to assess dietary status or to test associations between diet and some other variable such as blood cholesterol or serum lipids." If energy and energy-yielding nutrients are to be investigated, a 7-d record would be sufficient if an accuracy of plus or minus 10% standard error is acceptable. Vitamins, minerals, and fiber require longer periods of observation, at least 14 d, which does not have to be obtained over a single period of time. This could be 4-d periods of records over several months.

It is very difficult to obtain a valid estimate of habitual patterns and levels of food consumption for an individual.[123] The relative risk estimated in most studies of dietary factors and health outcomes are probably substantially underestimated.[124] For nutrients such as vitamin A and cholesterol, no meaningful results may be expected with 3- or 7-d records or recalls. Pennington[125] states that using food records, weighed intakes, and duplicate portions to assess dietary status distorts the usual eating patterns. The concern with diet histories, food frequencies, and 24-h recalls is the ability to remember food and quantities consumed.

Food intake survey reports in the literature should at least include information about the type of record used, instructions given to athletes for collecting this information, forms (if any) given to the athlete, and methods of measuring (or estimating) intake especially for meat, fish, and poultry, where there is a large variation in portion size. Food models are often used and these may increase the accuracy of estimating portion sizes.

C. Standards Used for Comparisons

After accumulating the results of a dietary analysis, a decision must be made about the standard to be used for a comparison. Comparing individual intake to the Recommended Dietary Allowance is open to criticism. "The Recommended Dietary Allowances (RDAs) are the levels of intake of essential nutrients that, on the basis of scientific knowledge, are judged by the Food and Nutrition Board to be adequate to meet the known nutrient needs of practically all healthy persons".[126] In the past these RDAs were presumed to be for group applications. However, the present RDA states that "a comparison of individual intakes, averaged over a sufficient length of time, to the RDA allows an estimate to be made about the probable risk of deficiency for that individual."

In any case, these recommendations are for "reference" people and adjustments must be made for athletes with increased physical activity, larger body size, and increased sweating leading to losses of water, salt, and other essential nutrients. Mature athletes, in many cases, are 100 or more pounds heavier and a foot or more taller than the median heights and weights provided with the RDA.

Most dietary surveys do, however, compare dietary intakes to the RDAs, but many years ago Leverton[127] warned that the RDAs are not for amateurs. The RDAs are a valuable tool for interpreting food consumption data but they can be misused. The effective application of the RDAs "requires understanding, skill, restraint, and even tolerance".

The requirements for protein in the RDAs is based on a requirement of 0.8 g of protein per kilogram of body weight (kg BW) per day. Various sports medicine scientists have stated that athletes need from 1 to 3 g of protein/kg BW/day.[128] These calculations for protein should be presented in the diet analysis results in order that the readers may judge for themselves if protein is adequate for the athletes.

The intake of several nutrients (such as protein) are based on body weight.[129] Depending upon the amount of fat and muscle, errors occur. The error in calculating recommended intakes on a body weight basis could be reduced by adjusting recommended intakes on the basis of actual lean body mass, or of lean body mass of a reference lean or obese body composition and expressed as a range. As body mass increases from normal to obese, the prevalence of deficiency for protein increased from 2 to 3% up to 93%. It is suggested that the recommendation for nutrients calculated on a body weight basis ideally be calculated on a lean body mass basis or at least on an estimated lean body mass of normal, underweight, and overweight reference persons.

If an individual maintains proper weight over time, the amount of food consumed reflects energy needs. Foods eaten to satisfy energy needs must include allowances for all other nutrients if the diet meets the person's requirements.[126] Nutrient density based on the concentration of each nutrient per 100 kcal of total dietary energy, has been published and is used as a comparison standard, especially for some of the B vitamins.[130]

D. Nutrient Intakes Considered Low

A cut-off point for "low" or "poor" intakes is usually indicated in nutritional surveys. Except for calories, the RDA is set two standard deviations above the mean to cover the needs of almost all individuals within the group. The RDA for caloric intake was set at the mean population requirement for each age group. "A margin of safety is included in the Recommended Dietary Allowances. Therefore average intake of a group does not have to equal the recommended allowance."[57] Using the value of a mean intake below 70% of the RDA, problem nutrients were identified in the Nationwide Food Consumption Survey of 1977 to 1978.[131] Other nutritional studies have classified nutrient intakes below two thirds of the RDA as low.[132]

E. Data Bases and Dietary Analysis

When selecting nutrient-calculation software packages, the quality of the nutrient data base is of prime importance.[133] Data base concerns include: completeness of foods and nutrients of interest to the researchers, specificity in order to accurately assess nutrients, current information on nutrients and foods including reformulations of existing products, quality control procedures to ensure accuracy. If the described food is not in the data base, a loss of dietary information results. Smaller data bases may appear to offer advantages but they include fewer foods and fewer nutrients. If the specific food were not found, then substitutions would have to be made. According to Hoover et al.[134] "If numerous substitutions are made, inaccurate diagnostic information may results, causing nutrient analysis to be an imprecise screening tool that does not provide a sound basis for nutrition guidance."

The United States Department of Agriculture's Nutrient Data Base contains data for energy and 28 components for over 5000 food items.[135] Data are based on the latest information from the National Nutrient Data Bank, the computer-based system used to update USDA's standard reference on food composition, Agriculture Handbook No. 8. The United States Department of Agriculture's Consumer Nutrition Center is responsible for maintaining the National Nutrient Data Bank.[136]

Large dietary data bases use, as their basis, electronic media containing current revisions of Agriculture Handbook No. 8, U.S. Department of Agriculture. A difference in nutrition data base information may be due to timing of the data base update and the use of industry, research, or other government food analysis figures, which most data base managers add for more complete information.

Data base users must realize that there are substantial gaps or holes in the tables of food composition. There is only a small amount of information available for some of the nutrients. The amounts of fiber, simple sugars, vitamins E, pyridoxine, folacin, B_{12}, and minerals zinc and copper may not reflect actual intake since not all foods have been analyzed for these nutrients. Readers of dietary intake surveys should take this into consideration when nutrient deficiencies are discussed.

Hoover and Perloff[137] have published a model for review of nutrient data base system capabilities to assist users to evaluate a nutrient data base and a system's performance and capabilities. This model allows data bank operators to check their system for errors or omissions. Karkeck[138] observed that coding food for large data bases takes time, precision, and frequent checking for accuracy. Many current computer programs avoid coding by using the actual description of the food.

Dwyer and Suitor[139] evaluated mail order and microcomputer diet analysis programs. They felt that the buyer should beware and listed problems that might be encountered, such as coding difficulties, unclear manuals, no method of correcting data, inappropriate standards, incomplete or no printout, and no way to uptake the data base.

At the very least, dietary survey reports should publish the type of computer program used, type of computer, data base, and method of indicating incomplete data in the foods and nutrients information. After considering all these points, an expert is needed to translate the computer output into dietary advice. The largest problem when looking at computer diet analysis is the hazard of "having an unqualified individual interpret the data".[140]

IV. SURVEYS OF ATHLETES' DIETARY INTAKES

Evaluating nutrition research is a difficult task. One researcher[141] believes that quality nutrition research studies should have at least 50 human subjects, appropriate control groups, controlled nutrient intake, adequate consumption data for pre- and postexperimental periods, a level of food consumption that is reasonable, and significant statistical results. Unfortunately, very few survey studies meet these specifications.

Evaluating sports nutrition research is even more difficult because of differences in various sports. Attempts to use survey data for comparison of athletes' intakes must consider the sport, specific event, times (minutes, hours, days to complete the event), climate, number of subjects surveyed, age, experience in the sport, supplements, and freedom of food choices. It is even difficult to compare the nutrient intake of members of the same team, especially if they play different positions. Sweeping statements about "all athletes" add little to sports nutrition research.

A. Surveys of a Variety of Teams

"Dietary surveys of athletes are useful not to set standards of nutrition but rather to discover deficiencies and thus to know what dietary corrections are needed."[142] Athletes engaged in endurance sports may have nutritional needs beyond that of other athletes. An endurance event is defined as lasting more than 1.5 h and ultraendurance as taking more than 6 h.[143] High-carbohydrate diets for endurance athletes are usually presented in terms of percent of calories from carbohydrate, when what is needed is an eating plan for athletes who are participating for longer than three continuous hours in their events.[144]

Grandjean[145] studied the macronutrient intake of athletes including Division I athletes, those participating in the United States Olympic Committee-sponsored competitions, and professional athletes and compared the athletes with a sample of the U.S. general population from a large government nationwide survey. These 237 athletes were competing in a variety of sports: wrestling, figure skating, distance running, judo, weightlifting, football, swimming, basketball, cycling, and baseball. The baseball players had the highest mean caloric intake and the wrestlers the lowest of the male athletes. The figure skaters were lowest in caloric intake while the cyclers were highest of the three female teams surveyed. Wrestlers had the highest percent of calories from carbohydrates (54%) and the lowest from protein (12%). The figure skaters had the lowest percent of calories from fat (34%). The baseball players and weightlifters had the highest percent of calories from protein (18%) and the basketball players had the highest percentage of calories from fat (41%). Grandjean points out that it is very difficult to calculate the amounts of the macronutrients needed for sports. She states that "either the majority of athletes are consuming less than desirable diets, the recommendations are not on target, or the recommendations are too unspecific."

Short and Short[146] collected data for 4 years on 554 athletes involved with ten men's and six women's athletic teams at Syracuse University. At various times during this period, 3-d records (14-d records for wrestlers), 24-h records, and weighed intakes were used to analyze men's basketball, bodybuilders, crew, football, gymnastic, lacrosse, mountain climbers, soccer, track and field, and wrestling teams, as well as women's basketball, crew, dancing, lacrosse, swimming, and volleyball teams. Diet records were kept by the football teams every semester, six different semesters by the wrestling teams, and less frequently by the members of other teams. The diets, which included snacks, were analyzed by a computer program written by one of the authors (W. Short) using a data base of 6076 foods and 37 nutrients. A combination of the energy program and the diet program was used for the more recent part of the study. The mean caloric intake for fall football team members was 5270, with a maximum intake of 14,000 kcal per day. On the other hand, the minimum for the wrestling and gymnastic teams was very low (400 kcal). Wrestlers cutting weight may eat nothing on the day before a match. During a season, this practice may lead to nutritional problems. All athletes, with the exception of the wrestlers and gymnasts (with minimal caloric intakes) were receiving enough protein when the intake was calculated on a per kilogram body weight basis, compared to the RDA, or on a per 1000 kcal basis. In a total study, more than one third of the teams surveyed had at least 20% of the members with low intakes of vitamin A. The athletes frequently had diets low in potassium. Wrestlers' diets were poor in calories, thiamin, riboflavin, vitamin A, niacin, and fiber. Women's teams were low in iron intake. A high proportion of calories in the football diet came from fat (38 to 42% with a maximum of 61%). It would be difficult to eat over 10,000 kcal (as the men on the football line frequently did) on a low-fat diet. Supplements taken by the football teams included mainly multivitamin pills and vitamin C tablets. This was also true of the wrestling team, except that their vitamin pills tended to be of higher potency. The cholesterol intake of the football teams was usually high. The mean intake was from 800 to 1200 mg of cholesterol with a maximum of over 3400 mg per day. These men ate large amounts of eggs for breakfast. During most of the semester, more than half of the men were eating over three times the protein RDA. Excluding the wrestling team, half of the men and over one fourth of the women were eating over three times the RDA for vitamin C. For all teams surveyed, the mean percent of calories from fat was fairly constant at 36 to 37% over the years. Snacks for some teams provided a large amount of calories. Some members of the football team ate an entire additional dinner at night after their training table dinner. The wrestling team ate a high-calorie meal late at night after a meet. The American Dietetic Association recommends that the "distribution of nutrients composing the athlete's diet should be about 15% protein, 25% to 30% fat, and 55% to 60% carbohydrate (and preferably more)."[147] For endurance sports, this may be unrealistic. They do not recommend supplements except to state that iron may be needed for female athletes, athletes who avoid red meat, endurance athletes, and adolescent male athletes.

Burke et al., in a series of articles, reported on the dietary intake of Australian male triathletes, marathon runners, football players, and weightlifters, and examined the food use patterns of the four groups.[148] Endurance athletes had a higher carbohydrate intake because of the higher amount of breads, cereals, and starchy vegetables used. The weightlifters had more protein because they used more meat, eggs, and dairy products (which was the reason for higher calcium and riboflavin intakes). The football players and weightlifters had a higher percent of calories from fat because they ate more fats and oils. These conclusions were not too surprising. The findings about the athletes' attitudes toward nutrition were interesting. The endurance athletes were most conscious of the importance of nutrition to their sport. The triathletes modified their eating habits to meet their specialized needs, but in so doing became unecessarily restrictive and focused on single nutrients. The football players seemed uninterested in nutrition, and did not believe it affected their performance except in a specific case, such as the pregame meal.

Midway through their competitive season and two weeks postseason, 24 college females from such diverse sports as field hockey (9), golf (5), cross country (6), and tennis (4) were grouped together to compare with 24 nonathletes using diet records.[149] Dietary intake changed very little across this time-span. The athletes' diets were very similar to the nonathletes. All were low in calories, iron, and calcium. It was suggested that the female athletes' wish to be thinner may influence their eating habits more than their exercise regimen.

Welch et al.[150] studied 39 female athletes (age 17 to 22) participating in intercollegiate basketball, cross-country running, field hockey, golf, softball, swimming, tennis, track and field, and volleyball teams. The women were divided into two groups. One group of 10 women had nutritional problems (such as weight, anemia, spastic colon) and the others served as a control. The first group was given two to five counseling sessions. Each athlete kept a 7-d diet record and interviewers obtained a 24-h diet recall from each athlete before and after the season. The counseled group improved their protein and vitamin A intake but not their iron. Calcium intake was only slightly improved. The average caloric intake of both groups was between 1700 and 1800 kcal. The counseled group went from 10 to 12% of calories from protein, from 42 to 29% of calories from fat, and from 48 to 59% from carbohydrate. The counseled group decreased fat significantly by increasing foods from the bread/cereal and dairy groups while decreasing foods high in fats, oils, and sweets.

Researchers from the German Democratic Republic determined the nutritional quality and quantity of food intake using data from other studies.[151] According to the authors, the great successes of East German athletes are the result of comprehensive training and proper nutrition. The caloric requirements in different types of sports was calculated to average 72 kcal/kg BW except for speed-strength sports (skating, sprint, gymnastics, jumping) which need 66 kcal/kg BW and strength sports (weightlifting and shotput) which need 76 kcal/kg BW. In training camps, the mean fat intake was 38 to 40% of caloric intake and the carbohydrate averaged 47%. The authors stated that with caloric intakes (over 5000 kcal), it would be difficult to increase the carbohydrate. The authors advocated adding carbohydrate-enriched beverages to the diets of these athletes. The types of studies performed or specific sports were not stated. The authors stated that strength or endurance athletes require 2 g/kg BW of protein per day, but the optimum could be higher (3 g/kgBW). The authors concluded that "athletes should have a sound knowledge and education in this important field of nutrition in training and contests".

As part of a study[25] evaluating bone densities of several groups of women, a 24-h dietary recall and a food frequency questionnaire were used with 14 college dancers and 13 college women on a track team to determine the high-calcium foods eaten. Calcium intake, as indicated by a 1-d recall, was not different for the dancers and track team. However, using a food frequency score, the dancers included fewer calcium-rich foods than the track team. Using a bone scan, no significant difference in bone density was found between these groups.

Mays and Scoular[152] studied 34 football, 16 basketball, and 10 track male collegiate team members (age 18 to 25). Food eaten was recorded and checked in the cafeteria line for 5 d each during preseason, in season, and post-season. The mean caloric intake for football started at 5030 preseason, and decreased to 4600 during the season, and was 3570 kcal post-season. Basketball intake started at 4200 kcal and went to 4630 post-season. The mean track intake preseason was 4300 and during the season was 4680 kcal. The percent caloric distribution was from 13 to 16% from protein, 42 to 46% from fat, and 38 to 44% from carbohydrate. The vitamin and mineral intake was in excess of the adjusted recommended allowances "with the possible exceptions of thiamine and ascorbic acid" which were felt to be less than calculated values "since food processing procedures affects them adversely".

At the University of Wisconsin, 12 basketball players, 6 swimmers, and 10 ice hockey players recorded their food intake for 2 weeks during season.[153] Diets were scored by giving points for the number of servings eaten from various food categories. Only 10 diets were rated good or excellent and the remaining 18 were judged to be fair or poor. Total caloric intake was low for athletes and the diets appeared to be low in vitamin A, vitamin C, and calcium. The carbohydrate content of the diets was low and came chiefly from simple sugars. The majority of the athletes skipped breakfast and one fourth frequently missed lunch. One fourth of the athletes took vitamin supplements. The amount and potency of supplements was not stated.

Australian Olympic athletes (66 males age 18 to 40 and 14 females age 14 to 28) were studied using 7-d records and dietary questionnaires.[154] Teams studied included swimming and diving, track and field, cycling, pentathlon, boxing, wrestling, weightlifting, rowing, canoeing, hockey, basketball, gymnastics, fencing, equestrian, shooting, and yachting. The male athletes were divided into three groups according to the amount of work required for participation in their sport. When the diet records were analyzed, it was found that the protein intake was 1.8 g/kg BW for men and 1.9 g/kg BW for women. The mean intake from fat was 43% of calories for males and 45% for females. The total caloric intake ranged from 2000 to over 6000 kcal. The mean intake of all micronutrients assessed was in excess of suggested allowances. A group of athletes who gained places in the finals (some winning medals), had significantly higher thiamin intakes when compared with a low-thiamin-intake group whose performances at the Games were indifferent. Over half of the athletes consumed a high-protein pregame meal 1.5 to 4 h before the competition. Over half of the athletes were taking some type of vitamin/mineral/food supplement. The author concluded that "it was apparent that most of the athletes had not received qualified dietary advice."

Four- or seven-day food diaries were obtained from 418 endurance, strength, and team athletes in The Netherlands.[155] The mean energy intake for the males was from 12 to 25 megajoules (MJ) or 2868 kcal to 5975 kcal. For females the intake was from 7 to 13 MJ (1673 to 3107 kcal). Thirty-five percent of the endurance athletes and 52% of the strengh athletes had energy intakes less than the World Health Organization standard for light activity. Carbohydrate contributed from 40 to 63% of energy. The athletes needed an energy intake of at least 13 MJ (3107 kcal) in order to meet the recommendation for iron (18 mg). When the energy intake of the athletes was more than 17 MJ (4063 kcal), the thiamin intake was insufficient for the athletes' needs.

A survey sent to 137 coaches of varsity teams in the "Big Ten" schools indicated that 22% of the coaches instructed the players to take vitamins, 7% told them to take minerals, and 2% advised taking protein supplements.[19] When asked if they dispensed these products, the reply was affirmative for vitamins (17%), protein (8%), and minerals (8%). Of 14 coaches responding to a question about measuring nutritional status of their athletes, two used dietary surveys, and the rest used no objective method. Thirty-nine percent of those coaching female teams and 26% of those coaching male teams prescribed diets for weight loss. Thirteen percent of the coaches regard steak and other high-protein meals as essential for the pre-event meal.

While surveying 2977 athletes in high school and college, Parr[16] found that 42% of the college athletes and 46% of the high school athletes took vitamin (mostly multivitamin) supplements. They also took single-vitamin supplements of vitamins A, B complex, C, or E. Nine percent of the college athletes and 15% of the high school athletes took mineral supplements, mostly iron, but some took zinc, multimineral, or calcium tablets. Only 6% of the college students and 10% of the high school players took protein supplements.

A study investigating factors influencing the use of nutritional supplements by college athletes found no relationship between exercise level and supplement use.[156] All of the men in the weightlifting group were taking megavitamins (more than 1000% of the U.S. RDA) and/or other "unorthodox products". Runners who were supervised by a coach used fewer supplements than the runners who were unsupervised.

As part of a questionnaire sent to 943 high school athletes, Douglas and Douglas asked how often foods in each of the four food groups were consumed.[51] Males had higher scores (better diets) than did the females. Athletes in cross-country, football, lacrosse, soccer, swimming, and track and field had higher scores than did athletes in other sports. Field hockey players and gymnasts earned the lowest scores. Replies to questions about vitamin supplementation elicited the information that 36% occasionally took vitamin pills, 19% regularly took vitamins, and 3% took vitamin supplements only during season. The authors found that the higher food practice scores could not be attributed to increased knowledge. The higher food practice scores of the men was attributed to the fact that they ate more food and were, therefore, more likely to consume the recommended number of servings of the food groups.

German endurance athletes (13 long-distance runners, age 25 to 41, and 8 cyclists, age 17 to 29), who had competed at national and international levels, recorded their food and fluid intakes for three to four successive days during training.[157] The average caloric intake of the runners was 3316 kcal with a water intake of 33 ml/kg BW. The cyclists ingested 6282 kcal with a water intake of 36 ml/kg BW. They reported frequent eating and drinking periods (from 8 to 10 a day). Forty-five percent of the total daily fluid intake of the groups occurred after eight o'clock in the evening. The authors concluded that the "proper time of food and fluid intake as well as the content and composition of the athlete's diet plays an important role in fitness."

It is unusual to find follow-up studies of former athletes, especially a long-term study. The Michigan State University Longevity Study[158] was started in 1952 with 625 varsity lettermen athletes and 557 age-matched male nonathletes. Questionnaires were sent at 8-year intervals. These men were put into six groups according to their caloric expenditure (group 1 members were expending almost no calories while group 6 was using 2500 or more calories). Groups 1 and 2, having the lowest aerobic exercise, had the highest death rates. Coronary vascular disease (CVD) was not related to age in this population. College athletic status and 1976 exercise level were not significantly related to mortality. A higher prevalence of CVD and high blood pressure (HBP) occurred at the lower exercise groups, but also was observed at the highest exercise group, "suggesting a moderate amount of aerobic activity as optimal''. It is disappointing that no nutritional intake data was included in this informative study.

Researchers at the Australian Institute of Sport studied the effect of vitamin and mineral supplementation over 7 to 8 months with 82 male and female athletes from basketball, gymnastics, rowing, and swimming divided into an experimental and a matched control group.[159] A 3-d record (two training days and one rest day) of food consumption was analyzed for each athlete to ensure that all athletes were receiving recommended daily intakes of vitamins and minerals from diet alone. The supplements were vitamins (in high dosage) and mineral tablets. Supplemented female basketball players (7 subjects) had an increase in body weight, skinfold sum, and jumping ability. It was concluded that this study provided little evidence of any positive effect of supplementation on athletic performance.

B. Basketball Players' Dietary Intakes

National Basketball Association (NBA) players on an all-star team were compared to those playing professional basketball, but not yet named all-star.[160] A 24-h recall was used for their dietary intake and only five males were in each group. The superstars were found to eat more carbohydrate and less fat and protein on game days than did the regular NBA players.

Hickson et al.[161] surveyed female intercollegiate basketball and gymnastic teams for dietary intake during their competitive seasons. The basketball players had higher mean energy intakes (1995 kcal) than did the gymnasts (1827 kcal), but the basketball players were heavier. If energy intake is expressed as kilocalories per day divided by kilograms of body weight (BW), the intake would be an average of 30 kcal/kg BW for basketball and 32 kcal/kg BW for the gymnasts. They found no significant difference in nutritional intake between the two teams. Marginal intakes (less than 70% of the RDA) for pyridoxine and magnesium, and intakes below 60% of the RDA for iron and zinc were reported. Food composition data, however, is not available for all foods for magnesium and zinc. Only 5% of the 22 subjects consumed more than 70% of the RDA for all nutrients. The authors concluded that exercise-enhanced energy intakes will not necessarily prevent occurrence of marginal nutrient intakes, as is commonly believed.

Johnson[162] studied 60 high school and college female basketball players at two high schools and two colleges (age 14 to 23 years). The 4-d diet records used for the athletes consisted of a home-game day, away-game day, practice-session day, and a weekend day. The mean caloric intake of the athletes was 2124 kcal, and no significant difference was found among the 4 d recorded by the athletes. The athletes were found to have low (less than two thirds of the RDA) intakes of calcium, phosphorus, iron, potassium, vitamin A, and greater than 300% of the RDA for vitamin C. Percentage of calories in the athletes' diet was divided into 15% from protein, 35% fat, 49.5% from carbohydrate, and 0.5% from alcohol. Protein intake calculated on a per kilogram of body weight basis averaged 1.36 g. Fifteen percent of the athletes took vitamin/mineral supplements.

In a study of college male and female basketball players, caloric intakes by the 16 men averaged twice those of the 10 women.[163] All nutrient intakes except vitamins A and D were higher for the men than for the women.

C. Cyclists' Diets

Competitive cycling is a lengthy endurance exercise which demands a high energy consumption. A high carbohydrate intake is critical.

Two elite cyclists traveling 2050 miles over dirt trails and highway recorded their food and beverage intake for 10 d.[164] The caloric intake averaged 7195 kcal, with 10% from protein, 26% from fat, and 64% from carbohydrate, of which 44% came from cookies, sugar drinks, and candy. Total fluid intake averaged 14.5 oz per hour of riding time, of which 54% was water. It was noted that when planning menus for endurance athletes, it is necessary to discover the athletes' food preferences.

Data was collected on 14 male university cyclists over 5 d of training and 3 d that included a racing weekend.[165] There were two collection periods within a month. Subjects were free-living and weighed their own food. It is unknown if these intakes were inspected in any way. The cyclists consumed up to nine meals or snacks per day. In diets averaging between 4152 and 4460 kcal per day, 58% to 61% came from carbohydrate, 26 to 27% came from fat, and 13 to 14% was from protein. The vitamin and mineral intake was far above the RDA, while cholesterol intake was low and fiber was high. Since the protein intake was not expressed as amount per kilogram of body weight, it was difficult to discern if the protein intake was sufficient.

An example of ultraendurance cycling is the Race across America (RAAM) which starts on the west coast and finishes on the east coast. This is a nonstop multiple-day race allowing for little rest time. Clark et al.[166] outlined tips for feeding the ultraendurance athlete and for training the backup crew. The case study followed the 31-year-old women's winner in her 2930-mile race. She cycled an average of 240 miles per day with a mean caloric intake of 420 kcal per hour and 7950 kcal per day. Eating more potassium-rich foods helped her through the fatigue she experienced by the fourth day. She had trouble taking in enough fluids and food toward the end of each day and by the seventh day, found it difficult to make decisions and stay awake. Primary food consumed included bananas, watermelon, baked potatoes, hot cereal, pasta, pretzels, saltines, wheat crackers, plus electrolyte and carbohydrate beverages. She finished in 12 d, 6 h, and 21 min, claiming that "Food made all the difference — no one can endure this much exercise without proper nutrition".

Lindeman[167] studied one 39-year-old male who finished the RAAM in 10 d, 7 h. Averaging the dietary intake over the time spent cycling showed 8429 kcal (78% from carbohydrate, 13% from protein, and 9% from fat). All other nutrient intake was very high. Glucose electrolyte solutions were used as well as high-fiber "sports bars". The cyclist had major gastrointestinal complaints which may have been due to being chronically hyperhydrated, a high fiber intake (57 g per day), large doses of ascorbic acid (3300 mg per day), a high concentration of the glucose electrolyte drink (23% diluted to 17%), and/or a high protein and amino acid intake from the electrolyte drink.

Slavin and McNamara[168] investigated the nutritional practices of 36 women elite racing cyclists (average age 27) and 76 recreational bicycle riders, average age 32. The cyclists filled out a questionnaire on cycling, menstrual, and nutritional information. Only eight of the racers submitted a 3-d food intake record. About one third of each group described themselves as moderate vegetarians (avoided red meat). More tourists than racing cyclists reported carbohydrate loading but this was described as just "eating more carbohydrate". More racers than tourists consumed megadoses of supplements including vitamin C (58% of racers), multivitamins (64%), iron (47%), and B complex vitamins (56%). About one third of the tourists took vitamin C supplements. The racers who completed their diet records had excellent nutrient intakes. Both groups reported that most of their nutrition information came from magazines, other cyclists, and coaches. Only 10% of tourists and 8% of the racers consulted a dietitian or nutritionist (qualifications not stated). About one third of the racers were amenorrheic, all of women were also vegetarians. However, some of the women racers with normal menstrual cycles were also vegetarians. Diet "histories" for racers indicated that they ate more than 2000 kcal per day. Iron was the only nutrient that was marginally low. Athletes received nutrition information mainly from coaches and sporting journals. The authors "believe that nutrition educators should familiarize themselves with these avenues if they wish to provide nutrition counseling to athletes".

While reporting on athlete's diets, it should be noted that some do not eat at all before an event.[169] It was theorized that fasting would raise plasma fatty acids and help spare glycogen. It was found, however, that after a fast, 10 competitive cyclists had a significantly decreased time to exhaustion as compared with normal diet conditions.

D. Dancers' Diets

Male and female dancers involved in ballet, jazz, and modern dance were mailed a brief (13 foods) food frequency (amount per week) questionnaire.[38] Over half of the 106 dancers consumed two servings of dairy food a day, but the mean intake of milk was one cup per day. Among the 77% who reported eating fresh fruit, the mean was 1.8 pieces per day. Almost the same percentage ate vegetables. When asked about fiber cereals and whole grain bread, almost half (46%) reported eating less than one serving per day. Most of the dancers ate some animal protein and this averaged 3 oz per day (ranging from 0 to 10 oz per day). The majority of dancers indicated that they ate more when not dancing. Many (60%) of the dancers took nutrition supplements which included multivitamin supplements, vitamin C, calcium, vitamin E, B complex vitamins, and iron plus miscellaneous other supplements such as potassium, yeast, and protein products. The ballet dancers averaged over four caffeinated beverages per day and almost 75% of all dancers drank alcoholic beverages — some as much as 20 drinks per week.

Calabrese et al.[170] studied the nutritional habits and menstrual abnormalities of 34 female classical ballet dancers. The dancers kept a 3-d record of food, drink, and nutritional supplements. The mean caloric intake was 1358 calories with a range of 550 to 2115 kcal. The mean protein intake of these dancers was 99% of the RDA. Vitamins A, D, B_{12}, and folic acid were low as well as iron, calcium, and phosphorus. Nutritional supplements were taken by 40% of the subjects. These were usually not multivitamin/mineral pills but were large doses of one or two nutrients. The nutritional histories and 1-d recalls were evaluated a year later with similar results. The authors concluded that these subjects knew little about basic nutritional concepts and were involved with a significant number of food fads. The mean percent of body fat was found to be 16.9% by hydrostatic weighing. Half of these women age 15 to 31 had menstrual abnormalities.

Brooks-Gunn et al.[171] surveyed 55 dancers performing in national and regional ballet companies in America and Western Europe. They found that one third of these professionally trained dancers had eating disorders. American Ballet Theatre dancers (10 men and 10 women with a mean age of 25) completed a 6-d food diary.[172] The mean caloric intake was almost 3000 kcal for men and almost 1700 for women. The protein intake averaged 122 g for men and 60 g for women. The percent of calories from carbohydrate was 38% for men and 50% for the women. Intakes below 25% of the RDA were most frequently noted for vitamin B_{12}, folic acid, biotin, and vitamin D. The mean for female iron intake was low (13.5 mg) and many were low in calcium. Most took daily multiple megavitamin supplements. The dancers' diets were judged to be monotonous and unbalanced. The women avoided red meat and milk. The men ate less salad, fruit, and vegetables than the women. Potatoes and pasta were eaten at pre-performance meals for energy. Factors that contributed to low nutrient intakes among these dancers were the women's low caloric intake, lack of correct nutrition information, avoidance of red meat and milk, and low carbohydrate intake as percent of total calories.

Evers measured and evaluated dietary intake and anorexia nervosa symptoms of 21 female students in university dance classes and compared them with 29 non-dance class students.[173] Three-day food-intake records were analyzed. There was no significant difference between the two groups in nutritional intake except for caloric intake and vitamin A intake. The control group had a mean caloric intake of 1931 kcal while the dancers were eating only 1775 kcal. The percent of subjects consuming less than two thirds of the RDA for energy was significantly higher in the dance group than in the controls. Dancers consumed more vitamin A (6166 IU) than did the controls (5294 IU). Both groups had members low in calcium and iron. Almost half of the subjects consumed some type of supplements. Evers concluded that almost half of the women were consuming iron-poor diets and were not taking iron supplements.

Benson et al. analyzed the diets of 92 female adolescent ballet dancers (age 12 to 17) enrolled in six different professional schools.[174] Three-day diet records from each dancer were analyzed with a data base program of 700 foods. The results indicated that a large number of dancers were consuming less than two thirds of the RDA for folacin, calcium, iron, and zinc. Almost half of the dancers had iron intakes less than two thirds of the RDA. The average caloric intake was 1890, but 11% ate less than 1200 calories per day. Average caloric intake from protein was 15.6%, 34.6% from fat, and 49.8% from carbohydrate. One fourth derived more than 40% of calories from fat. About 60% of the subjects took mineral or vitamin supplements but rarely did the supplement cover any nutritional deficiency the dancer might have.

Marching band majorettes have problems that are similar to dancers. They must maintain weights lower than average for women of the same height. Eating behaviors and the effect of nutritional counseling were studied with 11 varsity majorettes.[175] A physician obtained a 24-h diet history before football season. The 1-d caloric intakes for these women ranged from 690 to 1100 kcal. Along with calories, the majorettes were deficient in protein, iron, calcium, and potassium. These majorettes wanted advice about good nutritional habits but were pressured by faculty advisors and peers to be thin. A group counseling session was provided by a registered dietition and a physician. These women were interviewed again 8 weeks after the group counseling. An attempt was made to counsel the faculty advisor and majorette team captain about sensible dieting and weight control. The authors indicated that they had little success in counseling either students or faculty.

E. Field Hockey Players' Diets

Ready[176] evaluated the Canadian women's Olympic field hockey team of 19 athletes with an avearage age of 13 years. A 3-d dietary record was used, analyzed by computer and compared to the recommended values for Canadians, the Recommended Nutrient Intake (RNI). The mean energy intake was 1967 kcal; 42% as carbohydrate, 39% as fat, and 15% as protein. A significant number of these field hockey women did not meet the recommendations for vitamin A, B_6, B_{12}, or folate. Only 5 of the 19 women met the RNI for iron, and fiber intake was low. Over one fourth of the caloric intake came from fats, sweets, and alcohol. About 50% of the athlete's intake was consumed during the evening.

F. Football Player's Diets

Hickson et al.[177] surveyed the food intake of 134 high school football players (age 12 to 18 years). They used a 24-h recall method during training in August. The mean caloric and nutrient intakes for senior high (age 15 to 18) students met or exceeded the RDA and were greater than the junior high (age 12 to 14) students, except for vitamin A. The junior high school boys met or exceeded the RDA for nutrients analyzed, except they were low in calories and slightly low in zinc (87% RDA). The mean caloric intake for these boys was 2523 while that of the senior high boys was 3365 kcal. The distribution of energy was similar for both groups with 14 to 15% of caloric intake from protein, 45 to 46% from carbohydrate, and 38 to 40% from fat. They ate more from the dairy group and from the "other" group (fats, sweets, and beverages) than a sample of the same-age boys from a national survey. Meals were frequently skipped by these football players: 19% missed breakfast, 13% skipped lunch, and 3% did not eat dinner. The authors stated that the body weight of the senior high students indicated that they consumed enough fluid to prevent dehydration. However, during days six through nine of training the temperature reached

97°F in the morning with a relative humidity reading of 83. The mean body weight was 101 kg and their change of weight was from minus 2.9 to 0.3 kg which is close to a loss of 3% of body weight. This would not be conducive to peak performance or good health.

Gorman and Berning[178] described a nutrition program used with the Denver Broncos professional football team. Informal nutrition education seminars were presented to the players, coaching staff, and players' wives. Individual football players were provided with dietary counseling after a 3-d food record was analyzed. Diets were designed to fit the specific needs of each player.

Hickson and colleagues[179] studied 16 intercollegiate football athletes (19.6 years old) at training table over three consecutive weekdays during winter conditioning. Food items were weighed and plate waste was weighed or estimated at the dining hall. Snacks were reported by recall at the next meal. Dinner was the largest meal, providing 70% more energy than breakfast or lunch. The range of caloric intake was 2053 to 5464, with a mean of 22% from protein, 39% from fat, and 39% from carbohydrate. Meat consumption provided one third of the calories, two thirds of the protein, and 45% of the fat intake. The major source of carbohydrate intake came from the "other" food group (fats, sweets, beverages). The mean intake of 10 vitamins and minerals analyzed exceeded the RDA except for magnesium, folacin, and pyridoxine, which were low but not less than 70% of the RDA. It was noted that not all foods have been analyzed for these nutrients.

Zallen and Fitterhof[180] compared the nutrient intake of 33 East Carolina University football players with that of 35 male students. Both groups mailed 24-h records on three nights in successive weeks. The athletes consumed close to 5000 kcal while their protein intake was 165 g, fat was 190 g, carbohydrate 637 g, and liquid intake was 370 oz. Nutrients were mostly within 87% of recommendations. Since mail-in responses are difficult to check for memory failure or lack of information, methods used to verify the data should be stated.

Members of the Syracuse University football team who regularly played almost every game (33 men) were surveyed about their use of 23 different supplements.[181] A multivitamin pill (of the type containing no more than the RDA for vitamins) was the most used supplement (used by 50% of those surveyed). Single-vitamin use included vitamin E (used by 30%) and vitamin C (used by 20%). Twenty-four percent of the men took calcium supplements and 15% took iron pills. Only two men took protein supplements. The caffeine intake was extensive (88% of those surveyed drank two to three cans of soft drinks containing caffeine per day and 40% regularly drank coffee. Only three of those surveyed used smokeless tobacco. These men reported that they did not use bee pollen, desiccated liver, lecithin, biotin, ginseng, or spirulina. Brewers' yeast and amino acid preparations were taken by one man.

G. Gymnasts' Diets

The nutritional habits of 97 competitive female adolescent (age 11 to 17) gymnasts from six different gymnastic schools were evaluated by Loosli et al.[44] using 3-d records. The average caloric intake was low (1838 kcal) and 40% or more consumed diets low (less than two thirds of the RDA) in calcium, folate, vitamin E, pyridoxine, iron, and zinc. Forty percent of the gymnasts were low in calcium and 53% were low in iron intake. The average caloric intake from protein was 15%, from fat 36%, and from carbohydrate 49%. These athletes choose diets low in fiber (3.6 g/d). The use of vitamin or mineral supplements (43%) rarely compensated for their low nutrient intake.

Moffatt[182] examined the dietary status of 13 elite female high school (age 15) gymnastic team members by analyzing two 3-d food records. The records were collected over a 3-week period and analyzed using primarily 1963 food composition tables. Between 30 and 60% of the gymnasts consumed less than 50% of the RDA for pyridoxine, folic acid, calcium, iron, and zinc. Only three girls used supplements (two used vitamin C and one used a multivitamin preparation). These gymnasts had 10% less body fat (13%) than nonathletic girls of the same age, height, and body weight (23.5%). About 44% of the girls' caloric intake was provided by cakes, candy, soft drinks, butter, jelly, and jams.

Huber et al.[183] studied the nutritional status and body composition of eight college female gymnasts and seven college female cross-country runners using 3-d diet intakes, activity records, underwater weighing, and treadmill tests. The gymnasts had caloric intake of 1357 per day while the runners ate 1661 kcal. It was calculated that the gymnasts used 2855 kcal per day and the runners used 2651 kcal. More than 50% of both groups were low (less than 75% of the RDA) in calcium, iron, and vitamin A. The gymnasts were also low in thiamin and riboflavin. It was conluded that both the gymnasts and runners had a low percent of body fat, serious caloric intake deficiencies, and inadequate nutritional intake.

Female gymnasts (20 with an average age of 14.8 years) recorded their intake during a 3-d training period.[184] The diets were found to be low (less than 85% RDA) for vitamins A, D, folic acid, and calcium, phosphorus, magnesium, and zinc. Vitamin supplements were used by one fourth of the group. The mean intake of calories was 1744: 56 g of protein, 75 g of fat, and 218 g of total carbohydrate. It was concluded that although the female gymnasts were taking in 122% RDA for protein, this might not be enough for their low caloric input compared to amount of energy expended.

H. Ice Hockey Players and Figure Skaters

Thomson et al.[185] investigated the eating habits of 64 competitive male Canadian hockey players (age 10 to 14) and 40 less-skilled house league players at the same age. Estimation of the boys' eating habits and caloric intakes were determined by a 24-h recall during interviews in each boy's home. The total caloric intakes were not significantly different by age or competition group. The caloric intake calculated per kilogram body weight was similar between the two groups. The caloric intake ranged from 2468 to 3266 kcal per day. "Empty calories" supplied 20 to 23% of the total calories. Consumption of vegetables and fruits was low, meat intake was adequate, dairy intake was high. The rating score used by the authors to determine adequacy of food group and total food intake indicated that there was no significant difference among these boys by age group or sports league participation.

Competitive ice skaters, 17 male and 23 female figure skaters, were studied to find a relationship of body image and dietary intake.[186] The results indicated that there was more pressure on the females to be thin than on the males. The females' diets were low in energy, iron, vitamin B_{12}, and calcium. Dietary intake for the men was adequate in energy and most of the nutrients.

I. Diets for Outdoor Cold-Weather Exercise and Sports

Energy intakes and physical performance of eight men were studied for 31 d at moderate altitudes.[187] The authors developed a lightweight, energy-dense ration modified after one designed for use in sustained military field operations. Temperatures ranged from 5 to 35°C and the men climbed to 4300 m (14,104 ft). Mean energy intake averaged 2354 kcal before the expedition, 3430 during the 31 d, and 3384 after their return. Reduction in body fat was significant, and the energy deficit was estimated at between 473 and 963 kcal/d. It was concluded that when using a dehydrated ration, weight loss and gastrointestinal distress might be minimized by substituting some fat in place of the carbohydrate, which ranged between 65 to 67% of calories.

Data from a 1989 Mt. Everest expedition (ten climbers and five at base camp) is now being published.[188] Results indicated that the ten climbers burned an average of 5148 kcal per day at altitudes up to 29,000 ft. Some used up to 8000 kcal. The 15 men and women averaged 30% of kilocalories from fat, 52% from carbohydrate. It was suggested that their lower fat intake was because it takes less oxygen to obtain energy from carbohydrates than from fat. Both the climbers and those at the base camp ate only 50 to 60% of the calories that they used and averaged a 13% weight loss.

A study comparing energy balances of men on long and short sledging journeys in Antarctica found that the men could tolerate energy imbalances for short trips of 8 to 14 d; but during the Antarctic crossing of 74 d, the men increased their energy intake to keep body weight more constant.[189] The standard British Antarctic Survey rations provide 48% of the caloric content from fat.

The Leningrad Scientific Research Institute for Physical Culture conducted surveys of over 1000 athletes (age 11 to 25 years) involved in winter sports.[190] They concluded that the younger (11 to 14 years) group had lower intakes of thiamin, riboflavin, and vitamin C. A significant number of athletes were also iron deficient.

Ellsworth et al.[191] investigated the nutrient intake of 13 male (age 18 to 28 years) and 14 female (age 15 to 31) members of the United States Nordic Ski Team. Four sets of 3-d records were collected at 3- to 4-month intervals during a year of training and competition (cross country for all females and nine men and combined Nordic events for four men). Food intake was weighed and measured at the third session. The skiers consumed a diet high in fat, low in carbohydrate, and averaged more than the RDA for all the vitamins and minerals analyzed except iron. At the last session, 40% of the females ate less than 800 mg of calcium. The caloric intake was high, with 3492 to 5450 kcal (49 to 76 kcal/kg BW) for men and 2414 to 3960 kcal (42 to 71 kcal/kg BW) for women. The caloric needs for skiers have been calculated to be 90 kcal/kg BW but only two men consumed that many calories. The percentage of calories from the fuel nutrients ranged between 13 and 14% for protein for both men and women; 34 to 43% kcal from fat for men, and 34 to 41% for women; and 40 to 52% of calories from carbohydrate for men and 42 to 50% for women. Alcohol provided up to 3% of calories for men and 4.5% for women. The cholesterol intake ranged from 655 to 1210 mg for men and from 369 to 736 mg for women, which is far above any dietary guidelines. The fat consumption increased and carbohydrate intake decreased at training table as compared with at-home eating habits. This may suggest that training table menus need to be revised.

Campbell[192] reported a weighed-diet survey with six men (age 21 to 50) on a sledging expedition north of the Arctic Circle. The men traveled on foot and on skis hauling food and equipment on two sledges for 33 d. The diet was the same every day. Breakfast consisted of porridge; lunch of peanuts, raisins, and chocolate; and dinner of soup, meat, and vegetables. Biscuits, cheese, and margarine were available with all meals. The mean energy intake while traveling was 16.5 MJ (3943.5 kcal) consisting of 38% fat, 47% carbohydrate, and 15% protein. The mean caloric intake from the third week to the end was more than the first week's intake. All of the men lost weight (average of 2.3 kg, fat loss of 2.9 kg). Since they were hauling 8 to 10 h a day, this was hard traveling. Boredom with the food could also have been a factor limiting their intake. A summary of earlier Antarctic expeditions when traveling by dog sledge or manhauling indicated low caloric intakes averaging 13 MJ (3107 kcal). However, Antarctic expeditions had more lost time (less energy expended) because of bad weather than did the Arctic expedition. It was interesting to note that Campbell and Donaldson[193] published the daily energy intake of their 18 sledge dogs in Antarctica. During 12 weeks of traveling, the energy intake of the dogs averaged 13.9 MJ (3322 kcal) which was more than the intake of some of the men on the expedition.

Nutrition and heavy alpine physical performance in Switzerland was studied with six men (age 22 to 39) climbing at 3500 to 4000 m in a mean temperature of $-13°C$.[194] Four of the men were on a high-protein and -fat diet composed of 13.5% protein, 38.5% fat, and 48%

carbohydrate. The other two men were eating a high-carbohydrate diet of 61% carbohydrate, 30.5% fat, and 8.5% protein. They expended 800 kcal per hour during the steep climbing and an average of 3200 to 4500 kcal each day, and were in negative caloric balance. On various days, the men were only eating 35 to 70% of the energy they were using. The loss in body weight averaged from 2.1 to 4 kg. None of the climbers maintained a positive nitrogen balance. The food was low in water and they had a low fluid intake (1400 to 2100 ml/d) since they had to melt snow for drinking. An adequate fluid intake was calculated to be 3 to 4 l per day. Even though they were rated as excellent climbers, the men ate less than was offered because they were too tired to eat.

J. Rowers' Diets

Collegiate rowers (12 men and 10 women) were studied for 4 weeks to determine if the amount of carbohydrate in their diets would affect muscle glycogen and power output.[195] The Ohio State University researchers found that a diet high in carbohydrate (10 g carbohydrate kg^{-1} d^{-1}, which was 70% of energy intake) increased muscle glycogen levels and resulted in better time trials than the diets containing 5 g carbohydrate kg^{-1} d^{-1} in these rowers training twice a day for 4 weeks. However, the lower-carbohydrate diet maintained normal muscle glycogen and power during the same time period. The rest of the diet was reported as 2 g/kg of body mass of protein on both diets, 17% of caolories from fat on the higher-carbohydrate diet, and 43% of energy from fat on the lower-carbohydrate diet.

University champion rowers from The Netherlands were studied during training for the Olympics and 3 months after their training period.[196] Their food intake was analyzed from 7 d records. The caloric intake during extensive training (3 h/d) was calculated to be 4100 kcal (46 kcal/kg BW). Of this intake, 13% of kcal were from protein food sources, 43% from carbohydrate, and 43% from fat, less than 0.5% from alcohol. The protein intake averaged 1.6 g/kg BW which came mainly from animal protein food. When these same men were rowing recreationally, their intake was 37 kcal/kg BW. The calories were divided into 11% from protein food sources (1 g/kg BW), 43.5% from carbohydrate, 38% from fat, and 7.5% from alcohol. The quantity of milk, meat, vegetable, and fruit intake decreased during the recreational time of rowing which accounted for the decrease in caloric intake.

K. Runners' Diets

The term "runners" covers many types of events and a wide variety of energy expenditures, from sprints to ultramarathons and triathlons. Dietary intakes, obviously, will differ.

The dietary intakes, energy expenditures, and anthropometric characteristics of 44 junior high and high school female cross-country runners were studied in central New York State.[197] Pyridoxine, magnesium, and zinc intakes were below 76% of the RDA while iron and calcium intakes were about 80% of the RDA. Their mean energy intake was 84% of their calculated mean caloric needs, although there was not a progressive weight loss. It is not mandatory that students have a lunch period in New York State and eight of the athletes did not have time for lunch.

Amenorrheic and eumenorrheic (six each) adolescent runners completed 7-d dietary records and a questionnaire about health and exercise habits.[198] Amenorrheic runners ran more miles per week, consumed an average of 1912 kcal per day (15% protein, 50% carbohydrate, and 35% fat), and less than 70% of the iron RDA. The eumenorrheic runners ate 1644 kcal per day (14% protein, 50% carbohydrate, and 36% fat) and had less than 70% of the RDA for calcium, iron, magnesium, and zinc.

Some elite runners with low caloric intake seem to be able to maintain their weight and still run well. This was investigated with eight runners having a deficit of 1260 calories over a 3-month period and seven runners on a balanced energy diet.[199] Weights of both groups of runners were similar and did not change. The low calorie intake group ate 2585 calories, which were 47% carbohydrate, 34% fat, and 1.7 g protein per kilogram body weight. The balanced intake group ate 3833 calories, of which 50% was carbohydrate, 34% fat, and 2 g protein/kg BW. It was concluded that the low intake runners were "compromising carbohydrate intake".

Elite male distance runners (80) were questioned by mail about their nutritional practices.[200] Over 50% reported that they never restricted food intake and never (78%) exercised to control weight. Most of the men had breakfast, lunch, and dinner, although more skipped lunch than the other meals. Red meat was restricted by 35%, and 12% restricted milk intake. Stress fractures had occurred in 29%, of whom 41% had restricted red meat.

Three-day diet records were collected from 103 distance runners and compared with 74 age-matched inactive women.[201] The runners consumed more carbohydrate, less fat, protein, cholesterol, and more magnesium, thiamin, and fiber than the less active women.

Nutrient intakes and iron status were studied in 10 female (average age 34 years) long-distance runners during 9 weeks of training.[202] Three-day diet records collected during weeks one, four, and nine revealed that the caloric intake went from 2272 down to 1786. The percent of calories from protein (14%), carbohydrate (48 to 50%), and fat (36 to 38%) were similar over time. Dietary intakes of iron and vitamins B_6, B_{12}, and folacin were low but the blood tests were normal. It was suggested that if these deficiencies continued over a longer period of time, the women would show deficiency symptoms.

The diets of 15 male distance runners (age 25 to 47) were evaluated during eight consecutive days in the middle of the 1982 Great Hawaiian Footrace (500 km).[203] Each runner kept his own daily intake record. Of the 8 d recorded, 6 were race days (averaged 28 km/d) and 2 were rest days. The average body weigh and body fat (by skinfold calipers) increased by the end of the race, which seems unusual. The caloric intake averaged 4400 kcal (10% protein, 49% carbohydrate, 26% fat, 15% alcohol) and 4336 kcal for rest days. All nutrient intakes met or exceeded the RDA except zinc and magnesium. Zinc values were slightly low during race days and magnesium vales were low during rest days. Twelve of the runners took nutrition supplements. This evidence does "not support excessive (i.e., twice the RDA) supplementation for a male distance runner's diet."

Twelve men (age 23 to 60) entered in the 1979 Great Hawaiian Footrace kept daily records of their dietary intakes.[204] Caloric intakes were estimated to average 4800 kcal per day while they were running 28 km/d. Their morning body weight and percent body fat did not change significantly during the race. Blood samples were taken on eight different days to analyze nine different minerals. All nine blood mineral values were within normal clinical values, although they changed at various times during the race. It was unclear how the diet records were analyzed. The authors stated that "according to the basic four food plan, the reported diets on all subjects should have provided the essential nutrient requirements." They concluded that using the daily food plan might be all that is required to prevent mineral deficiency in health athletes. In this study, beer accounted for 60% of the total fluid intake and 22% of total calories. Large amounts of alcohol are usually not associated with the diets of endurance athletes during events.

The dietary characteristics and performance training of 16 American and 12 Japanese wheelchair marathoners were investigated.[205] Americans consumed 1909 calories per day while the Japanese had 1627 kcal. However, the two groups had a similar percent of calories from protein (20%), carbohydrate (53%), and fat (26%). Americans did more weight training, swimming, and kayaking while training. The Japanese spent more time using wheelchair rollers and road pushing.

Three-day diet records, blood tests, and skinfold thickness were used by Deuster et al.[206] to assess the nutritional intake and status of 51 women (age 19 to 43) who had trained and qualified for the First Women's Olympic Marathon Trials. Their mean caloric intake was 2397 kcals (range of 1067 to 4271) which was low for their activity (running 30 to 98 miles per week). Their caloric intake was divided into averages of 13% from protein, 32% from fat, and 55% from carbohydrate. The mean intake of crude fiber was 7.5 g (1.8 to 28.7). The mean intakes of calcium, magnesium, iron, and copper met or exceeded the RDA or suggested range. However, 23% of the women had lower than recommended amounts of calcium and magnesium, 43% were consuming less than the RDA for iron, more than 62% were consuming less copper than the lower suggested range, and 76% were low in zinc. The concentration of serum ferritin and plasma zinc indicated marginal iron and zinc status. Assuming that less than 12 ng/ml serum ferritin concentration indicated absent iron stores, 35% of these women had low iron stores. Nutrition supplements taken by 53% of these runners contributed more to the total intake than did the nutrients from food.

Female runners, who had competed nationally, answered survey questions about their eating habits and nutrition knowledge.[207] Over 40% of the 93 women did not eat red meat. Of this group more were amenorrheic and anemic, and had low protein, iron, and zinc intakes.

Barr[42] found that 75% of the 104 female marathon runners and 65% of the 105 fitness class women reported using an average of two to three supplements per day. These were mainly multivitamin/mineral supplements, followed by iron and vitamin C. Supplement use was most common among the 38% of women who were semivegetarians.

Heavey[208] divided runners into a group of 14 high-mileage (averaging 32 miles per week) runners and a moderate-mileage group of 12, who averaged 14 miles per week. The moderate-mileage runners ate more eggs, fruits, vegetables, less whole milk, but more skim milk than the high-mileage runners.

Blair et al.[209] studied 34 middle-aged (35 to 59 years old) men and 27 women long-distance runners (averaging 55 to 65 km per week). They compared runners with controls and found that runners had higher caloric intakes (40 to 60% higher on a weight-adjusted basis), ate more fat and carbohydrates, and were more likely to consume alcoholic beverages than the controls. The runners ate less protein (when expressed as a percent of total caloric intake) than controls and obtained a larger percentage of carbohydrate calories from sources other than starch.

Snyder et al.[210] studied the dietary patterns and iron parameters of middle-aged (average of 38 to 39 years) female runners. They used 3-d dietary intake analyses to compare nine women who consumed a modified vegetarian diet with nine women who ate red meat. They found a marked decrease in ferritin in the vegetarian women which they felt was due to the low iron bioavailability.

Haymes and Spillman[211] analyzed 3-d food diaries of 11 women distance runners, 12 sprinters, and 11 moderately active women. Differences in dietary iron, hemoglobin, plasma iron, and transferrin were not significant among the three groups. Almost half of the distance runners had ferritin levels suggestive of iron depletion. The authors concluded that low ferritin levels were more common among women distance runners than sprinters and that this difference was not due to differences in dietary iron intake.[212] They also reported that the caloric intake of middle-distance runners (1823 kcal), sprinters (2018 kcal), and field event university female athletes (1731 kcal) was not significantly different from controls (1845 kcal). The sprinters' diets were highest in fat (85 g) but lowest in carbohydrates (220 g). The sprinters had a low thiamin intake, riboflavin and niacin intakes were less than the RDA for the runners. All groups were low in iron, and all except the runners had low calcium intakes. The athletes' intake of sodium was less than the controls.

Clement and Asmundson[213] looked at the nutritional intake of 35 male and 17 female distance and middle-distance college runners (average age 21 to 22). A 7-d record of weighed food showed that the average caloric intake of the men was 3020 kcal and that of the women was 2026. Ninety-one percent of the women and 2.6% of the men had inadequate intakes of iron according to the Canadian recommended daily nutrient intake (10 mg for men and 14 for women). There was little evidence of clinical anemia, but almost 30% of the men and over 82% of the women had ferritin concentrations indicating a risk for iron deficiency.

Besenfelder et al.[214] studied the iron status of five long-distance female runners during a 9-week training period. Three-day diet records were collected at weeks one, four, and nine. The mean intake of calories ranged from 2073 to 2513, protein from 83 to 110 g, vitamin C from 164 to 199 mg, and iron from 17 to 21 mg. Although the iron intake was satisfactory according to the RDA, blood iron status decreased from week one to week four and then stabilized. This appeared to be independent of iron intake and might decrease physical performance.

Hartung et al.[215] studied the effect of diet on high-density lipoprotein (HDL) cholesterol in 59 middle-aged (35 to 66 years old) marathon runners, 85 joggers, and 74 inactive men. Diet information was collected using a questionnaire which asked how many servings of 25 foods or groups of foods the subject ate daily, weekly, monthly, or yearly. The authors admitted that this method was not the best for obtaining diet information but referenced several epidemiologic studies using this method (references mostly from the 1960s). A food knowledge examination was given to the subjects but there was no indication of the specific questions or methods used to validate the examination. The marathon runners and joggers did not differ substantially from the inactive men in reported diets, but the active men had higher HDL cholesterol. The runners and joggers reported eating less meat than the inactive men. The marathoners ate more cottage cheese and the joggers consumed less sugar than the inactive subjects. The marathoners drank less whiskey than the joggers. The authors did not attribute the difference in cholesterol levels to dietary factors but to the distances run by the marathoners and joggers.

Thompson et al.[216] reported that 10 male distance runners (16 km/d) at 3587 kcal/d, of which 53% was carbohydrate, 15% protein, and 32% fat, for 21 d. Their HDL cholesterol decreased 6 mg/dl during the first 2 weeks, and then there was no change in HDL.

Bassler,[217] a former member of Pritikin's advisory board, reported on the hazards of restrictive diets for runners. He cited cases of 14 men (age 18 to 60) whose death was associated with low body fat, high training mileage, and dietary restriction. Eleven of these men were restricting an average of six of the following foods: beef, eggs, milk, other animal protein, salt, sugar, alcohol, caffeine, and vegetable oil. Bassler proposed the term "nutritional arrhythmia" for cases of diet restriction and unexplained sudden death in runners. He pointed out that those who advocate such diets should be aware of the possible dangers and stated that "cachectic vegetarian athletes should be encouraged to eat a balanced diet including ample foods from all food groups."

Lampe et al.[218] evaluated the iron status of nine female marathon runners (age 27 to 34) during 11 weeks of training for a marathon and following the race. The results of a 3-d food diary recorded midway in the training indicated that the average for energy, protein, vitamin C, were all near or above the RDA. The mean intake of iron, however, was 14 mg (78% RDA), ranging from 7 to 20 mg. Three subjects took iron and vitamin C supplements. The authors noted that although the iron status was poor, serum ferritin levels were elevated for 3 d after the marathon. Therefore, these levels may not adequately reflect iron stores.

Grace and Jeffrey[219] measured trace mineral intakes for 13 members of a college women's track team (age 18 to 22 years) and 13 sedentary female college studies of the same age. Iron, zinc, and copper intakes were measured by analysis of 1-d duplicate-portion composites, 4-d weighed food records, and 24-h recalls. The iron and zinc intakes were lowest in the duplication-portion analysis. Copper intake means were higher by analysis and by 24-h dietary recall than by the other methods. The calculated average caloric intakes of the athletes was 1668. Almost half (46%) of the athletes and 85% of the nonathletes consumed less than two thirds of the RDA for iron and for zinc.

Lathan and Cantwell[220] described, perhaps, the ultimate in distance running. This was a case study report of a male trans-American ultramarathoner. In 1979 at age 38, he established a 24-h distance record and went into training (130 to 140 miles per week) for a run across in the U.S. His normal diet consisted mainly of fruits, vegetables, chicken, and fish. When he began the run his total cholesterol was 119 mg/dl and his HDL cholesterol was 37 mg/dl. He started running from New York city and arrived at the Golden Gate Bridge 48 d, 1 h, and 48 min later. His support crew provided him with fluids consisting of a combination of fructose, potassium, sodium chloride, and citric acid plus three to four high-carbohydrate meals a day.

L. Soccer Players' Diets

Dietary analysis of the Puerto Rico National Soccer Team for two 6-d periods showed a dietary intake close to 4000 kcal per day.[221] Their protein intake averaged 2.3 g per kg of body weight, carbohydrates were 53% of calories, fats contributed 32% of total energy, and cholesterol intake was 591 mg. All micronutrients exceeded the RDA for these athletes (age 17), with the exception of calcium. It was recommended that carbohydrate intake be increased and fat reduced in the diet of these athletes.

Hickson et al.[222] investigated 18 members of a men's intercollegiate soccer team during preseason conditioning and fall competition season. The athletes' preseason intake was observed and recorded at the university cafeteria training table over three consecutive week-days. During the competitive season, players kept food intake records over two to three weekdays. The caloric intake for preseason was 4492 kcal and 3346 during the season. The percent of total calories during preseason was 14% from protein, 33% fat, and 52% car-bohydrate. During the competitive season, the caloric intake was divided into 17% from protein, 37% fat, and 46% carbohydrate. The mean intake of six vitamins and four minerals exceeded the RDA during preseason and during the competitive season. The carbohydate intake may have been below that recommended to be best for sports performance. The authors stated that high carbohydrate intake is not the only factor in winning soccer com-petitions, since the team won the NCAA Division I championships.

Tater et al.[223] reported on the lipoprotein status in professional soccer players after a vacation time and 1 month after the start of an intensive training. A 7-d diet recall was taken by a dietitian the first day and a month later. The athletes were consuming over 3900 kca; 130 g of protein, 482 g of carbohydrates, 163 g of total fat, 675 g of cholesterol, and had a polyunsaturated:saturated fat (P/S) ratio of .33. The low-density lipoprotein (LDL) cho-lesterol was constant throughout this period and was lower than the controls. The HDL cholesterol, which was higher than the controls, decreased after intensive training.

M. Swimmers' Diets

The dietary intakes of 14 members of a collegiate women's swim team was studied.[224] They completed a 3-d food intake record and trained for a minimum of 2 h per day. The swimmers' diets met the RDA for all nutrients evaluated except calcium. Their energy intake range from 1576 to 3131 kcal and their carbohydrate and fat intake was "close to recom-mendations".

United States Swimming, International Center for Aquatic Research selected 22 male and 21 female swimmers (age 14 to 18) to participate in a training camp.[225] Swimmers' 5-d dietary records showed a caloric intake of 5221 kcal for males and 3572 for females. Their diets were high in fat and low in carbohydrates. The female swimmers did not meet the

RDA for calcium and iron. The authors point out that, although a group of athletes may have an adequate diet, individual athletes may have poor intakes.

All members of a university men's (13) and women's (16) swim teams provided 7-d dietary records before and at the end of a competitive season as part of a study of copper, iron, and zinc status.[226] Caloric intake increased post-season for both men and women. It was found that copper, iron, and zinc statuses were not adversely affected by intensive training when dietary intakes were adequate.

Earlier, the same authors studied the copper, zinc, and iron status of 12 female university swim team members before and at the end of the competitive season.[227] Self-reported 7-d records were used for dietary analysis. The caloric intake increased during training because of an increase in carbohydrate in the diet. As long as the dietary intake was adequate, the trace mineral status was not affected by strenuous training. The average energy intake at the start of the season was 2030 kcal and at the end, the athletes were eating 2269 kcal per day.

Berning[45] surveyed the dietary intake of male (mean age of 16) and female (mean age of 15) elite national swimmers. The total number of subjects was not stated. It was found that these swimmers had 46 to 48% of calories from carbohydrate, 12 to 13% of intake from protein, and 41 to 43% was fat. These athletes were more than meeting the requirements for vitamins calculated. The average calcium and iron intakes met the RDAs, but half of the girls were low in calcium and in iron, while 14% of the boys were low in calcium. The majority (63%) took vitamin/mineral supplements, which most commonly was vitamin C, followed by multivitamin pills, iron, and calcium pills. The consumption of lecithin, amino acids, bee pollen, RNA, and DNA was noted. The timing of the pre-event meal varied. Eleven percent of these swimmers ate up to 30 min before swimming, 12% ate 31 to 60 min before, and 77% of the subjects ate 1 to 1.5 h before swimming. The meals were composed mostly of complex carbohydrate food.

Campbell and MacFayden[228] looked at the dietary practices of 101 Canadian adolescent male and female competitive swimmers. They grouped these swimmers into 15- to 16-year olds, 16- to 18-year-olds, and 20-year-olds who could meet time standards set in two events of 100 m or over and in one event of 50 m or over. Three-day food records were collected and compared to the 1975 Canadian Dietary Standard Committee for revision of the Canadian Dietary Standard.[229] The 3-d mean intake of calories and nutrients met the Canadian Dietary Standard recommendations for all ages and for both boys and girls; however, some swimmers ate less than the recommended amounts of calories, iron, and vitamin A. A higher percentage of calories and nutrients were consumed at home than away from home by all age and sex groups. The evening snack provided almost the same percentage of calories and nutrients as the breakfast meal, and in some cases, the luncheon meal. About 40% or more of the total calorie and nutrient intake was provided by the dinner and evening snack. More swimmers took supplements during training than before competition. The most frequently eaten foods for pregame meals were cereals and carbohydrate foods. The foods most frequently avoided during the pregame period were fatty foods, "heavy foods", and pizza.

Nine female competitive swim team members and 15 synchronized swim team members, age 19 to 20, were compared with 10 sedentary females to explore exercise intensity, dietary intake, and plasma cholesterol levels.[230] Four-day diet records were kept for comparison four times during a 24-week period. The competitive swimmers consumed 7.5% more calories than the synchronized swimmers and 21.5% more than the sedentary females. The percentage of calories from protein, fat, and carbohydrate and the cholesterol intake was similar among all groups. The results of this study indicated that plasma HDL cholesterol was significantly increased in these women who participated in an intensive, but not moderate, exercise program.

Adams et al.[231] studied the effects of a liquid dietary supplement on the dietary intake of 12 female collegiate swim members, age 18 to 21. A 1-d record was used every fourth day for 7 weeks to compare seven subjects consuming self-selected diets with five swimmers who consumed two 8-oz cans of liquid diet supplement (250 kcal per 8 oz) between meals plus their self-selected diets. All athletes' mean dietary intake was more than the RDA for energy (control was 2479 kcal, experimental was 2873 kcal), protein, vitamins A, C, thiamin, niacin, and phosphorus. Mean intakes for both groups were below the RDA for vitamin D and iron, and close to the RDA for calcium. Those consuming supplements had more protein, calcium, phosphorus, iron, and potassium than the controls and ate more frequently. One reason for the low calcium intake was that many swimmers chose soft drinks rather than milk at all meals except breakfast.

Houston[232] studied the diet, training, and sleep habits of 8 male and 12 female elite Canadian swimmers. Total swim distances completed in this beginning training was similar for males (average age 18) and for females (average age 17). Three-day records of weighed food were used to assess dietary intake. Female swimmers' intake was low for food from the meat and milk group, suggesting that too little calcium, iron, and perhaps protein was consumed. Sixty percent of these athletes were taking vitamin or mineral supplements. The food intake of the men was twice that of the women. Women had an inadequate caloric intake. The males averaged five meals per day and the females ate four meals per day. Those who ate four meals a day were likely to skip the meal before morning training or snack before bed.

N. Triathletes' Diets

The triathlon may refer to a combination of any three athletic events, but usually combines swimming, cycling, and running. The Ironman World Triathlon Championship is a race consisting of a 2.4-mile swim, a 112-mile bicycle course, and a 26.2-mile run. A half-triathlon involves 1.9 km of swimming, 90 km of bicycling, and 21.1 km of running.

A study of the dietary habits of 52 triathletes at various times during competition indicated that almost half of the survey respondents had no dietary change 1 to 3 d before the event.[233] The last meal before the event for 60% of the subjects was breakfast. Most of them drank water 1 h before the event, 98% drank fluids (mostly water) during the event, after the event all drank fluids (mostly water), and 73% ate a high-carbohydrate meal. Since this was a short-course triathlon, only 19% reported eating solid food during the event, although 30% said they ate solid food in longer triathlons. Traditional carbohydrate loading (with a depletion phase) was rarely practiced, but over 40% used a modified carbohydrate loading (70% or more calories from carbohydrate). In the precompetition diet, from 58 to 76% of the triathletes omitted some of the following foods from the diet: dairy, meat and meat substitutes, sweets, fat, convenience foods, snacks, supplements, and beverages such as carbonated drinks, alcohol, coffee, and tea.

Triathletes were studied to determine gastrointestinal complaints and dietary patterns.[40] All 21 females and 50 males studied finished the triathlon (1.5-km swim, 40-km bike, 10-km run). The 3-d dietary intake was self-recorded during a training periods within 6 weeks after the triathlon. The average caloric intake was 10,835 kJ/d (2590 kcal) with 54% from carbohydrate, 30% from fat, 15% from protein, and 3.4% from alcohol. The protein intake averaged 1.4 g/kg BW. The mean intakes for vitamins, except vitamin E, were above the RDA, but some individuals were low. Almost 40% of the athletes took a vitamin/mineral supplement evey day; but even with supplements, more than half were low in folacin and vitamin E. Mean total intakes of minerals from food were above the RDA, but more than 40% consumed less than the RDA for magnesium and zinc. Copper intake was also low. Even when iron from supplements was calculated, 43% of the women and 2% of the men were below the RDA for iron. Most of the athletes preferred water as a beverage, but glucose-polymer drinks were used by 29% of the women when biking, 19% when running, and by more than 50% of the men while biking and running.

Nutritional problems confronting ultraendurance athletes (including triathletes) were discussed in two articles by the same author.[234,235] Carbohydrate intake is of prime importance for these athletes. In order to meet carbohydrate needs, low intake of protein may result, especially with women athletes on low caloric intakes. It was stated that protein intake should be from 15 to 18% of total calories.

Gastrointestinal complaints in relation to dietary intakes in triathletes (half-triathlon) were studied in The Netherlands and Belgium.[236] More gastrointestinal problems were reported by the 55 male athletes during the running part of the event than the swimming or cycling. Those athletes who ate diets with higher amounts of protein, fat, and increased beverage osmolality had more gastrointestinal problems, probably since these substances have all been reported to delay gastric emptying time. All athletes who vomited had eaten in the last half hour before the event. Solid foods and beverages were self-reported as those eaten before, during, and after the competition. The diets were analyzed, but the nutrient content was not reported. The authors concluded that increased intake of fat, protein, dietary fiber, and hypertonic beverages >325 mOsm/kg should be discouraged, while a diet low in fiber, fat, and protein, and high in carbohydrate should be urged.

Burke and Read[237] described the self-reported diets of 25 Australian male triathletes (age 19 to 46). During training, diet histories and food frequency techniques were used to collect dietary intake information. Twenty subjects completed 7-d food diaries. Skinfold and other anthropometric measurements were performed and blood samples were taken to measure iron status. The athletes indicated that the foods they used during triathlons (lasting from 3 h) up to the Ironman (takes 9 to 17 h to complete) were fresh and dried fruit, cookies, sandwiches, water, electrolyte drinks, soft drinks, 2 to 5% glucose/fructose polymer drinks during the cycling phase and cookies with the same liquids during the running phase of the event. Foods using during a training week included (per day): 18 servings of breads/cereals, 9 servings of fruit/starchy vegetables, 5 servings of high-sugar foods, and from 1 to 3 servings from other food groups. Over 80% of the men carbohydrate-loaded 2 to 4 d before the race. The mean energy intake of the training diet was 4095 kcal (59 kcal/kg body mass) with 59.5% coming from carbohydrate, 13% from protein (2 g/kg BW), 27% from fat, and 0.5% from alcohol. The intake of five vitamins and two minerals was above the Australians' nutrient recommendations. The intake of iron was calculated to be 30 mg (three times the recommendation). All iron status measurements were normal. These triathletes had frequent snacks and multiple meals to increase caloric intake. At the pre-event meal, all reported drinking extra liquids and all but two men had high-carbohydrate meals. All subjects recognized the importance of fluids before and during the triathlon.

Marquart et al.[238] evaluate serum zinc status among triathletes low and moderate in body fat, and male controls. They used a 7-d food record and found the energy intake was significantly higher for the low-body-fat group (3208 kcal/kg) than for the medium-fat group (2204 kcal) or the controls (2318 kcal/d). The zinc intake was higher for the low-body-fat group than for the medium-body-fat group. Over 80% of the medium-body-fat triathletes and 45% of the low-body-fat athletes had marginal serum zinc levels (less than 80 μg %). The authors believe that these men who restrict caloric intake to reduce body fat may be at an increased risk of developing marginal zinc status.

Bazzarre et al.[239] evaluated the nutritional status of 32 men and 5 women triathletes, 17 men and 11 women endurance athletes (runners, swimmers, and/or cyclists), and 12 men and 16 women controls (age 14 to 51 years) using 7-d food records. Males had a greater intake of calories and 17 out of 28 nutrients than did females. The mean intake of all male subjects was greater than the RDA for all nutrients except zinc and folic acid. The females in all groups were low in iron, zinc, pyroxidine, folic acid, and magnesium. The nutritional status blood measurements showed that females had poor iron levels but acceptable levels of zinc, copper, and vitamin C. The female triathletes and endurance athletes reported more cases of fatigue than did the other groups.

Novak[240] of Czechoslovakia descibed studies performed with ten males competing in the super ironman event. This event involves swimming 5 km, bicycling 103 km, and running 50 km. The subjects did not use carbohydrate-loading techniques and their carbohydrate stores were depleted by the end of the event. The author reported that in another study of an ironman competition, it was determined that the food intake could never cover the endurance performance kilocalorie requirements of approximately 40,000 kcal.

O. Volleyball Players' Diets

Perron and Endres[46] used a 24-h recall and 48-h record to evaluate the diets of 31 female adolescent volleyball players. They found that these athletes' diets were low in energy, calcium, and iron. These young women ate an average of almost five times a day, eating 13 servings of food a day. The largest percent of the total servings came from desserts, beverages, sugar, and salty snacks.

P. Diets for Weightlifters, Bodybuilders, and Strength Training

Bodybuilding is unlike most of the other sports in that body appearance is being judged, not strength, speed, or endurance. Bodybuilders want muscle size and very little body fat, and they have fixed ideas on how their diet can help promote this appearance. A review of the nutrition beliefs of bodybuilders has been published which includes a discussion of the adverse effects of some diet and training practices, including use of growth hormone, protein, energy restriction, dehydration, and supplements.[241]

The nutrient intake and lipid profiles of 19 male and 8 female bodybuilders competing in the National Physique Committee's USA Bodybuilding Championships were studied.[242] A 7-d food record was completed 1 week before the competition by 19 males and 8 females. The mean caloric intake for males was low, at 2015, while female intake was higher, at 2660 kcal. The percent of calories from protein was high, at 34% for males and 37% for females. Fat intake was very low, at 14% for males and 13% for females. Calcium and zinc intakes were low and cholesterol intake was high, although the total blood cholesterol level was within desirable range for 69% of the bodybuilders.

Six male and two female bodybuilders preparing for an Alabama state championship competition had their diets monitored 12 weeks, 6 weeks, and 1 week before the competition.[243] During this time period, the males decreased their caloric intake down to 2041 kcal, while women maintained theirs at 1276 kcal. The percent of calories from fat decreased to 9.8% and the percent of calories from protein increased to 33.3% for both males and females. Intake of the other nutrients determined from food intake was found to be below 70% of the RDA for calcium and zinc for the males at 1 week before competition. All during the study, females were below 70% of the RDA for folacin, vitamin E, calcium, potassium, and zinc.

The dietary practices of 13 male bodybuilders was investigated from self-reported 7-d intakes.[244] The mean intake for calories was 3369 kcal, of which 22% was from protein, carbohydrate 50%, and fat 28%. Protein intake was more than twice the RDA. It was suggested that those working with bodybuilders should realize that these athletes have a "bulking out" phase and a "leaning out" phase, and provide appropriate counseling.

A 25-year-old male bodybuilder preparing for an East Coast bodybuilding contest was followed over a 6-month period.[245] He started at 190 pounds and entered the competition at 168 pounds. During the off-season his caloric intake was 4193 kcal, with 23% of calories from protein and 24% from fat. During the precontest days his caloric intake dropped to 1936 kcal, with 64% of calories coming from protein, and 6% from fat. Three weeks before the event, haddock, rice, or potato were eaten every 2 h at least 10 times a day. Numerous supplements were taken, including amino acids, multivitamins, and minerals plus a complicated drug regimen. It was pointed out that "an athlete is often more motivated to make a change based on a performance argument rather than a health argument."

The food selection patterns of 7 male and 12 female bodybuilders were described as they prepared for competition.[246] Noncompetition diets (12 weeks before competition) and precompetition (3 d before) were examined using 3-d records, exchange lists, and nutrient density data. It was found that the variety of food in the diet decreased as the athletes drew close to competition time with protein in the diet increasing and fat decreasing drastically. Calcium and zinc were low in these diets.

Several years earlier, the same authors also studied bodybuilders (five males and six females) 24 to 48 h prior to the contest.[247] The precompetition diets were low in calories, fat, calcium, and iron (women only), and high in protein.

Ten female bodybuilders (age 18 to 30 years) participated in a study to look at dietary and exercise practices.[248] Six of the subjects were entered in the competition and others were not. Three-day food records were collected on four separate times representing precompetition and the weekend during competition. The competitors reduced their caloric intake more than the noncompetitors during the time before the event. All diets were high in protein and low in fat. The competitors were very low in fat (17% of calories from fat). Mean intake for vitamins B_{12}, D, E, folic acid, calcium, and zinc were below 66% of the RDA for the competitors.

An article written in 1981 was not published until 1991 in the Soviet Sports Review on controlling body weight in weightlifters.[249] The diet completely eliminated fats from the diet, decreased carbohydrates, kept protein constant, and decreased salt. Methods of losing weight included restriction of food and beverages, use of laxatives, diuretics, and sessions in heat rooms. It was difficult to ascertain if this was the recommendation or methods athletes were using. Intake the day before a competition suggested having 100 to 200 g of nonfat cheese, 100 to 150 g of meat, 2 eggs, and 1 to 2 glasses of sweet tea divided into four or five meals.

College students (333) were divided into three groups: sedentary, exercisers, and athletes, to determine the use of nutritional supplements.[250] All men who took "megavitamins and/ or other unorthodox products were weightlifters".

Celejowa and Homa[251] studied the food intake of ten Polish weightlifters (age 20 to 35) during training camp for champion competitors ranking just below the Olympic team. For 11 d, the food intake of these athletes was weight and representative samples assayed for total solids, protein, fat, and carbohydrate content. Micronutrients were determined by calculations from food composition tables. Intake of all the vitamins and minerals met or exceeded nutrient recommendations. The mean intake for iron was 29 mg and for calcium was 2.3 g. The athletes ate from 3200 to 4700 kcal per day which consisted of an average of 14% protein, 37% fat, and 49% carbohydrate. The average protein intake corresponded to 2 g of protein per kilogram of body weight. Results of nitrogen balance studies indicated that the amount of protein required ranged from 2.0 to 2.2 g/kg BW. The energy expended in 24 h, including the weightlifting sessions, ranged from 2829 to 4604 kcal.

Laritcheva et al[252] published studies of protein needs with champion weightlifters (age 21 to 34) in the former U.S.S.R. Energy expenditure for 24 h ranged from 3800 to 4500 kcal, but at high loadings (about 17,320 kg per 24 h) it ranged from 5000 to 5200 kcal. Caloric intakes corresponded to energy expenditure. Of the total caloric intake, 14 to 18% of calories came from protein, 45 to 48% from fat, and 37 to 41% from carbohydrates. During preparation for top-level contests, protein intake corresponded to 2.2–2.6 g/kg BW per day. At protein levels less than 2 g/kg BW during intensive training, a negative nitrogen balance was observed. During less stressful training, 2 g/kg BW sustained nitrogen balance. According to the authors, protein metabolism was determined from experiments on nitrogen assimilation and balance and excretion of nitrogen metabolism (urea, creatinine, creatine, amino nitrogen, and ammonia) in urine and sweat.

Q. Wrestlers' Diets

Because wrestlers believe that food intake has little effect on performance, nutritional practices may be poor.[253] Nutrition advice comes, not from sports nutritionists, but from fellow wrestlers who may recommend from 0 to 500 kcal per day. The wrestler may need from 1500 to 2200 kcal per day. Food restriction and fluid restriction are all too frequent weight-loss techniques.[254]

Steen and McKinney[49] collected data from two college wrestling teams (42 wrestlers, age 18 to 23 years old) using 24-h diet recall preseason, 4-d food record midseason, and a 1-d report 3 to 4 weeks after the last match. Thirty-seven percent of the wrestlers did not meet the caloric RDA for the "average person" and 15% had low protein intakes. Including supplements, 25% of these men consumed less than two thirds of the RDA for vitamin C, thiamine, and iron. Almost half were low in vitamin A, while more than half were below two thirds of the RDA for pyridoxine, zinc, and magnesium. The percentage of calories from protein and fat was higher than that recommended for athletes and much lower in carbohydrates. Caloric intake of alcohol (12% of caloric intake) was highest on day three of midseason, which may have been because this was a Saturday. All but 5% of the subjects used alcohol during the season. Food and fluid intake was low and sometimes nothing was taken by mouth for 2 d before a match.

Wrestlers' dietary intake was studied at Iowa State University.[255] Eleven wrestlers kept food intake records for five consecutive days twice during the season and once post-season. Dietary intakes were found to be low in vitamin A and thiamin without calculating supplement intake. Even after season, vitamin A was low in the wrestlers' diets.

Schwarzkopf and Jensen[256] reported on the effects of dietary control on making weight in seven collegiate wrestlers. The varsity wrestlers were given food containing 60% carbohydrate, 1 g of protein per kilogram body weight, and caloric deficiency (equal to, or more than, 1200 kcal) to reach a target weight in 6 weeks. Teammates (11 men) were assigned a target weight but given no dietary guidance. The wrestlers provided with the diet lost 6 lbs (the control group lost 1.4 lbs), reached target weight, and decreased lean weight 1 lb (controls decreased 1.4 lbs). There was a trend for greater improvement in performance by the wrestlers who had been given dietary guidance.

Steen and Brownell[257] collected information on 69 collegiate wrestlers at the Eastern Intercollegiate Wrestling Association Championships. The mean age at which they started wrestling was 10.9 years and were "cutting weight" at age 13.5 years. The average wrestler lost weight 15 times during a season with the average of most weight lost reported to be 15.8 lbs. Thirty-seven percent reported a weight loss of 11 to 20 lbs every week of the season. At this tournament, 89% of the wrestlers (excluding the heavyweight wrestlers) had to lose weight to qualify. The average weight lost was almost 10 lbs in less than 3 d.

It is difficult to follow college athletes after they graduate, but researchers persuaded 51 exwrestlers and 39 nonwrestlers to return questionnaires about their health.[258] Exwrestlers were found to have a greater incidence of overweight and obesity than nonwrestlers. Although not significant, exwrestlers had more hypertension and hypercholesteremia than did the nonwrestlers, indicating that some practices of wrestlers increase their risk of developing heart disease in later life.

Sumo wrestlers are huge and are as concerned about caloric intake as physical training.[259] They average 268 lbs in weight (height 70.8 in.), and may eat 5000 calories per day in only two meals. However, results of physical fitness tests are lower than other Japanese athletes and their life expectancy averages 10 years less than the average Japanese male, according to this article written many years ago. Sumo wrestlers may be heavier now, since an American-born top-ranking sumo wrestler is reported to weigh 580 lbs.[260]

V. CONCLUSIONS

It is a sad commentary that the conclusions from this review have changed little since the first edition. Most surveys of athletes' dietary intake have a long way to go to meet scientific criteria. Results of nutrition knowledge surveys indicate that athletes and their coaches think nutrition is important, have less than sufficient nutrition knowledge, but are doing little to learn more. Perhaps they do not care. I hope that is not true. Elite athletes have position coaches, strength coaches, trainers, and sports psychologists, but rarely do they have enough time with professsional sports nutritionists. The newest technology is put to use to cut a few seconds from timed events or to make super athletes. However, it seems that coaches and athletes are not concerned about the fuel (nutrition) they need to be winners.

Most surveys indicate that athletes of all ages do not know enough to apply scientific principles of sports nutrition to their diet. Most coaches do not have this information, and this is not their job. Most trainers have had some nutrition education, but they are too busy doing their job. Qualified sports nutritionists are needed wherever athletes are being trained. When will this happen? When the coaches and directors of athletes think proper diet is important, then dietitians specializing in sports nutrition will be hired. It should be noted that all other professionals taking care of athletes are paid for their expertise; sports nutritionists should not be volunteers.

Maybe it is true that it is impossible to find out, with any accuracy, what an individual athlete regularly eats and drinks without changing his/her dietary habits. It certainly is a much more difficult job than can be imagined by those who have never tried to collect dietary information. There is no standardization of dietary intake studies. The use of 24-h recalls continues when all evidence points to it being useless for individual diet collections. How can the RDAs or even dietary guidelines be used when these were set up for the general public? Athletes are not average people. They work harder, longer, have more muscle, and in some cases are 100 lbs heavier and over a foot taller than the so-called "reference person". In many cases, advice given to athletes is unrealistic. How can an athlete who needs 5,000 or 10,000 kcal go on a low-fat diet? Why should athletes whose event lasts only a few minutes carbohydrate-load before the event?

Surveys of what athletes are eating are, in many cases, not scientifically sound. What is learned from a dietary survey of sports when too few subjects are used, when various teams are combined to produce a "result", when improper methods are used to elicit dietary information, or when conclusions are reached after using all the wrong methods? Even if all the right things are done to find out what nutrients are low or too high in the diet, who is going to translate this into a proper diet, see that the athletes have the food available, and stay with them to see if the new diet is followed over a period of time?

Teams or groups having to "make weight" (gymnasts, wrestlers, dancers, some others) are most at risk for nutritional problems. Members of other teams may eat so much to replace energy used that they have all needed nutrients. Athletes may be low in nutrients even if slightly high in calories. Usually if the diets are very high in calories, the nutrient intake meets most standards. Snacks need to be reported, since many times they are high in calories, fat, sugar, and alcohol. Supplements need to be reported.

Brotherhood,[261] in his excellent article on nutrition and sports, concluded that "any athlete who expects to expend more than 9 MJ (2000 kcal) per day in training requires nutritional knowledge and support that matches his or her physical endeavors.'' Williams,[262] in his textbook, stated that ''Prudent nutritional recommendations for enhancement of health or athletic performance are based upon reputable research.''

In summary, there is no answer to the question of optimal diet for an athlete since each diet should be individualized for the sport, position played, body composition, and many other factors. It is impossible to condense nutrition advice for ''all athletes''. Even for a specific sport, dietary intakes vary and advice must be individualized. Devising the best diet should be left in the hands of a registered dietition specializing in sports nutrition.

Coaches, trainers, and especially the athletes need more effective nutrition education. Not only do they need to know more about diet for fitness and sports, but they need to be warned about buying useless, or even dangerous, pills and other products. Very few realize that the fad products sold as food supplements are not monitored for efficacy or safety. Athletes should be warned about nutrition information presented by unqualified people attempting to sell a product. More emphasis is needed on scientific nutrition education.

Nutrition is not going to make an Olympian from someone who has not trained; but nutrition is an essential part of all athletes' training. Let us hope that all health professionals, including qualified sports dietitians, will be able to work together for the good of each athlete.

REFERENCES

1. **Schultz, H. W.,** *Food Law Handbook,* AVI Publishing, Westport, CT, 1981, 496.
2. Pub.L. 94-278, sec 501 (a), which added section 411 to the Federal Food, Drug, and Cosmetic Act.
3. **Dykstra, G.,** *FDA and Dietary Supplement Regulation* Presented by the Deputy Associate Commissioner for Regulatory Affairs by video link to the National Foods Association meeting, Nashville, TN, July 27, 1992.
4. **Council on Practice,** The American Dietetic Association, 216 W. Jackson Blvd., Chicago, IL.
5. **Lombardo, J. A.,** Sports medicine: a team effort, *Phys. Sportsmed.,* 13, 72, 1985.
6. **Durnin, J. V. G. A.,** The influence of nutrition, *Can. Med. Assoc. J.,* 96, 715, 1967.
7. **Storlie, J.,** Nutrition assessment of athletes: a model for integrating nutrition and physical performance indicators, *Int. J. Sports Nutr.,* 1, 192, 1991.
8. **McCutcheon, M. L.,** The athlete's diet: a current view, *J. Family Pract.,* 16, 529, 1983.
9. **Selby, R., Weinstein, H. M., and Bird, T. S.,** The health of university athletes, attitudes, behaviors, and stressors, *J. Am. College Health,* 39, 11, 1990.
10. **Lessler, J. T. and Sirken, M. G.,** Laboratory-based research on the cognitive aspects of survey methodology: the goals and methods of the national center for health statistics study, *Milbank Memorial Fund Q. Health Soc.,* 63, 565, 1985.
11. **Corley, G., Demarest-Litchford, M., and Bazzarre, T. L.,** Nutrition knowledge and dietary practices of college coaches, *J. Am. Diet. Assoc.,* 90, 705, 1990.
12. **Graves, K. L., Farthing, M. C., Smith, S. A., and Turchi, J. M.,** Nutrition training, attitudes, knowledge, recommendations, responsibility and resource utilization of high school coaches and trainers, *J. Am. Diet. Assoc.,* 91, 321, 1991.
13. **Spear, B. A., Lummis, B., and Craig, C. B.,** Nutrition knowledge survey of high school coaches in Alabama, *J. Am. Diet. Assoc.,* 91, A-45, 1991.
14. **Pelzer, M. K., Hemmersbach, L. M., Valencic, C. A., and Vokaty, L. L.,** Implementing nutrition education with coaches of adolescents, *J. Am. Diet. Assoc.,* 91, A-96, 1991.
15. **Lapin, C. S., Cashman, L. K., Wright, D. E., and Stone, K. A.,** Nutrition recommendations made by Texas high school coaches to athletes, *J. Am. Diet. Assoc.,* 90, 774, 1990.
16. **Parr, R. B., Porter, M. A., and Hodgson, S. C.,** Nutrition knowledge and practice of coaches, trainers, and athletes, *Phys. Sportsmed.,* 12, 127, 1984.
17. **Anon.,** Dietary guidelines for Americans, eat a variety of foods, Home and Garden Bull. No. 232-1, U.S. Department of Agriculture, Washington, D.C., April, 1986.
18. **Bedgood, B. L. and Tuck, M. B.,** Nutrition knowledge of high school athletic coaches in Texas, *J. Am. Diet. Assoc.,* 83, 672, 1983.

19. **Wolf, E. M. B., Wirth, J. C., and Lohman, T. G.,** Nutritional practices of coaches in the Big Ten, *Phys. Sportsmed.,* 7, 113, 1979.

20. **Cho, M. and Fryer, B. A.,** Nutritional knowledge of collegiate physical education majors, *J. Am. Diet. Assoc.,* 65, 30, 1974.

21. **Bentivegna, A., Kelley, E. J., and Kalenak, A.,** Diet, fitness, and athletic performance, *Phys. Sportsmed.,* 7, 99, 1979.

22. **Soper, J., Carpenter, R. A., and Shannon, B. M.,** Nutrition knowledge of aerobic dance instructors, *J. Nutr. Educ.,* 24, 59, 1992.

23. **Leeds, M. J. and Denegar, C.,** Nutrition knowledge and food practices of collegiate athletes compared to nonathletes, *J. Am. Diet. Assoc.,* 91, A-13, 1991.

24. **Updegrove, N. A. and Achterberg, C. L.,** The conceptual relationship between training and eating in high school distance runners, *J. Nutr. Educ.,* 23, 18, 1990.

25. **Frederick, L. and Hawkins, S. T.,** A comparison of nutrition knowledge and attitudes, dietary practices, and bone densities of postmenopausal women, female college athletes, and nonathletic college women, *J. Am. Diet. Assoc.,* 92, 299, 1992.

26. **Foley, M. S., Yi, K., and Briones, E. R.,** Nutrition knowledge of wheelchair athletes, *J. Am. Diet. Assoc.,* 91, A-107, 1991.

27. **Shearer, J. D., Yadrick, M. K., Loudreaux, L. J., and Norris, P. A.,** Nutritional assessment of college freshman athletes, *J. Am. Diet. Assoc.,* 91, A-110, 1991.

28. **Landry, R. V., Oppliger, R. A., Estwanik, J., and Landry, G. L.,** Nutrition knowledge and weight control practices in adolescent wrestlers and boxers: a comparative study, *Med. Sci. Sports Exercise,* 23, S52, 1991.

29. **Gollman, B. S. and Carlyle, T. L.,** Nutrition knowledge and eating practice survey of exercising adults, *J. Am. Diet. Assoc.,* 90, A-121, 1990.

30. **Potter, G. S. and Wood, O. B.,** Comparison of self- and group instruction for teaching sports nutrition to college athletes, *J. Nutr. Educ.,* 23, 288, 1991.

31. **Furtado, M. M., Keane, M. W., Curry, K. R., and Johnson, P. M.,** The effect of nutrition education on nutrition knowledge and body composition of Little League cheerleaders, *J. Am. Diet. Assoc.,* 90, A-19, 1990.

32. **Trent, L. K.,** Nutrition knowledge of active-duty Navy personnel, *J. Am. Diet. Assoc.,* 92, 724, 1992.

33. **Weber, D.,** Navy Nutrition and Weight Control Guide, Publication NAVPERS 15658 (A), Naval Military Personnel Command, Washington, D.C., 1989.

34. **Walantas, S. D.,** Implementing a sports nutrition education program for the corps of cadets at the United States Military Academy, West Point, NY, *J. Am. Diet. Assoc.,* 90, A-129, 1990.

35. **Bermudez, M. G., Keane, M. W., Curry, K. R., and Lopez, R.,** The effect of nutrition education on the nutrition knowledge of college athletes, *J. Am. Diet. Assoc.,* 91, A-47, 1991.

36. **Reed-Wiesner, A. K. and Read, M. H.,** Health beliefs, nutrition knowledge and nutrient intake of university athletes, *J. Am. Diet. Assoc.,* 90, A-103, 1990.

37. **Barr, S. I.,** Nutrition knowledge of female varsity athletes and university students, *J. Am. Diet. Assoc.,* 87, 1660, 1987.

38. **Stensland, S. H. and Sobal, J.,** Dietary practices of ballet, jazz, and modern dancers, *J. Am. Diet. Assoc.,* 92, 319, 1992.

39. **Frederick, L. and Hawkins, S. T.,** A comparison of nutrition knowledge and attitudes, dietary practices, and bone densities of postmenopausal women, female college athletes, and nonathletic college women, *J. Am. Diet. Assoc.,* 92, 299, 1992.

40. **Worme, J. D., Doubt, T. J., Singh, A., Ryan, C. J., Moses, F. M., and Deuster, P. A.,** Dietary patterns, gastrointestinal complaints, and nutrition knowledge of recreational triathletes, *Am. J. Clin. Nutr.,* 51, 690, 1990.

41. **Shoaf, L. R., McClellan, P. D., and Birskovich, K. A.,** Nutrition knowledge, interests and information sources of male athletes, *J. Nutr. Educ.,* 18, 243, 1986.

42. **Barr, S. I.,** Nutrition knowledge and selected nutritional practices of female recreational athletes, *J. Nutr. Educ.,* 18, 167, 1986.

43. **Walsh, V. R.,** Health beliefs and practices of runners versus nonrunners, *Nursing Res.,* 34, 353, 1985.

44. **Loosli, A. R., Benson, J., Gillien, D. M., and Bourdet, K.,** Nutrition habits and knowledge in competitive adolescent female gymnasts, *Phys. Sportsmed.,* 14, 118, 1986.

45. **Berning, J.,** Swimmers' nutrition knowledge and practice, *Sports Nutr. News,* 4, 1, 1986.

46. **Perron, M. and Endres, J.,** Knowledge, attitudes, and dietary practices of female athletes, *J. Am. Diet. Assoc.,* 85, 573, 1985.

47. **Grandjean, A. C., Hursh, L. M., Majure, W. C., and Hanley, D. F.,** Nutrition knowledge and practices of college athletes, *Med. Sci. Sports Exercise,* 13, 82, 1981.

48. **Grandjean, A. C.,** Profile of nutritional beliefs and practices of the elite athlete, in *The Elite Athlete,* Butts, N. K., Gushiken, T. T., and Zarins, C., Eds., Spectrum, Jamaica, N.Y., 1985.

49. **Steen, S. N. and McKinney, S.,** Nutrition assessment of college wrestlers, *Phys. Sportsmed.,* 14, 100, 1986.

50. **Holler, H. J. and Hilliker, M. L.,** Nutrition education for high school wrestlers, *J. Am. Diet. Assoc.,* 91, A-79, 1991.

51. **Douglas, P. D. and Douglas, J. G.,** Nutrition knowledge and food practices of high school athletes, *J. Am. Diet. Assoc.,* 84, 1198, 1984.

52. **Werblow, J. A., Fox, H. M., and Henneman, A.,** Nutrition knowledge, attitudes, and food patterns of women athletes, *J. Am. Diet. Assoc.,* 73, 242, 1978.

53. **Campbell, M. L. and MacFadyen, K. L.,** Nutritional knowledge, beliefs and dietary practices of competitive swimmers, *Can. Hom. Econ. J.,* 34, 47, 1984.

54. **Day, P. J. and Arnold, R. K.,** Nutrition knowledge among male and female participants of four distinct health/fitness facilities, *J. Am. Diet. Assoc.,* 90, A18, 1990.

55. **Auld, G. W., Smiciklas-Wright, H., and Shannon, B. M.,** School health interventions for adolescents at nutritional risk: a survey of health teachers, nurses, and coaches, *J. Nutr. Educ.,* 20, 319, 1988.

56. **Murphy, P.,** Youth sports coaches: using hunches to fill a blank page, *Phys. Sportsmed.,* 13, 136, 1985.

57. **Jobe, F. W. and Moynes, D.,** *The Official Little League Fitness Guide,* Simon & Schuster, New York, 1984.

58. **Schapira, D. V., Kumar, N. B., Lyman, G. H., and McMillan, S. C.,** The value of current nutrition information, *Preventive Med.,* 19, 45, 1990.

59. **Feinberg, S. E., Loftus, E. F., and Tanur, J. M.,** Cognitive aspects of health surveys for public information and policy, *Milbank Memorial Fund Q. Health Soc.,* 63, 598, 1985.

60. **Worthington-Roberts, B.,** Nutrition and athletic performance, *Nutr. Int.,* 2, 1, 1986.

61. **Phinney, S. D.,** Nutrition science and the individual athlete, *Nutr. Int.,* 2, 69, 1986.

62. **Gibson, R. S.,** *Principles of Nutritional Assessment,* Oxford University Press, New York, 1990.

63. **Anderson, S. A.,** Guidelines for use of dietary intake data. *J. Am. Diet. Assoc.,* 88, 1258, 1988.

64. **Basiotis, P. P., Welsh, S. O., Cronin, F. J., Kelsay, J. L., and Mertz, W.,** Number of days of food intake records required to estimate individual and group nutrient intakes with defined confidence, *J. Nutr.,* 117, 1638, 1987.

65. **Medlin, C. and Skinner, J. D.,** Individual dietary intake methodology: a 50-year review of progress, *J. Am. Diet. Assoc.,* 88, 1250, 1988.

66. **Marr, J. W. and Heady, J. A.,** Within- and between-person variation in dietary surveys: number of days needed to classify individuals, *Hum. Nutr.,* 40, 347, 1986.

67. **Bolland, J. E., Yuhas, J. A., and Bolland, T. W.,** Estimation of food portion sizes: effectiveness of training, *J. Am. Diet. Assoc.,* 88, 817, 1988.

68. **Thompson, F. E., Larkin, F. A., and Brown, M. B.,** Weekend-weekday differences in reported dietary intake: the nationwide food consumption survey, 1977–78, *Nutr. Res.,* 6, 647, 1986.

69. **Marr, J. W.,** Individual dietary surveys: purposes and methods, *World Rev. Nutr. Diet,* 13, 105, 1971.

70. **Kim, W. W., Mertz, W., Judd, J. T., Marshall, M. W., Kelsay, J. L., and Prather, E. S.,** Effect of making duplicate food collections on nutrient intakes calculated from food records, *Am. J. Clin. Nutr.,* 40, 1333, 1984.

71. **Kretsch, M. J. and Fong, A. K. H.,** Validation of a new computerized technique for quantitating individual dietary intake: the Nutrition Evaluation Scale System (NESSy) vs the weighed food record, *Am. J. Clin. Nutr.,* 51, 477, 1990.

72. **Livingstone, M. B. E., Prentice, A. M., Strain, J. J., Coward, W. A., Black, A. E., Barker, M. E., McKenna, P. G., and Whitehead, R. G.,** Accuracy of weighed dietary records in studies of diet and health, *Br. Med. J.,* 300, 708, 1990.

73. **Anon.,** Errors in reporting habitual energy intake, *Nutr. Rev.,* 49, 215, 1991.

74. **Ahluwalia, N. and Lammi-Keefe, C. J.,** Estimating the nutrient intake of older adults: components of variation and the effect of varying the number of 24-hour dietary recalls, *J. Am. Diet. Assoc.,* 91, 1438, 1991.

75. **Woteki, C. E.,** Methods for surveying food habits: how do we know what Americans are eating? *Clin. Nutr.,* 5, 9, 1986.

76. **Karvetti, R. and Knuts, L.,** Validity of the 24-hour dietary recall, *J. Am. Diet. Assoc.,* 85, 1437, 1985.

77. **Todd, K. S., Hudes, M., and Calloway, D. H.,** Food intake measurement: problems and approaches, *Am. J. Clin. Nutr.,* 37, 139, 1983.

78. **Guthrie, H. A. and Crocetti, A. F.,** Variability of nutrient intake over a 3-day period, *J. Am. Diet. Assoc.,* 85, 325, 1985.

79. **Pao, E. M., Sykes, K. E., and Cypel, Y. S.,** USDA Methodological Research for Large Scale Dietary Intake Surveys, 1975–88, Home Economics Research Report No. 49, *United States Department of Agriculture, Human Nutrition Information Services,* Washington, D.C., December, 1989, p. 380.

80. **Gersovitz, M., Madden, J. P., and Smiciklas-Wright, H.,** Validity of the 24-hour dietary recall and seven-day record for group comparisons, *J. Am. Diet. Assoc.,* 73, 48, 1978.

81. **Pao, E. M., Mickle, S. J., and Burk, M. C.,** One-day and 3-day nutrient intakes by individuals — Nationwide Food Consumption, Survey findings, spring 1977, *J. Am. Diet. Assoc.,* 85, 313, 1985.

82. **St. Jeor, S. T., Guthrie H. A., and Jones, M. B.,** Variability in nutrient intake in a 28-day period, *J. Am. Diet. Assoc.,* 83, 155, 1983.

83. **Payette, H. and Gray-Donald, K.,** Dietary intake and biochemical indices of nutritional status in an elderly population with estimates of the precision of the 7-d food record, *Am. J. Clin. Nutr.,* 54, 478, 1991.

84. **Freudenheim, J. L., Johnson, N. E., and Wardrop, R. L.,** Misclassification of nutrient intake of individuals and groups using one-, two-, three-, and seven-day food records, *Am. J. Epidemiol.,* 126, 703, 1987.

85. **Mertz, W., Tsui, J. C., Judd, J. T., Reiser, S., Hallfrisch, J., Morris, E. R., Steele, P. D., and Lashley, E.,** What are people really eating? The relation between energy intake derived from estimated diet records and intake determined to maintain body weight, *Am. J. Clin. Nutr.,* 54, 291, 1991.

86. **Larkin, F. A., Metzner, H. L., and Guire, K. E.,** Comparison of three consecutive-day and three random-day records of dietary intake, *J. Am. Diet. Assoc.,* 91, 1538, 1991.

87. **Edington, J., Thorogood, M., Geekie, M., Ball, M., and Mann, J.,** Assessment of nutritional intake using dietary records with estimated weights, *J. Hum. Nutr. Diet.,* 2, 407, 1989.

88. **Miller, J. Z., Kimes, T., Hui, S., Andon, M. B., and Johnson, C. C., Jr.,** Nutrient intake variability in a pediatric population: implications for study design, *J. Nutr.,* 121, 265, 1991.

89. **Basch, C. E., Shea, S., Arliss, R., Contento, I. R., Rips, J., Gutin, B., Irigoyen, M., and Zybert, P.,** Validation of mothers' reports of dietary intake by four to seven year-old children, *Am. J. Public Health,* 81, 1314, 1990.

90. **Rizek, R. L. and Pao, E. M.,** Dietary intake methodology. I. USDA surveys and supporting research, *J. Nutr.,* 120, 1525, 1990.

91. **Burke, B. S.,** The dietary history as a tool in research, *J. Am. Diet. Assoc.,* 23, 1041, 1947.

92. **Block, G., Woods, M., Potosky, A., and Clifford, C.,** Validation of a self-administered diet history questionnaire using multiple diet records, *J. Clin. Epidemiol.,* 43, 1327, 1990.

93. **McDonald, A., Van Horn, L., Slattery, M., Hilner, J., Bragg, C., Jacobs, D., Jr., Hubert, H., and Betz, E.,** The CARDIA dietary history: development, implementation, and evaluation, *J. Am. Diet. Assoc.,* 91, 1104, 1991.

94. **Block, G. and Hartman, A. M.,** Issues in reproducibility and validity of dietary studies, *Am. J. Clin. Nutr.,* 50, 1133, 1989.

95. **Horwath, C. C.,** Food frequency questionnaires: a review, *Aust. J. Nutr. Diet.,* 47, 71, 1990.

96. **Thompson, F. E., Metzner, H. L., Lamphiear, D. E., and Hawthorne, V. M.,** Characteristics of individuals and long term reproducibility of dietary reports: the Tecumseh diet methodology study, *J. Clin. Epidemiol.,* 43, 1169, 1990.

97. **Eck, L. H., Hanson, C. L., Slawson, D., and Lavasque, M. E.,** Measuring short-term dietary intake: development and testing of a 1-week food frequency questionnaire, *J. Am. Diet. Assoc.,* 91, 940, 1991.

98. **Eck, L. H. and Willett, W. C.,** Considerations in modifying a semiquantitative food frequency questionnaire, *J. Am. Diet. Assoc.,* 91, 979, 1991.

99. **Clapp, J. A., McPherson, R. S., Reed, D. B., and Hsi, B. P.,** Comparison of a food frequency questionnaire using reported vs standard portion sizes for classifying individuals according to nutrient intake, *J. Am. Diet. Assoc.,* 91, 316, 1991.

100. **Kristal, A. R., Abrams, B. F., Thornquist, M. D., Disogra, L., Croyle, R. T., Shattuck, A. L., and Henry, H. J.,** Development and validation of a food use checklist for evaluation of community nutrition interventions, *Am. J. Public Health,* 80, 1318, 1990.

101. **Smucker, R., Block, G., Coyle, L. Harvin, A., and Kessler, L.,** A dietary and risk factor questionnaire and analysis system for personal computers, *Am. J. Epidemiol.,* 129, 445, 1989.

102. **Francescato, M. P., Cok, O., and de Bernard, R. B.,** Analysis of the degree of precision of computer-assisted dietary survey method, *J. Hum. Nutr. Diet.,* 1, 321, 1988.

103. **Connor, S. L., Gustafson, J. R., Sexton, G., Becker, N., and Aaartnaud-Wild, S., and Connor, W. E.,** The diet habit survey: a new method of dietary assessment that relates to plasma cholesterol changes, *J. Am. Diet. Assoc.,* 92, 41, 1992.

104. **Briefel, R. R., Flegal, K. M., Winn, D. M., Loria, C. M., Johnson, C. L., and Sempos, C. T.,** Assessing the nation's diet: limitations of the food frequency questionnaire, *J. Am. Diet. Assoc.,* 92, 959, 1992.

105. **Block, G. and Subar, A. F.,** Estimates of nutrient intake from a food frequency questionnaire: the 1987 national health interview survey, *J. Am. Diet. Assoc.,* 92, 969, 1992.

106. **Frank, G. C., Nicklas, T. A., Webber, L. S., Major, C., Miller, J. F., and Berenson, G. S.,** A food frequency questionnaire for adolescents: defining eating patterns, *J. Am. Diet. Assoc.,* 92, 313, 1992.

107. **Zulkifli, S. N. and Yu, S. M.,** The food frequency method for dietary assessment, *J. Am. Diet. Assoc.,* 92, 681, 1992.

108. **Suitor, C. W. and Gardner, J. D.,** Development of an interactive, self-administered computerized food frequency questionnaire for use with low-income women, *J. Nutr. Educ.,* 24, 82, 1992.

109. **Block, G., Thompson, F. E., Hartman, A. M., Larkin, F. A., and Guire, K. E.,** Comparison of two dietary questionnaires validated against multiple dietary records collected during a 1-year period, *J. Am. Diet. Assoc.,* 92, 686, 1992.

110. **Crockett, S. J., Potter, J. D., Wright, M. S., and Bacheller, A.,** Validation of a self-reported shelf inventory to measure food purchase behavior, *J. Am. Diet. Assoc.,* 92, 694, 1992.

111. **Monsen, E. R.,** Controversy: what are appropriate uses of food frequency questionnaire data?, *J. Am. Diet. Assoc.,* 92, 959, 1992.

112. **Simons-Morton, B. G., Forthofer, R., Huang, I. W., Baranowski, T., Reed, D., and Fleishman, R.,** Reliability of direct observation of schoolchildren's consumption of bag lunches, *J. Am. Diet. Assoc.,* 92, 219, 1992.

113. **Heaney, R. P., Davies, K. M., Recker, R. R., and Packard, P. T.,** Long-term consistency of nutrient intakes in humans, *J. Nutr.,* 120, 869, 1990.

114. **Gibson, R. S.,** Validity in dietary assessment: a review, *J. Can. Diet. Assoc.,* 51, 275, 1990.

115. **Roberts, S. B., Ferland, G., Young, V. R., Morrow, F., Heyman, M. B., Melanson, K. J., Gullans, S. R., and Dallal, G. E.,** Objective verification of dietary intake by measurement of urine osmolality, *Am. J. Clin. Nutr.,* 54, 774, 1991.

116. **Hulten, B., Bengtsson, C., and Isaksson, B.,** Some errors inherent in a longitudinal dietary survey revealed by the urine nitrogen test, *Eur. J. Clin. Nutr.,* 44, 169, 1990.

117. **Schoeller, D. A.,** How accurate is self-reported dietary energy intake?, *Nutr. Rev.,* 48, 273, 1990.

118. **Rising, R., Alger, S., Boyce, V., Seaagle, H., Ferraro, R., Fontvielle, A. M., and Ravussin, E.,** Food intake measured by an automated food-selection system: relationship to energy expenditure, *Am. J. Clin. Nutr.,* 55, 343, 1992.

119. **Sevenhuysen, G. P. and Zacharias, E.,** Comparison of food intake assessments obtained with recall interviews and photographic records, *Nutr. Rep. Int.,* 40, 49, 1989.

120. **Sevenhuysen, G. P., Staveren, W. V., Dekker, K., and Spronck, E.,** Estimates of daily intakes by food image processing, *Nutr. Res.,* 10, 965, 1990.

121. **Gines, D. J.,** Computer graphics increase accuracy of estimates of sizes of servings of food in dietary assessment, *J. Am. Diet. Assoc.,* 91, A19, 1991.

122. **Bingham, S. A.,** The dietary assessment of individuals; methods, accuracy, new techniques and recommendations, *Nutr. Abstr. Rev.,* 57, 1, 1987.

123. **Borrelli, R.,** Collection of food intake data: a reappraisal of criteria for judging methods, *Br. J. Nutr.,* 63, 411, 1990.

124. **Anon.,** Estimating usual dietary intake of individuals: some additional considerations, *Nutr. Rev.,* 49, 252, 1991.

125. **Pennington, J. A. T.,** Associations between diet and health: the use of food consumption measurements, nutrient databases, and dietary guidelines, *J. Am. Diet. Assoc.,* 88, 1221, 1988.

126. **Subcommittee on the Tenth Edition of the RDAs, Food and Nutrition Board, Commission on Life Sciences, National Research Council,** *Recommended Dietary Allowances,* 10th ed., National Acadmy Press, Washington, D.C., 1989.

127. **Leverton, R. M.,** The RDAs are not for amateurs, *J. Am. Diet. Assoc.,* 66, 9, 1975.

128. **Williams, M. H.,** *Nutritional Aspects of Human Physical and Athletic Performance,* 2nd ed., Charles C. Thomas, Springfield, IL, 1985.

129. **Johnston, J. L. and Morin, L.,** Limitations of nutrient requirement estimates based on body weight, *J. Can. Diet. Assoc.,* 51, 33, 1990.

130. **Hanson, R. G. and Wyse, B. W.,** Expression of nutrient allowances per 1,000 kilocalories, *J. Am. Diet. Assoc.,* 76, 223, 1980.

131. **Pao, E. M. and Mickle, S. J.,** Problem nutrients in the United States, *Food Technol.,* 35, 58, 1981.

132. **Stuff, J. E., Garza, C., Smith, E. O., Nichols, B. L., and Montandon, C. M.,** A comparison of dietary methods in nutritional studies, *Am. J. Clin. Nutr.,* 37, 300, 1983.

133. **Buzzard, I. M., Price, K. S., and Warren, R. A.,** Considerations for selecting nutrient-calculation software: evaluation of the nutrient database, *Am. J. Clin. Nutr.,* 54, 7, 1991.

134. **Hoover, L. W., Dowdy, R. P., and Hughes, K. V.,** Consequences of utilizing reduced nutrient data bases for estimating dietary adequacy, *J. Am. Diet. Assoc.,* 85, 298, 1985.

135. **Perloff, B. P., Rizek, R. L., Haytowitz, D. B., and Reid, P. R.,** Dietary intake methodology. II. USDA's nutrient data base for nationwide dietary intake surveys, *J. Nutr.,* 120, 1530, 1990.

136. **Hepburn, F. N.,** The USDA National nutrient data bank, *Am. J. Clin. Nutr.,* 35, 1297, 1982.

137. **Hoover, L. W. and Perloff, B. P.,** *Model for Review of Nutrient Data Base System Capabilites,* 2nd ed., University of Missouri, Columbia, MO, 1984.

138. **Karkeck, J. M.,** Improving the use of dietary survey methodology, *J. Am. Diet. Assoc.,* 87, 869, 1987.

139. **Dwyer, J. and Suitor, C. W.,** Caveat emptor: assessing needs, evaluating computer options, *J. Am. Diet. Assoc.,* 84, 302, 1984.

140. **Guthrie, H. A.,** *Introductory Nutrition,* 5th ed., C. V. Mosby, St. Louis, MO, 1983.

141. **Ink, S. L.,** Evaluating nutrition research, presented at the *Food Health Claims Symposium,* sponsored by Tufts University and the Food and Drug Administration, March 29, 1990, Boston, MA.

142. **Leaf, A. and Frisa, K. B.,** Eating for health or for athletic performance?, *Am. J. Clin. Nutr.,* 49, 1066, 1989.

143. **Lindeman, A. K.,** Eating for endurance and ultraendurance, *Phys. Sportsmed.,* 20, 87, 1992.

144. **Hoffman, C. J. and Coleman, E.,** An eating plan and update on recommended dietary practices for the endurance athlete, *J. Am. Diet. Assoc.,* 91, 325, 1991.

145. **Grandjean, A. C.,** Macronutrient intake of US athletes compared with the general population and recommendations made for athletes, *Am. J. Clin. Nutr.,* 49, 1070, 1989.

146. **Short, S. H. and Short, W. R.,** Four-year study of university athletes' dietary intake, *J. Am. Diet. Assoc.,* 82, 632, 1983.

147. **Marcus, J. B., Ed.,** Sports nutrition, a guide for the professional working with active people, Sports and Cardiovascular Nutritionists (SCAN), a dietetic practice group of The American Dietetic Association, Chicago, IL, 1986.

148. **Burke, L. M., Gollan, R. A., and Read, R. S. D.,** Dietary intakes and food use of groups of elite Australian male athletes, *Int. J. Sport Nutr.,* 1, 378, 1991.

149. **Nutter, J.,** Seasonal changes in female athletes' diets, *Int. J. Sport Nutr.,* 1, 395, 1991.

150. **Welch, P. K., Zager, K. A., Endres, J., and Poon, S. W.,** Nutrition education, body composition, and dietary intake of female college athletes, *Phys. Sportsmed.,* 15, 63, 1987.

151. **Strauzenberg, S. E., Schneider, F., Donath, R., Zerbes, H., and Kohler, E.,** The problem of dieting in training and athletic performance, *Bibl. Nutr. Diet.,* 27, 133, 1979.

152. **Mays, R. W. and Scoular, F. I.,** Food eaten by athletes, *J. Am. Diet. Assoc.,* 39, 225, 1961.

153. **Bobb, A., Pringle, D., and Ryan, A. J.,** A brief study of the diet of athletes, *J. Sports Med.,* 9, 255, 1969.

154. **Steel, J. E.,** A nutritional study of Australian Olympic athletes, *Med. J. Austr.,* 2, 119, 1970.

155. **van Erp-Baart, A. M. J., Saris, W. H. M., Binkhorst, R. A., Voos, J. A., and Brouns, F.,** A nationwide survey on nutritional habits in athletes, *Med. Sci. Sports Exercise,* 19, S21, 1987.

156. **Minessale, R. A. and Schulz, L. O.,** Factors influencing the use of nutritional supplements by college athletes, *Am. J. Clin. Nutr.,* 46, 529, 1987.

157. **Kirsch, K. A. and von Ameln, H.,** Feeding patterns of endurance athletes, *Eur. J. Appl. Physiol.,* 47, 197, 1981.

158. **Quinn, T. J., Sprague, H. A., Van Huss, W. D., and Olson, H. W.,** Caloric expenditure, life status, and disease in former male athletes and non-athletes, *Med. Sci. Sports Exercise,* 22, 742, 1990.

159. **Telford, R. D., Catchpole, E. A., Deakin, V., Hahn, A. G., and Plank, A. W.,** The effect of 7 to 8 months of vitamin/mineral supplementation on athletic performance, *Int. J. Sport Nutr.,* 2, 135, 1992.

160. **Fujioka, K., Kain, D., Mackenzie, R. B., and Gray, D. S.,** Increased carbohydrate intake of national basketball association superstar athletes, *Am. J. Clin. Nutr.,* 54, S32, 1991.

161. **Hickson, J. F., Schrader, J., and Trischler, L. C.,** Dietary intakes of female basketball and gymnastic athletes, *J. Am. Diet. Assoc.,* 86, 251, 1986.

162. **Johnson, E. B.,** An Analysis of the Nutrient Intake of High School and College Female Basketball Players, Masters Thesis, Syracuse University, New York, 1982.

163. **Nowak, R. K. and Schulz, L. O.,** Body composition and nutrient intakes of college men and women basketball players, *J. Am. Diet. Assoc.,* 88, 575, 1988.

164. **Gabel, K. A. and Aldous, A.,** Dietary and hematological assessment of elite cyclists during ten day 2050 mile ride, *J. Am. Diet. Assoc.,* 90, A107, 1990.

165. **Jensen, C. D., Zaltas, E. S., and Whittam, J. H.,** Dietary intakes of male endurance cyclists during training and racing, *J. Am. Diet. Assoc.,* 92, 986, 1992.

166. **Clark, N., Tobin, J., and Ellis, C.,** Feeding the ultraendurance athlete: practical tips and a case study, *J. Am. Diet. Assoc.,* 92, 1258, 1992.

167. **Lindeman, A. K.,** Nutrient intake of an ultraendurance cyclist, *Int. J. Sport Nutr.,* 1, 79, 1991.

168. **Slavin, J. L. and McNamara, E. A.,** Nutritional practices of women cyclists, including recreational riders and elite racers, in *Sport, Health and Nutrition,* Vol. 2, Human Kinetics Publishing, Champaign, IL, 1986.

169. **Loy, S. F., Conlee, R. K., Winder, W. W., Nelson, A. G., Arnall, D. A., and Fisher, A. G.,** Effects of 24-hour fast on cycling endurance time at two different intensities, *J. Appl. Physiol.,* 61, 654, 1986.

170. **Calabrese, L. H., Kirkendall, D. T., Floyd, M., Rapoport, S., Williams, G. W., Weiker, G. G., and Bergfeld, J. A.,** Menstrual abnormalities, nutritional patterns, and body composition in female classical ballet dancers, *Phys. Sportsmed.,* 11, 86, 1983.

171. **Brooks-Gunn, J., Warren, M. P., and Hamilton, L. H.,** The relation of eating problems and amenorrhea in ballet dancers, *Med. Sci. Sports Exercise,* 19, 41, 1987.

172. **Cohen, J. L., Potosnak, L., Frank, O., and Baker, H.,** A nutritional and hematologic assessment of elite ballet dancers, *Phys. Sportsmed.,* 13, 43, 1985.

173. **Evers, C. L.,** Dietary intake and symptoms of anorexia nervosa in female university dancers, *J. Am. Diet. Assoc.,* 87, 66, 1987.

174. **Benson, J., Gillien, D. M., Bourdet, K., and Loosli, A. R.,** Inadequate nutrition and chronic calorie restriction in adolescent ballerinas, *Phys. Sportsmed.,* 13, 79, 1985.

175. **Humphries, L. L. and Gruber, J. J.,** Nutrition behaviors of university majorettes, *Phys. Sportsmed.,* 14, 91, 1986.

176. **Ready, A. E.,** Nutrient intake of the Canadian women's Olympic field hockey team (1984), *Can. Home Econ. J.,* 37, 29, 1987.

177. **Hickson, J. F., Duke, M. A., Risser, W. L., Johnson, C. W., Palmer, R., and Stockton, J. E.,** Nutritional intake from food sources of high school football athletes, *J. Am. Diet. Assoc.,* 87, 926, 1987.

178. **Gorman, I. and Berning, J.,** Nutrition education in a strength and conditioning program?, *Natl. Strength Cond. Assoc. J.,* 7, 68, 1985.

179. **Hickson, J. F., Wolinsky, I., Pivarnik, J. M., Neuman, E. A., Itak, J. F., and Stockton, J. E.,** Nutritional profile of football athletes eating from a training table, *Nutr. Res.,* 7, 27, 1987.

180. **Zallen, E. M. and Fitterhof, W. F.,** Nutrition knowledge and nutrient intake of football players in training compared to male students not in training, Abstr., Am. Diet. Assoc. 70th Annual Meeting, Atlanta, GA, 1987, 144.

181. **Stoeppel, C.,** Survey of Supplement Use by Syracuse University Football Team Members, unpublished paper, Syracuse University, Fall, 1986.

182. **Moffatt, R. J.,** Dietary status of elite female high school gymnasts: inadequacy of vitamin and mineral intake, *J. Am. Diet. Assoc.,* 84, 1361, 1984.

183. **Huber, L. H., Zeigler, P., Congdon, K., Lindholm, S., and Manfredi, T. G.,** Nutritional status of college female gymnasts and cross-country runners, *Med. Sci. Sports Exercise,* 18, S64, 1986.

184. **Calabrese, L. H.,** Nutritional and medical aspects of gymnastics, *Clin. Sports Med.,* 4, 23, 1985.

185. **Thomson, M. J., Cunningham, D. A., and Wearring, G. A.,** Eating habits and caloric intake of physically active young boys, ages 10 to 14 years, *Can. J. Appl. Sports Sci.,* 5, 9, 1980.

186. **Rucinski, A.,** Relationship of body image and dietary intake of competitive ice skaters, *J. Am. Diet. Assoc.,* 89, 98, 1989.

187. **Worme, J. D., Lickteig, J. A., Reynolds, R. D., and Deuster, P. A.,** Consumption of a dehydrated ratio for 31 days at moderate altitudes: energy intakes and physical performance, *J. Am. Diet. Assoc.,* 91, 1543, 1991.

188. **Howard, M. P. and Reynolds, R. D.,** in *Quarterly Report of Selected Research Projects,* Agricultural Research Service, U.S. Department of Agriculture, Washington, D.C., Jan–Mar, 1992, p. 16.

189. **Duncan, R.,** A comparison between the energy balance of men on long and short sledging journeys, *Nutrition,* 4, 357, 1988.

190. **Morozov, V. I., Priyatkin, S. A., Rogozkin, V. A., Shishina, N. N., and Fedorova, G. P.,** Vitamin supply, iron status and the state of nonspecific resistance system in athletes of different ages and sexes, *Soviet Sports Rev.,* 23, 152, 1988 (Transl).

191. **Ellsworth, N. M., Hewitt, B. F., and Haskell, W. L.,** Nutrient intake of elite male and female Nordic skiers, *Phys. Sports Med.,* 13, 79, 1985.

192. **Campbell, I. T.,** Energy intakes on sledging expeditions, *Br. J. Nutr.,* 45, 89, 1981.

193. **Campbell, I. T. and Donaldson, J.,** Energy requirements of antarctic sledge dogs, *Br. J. Nutr.,* 45, 95, 1981.

194. **Hartmann, G. and Oberli, H.,** Nutrition and heavy Alpine physical performance, *Bibl. Nutr. Diet.,* 27, 126, 1979.

195. **Simonsen, J. C., Sherman, W. M., Lamb, D. R., Dernback, A. R., Doyle, J. A., and Strauss, R.,** Dietary carbohydrate, muscle glycogen, and power output during rowing training, *J. Appl. Physiol.,* 70, 1500, 1991.

196. **de Wijn, J. F., Leusink, J., and Post, G. B.,** Diet, body composition and physical condition of champion rowers during periods of training and out of training, *Bibl. Nutr. Diet.,* 27, 143, 1979.

197. **Bergen-Cico, D. K., and Short, S. H.,** Dietary intakes, energy expenditures, and anthropometric characteristics of adolescent female cross-country runners, *J. Am. Diet. Assoc.,* 92, 611, 1992.

198. **Baer, J. T. and Taper, L. J.,** Amenorrheic and eumenorrheic adolescent runners: dietary intake and exercise training status, *J. Am. Diet. Assoc.,* 92, 89, 1992.

199. **Manore, M. M., Thompson, J. L., and Skinner, J. S.,** Nutrient intakes in elite male runners with low and balanced (BAL) energy intakes, *Med. Sci. Sports Exercise,* 23, S75, 1991.

200. **Clark, N. and Snyder, A.,** Nutritional practices of elite male runners, *J. Am. Diet. Assoc.,* 90, A31, 1990.

201. **Pate, R. R., Sargent, R. G., Baldwin, C., and Burgess, M. L.,** Dietary intake of women runners, *Int. J. Sport Med.,* 11, 461, 1990.

202. **Manore, M. M., Besenfelder, P. D., Carroll, S. S., and Hooker, S. P.,** Nutrient intakes and iron status in female long distance runners during training, *J. Am. Diet. Assoc.,* 89, 257, 1989.

203. **Peters, A. J., Dressendorfer, R. H., Rimar, J., and Keen, C. L.,** Diets of endurance runners competing in a 20-day road race, *Phys. Sportsmed.,* 14, 63, 1986.

204. **Dressendorfer, R. H., Wade, C. E., Keen, C. L., and Scaff, J. H.,** Plasma mineral levels in marathon runners during a 20-day road race, *Phys. Sportsmed.,* 10, 113, 1982.

205. **Lally, D. A., Wang, J. H., Goebert, D. A., Quigley, R. D., and Hartung, G. H.,** Performance, training, and dietary characteristics of American and Japanese wheelchair marathoners, *Med. Sci. Sports Exercise,* 23, S101, 1991.

206. **Deuster, P. A., Kyle, S. B., Moser, P. B., Vigersky, R. A., Singh, A., and Schoomaker, E. B.,** Nutritional survey of highly trained women runners, *Am. J. Clin. Nutr.,* 44, 954, 1986.

207. **Clark, N., Nelson, M., and Evans, W.,** Nutrition education for elite female runners, *Phys. Sportsmed.,* 16, 124, 1988.

208. **Heavey, A. C.,** Food frequency comparisons between high mileage and moderate mileage runners, SCAN's Pulse, the Am. Diet. Assoc. practice group, *Sports Cardiovasc. Nutr. Newsl.,* 4 (Spring), 3, 1985.

209. **Blair, S. N., Ellsworth, N. M., Haskell, W. L., Stern, M. P., Farquhar, J. W., and Wood, P. D.,** Comparison of nutrient intake in middle-aged men and women runners and controls, *Med. Sci. Sports Exercise,* 13, 310, 1981.

210. **Snyder, A. C., Dvorak, L. L., and Roepke, J. B.,** Dietary patterns and iron parameters of middle aged female runners, *Med. Sci. Sports Exercise,* 19, S38, 1987.

211. **Haymes, E. M. and Spillman, D. M.,** Iron status of women distance runners, sprinters, and moderately active women, *Med. Sci. Sports Exercise,* 19, S20, 1987.

212. **Spillman, D. M. and Haymes, E. M.,** Nutrient intake of an elite collegiate women's track team, Am. Diet. Assoc. National Meeting Abstracts, 70th Annual Meeting, Atlanta, GA, October 1987, p. 91.

213. **Clement, D. B. and Asmundson, R. C.,** Nutritional intake and hematological parameters in endurance runners, *Phys. Sportsmed.,* 10, 37, 1982.

214. **Besenfelder, P. D., Manore, M. M., and Wells, C. L.,** Effect of training on iron status in female long-distance runners, Abstracts, The Am. Diet. Assoc. 69th Annual Meeting, Las Vegas, NV, October 1986, p. 122.

215. **Hartung, G. H., Foreyt, J. P., Mitchell, R. E., Vlasek, I., and Gotto, A. M.,** Relation of diet to high-density-lipoprotein cholesterol in middle-aged marathon runners, joggers, and inactive men, *N. Engl. J. Med.,* 302, 357, 1980.

216. **Thompson, P. D., Cullianame, E., Eshleman, R., and Herbert, P. N.,** Lipoprotein changes when a reported diet is tested in distance runners, *Am. J. Clin. Nutr.,* 39, 368, 1984.

217. **Bassler, T. J.,** Hazards of restrictive diets, *JAMA,* 252, 483, 1984.

218. **Lampe, J. W., Slavin, J. L., and Apple, F. S.,** Poor iron status of women runners training for a marathon, *Int. J. Sport Med.,* 7, 111, 1986.

219. **Grace, S. J. and Jeffrey, D. M.,** Iron, zinc, and copper intakes of women track team members, *Fed. Proc.,* 42, 803, 1983.

220. **Lathan, S. R. and Cantwell, J. D.,** A run for the record, studies on a trans-American ultramarathoner, *JAMA,* 245, 367, 1981.

221. **Rico, J., Frontera, W. R., Rivera, M. A., Mole, P. A., and Meredith, C. N.,** Nutritional habits and body composition of elite soccer players, *Med. Sci. Sports Exercise,* 24, S288, 1992.

222. **Hickson, J. F., Schrader, J. W., Pivarnik, J. H., and Stockton, J. E.,** Nutritional intake from food sources of soccer athletes during two stage of training, *Nutr. Rep. Int.,* 34, 85, 1986.

223. **Tater, D., Leglise, D., Person, B., Lambert, D., and Bercovici, J. P.,** Liproproteins status in professional football players after period of vacation and one month after a new intensive training program, *Horm. Metab. Res.,* 19, 24, 1987.

224. **Barr, S. I.,** Relationship of eating attitudes to anthropometric variables and dietary intakes of female collegiate swimmers, *J. Am. Diet. Assoc.,* 91, 976, 1991.

225. **Berning, J. R., Troup, J. P., VanHandel, P. J., Daniels, J., and Daniels, N.,** The nutritional habits of young adolescent swimmers, *Int. J. Sport Nutr.,* 1, 240, 1991.

226. **Lukaski, H. C., Hoverson, B. S., Gallagher, S. K., and Bolonchuk, W. W.,** Physical training and copper, iron and zinc status of swimmers, *Am. J. Clin. Nutr.,* 51, 1093, 1990.

227. **Lukaski, H. C., Hoverson, B. S., Milne, D. B., and Bolonchuk, W. W.,** Copper, zinc, and iron status of female swimmers, *Nutr. Res.,* 9, 493, 1989.

228. **Campbell, M. L. and MacFadyen, K. L.,** Nutritional knowledge, beliefs and dietary practices of competitive swimmers, *Can. Home Econ. J.,* 34, 47, 1984.

229. **Dietary Standard of Canada,** Ottawa Department of National Health and Welfare, 1975.

230. **Smith, M. P., Mendez, J., Druckenmiller, M., and Kris-Etherton, P. M.,** Exercise intensity, dietary intake, and high density lipoprotein cholesterol in young female competitive swimmers, *Am. J. Clin. Nutr.,* 36, 251, 1982.

231. **Adams, M. M., Porcello, L. P., and Vivian V. M.,** Effect of a supplement on dietary intakes of female collegiate swimmers, *Phys. Sportsmed.,* 10, 122, 1982.

232. **Houston, M. E.,** Diet, training and sleep: a survey study of elite Canadian swimmers, *Can. J. Appl. Sport. Sci.,* 5, 161, 1980.

233. **Lindman, A. K.,** Eating and training habits of triathletes: a balancing act, *J. Am. Diet. Assoc.,* 90, 991, 1990.

234. **Applegate, E. A.,** Nutritional concerns of the ultraendurance triathlete, *Med. Sci. Sports Exercise,* 21, S205, 1989.

235. **Applegate, E. A.,** Nutritional considerations for ultraendurance performance, *Int. J. Sport Nutr.,* 1, 118, 1991.

236. **Reher, N. J., van Kemenade, M., Meester, W., Brouns, F., and Saris, W. H. M.,** Gastrointestinal complaints in relation to dietary intakes in triathletes, *Int. J. Sport Nutr.,* 2, 48, 1992.

237. **Burke, L. M. and Read, R. S. D.,** Diet patterns of elite Australian male triathletes, *Phys. Sportsmed.,* 15, 140, 1987.

238. **Marquart, L. F., Wu, S. M., Izurieta, M. I., and Bazzarre, T. L.,** Zinc status among low fat and moderate fat tirathletes and controls, *Med. Sci. Sports Exercise,* 19, S21, 1987.

239. **Bazzarre, T. L., Marquart, L. F., Izurieta, M., and Jones, A.,** Incidence of poor nutritional status among triathletes, endurance athletes and control subjects, *Med. Sci. Sports Exercise,* 18, S90, 1986.

240. **Novak, J.,** Super iron-man competitions, *Nat. Strength Cond. Assoc. J.,* 7, 66, 1985.

241. **DeBruyne, L. K.,** Nutrition notions of bodybuilders, *Nutr. Clin.,* 6, 1, 1991.

242. **Bazzarre, T. L., Kleiner, S. M., and Litchford, M. D.,** Nutrient intake, body fat, and lipid profiles of competitive male and female bodybuilders, *J. Am. Coll. Nutr.,* 9, 136, 1990.

243. **Newton, L. E., Hunter, G. R., Bammon, M. M., and Roney, R. K.,** The effects of 12 weeks precompetition preparation on diet and body composition in bodybuilders, *Med. Sci. Sports Exercise,* 23, S29, 1991.

244. **Freed, T. M. and McGinnis, M.,** The dietary practices of a sample of serious male body builders, *J. Am. Diet. Assoc.,* 90, A36, 1990.

245. **Steen, S. N.,** Precontest strategies of a male bodybuilder, *Int. J. Sport Nutr.,* 1, 69, 1991.

246. **Sandoval, W. M. and Heyward, V. H.,** Food selection patterns of bodybuilders, *Int. J. Sport Nutr.,* 1, 61, 1991.

247. **Sandoval, W. M., Heyward, V. H., and Lyons, T. M.,** Comparison of body composition, exercise and nutritional profiles of female and male body builders at competition, *J. Sports Med.,* 29, 63, 1989.

248. **Lamar-Hildebrand, N., Saldanha, L., and Endres, J.,** Dietary and exercise practices of college-aged female bodybuilders, *J. Am. Diet. Assoc.,* 89, 1308, 1989.

249. **Vorobiev, A. N.,** Controlling body weight (weightlifters), Weightlifting, 234, 1981 in *Soviet Sports Rev.,* 26, 62, 1991.

250. **Schulz, L. O.,** Factors influencing the use of nutritional supplements by college students with varying levels of physical activity, *Nutr. Res.,* 8, 459, 1988.

251. **Celejowa, I. and Homa, M.,** Food intake, nitrogen and energy balance in Polish weight lifters, during a training camp, *Nutr. Metab.,* 12, 259, 1970.

252. **Laritcheva, K. A., Yalovaya, N. I., Shubin, V. I., and Smirnov, P. V.,** Study of energy expenditure and protein needs of top weight lifters, in *Nutrition, Physical Fitness and Health,* Parizkova, J. and Rogozkin, V. A., Eds., University Park Press, Baltimore, MD, 1978.

253. **Barnes, L.,** How physicians can help high school wrestlers control weight, *Phys. Sports Med.,* 15, 166, 1987.

254. **Tipton, C. M.,** Commentary: physicians should advise wrestlers about weight loss, *Phys. Sports Med.,* 15, 160, 1987.

255. **Larson, D. J.,** Relationship of Dietary Intake to Index Leanness-Fatness in Wrestlers in Training, unpublished thesis, Iowa State University, 1978.

256. **Schwarzkopf, R. and Jensen, D.,** The effects of dietary control on making weight in collegiate wrestlers, *Med. Sci. Sports Exercise,* 19, S69, 1987.

257. **Steen, S. N. and Brownell, K. D.,** Weight loss patterns and nutrition practices of collegiate wrestlers, Abstracts, The Am. Diet. Assoc. 69th Annual Meeting, Las Vegas, NV, October 1986, p. 125.

258. **Gunderson, H. K. and McIntosh, M. K.,** An increased incidence of overweight, obesity, and indicators of chronic disease among ex-collegiate wrestlers, *J. Am. Diet. Assoc.,* 90, A121, 1990.
259. **Manley, M.,** Sumo wrestlers: making gluttony pay, *Phys. Sportsmed.,* July 61, 1974.
260. **Lidz, F.,** Meat bomb, *Sports Illustrated,* May 18, 1992, p. 69.
261. **Brotherhood, J. R.,** Nutrition and sports performance, *Sports Med.,* 1 (Sept–Oct), 350, 1984.
262. **Williams, M. H.,** *Nutrition for Fitness and Sport,* 3rd ed., Wm. C. Brown, Dubuque, IA, 1992.

Chapter **17**

NUTRITION AND STRENGTH

Terry L. Bazzarre
(with technical assistance from
Anthony Scarpino and David S. Chance)

CONTENTS

0-8493-7911-3/94/$0.00+$.50
© 1994 by CRC Press, Inc.

I. INTRODUCTION

Short[1] has reviewed the literature on the food intake of athletes and working populations. Little information is available on the food/nutrient intake of athletes engaged in strength-training activities. Most of the research cited in this review is based on study populations of athletes who are primarily involved in strength training, such as weightlifters, powerlifters, and bodybuilders. Because of the sparsity of data, information on wrestlers and football players, who also devote a considerable portion of their training program to gaining strength, has been included. In fact, many other athletes, such as gymnasts, skiers, basketball players, and tennis players now devote a significant portion of their training program to weight-training activities. Many trainers now recognize the importance of strong muscles in the prevention of fatigue and injuries, and in the promotion of muscular endurance. Consequently, strength training has become an integral component of the training program for athletes from a wide variety of sports. Strength training is also a major component of many fitness programs offered in a variety of settings.

Finally, it is important to recognize that while some athletes engage only in strength-training activities, many other athletes have balanced their gains in strength by incorporating stretching and flexibility exercises into their training programs. Other strength-trained athletes also include aerobic training into their schedules. For example, some bodybuilders now use aerobic training such as cycling as a means of increasing muscular definition in the final stages of their preparation for competition. Thus, the overall training programs of the populations cited in this review reflect observations based on individuals who presumably devote a considerable part of their training to the development of muscular strength, but these athletes may also engage in other beneficial forms of physical training.

II. METHODOLOGICAL CONSIDERATIONS

In reviewing the literature on the food and nutrient intake of strength-trained athletes, it is important to recognize that the measurement of food intake is only one component of evaluating the nutritional status of an individual or a population.[2] The four major components of evaluating nutritional status include the measurement of food intake, anthropometric assessment of body composition and other physical dimensions of the body, the evaluation of clinical signs and symptoms of poor nutritional status, and, finally, biochemical or laboratory assessments of various tissues of the body.

The adequacy of evaluating nutritional status is always dependent upon the use of ancillary information on the demographic characteristics of an individual and some knowledge about both the personal and familial medical history of the individual or population. This information is particularly useful in the selection of the normative data or reference standards that will be used to compare or evaluate the data obtained from the individual or population being screened for nutrition problems.

To date, there are no known reference data for athletes in general, nor for any specific group of athletes. Furthermore, it is not clear if such data are needed. Nevertheless, caution is warranted in the selection and use of population-based reference standards obtained from various segments of the general population with individual data for athletes. The body mass index (BMI) for example, which is often used as an index of excess adiposity in the general population, may be entirely inappropriate for athletes, especially strength-trained athletes, for whom high BMI values would reflect increased lean body mass (LBM) rather than increased adiposity. In addition, the use of the BMI or even body weight in calculating correlations between body composition and selected risk factors or performance variables may result in the identification of relationships which are opposite to those observed in the general population or in obese populations.

The collection of food intake information may be achieved by using various methods which generally reflect the need to collect data for a specific day or period of time (i.e., food records or 24-h dietary recalls) while other methods such as diet histories and food frequency questionnaires can be used to assess usual food intake.[3,4] The methods used to assess food intake information in studies of athletes have not always been described, and the lack of familiarity with the various methods/terminology has occasionally resulted in false information about the method that was actually used (e.g., some investigators have reported using a diet history when they actually used a food record or a 24-h recall). Generally, 3- to 7-d food records are considered more valid and reliable estimates of actual food intake for individuals and groups than 24-h recalls and diet histories, which are subject to problems related to memory.[3,4] Diet histories are generally a more reliable estimate of usual intake than the 24-h recall, because a single day's food intake may not be representative of the wide variety of food choices that an individual makes during the period of a year.[3,4] Therefore, caution is warranted in generalizing about the information collected on small samples, especially when the data are based on the 24-h recall method. The interpretation of nutrient intakes must also be made with caution if little or no information is provided about the food composition data base used in analyzing the nutrient content of an athlete's diet. Some food composition tables/software have a limited number of food items, while other tables may not be complete for all nutrients.[3] Thus, it is possible that the amount of a nutrient ingested by an individual may be greater than the reported intake because the amount of the nutrient present in all foods consumed was not accounted for. Care must also be taken in interpreting the data because food tables generally use a weighted average for the value listed for a specific food; however, the actual amount of nutrient present in the food may vary widely depending on differences in soil and water content (especially minerals). Food preparation methods may affect biological availability of nutrients. For example, vitamin C levels may decrease rapidly as a result of exposure to heat from cooking or from light. For these reasons, measures of variability are also important considerations in interpreting mean intakes.

Some investigators report the distribution of nutrient intakes among populations as well as mean values in order to provide a more comprehensive evaluation of nutritional status. Investigators also use a wide variety of descriptive information in reporting their findings which has prevented a direct comparison of the data from one study to another. For example, some investigators report energy intakes provided by protein, fat, and carbohydrate in total grams per day or in total grams per kilogram body weight, while other investigators may report intakes as a percent of total calories consumed. Studies on the nutrient intakes of athletes or other groups of individuals who have unusual body proportions, such as 7-ft-tall basketball players or 5-ft-tall jockeys, may need to adjust their values to reflect the effects of these differences in body composition. An evaluation of dietary intakes of bodybuilders is an example of the need to consider differences in body types within a group of athletes, as competitive male bodybuilders in the lightweight division are frequently under 5′6″ while those in the heavyweight division are often well over 6′0″. The relatively low body fat, high lean body mass of competitive bodybuilders represents another reason for carefully considering the descriptive units used to report nutrient intakes.

The interpretation of data collected from athletes living in foreign countries is also an important consideration. Food composition tables and reference standards such as dietary allowances vary from country to country. Cultural food practices and differences in food availability may also account for differences in nutrient intakes among athletes in different countries. Fresh fruits and vegetables are not always available or economical for many populations. Individuals evaluated in institutional settings or sports academies may also consume foods based on what is available rather than on the basis of individual food preferences.

In evaluating biochemical indices of nutritional status of athletes, it is important to recognize that the effects of hemoconcentration due to excessive sweating or as a potential reflection of consuming "excessive" intakes of protein and other constituents of the blood may alter the interpretation of blood values. The hypervolemia of endurance training which is associated with an increase in total blood volume represents a pseudo-dilutional anemia in endurance-trained athletes; however, an expansion of blood volume due to increased strength training has not been reported. Thus, the interpretation of blood concentrations of nutrient metabolites may vary from one population of athletes to the next, and may vary with changes in the training program of a given individual. Care must also be taken in the collection of plasma and serum samples as hemolysis of red blood cells (RBC) may significantly increase plasma/serum concentrations. The concentration of some constituents in erythrocytes (RBC) may be falsely elevated because of the increased concentrations in RBC compared to plasma or serum.[2]

Finally, it is important to recognize that blood concentrations of many nutrients do not generally change until tissue stores are either depleted or, alternatively, until tissue stores become saturated. Thus, the inadequate or excessive intake of foods and nutrients may be the only component of nutritional assessment that would reflect the potential development of nutrition problems in the future.

III. FOOD INTAKE AND NUTRITIONAL STATUS OF STRENGTH-TRAINED ATHLETES

A. Bodybuilders

A report by Short and Short[5] of the nutrient intakes of Syracuse University athletes represents one of the earliest efforts to measure food intake of athletes in a comprehensive and systematic manner. Their report, based on measuring dietary intakes of 554 male and female athletes who averaged at least 2 h of training on a daily basis, included data for six male bodybuilders. Anthropometric, biochemical, and training information about this population, which would be helpful in evaluating the nutrient intakes of this population and in comparing these results, were not included in their 4-year study. The data are, nevertheless, useful as a starting point for a review and discussion of the dietary intake of bodybuilders.

A total of seven studies on male bodybuilders[5-11] and three studies of female bodybuilders[6,7,13] have been reported in the literature (Table 1). Fogleholm et al.[14] evaluated dietary, anthropometric, and biochemical data for 25 Finnish weightlifters and 34 wrestlers; however, all of these data were reported in a larger sample of 147 athletes classified as "moderate energy expenditure" athletes. Unfortunately, because of collapsing their data into the larger sample which included athletes engaged in "sprinting" and "throwing", none of their results are reported in this chapter.

The sample size of the individual studies has been quite small. The total sample ranged from 6 to 35 subjects, except for a group of 76 South African bodybuilders studied by Faber et al.[8] Thus, data are available on a total of 173 male and 29 female bodybuilders. Most subjects were between 18 and 30 years of age.

Kleiner et al.[9] conducted a 6-month longitudinal study of 18 steroid-using (SU) and 17 non-steroid-using (NSU) bodybuilders while Lamar-Hildebrand et al.[13] monitored 6 competitive and 4 noncompetitive female bodybuilders during a 12-week period. All other studies represent cross-sectional data. Measures of food intake were generally based on food records collected by subjects ranging in length from 3 to 7 d. Hurley et al.[10] used both the 24-h recall and diet history methods, while Spitler et al.[11] included a "recall diet history". Different versions of food composition information were used in these studies. None of the reports on nutrient intake include intakes reflecting supplement use, although supplements are widely used by bodybuilders.

Kleiner et al.[9] and Lamar-Hildebrand et al.[13] demonstrated that significant changes in food intake occur during the training period leading up to competition. The data published by Kleiner et al.[9] and others do not represent nutrient intakes of athletes at or near the time of competition, while data reported by Bazzarre et al.[6,7] and Lamar-Hildebrand et al.[13] include data for nutrient intakes within 1 week of competition. Thus, differences in reported intakes among these studies may reflect differences in food intake associated with changes in training. Additionally, the data reported by Bazzarre et al.[6,7] represent information on elite bodybuilders at the time of national competition.

Some of the reported dietary information obtained from male bodybuilders is very limited. For example, Spitler et al.[11] and Hurley et al.[10] only reported the distribution of energy intake provided by protein, fat, and carbohydrate, but did not report mean energy intake. Only four of the seven studies on male bodybuilders provided any information about vitamin and mineral intakes.[5-7,9] Few investigators reported any information about the prevalence of vitamin/mineral supplement use among these populations.[9] In general, the nutrient intakes of the strength-trained athletes in each of the studies listed in Table 1 show wide interindividual variability.

Energy intakes ranged from 2015 ± 1060 to 4143 ± 1088 kcal in these studies (see Table 1). Mean energy intake was lower among elite male bodybuilders at the time of national competition[6,7] than those measured during some phase of the training season.[5,8,9]

Energy intakes of 76 South African bodybuilders reported by Faber et al.[8] were quite variable; however, the intake of those bodybuilders, who consumed no eggs (3187 ± 1027 kcal), was considerably less than that of bodybuilders who consumed an average of 12 eggs daily (4143 ± 1088 kcal). Differences in egg intake appeared to alter significantly the distribution of energy intake provided by protein, fat, and carbohydrate in these South African bodybuilders, accounting for a 12% increase in the proportion of calories provided by both protein and fat, and a 22% decrease in the proportion of calories provided by carbohydrate. These differences illustrate the important contribution of differences in food selection on the nutrient composition of these athletes' diets.

Protein intake in these studies was in excess of the Recommended Dietary Allowances (RDA),[15] averaging well over 100 g daily. Protein provided from 19 to as much as 85% of total energy intake. Protein intake of male bodybuilders averaged 34 to 40% of total energy intake at the time of competition;[6,7] bodybuilders at the more senior competitive level consumed more protein and less fat than their "junior"-level counterparts. Similar differences were also observed for competitive female bodybuilders, although the magnitude of these differences between the "senior" ladies and their "junior" counterparts was much less impressive.

The distribution of energy intake provided by protein, fat, and carbohydrate was relatively similar for both male and female bodybuilders at the time of national competition.[6,7] These data may suggest that both male and female bodybuilders tend to develop similar goals in regulating the qualitative energy content of their diets as they prepare for competition although large interindividual variability clearly exists. Protein as a percent of total energy intake is about 20% above the levels reported for the U.S. population, while fat intake has been reduced to remarkably low levels of about 10 to 15% of total energy intake. Thus, the high carbohydrate content of the diet of bodybuilders at the time of competition is quite similar to the high carbohydrate content of the diet of endurance athletes during their "carbohydrate-loading" regimens.

At the time of competition, dietary fat intake was quite low for male and female bodybuilders, ranging from a total of 33 ± 19 to 40 ± 51 g daily for males, compared to a range of 22 ± 17 to 33 ± 17 g daily for females.[6,7] Competitive bodybuilders consumed very little fat as a percent of total calories (10 to 15%) compared to the data for bodybuilders reported in other studies (34 to 50% for males).[5,9,10] Fat, as a percent of total calories, provided 20% and 27% of total calories for competitive and noncompetitive female bodybuilders, respectively, evaluated by Lamar-Hildebrandt et al.[13]

TABLE 1 Nutrient Intakes of Athletes Engaged in Strength-Training Activities

Investigators	Sample	Age	Method	% Body Fat	Energy (kcals)	PRO (g,%kcals)	FAT (g,%kcals)	CHO (g,%kcals)	P/S ratio	Cholesterol (mg/d)	Fiber (g/d)
Male Bodybuilders											
Faber, 1986[8]	76 males	27 ± 6	7-d FR	16.0 ± 2.6	3187 ± 1027[a]	19%	36%	42%	0.62 ± 0.24	509 ± 151	17 ± 10
Kleiner et al., 1989[9] (longitudinal)	18 male SU	30	3-d FR	14.9 ± 2.5	4143 ± 1088[b]	31%	46%	20%	0.55 ± 0.19	2823 ± 542	18 ± 11
	17 male NSU	26		13.1 13.8	5739 ± 2500	22%	34%	44%	0.6 ± 0.3	1413 ± 1151	—
Bazzarre et al., 1990[7]	19 males	28 ± 4	7-d FR	6.0 ± 1.8	2015 ± 1060	169 ± 94; 34 ± 12%	40 ± 51; 15 ± 9%	243 ± 121; 50 ± 13%	2.4 ± 1.1	513 ± 582	18 ± 12
Bazzarre et al., 1992[6]	19 males	30	3-d FR	4.9 ± 1.6	2620 ± 803	247 ± 105; 40 ± 15%	33 ± 19; 11 ± 5%	334 ± 194; 49 ± 21%	1.0 ± 1.0	444 ± 318	9 ± 7
Spitler et al.[11]	10 males	30	NR	9.9	—	85%	10%	5%	—	—	—
Hurley et al., 1984[10]	8 males	29 ± 1	24-h DR and diet history	12.0 ± 1.0	—	20%	40–50%	30–35%	—	—	—
Short and Short, 1983[5]	6 males	—	3-d FR	—	3962	197; 19%	176; 39%	350; 36%	0.27	1271	—
Female Bodybuilders (BB) and Weightlifters (WL)											
Morgan et al., 1986[12]	9 female WL	36	3-d FR	21.3 ± 1.5 BMI	1549 ± 430	85 ± 30; 23 ± 8%	57 ± 34; 32 ± 13%	182 ± 63; 47 ± 10%	1.2 ± 0.7	317 ± 124	—
Bazzarre et al., 1990[7]	8 female BB	28 ± 4	7-d FR	9.8 ± 1.5	2260 ± 2660	162 ± 93; 37 ± 16%	33 ± 41; 13 ± 9%	332 ± 525; 49 ± 18%	3.8 ± 1.9	462 ± 631	13 ± 7
Bazzarre et al., 1992[6]	11 female BB	29	3-d FR	9.1 ± 1.4	1597 ± 614	143 ± 45; 39 ± 13%	22 ± 17; 12 ± 5%	206 ± 120; 48 ± 16%	1.0 ± 1.0	223 ± 138	7 ± 5
LaMar-Hildebrand[13] (longitudinal)	6 comp. BB	18–30	3-d FR	53 ± 6 kg	2228 ± 1192	57 ± 25	49 ± 48	359 ± 194	—	148 ± 104	—
	4 noncomp. BB			60 ± 5 kg	1873 ± 393	82 ± 25	56 ± 28	284 ± 48	—	332 ± 316	—

Weightlifters (WL) and Wrestlers (WRE)

Reference	Subjects	Age	Method	Weight							
Chen et al.[17]	10 elite WL	21 ± 2	3–5-d FR	80 ± 19 kg	4597 ± 604 57 ± 6/kg BW	257 ± 47 22 ± 4%	205 ± 33 40 ± 7%	431 ± 96 38 ± 8%	—	—	—
	5 amateur WL	16 ± 1		71 ± 2 kg	4113 ± 555 58 ± 8/kg BW	143 ± 20 14 ± 2%	203 ± 21 44 ± 5%	430 ± 115 42 ± 11%	—	—	—
Heinemann and Zerbes, 1989[18]	15 WL	15–19	3-d FR	95 kg	79/kg BW	15% kcals	46% kcals	39% kcals	—	—	—
	20 WRE	19–22		85 kg	52/kg BW	18% kcals	38% kcals	44% kcals			
Football Players											
Hickson et al., 1987[20]	88 H.S.	15–18	24-h DR	76 ± 14 kg	3365 ± 1592 48 ± 21/kg BW	133 ± 77 1.9 ± 1.0 g/kg	154 ± 90	366 ± 170	—	—	—
	46 Jr. H.S.	12–14		61 ± 12 kg	2523 ± 936 43 ± 16/kg BW	91 ± 34 1.5 ± 0.6 g/kg	109 ± 59	302 ± 125	—	—	—
Hickson et al., 1987[21]	11 College	19.6 ± 0.4	3-d FR	108 ± 3 kg	3593 ± 217	190 ± 10 22 ± 1%	158 ± 12 39 ± 1%	329 ± 26 39 ± 1%	—	—	—

[a] Consumed <1.5 eggs per day.
[b] Consumed >6 eggs per day.

Note: SU, Steroid users; NSU, non-steroid users; FR, food record; NR, not recorded; DR, diet record.

The polyunsaturated–saturated fat (P/S) ratio in the diets of bodybuilders is quite variable among the reported studies (Table 1). P/S ratios ranged from lows of 0.27 reported by Short and Short[5] to 0.6 ± 0.3 in 35 male bodybuilders evaluated in the longitudinal study of Kleiner et al.[9] to highs of 2.4 ± 1.1 for male bodybuilders[7] and 3.8 ± 1.9 for female bodybuilders.[7]

Mean dietary cholesterol intakes have ranged from 444 ± 318 to 2823 ± 542 mg daily for male bodybuilders (Table 1). Mean dietary cholesterol intakes for female bodybuilders ranged from 148 ± 104 to 462 ± 631 mg daily. Thus, dietary cholesterol intakes tend to be higher among males than females, and many bodybuilders appear to consume higher amounts of cholesterol than recommended according to the National Cholesterol Education Program Guidelines (NCEP).[16] One subject consumed as many as 81 eggs per week.[8]

Dietary fiber intake (Table 1) among "senior"-level elite male and female bodybuilders[6] was approximately half that of their "junior"-level male and female counterparts.[7] The low intakes of 9 ± 7 and 7 ± 5 g daily among the senior-level males and females, respectively, in comparison to the junior-level males and females may reflect differences in food choices or differences in food composition tables. Since carbohydrate intake as a percent of total calorie intake was relatively similar among both groups, while total energy intake was approximately 600 calories less among senior-level vs. junior-level competitors, these differences may simply reflect differences in absolute carbohydrate intake. Dietary fiber intake among 76 South African bodybuilders averaged 18 ± 9 g daily, and did not vary significantly between bodybuilders who consumed a large quantity of eggs per week compared to those bodybuilders who consumed few eggs.[8] Longitudinal data are needed in order to determine if the usual fiber intakes of elite bodybuilders are also low. Such data combined with other biochemical data would be needed in order to assess the physiological consequences of a low fiber intake. Data are also needed on the types (soluble and insoluble) of fiber, and the amounts of each in order to evaluate the potential role of fiber on blood lipids and blood pressure of bodybuilders as well as other populations of interest.

Vitamin and mineral intakes (Table 2) have not been reported in several of the studies in which food intake information was collected.[10,11] Vitamins A and C intakes were generally well above the RDA. Intakes for thiamin and other B vitamins also appear to be above the RDA. Vitamin D intake was nil for competitive female bodybuilders evaluated by Bazzarre et al.[6] The vitamin D intake varied widely among competitive male bodybuilders in the same study, which reflected differences in the consumption of dairy products. Avoidance of dairy products is commonplace among bodybuilders as they prepare for competition; however, the scientific basis for this practice is unknown.

Dietary calcium intakes varied among the studies ranging from 605 ± 586 to 2987 ± 1825 mg among male bodybuilders and from 293 ± 231 to 962 ± 544 mg among female bodybuilders (Table 2). Lower intakes were consistently observed for study populations evaluated at the time of competition compared to other study populations. Low calcium intakes reflected the restriction of milk and dairy products. While low calcium intakes among female endurance athletes with amenorrhea has created concern about their increased risk of osteoporosis, it is not clear if reduced bone density is a problem for strength-trained female athletes who also have low calcium and vitamin D intakes.

Iron intakes were well above the RDA for male bodybuilders,[5-7,9] and for competitive female bodybuilders.[6,7] Competitive female bodybuilders studied by Lamar-Hildebrand et al.[13] consumed about 20% less iron than their noncompetitive counterparts. Magnesium intakes for competitive male bodybuilders were well above the RDA while magnesium intakes for competitive female bodybuilders tended to be at or above the RDA.[6,7]

Zinc intakes were lower than the RDA for competitive male and female bodybuilders,[6,7] while male bodybuilders studied by Kleiner et al.[9] averaged 44 ± 31 mg daily. Zinc intake

TABLE 2 Mineral and Vitamin Intakes of Athletes Engaged in Strength-Training Activities

Investigators	Sample	Calcium (mg)	Magnesium (mg)	Iron (mg)	Zinc (mg)	Copper (mg)	Vitamins A (RE)	C (mg)	D (mg)	Thiamin (mg)
Male Bodybuilders										
Faber et al., 1986[8]	76 males	1508 ± 664	447 ± 153	24 ± 8	24 ± 9	2.9 ± 1.4	3476 ± 2364	178 ± 112	—	2.1 ± 0.7
Kleiner et al., 1989[9]	18 steroid users	2987 ± 1825	—	44 ± 31	40 ± 31	—	5366 ± 9087	493 ± 326	—	9 ± 14
	17 nonusers									
Bazzarre et al., 1990[7]	19 males	605 ± 586	385 ± 214	16 ± 9	11 ± 6	2.5 ± 1.8	—	272 ± 258	—	—
Bazzarre et al., 1992[6]	19 males	917 ± 953	700 ± 318	24 ± 6	14 ± 5	2.1 ± 1.4	—	—	93 ± 287	—
Short and Short, 1983[5]	6 males	1786	—	29	—	—	1210	185	—	—
Female Bodybuilders										
Bazzarre et al., 1990[7]	8 females	293 ± 231	254 ± 107	24 ± 40	9 ± 5	1.9 ± 1.6	—	196 ± 168	—	—
Bazzarre et al., 1992[6]	11 females	418 ± 198	424 ± 158	17 ± 10	9 ± 5	1.1 ± 0.6	—	—	0	—
Lamar-Hildebrand[13]	6 comp.	709 ± 662	—	12 ± 6			—			
	4 noncomp.	962 ± 544	—	15 ± 5						
Weightlifters (WL), Wrestlers (WRE), and Football Players (FB)										
Chen et al., 1989[17]	10 elite WL	1597 ± 195	777 ± 304	50 ± 9	—	—	1547 ± 99	93 ± 35	—	1.8 ± 0.3
	5 amateur WL	908 ± 144	374 ± 141	46 ± 6	36 ± 11	5.5 ± 1.2	1199 ± 172	52 ± 13	—	2.4 ± 0.4
Heinemann and Zerbes, 1989[18]	15 WL	—	—	—	—	—	—	260	—	—
	20 WRE	—	—	—	—	—	—	230	—	—
Hickson et al., 1987[20]	46 Jr. HS FB	1261 ± 655	482 ± 287	15 ± 11	13 ± 8	—	6063 ± 6130	103 ± 93	—	1.5 ± 1.0
	88 HS FB	1737 ± 1359	634 ± 437	20 ± 12	17 ± 12	—	8025 ± 8658	180 ± 239	—	2.2 ± 1.6
Hickson et al., 1987[21]	11 college FB	110% RDA	79% RDA	231% RDA	166% RDA	—	108% RDA	265% RDA	—	133% RDA

among South African bodybuilders averaged 24 ± 9 g daily compared to 31 ± 17 g daily when supplements were included in estimating daily intakes.[8] Copper intakes for competitive male bodybuilders[6,7] were well within the Estimated Safe and Adequate Daily Dietary Intake (ESADDI).[15] Copper intakes ranged from 1.1 ± 0.6 to 1.9 ± 1.6 mg daily in competitive female bodybuilders evaluated by Bazzarre et al.[6,7] which would be considered below the ESADDI level in one group[6] and slightly above the ESADDI level for the other group.[7] Copper intakes among South African bodybuilders was 2.9 ± 1.4 mg daily; and 4.2 ± 2.6 mg daily when supplements were included.[8]

Lower vitamin/mineral intakes among females tend to reflect lower calorie/food intakes compared to males, which follows the general patterns usually observed between males and females. The lower intakes of vitamins and minerals among the competitive male bodybuilders[6,7] compared to other bodybuilders also reflect lower energy/food intakes.

B. Weightlifters and Wrestlers

Five studies on the dietary intakes of weightlifters and wrestlers have been reported in the literature.[10,12,17-19] The data reported by Chen et al.[17] are based on a comparison of the intakes of ten elite weightlifters 21 ± 2 years of age compared to five amateur weightlifters 16 ± 1 year of age.[17] It is important to recognize that the latter data reflect the cultural food patterns of Chinese athletes, and that the data do not account for a 10-kg weight difference as well as potential differences in training dose (volume and intensity) that might account for differences in intakes between the amateur and elite groups.

Using the 24-h recall method of estimating nutrient intake, Warren et al.[19] reported average daily energy intakes greater than 3714 ± 1573 kcal d^{-1} and protein intakes above 2.0 g d^{-1} in a group of 28 male Olympic weightlifters. Hurley et al. compared the dietary intakes of 8 male bodybuilders to that of 8 male powerlifters[10] while Heinemann and Zerbes[18] measured the dietary intakes of 15 weightlifters and 20 wrestlers. The latter study included data obtained for other groups of athletes not reported here, and also reflects cultural food practices of German athletes.[18] In addition to the need to consider the potential impact of differences in the training regimens of wrestlers vs. weightlifters, it is also important to recognize that the weightlifters' body weight averaged 95 kg compared to 85 kg for the wrestlers. Morgan et al.[12] reported the only data for a group of 9 females engaged in a wide variety of strength-training regimens which were compared to a control group of 9 sedentary females and a groups of 9 female endurance athletes.

Energy intake among the elite Chinese weightlifters was approximately 500 calories more per day than their amateur counterparts.[17] The lower intake among the amateur weightlifters might be explained by their lower body weights and/or by a presumed decrease in physical training effort in comparison to their elite counterparts. Similarly, the 27-calorie per kilogram body weight (BW) difference between the wrestlers and weightlifters may be accounted for by the 10-kg difference in body weight as well as, perhaps, a greater need for wrestlers to maintain a reduced body weight compared to weightlifters.[18] Energy intake per kilogram body weight was fairly similar among Chinese amateur and elite weightlifters and German wrestlers (52 to 58 kcal/kg BW), but much less than that of German weightlifters (79 kcal/kg BW).

Hurley et al.[10] combined the data for both bodybuilders and weightlifters, and only reported information on the percent of total calories provided by protein, fat, and carbohydrate. These combined intakes were similar to the distributions reported by Chen et al.[17] for elite weightlifters (20 to 22% of kilocalories by protein). The amount of protein consumed as a percent of total calories among the amateur Chinese weightlifters (14%) was similar to that of German weightlifters and wrestlers (15 to 18%).

The female "weightlifter" group reported by Morgan et al.[12] consumed 23, 32, and 47% of calories as protein, fat, and carbohydrate, respectively. The carbohydrate intake as a percent of calories was somewhat similar to that of elite female bodybuilders (48 to 49%).[6,7] However, elite female bodybuilders were consuming about 37 to 39% of total calories as protein at the time of competition, but only 12 to 13% of total calories as fat.

Calcium and magnesium intakes of elite Chinese weightlifters were almost twice that of their amateur weightlifting counterparts; however, no explanations for these differences were provided by the authors.[15] Differences in food choices represent the most likely explanation for these differences in nutrient intakes as energy intakes were quite similar on a per kilogram body weight basis. Chinese weightlifters had the highest iron intakes of any of the populations studied (50 ± 9 and 46 ± 6 mg daily for elite and amateurs, respectively). Unusually high zinc and copper intakes were also reported for amateur Chinese weightlifters (no data were reported for elite weightlifters). Vitamin C intakes were lower for Chinese strength-trained athletes than for any other population evaluated; and, averaged only 52 ± 13 mg daily for amateur weightlifters.

C. Other Strength-Trained Populations (Football Players)

Hickson et al. studied 11 collegiate football players, 88 high school football players, and 46 junior high school football players (Table 1).[20,21] Short and Short[5] studied the dietary intakes of football players over a 4-year period during which the sample ranged from as few as 10 players to as many as 34 subjects (data not included in Table 1).[5] They also reported data for football players categorized as defensive backs, offensive team, and defensive team. We are not aware of any available information on the dietary intakes of professional football players.

Energy intake increased with age and body size in the football players evaluated by Hickson et al.[20,21] Mean energy intakes among the Syracuse University football team ranged from 4470 to 6149 calories during the 4-year period.[5] Individual intakes ranged from as low as 1990 to as much as 11,020 calories.[5] Energy intakes appeared to be less during the spring training period than during the competitive fall season. Protein, fat, and carbohydrate intakes as a percent of total energy intakes were 22, 39, and 39%, respectively, for the 11 college football players studied by Hickson et al.[21] compared to 16, 38 to 41, and 43 to 45%, respectively, for the Syracuse football players.[5]

Mean dietary cholesterol intakes among Syracuse University football players (Table 1) were extremely high, ranging from 626 to 1425 mg daily.[5] Individual intakes ranged from a low of 296 mg daily to a high of 3584 mg. The P/S ratio of the diets consumed by these same football players was exceptionally low, ranging from a mean of 0.23 to a high of 0.38. The P/S ratio of the diet of individual athletes was also quite low, reaching values of 0.07, 0.08, and 0.09 among different groups of players. The highest P/S ratios among individual football players were 0.50, 0.57, and 0.72. The P/S ratios of the diets of these athletes were not even close to the 1:1 ratio. A good number of athletes apparently consumed more than 300 g of fat on a daily basis. Clearly, the dietary intakes of these football players would place some athletes into a high risk group for cardiovascular disease. Data on the blood lipid profiles, blood pressure, and body fat levels are clearly needed. Since many collegiate linemen also demonstrated considerable abdominal obesity, the assessment of cardiovascular risks among this group is warranted.

Mean dietary intakes for calcium, magnesium, and iron (Table 2) were greater than the RDA for junior high school, senior high school, and collegiate football players studied by Hickson et al.[20,21] Mean zinc intakes were above the RDA for senior high school and collegiate players, but not for their junior high school counterparts. The higher food/energy intakes of the older players contributed to the high intakes of vitamins and minerals among these groups. The high food/energy intakes reported by Short and Short[5] for the Syracuse University football players also contributed to the high level of adequacy for vitamins and minerals among this group.

D. Recreational Strength-Trained Athletes

Little information has been reported on the nutritional status of individuals involved in recreational strength training. Lamar-Hildebrand et al.[13] reported data on six noncompetitive females involved in bodybuilding who might be classified as recreational, strength-trained athletes. The nine females evaluated by Morgan et al.[12] might also be classified as recreational athletes. Because of the sparsity of data on females, the data from all studies for females engaged in any form of strength training were grouped together. Bazzarre et al.[22] conducted a 24-week longitudinal study of endurance athletes which included a group of 12 control males who regularly engaged in strength training, and who maintained a relatively constant training program during the 24 week study. Age, heights, body weights, and body fat levels were not significantly different between the recreational strength-trained males and a group of 17 recreational endurance athletes. Although the male strength-trained athletes (controls) consumed about 150 kcal more per day than the endurance athletes, these differences were not statistically significant. The protein, fat, and carbohydrate intakes were relatively similar between these two groups at 14, 31–34, and 46–50%, respectively.

The energy intake of these recreational strength athletes was similar to that of bodybuilders at the time of competition, but less than that reported for other bodybuilders, wrestlers, and weightlifters, as well as high school and college age football players. Protein as a percent of total kilocalories was similar to that of amateur Chinese athletes (14%) evaluated by Chen et al.,[17] but much less than that reported in other studies (Table 1). These data may suggest that more highly trained strength athletes consume more energy and more protein than their recreational or amateur counterparts.

Dietary cholesterol (453 ± 57 mg) intake was within the range reported for competitive male bodybuilders,[6,7] but much less than reported by Kleiner et al.[9] and Faber et al.[8] Fiber intake (6.2 ± 0.9 g) was lower than reported for competitive male bodybuilders (9 to 18 g daily).

The mean intakes for vitamins A, C, pyridoxine, B_{12}, thiamin, and riboflavin (but not niacin) were above RDA levels.[15] Mean intakes for calcium, phosphorus, magnesium, and iron were also at or above RDA levels, while dietary zinc and copper intakes (13.9 ± 1.4 and 1.3 ± 0.6 mg daily, respectively) were below RDA levels. Thus, low zinc intakes appear to be common among both recreational strength-trained athletes as well as male and female bodybuilders at the time of competition.

E. Biochemical Indices of Nutritional Status

Few of the studies on strength-trained athletes measured biochemical indices of nutritional status in the populations surveyed.[6,17,22,74] Since the mean dietary intakes of these subjects appeared to be adequate, it is not surprising that the mean biochemical indices for iron (hemoglobin, hematocrit, and serum ferritin), zinc, copper, magnesium, and calcium were all within normal ranges. Vitamin C levels were low in five recreational strength-trained athletes evaluated by Bazzarre et al.,[22] which was consistent with relatively low vitamin C intakes observed in this group. Fogleholm et al.[14] conducted extensive biochemical tests of nutritional status in their large sample of Finnish athletes, and found that the incidence of nutritional deficiency was less than 0 to 5% of the population for hemoglobin, ferritin, magnesium, zinc, and vitamin C. Three to four percent of the population of athletes had low erythrocyte transketolase activity, suggesting marginal or deficient thiamin status in these athletes.

IV. STUDIES OF PROTEIN REQUIREMENTS OF STRENGTH-TRAINED ATHLETES

While much research has been conducted on the energy required to perform different types and amounts of work, relatively few investigations have examined the nutrient requirements of subjects relative to increased amounts of work (i.e., increased energy expenditure). The protein requirements of athletes has been the focus of most studies that have examined the effects of physical training on nutrient needs. Results for at least 25 investigations on the protein requirements of athletes have been published in the literature.[23-47] Many investigators have examined the effects of protein requirements on sedentary or untrained subjects, while other investigators have examined the protein needs of endurance-trained athletes.

Most published review articles on the nutrient needs of athletes include sections on protein and energy. Most authors of review papers cited prior to 1975 drew conclusions based on assumptions about the protein needs of athletes. Unfortunately, the assumptions made in these early review papers (i.e., the protein needs of athletes/laborers are no different than the protein needs of the general population) were not based on any specific research conducted on athletes. The authors of these review articles simply made extrapolations based on the Recommended Dietary Allowances.[15] These review articles have, unfortunately, been cited all too frequently. The lack of awareness of the existing research data base may explain why so little research has been conducted on this topic.

This discussion has been organized according to the kinds of methods used to evaluate the protein needs of individuals including athletes engaged in strength training. These methods include complete nitrogen balance (NBAL) investigations (i.e., investigations which collected 24-h urine, fecal, and sweat excretions), investigations which measured only urinary output, and a single investigation in which only sweat nitrogen (N) losses were measured.[48]

Major limitations of many investigations include the extremely small sample size and the large interindividual variation. Kraut et al.[37] and Mole and Johnson[41] studied only two and three subjects, respectively, while Gontzea et al.[34] evaluated 30 subjects. Most investigators evaluated the N needs/metabolism of six or fewer subjects. We are unaware of any reports in the literature which contain complete NBAL data for females engaged in high levels of physical energy output, and little research has been conducted to date on the potential effects of differences in age on N needs relative to similar levels of work performance. Thus, important research questions on the role of gender and age on the protein needs of strength-trained athletes remain to be examined.

A. Nitrogen Balance Studies

At least 25 investigations are known in the literature which provide NBAL data on subjects performing various kinds of work/physical activity. Some of these investigations are reported in journals for which either complete bibliographic information and/or results were not available.

Increased physical training/increased energy expenditure appears to increase protein needs regardless of the form of exercise (i.e., muscular vs. endurance) although increased requirements appear to be greater for endurance-trained athletes than strength-trained athletes. Recent research by Murdoch and colleagues[47] suggests that the protein needs of highly trained endurance athletes were well above the RDA of 0.8 g/kg BW per day, as only 78% of subjects were in NBAL while consuming diets that provided at least 1.6 g protein per kilogram body weight per day, and at least 2800 kcal daily. These findings are consistent with reports by Tarnopolsky et al.[44] and others.[40,41] On the basis of multiple regression analysis, Tarnopolsky et al.[44] calculated that endurance athletes would be in NBAL at an intake of 1.4 g protein per kilogram body weight per day and a daily intake of approximately 4500 kcal. In this same study, Tarnopolsky et al. reported that the protein needs of endurance athletes and bodybuilders were 1.67 and 1.12 times greater than sedentary control subjects consuming 0.7 g of protein per kilogram body weight per day and 3200 kcal daily.

Consolazio et al.[31] reported marginal NBAL data for eight subjects during a rigorous physical training program. These subjects were participating in two 40-d NBAL studies separated into four 10-d periods each. In the first experiment, subjects received 3084 kcal and 1.4 g protein/kg BW daily, whereas in the second experiment, the subjects received 3500 kcal and 2.8 g protein/kg BW daily. Although no measures of variance were reported, mean NBAL during the four 10-d periods ranged from +0.26 to +0.71 g daily in experiment A, and from +0.14 to +3.24 g daily in experiment B. Assuming that the variance in these subjects was similar to that observed in other studies, it does not appear that all subjects in these two series of experiments were in NBAL. Consolazio et al.[31] noted that failure to measure or correct for "sweat [N] losses could seriously invalidate the accuracy of metabolic balance studies." Furthermore, these investigators recommended that individuals engaged in vigorous physical training programs consume at least 100 g protein daily.

Gontzea et al.[34,35] conducted two studies on NBAL of athletes cycling approximately 2 h daily. In the first study, 29 of 30 athletes were in NBAL at a daily intake of 1.0 g protein/kg BW, whereas only 2 of 6 subjects were in NBAL at a daily intake of 1.5 g protein/kg BW. It is not clear if the energy intake and exercise prescriptions in these two studies were the same.

Mole and Johnson[41] reported that three untrained subjects were in NBAL (N intake was 7% greater than N excretion) when consuming a diet that provided 2.0 g protein and 46 kcal/kg BW daily. When these subjects were exercised on a treadmill in which the workouts expended 500 and 1000 kcal (which were balanced by increased energy intake of 500 and 1000 kcal, respectively), N retention increased. Mole and Johnson[41] did not account for either sweat or miscellaneous N losses, and they included rest and exercise days within each 9-d study period, thus the validity of their observations is questionable.

Relatively recent studies on the protein requirements of bodybuilders suggest that muscular strength training increased protein needs, but the exact lower limits have not been well established. Tarnopolsky et al.[44] and Celejowa and Homa[30] reported positive NBAL among bodybuilders receiving between 1.05 and 2.77 g protein/kg BW daily. However, four of the ten weightlifters studied by Celowjowa and Homa[30] were in negative NBAL even when fed 2.0 g protein/kg BW per day. Marable et al.[40] reported marginal NBAL among bodybuilders consuming 2.0 g protein/kg BW daily while Laritcheva et al.[38] reported negative NBAL data for athletes consuming 2700 kcal and 2.7 g protein/kg BW or 1800 kcal and 1.3 g protein/kg BW daily.

Walberg et al.[46] reported that seven bodybuilders were in negative NBAL (−3.19 g) while consuming 0.8 g/kg BW protein daily, but they achieved a positive NBAL when protein intake was increased to 1.6 g protein. These bodybuilders trained 90 to 120 min daily, 6 d each week. The negative NBAL observed in these bodybuilders reflected the importance of total energy intake as well as the importance of the protein content. Both groups of bodybuilders consumed hypoenergetic diets (18 kcal/kg BW). Even though the low energy intake was held constant, a twofold increase in protein intake was associated with positive NBAL.

There has been some question as to whether individuals can maintain large positive NBAL over long periods of time. Oddoye and Margen[23] demonstrated that individuals placed on high-protein diets (following a prolonged period of negative NBAL) do indeed maintain large positive NBAL for prolonged periods of time (i.e., 20 to 50 d). These data suggest the potential for individuals involved in strength training to theoretically benefit from high protein intakes. Nitrogen retention was higher in strength- and endurance-trained subjects (32.4 vs. 7.1 g, respectively) consuming 2.8 g vs. 1.4 g protein/kg BW per day during a 40-d study conducted by Consolazio et al.[24] The men consuming the higher protein intake also increased their body weight (3.3 kg) more than the men on the lower intake (1.2 kg).

The outcome of increased NBAL on increased body weight (and preferentially, increased lean body mass, LBM) has been evaluated in some, but not all, NBAL studies of strength-trained athletes. Marable et al.[40] did not observe any significant differences in weight gains of men consuming 300% of the RDA for protein compared to men consuming the RDA. Dragan et al.[25] reported 6% gains in LBM (and 5% gains in strength) in Romanian weightlifters when they increased their dietary protein intake from 275 to 438% of the RDA over a period of several months. Frontera et al.[26] reported that 0.33 g protein/kg BW per day consumed daily for a period of 12 weeks resulted in significant increases in thigh muscle mass and urinary creatinine compared to strength training alone. Lemon and colleagues[27] have also reported increased muscle mass among participants consuming a high-protein diet (334% RDA) compared to 124% RDA among novice bodybuilders during a 6-d per week intensive training program; however, the increased nitrogen retention did not significantly affect increased muscle mass or muscle strength during the initial month of training. The latter studies also suggest the potential benefits of prolonged use of a high-protein diet on increased muscle mass and strength by maintaining a high NBAL during periods of adaptation to intensive training.

Butterfield[49] has criticized many NBAL studies of athletes because researchers failed to provide adequate calories or they did not allow for an adequate period of adjustment to the diet and/or training regimens. Ideally, investigators should provide at least 7 to 10 d for adjustment for changes in diet and/or training prescription. Many NBAL studies were conducted for periods of only 2 to 3 d each.

Not all studies have demonstrated increased protein needs of athletes. Polykov[42] reported that an unknown number of athletes went into positive NBAL after 15 d of a 30-d NBAL study in which the subjects consumed 0.57 g protein/kg BW per day while participating in a 500-kcal workout training program.

Butterfield and Calloway,[29] Todd et al.,[45] and Goranzon and Forsum[33] conducted studies in which subjects were fed 0.57 g protein/kg BW. Todd et al.[45] reported that subjects were in positive NBAL when energy intake exceeded energy expenditure, but subjects were in negative NBAL when energy intake was either low or when energy intake was less than expenditure. Goranzon and Forsum[33] reported that their subjects were in negative NBAL.

The subjects evaluated by Todd et al.[45] were not given a high work load (e.g., cycling at 40% of $\dot{V}O_2$ max for 1 h) and were previously untrained. It is unlikely that these subjects received any significant training effect from the exercise prescription used in this study. Thus, it seems inappropriate to use these data for drawing inferences about the protein needs of strength-trained athletes or highly trained endurance athletes.

The large group variation reported in these subjects[45] whose mean NBAL was positive also merits consideration. For example, at a level of 0.85 g protein/kg BW per day, the subjects' mean NBAL was 0.42 ± 0.73 g. The large standard deviation suggests that some of the subjects were in negative NBAL. These subjects were in more positive NBAL at higher levels of energy intake, i.e., 0.82 ± 0.58 g N per day.

The research by Todd et al.[45] is also unique because the only protein source used in this study was egg white fed in a liquid purified diet. Since egg white has the highest biological value of all food proteins, and since most individuals in a free-living population do not subsist on this kind of diet, it is important to note that more protein would be needed to achieve NBAL if the subjects were fed a mixed diet. The amount of protein would be approximately 25% higher if the subjects were fed a vegetarian diet in comparison to a mixed diet containing meat and dairy products. Other researchers have also used liquid formula diets or liquid formula diets in conjunction with solid foods.[44,46]

The differences in the data reported and the apparent lack of a rigorous design in some of these studies are reflected in the research reported in the literature. These investigations demonstrate the need to carefully examine the details of each study as these design factors may account for many of the differences observed across the studies. For example, some investigations did not account for or measure the amount of work performed, the energy intake of the subjects was not reported in other investigations, variable levels of energy were used relative to energy expenditure, and the source of dietary protein has varied widely.

Previous training status of strength athletes may also affect the protein needs as a reflection of the process of adaptation to the training load/stimulus. For example, Tarnopolsky et al.[28] showed that protein requirements of bodybuilders with more than 3 years of training experience averaged 0.9 g/kg BW per day in contrast to 1.5 g for novice bodybuilders during their first month of training.

Future investigations of the protein requirements of athletes may need to examine the protein/energy requirements relative to the potential confounding effects of increased adiposity. As noted in the study by Murdoch et al.,[47] the subjects with the lowest energy needs had higher body fat levels than all of the other subjects, and two of these individuals had the highest NBAL data observed. Thus, it is conceivable that untrained subjects such as those used by Todd et al.[45] and others might have lower protein needs as a result of increased energy efficiency concomitant with greater levels of adiposity. This relationship may be relative, as none of the research subjects studied by Murdoch et al.[47] would be considered obese. The inverse associations between energy intake and NBAL ($r = .39$) and between energy intake and percent body fat support the hypothesis that relative adiposity concomitant with increased energy efficiency (i.e., decreased energy needs) might contribute to decreased protein needs. The extremely low body fat levels achieved by highly competitive bodybuilders, and the large fluctuations in body fat levels during the year among bodybuilders, suggest that the protein needs of these athletes may shift during the year in response to changes in training, body fat levels, and with variations in the amount and source of protein-energy foods as well as supplements.

B. Nitrogen Needs of Athletes Based on Urinary Excretion Studies

Several investigations have been reported in the literature which assessed the N/protein needs of athletes based on urinary excretion only. The primary assumption in using 24-h urine samples is based on the premise that fecal N losses are relatively constant on a controlled diet, and that changes in urinary N excretion accurately reflect a decrease or increase on protein utilization if diet and other sources of N losses are kept constant.

Mole and Johnson[41] estimated that protein needs of athletes could be met by a diet containing 2.0 g protein and 46 kcal/kg BW per day. Marable et al.[40] noted that urinary N excretion decreased 7% when subjects consumed 0.8 g protein/kg BW per day, but decreased 22% when subjects were fed 2.4 g protein/kg BW per day, suggesting that the subjects were in more positive NBAL at the higher level of protein intake.

In a well-controlled study, Hickson et al.[36] reported that a single bout of strength training of 1 h duration did not significantly alter urinary N excretion. Given the need for a biologically significant dose of work, and the short duration of the latter study, combined with the limitations of the NBAL technique, it was not surprising that the single hour of strength training had no apparent effect on 24-h urinary N excretion or on urinary excretion measured during any portion of the 24-h period following the training stimulus. Furthermore, there may have been a lag period between the exercise stimulus and the time at which a change in urinary N excretion would be observed (i.e., more than 24 h of time).

C. Studies on Amino Acids

Dohm et al.[50] and Evans et al.[51] suggest that protein probably contributes 5 to 15% of total energy needs during exercise. This assumption is based on studies of relatively short duration (e.g., about 1 h) and reflects the effects of aerobic work. Similar studies based on individuals engaged in strength training have not been reported to date.

Evans et al.[51] reported that a single bout of exercise performed at 55% of $\dot{V}O_2$ max for 2 h increased total leucine oxidation 240% over the values observed over a 2-h period at rest. In this study, which used stable leucine, the investigators estimated that the amount of work performed during this 2-h period at a relatively low intensity of effort represented the oxidation of 853 mg of leucine (i.e., approximately 90% of the total daily requirement for this amino acid). Matthews et al., (1981) cited by Evans et al.,[51] reported that greater increases in energy expenditure increase both the rate and total amount of leucine oxidation. The work of Evans et al.[51] is consistent with the data reported by Hagg et al.,[52] who also reported an increase in leucine oxidation and a decrease in the rate of leucine utilization to support net protein synthesis. The twofold increase in leucine oxidation was paralleled by a twofold increase in plasma lactate and alanine, although blood concentrations of leucine and other amino acids remained unchanged. Thus, it is possible that the increased oxidation of specific amino acids as energy substrates might lead to an imbalance in the ratio of essential to nonessential amino acids, and consequently increase an athlete's risk of negative NBAL when energy and protein intakes are marginal. It is not clear if strength training would result in similar levels of leucine oxidation to that observed among subjects performing aerobic exercises.

Although the number of reports in the literature is relatively few, and although much of the research reported to date is based on relatively small samples, the data collected thus far suggest that protein needs may increase in response to increased energy expenditure or work. Unfortunately, little research has been reported that has evaluated the effects of work on the protein needs of females. Additionally little work has been reported on the effects of age on the protein needs of individuals performing similar levels of work. Variations on the effects of different amounts and types of strength training (i.e., powerlifting vs. body-building), differences in body fat, and energy source are needed. Since many bodybuilders often consume liquid protein supplements, the effects of liquid protein supplements vs. diets based on mixtures of solid foods are also needed.

More research is also needed in order to develop guidelines for dietary planning of individuals and groups of individuals who are performing large volumes of work. Many highly dedicated bodybuilders and powerlifters train 3 h per day or longer for 5 to 7 d each week. Thus, in developing guidelines, nutrition scientists must recognize that most of the research reported to date does not make an allowance for the potential effects of the large training prescriptions achieved by these elite athletes.

Lemon[53] suggests that on the basis of present data, strength athletes should be consuming at least 12 to 15% of their total energy requirements as protein. This amount would translate to about 1.5 to 2.0 g protein/kg BW per day, which is almost two times the RDA.

It is also important for nutritionists and athletes to recognize that even though the RDAs are based on protein intakes, the requirement is a reflection of the biological metabolism of specific amino acids. Young et al.[54] have published provocative findings on their estimates of amino acid needs using metabolic tracer techniques, noting that the requirements for some amino acids may be 23 to 178% greater than the estimates based on balance studies.

Bazzarre et al.[55] have recently measured changes in plasma amino acids in response to two successive bouts of exercise to exhaustion in triathletes using high-performance liquid chromatography (HPLC) analysis. Alanine, glycine, isoleucine, serine, valine, threonine, and tyrosine decreased significantly ($p \leq .05$) in response to the initial exercise to exhaustion challenge while taurine increased significantly. At the end of the 20-min recovery period following the first exhaustion, leucine, isoleucine, ornithine, phenylalanine, tyrosine, urea, and valine increased significantly. Alanine, glycine, isoleucine, leucine, valine, ornithine, serine, phenylalanine, threonine, and tyrosine decreased significantly in response to the second exercise to exhaustion. Using adjusted mean change scores, carbohydrate replacement had no effect on any amino acid from exhaustion to the end of recovery; however, from the end of the recovery period to the end of the second exhaustion, the changes in serine, glycine, and threonine were significantly different from the placebo (artificially sweetened water). Unfortunately, data on the effects of changes in amino acids in response to strength training to exhaustion have not been conducted.

V. STUDIES OF NUTRITIONAL ERGOGENIC AIDS ON STRENGTH PERFORMANCE

Although considerable anecdotal evidence, such as muscle/strength magazine articles and advertisements, suggests that bodybuilders use a wide variety of nutrition supplements, little research has been published on the effects of specific supplements on muscular performance and development. The potential benefits, if any, of many of the supplements consumed by bodybuilders and powerlifters may be difficult to evaluate if nutrient intake (and hence, nutritional status) is adequate. An assessment of the potential benefits of supplements would also be exacerbated by the fact that many athletes engaged in strength training use more than one kind of supplement.

Bucci[58] and Williams,[59] among others, have extensively reviewed the literature on nutritional ergogenic aids. Both authors have indicated that much of the research conducted to date has not been rigorously designed. The small sample size of many studies, combined with failure to use double-blind cross-over designs, and failure to use control subjects or to account for possible training effects has made it difficult to interpret many of the reported findings. Many of the studies that have demonstrated favorable benefits have been based on animals or humans that were deficient in the nutrient under investigation.

Fluid and electrolyte losses associated with heavy sweat losses are associated with increased muscular fatigue and decreased performance. Large imbalances affect the nervous system and can lead to ventricular fibrillation and even death. Chan et al.[60] showed that glucose–potassium loading (20 mmol [mEq]/500 ml glucose) of eight undernourished, hospitalized patients significantly increased the force–frequency characteristics and the maximal relaxation rate of the adductor pollicis muscle.

With the exception of amino acid supplements, most studies on the effects of various nutrient supplements have been conducted on athletes other than bodybuilders or powerlifters. The results of such studies are summarized in several other chapters. Warren et al.[19] did not find any significant improvement as a consequence of amino acid supplementation in snatch performance or other biochemical indices (lactate, ammonia, testosterone, cortisol, and growth hormone) in a group of 28 male Olympic-style weightlifters divided into experimental and placebo groups using a double-blind, cross-over design. The authors postulated that the absence of any significant effect may have been masked by the high protein intake of the subjects, which averaged more than 2.0 g/kg BW per day.

According to Bucci,[58] the stimulation of growth hormone and prolactin by arginine may have an anabolic effect on muscular development. Arginine may also increase creatine stores and may reduce ammonia levels. Bucci[58] reported anecdotal findings, stating that ingestion of 4 to 8 g of a 50:50 mixture of ornithine and arginine was associated with decreased muscular fatigue and post-workout muscle soreness in well-trained and steroid-free bodybuilders.

Using a double-blind design, Hawkins et al.[61] did not observe any benefit of oral arginine supplementation (1.0 g arginine/kg BW per day) in a group of 13 experienced male weightlifters divided into placebo and experimental groups on body composition changes during a weight loss program or on peak torque and endurance. During the 10-d low-calorie diet period, subjects lost an average of 3.2 kg BW and 2.0% body fat, peak torque declined ($p < .05$) while muscle endurance increased (significantly for biceps, but not quadriceps).

Howald et al.[62] found no significant difference in PWC 170 work performance (total amount of work performed) between placebo and vitamin C treatments (1 g/d in the morning) of 13 athletes, but heart rates were significantly lower in this double-blind, cross-over study. Blood glucose concentrations were significantly lower while free fatty acid concentrations were significantly higher during the PWC test for the vitamin C vs. the placebo treatments. An acute double-blind, cross-over study on the effects of 600 mg vitamin C or placebo administered 4 h prior to testing by Keith and Merrill[63] revealed no significant differences between placebo and experimental treatments on maximum grip strength nor on muscular endurance using a hand dynamometer.

Bramich and McNaughton[64] conducted a double-blind test on the muscular strength of pectoral and quadriceps muscles, muscle endurance, and $\dot{V}O_2$ max of 24 subjects given acute doses of vitamin C (500 or 2000 mg 4 h prior to testing) and after 1 week of supplementation. No significant changes in response to the 2000-mg acute dose were observed for muscular strength, endurance, or $\dot{V}O_2$ max; however, the 500-mg acute dose was associated with a significant increase in quadriceps strength and a decrease in $\dot{V}O_2$ max. At the end of the 7-d supplementation periods, the 2000-mg dose was associated only with a significant reduction in $\dot{V}O_2$ max, while the 500-mg dose was associated with significant increases in both quadriceps and pectoral strength, but decreased muscular endurance of both muscle groups as well as a significant decrease in $\dot{V}O_2$ max.

Bucci[58] has summarized research on the potential ergogenic benefits of alkalinizers. Alkalinizers theoretically reduce fatigue associated with anaerobic performance by maintaining blood and muscle pH. Decreased pH inhibits phosphofructokinase, the rate-limiting step in glycolysis. The majority of investigators who have measured anaerobic, short-term exercise performance times after large doses of bicarbonate of about 0.2 to 0.3 g/kg BW approximately 1 to 3 h before exercise have reported increased time to fatigue. Bucci[58] cautions about the possible adverse effects of excessive bicarbonate use, which include nausea, vomiting, flatulence, diarrhea, and muscle cramps. He also notes that although carbonate loading is not currently banned by any sports government agency, that this form of loading can be detected easily by simple urinalysis.

Apparently, little or no research has been reported to date that evaluated the effects of alkalinizers of anaerobic performance of weightlifters. Bucci[58] also notes the need to explore the potential benefits of nutrient antioxidants on the reduction of free radical damage associated with exercise. Supplements containing superoxide dismutase and catalase have been marketed for athletes, but the research on their benefits is lacking.

Supplement use was reported infrequently in the studies cited in the section on food intake of strength-trained athletes.[9,13,74] A wide range of supplements were used in the studies that evaluated supplement use. Supplement use generally ranged from about 60 to 100% of the athletes evaluated.

VI. HEALTH STATUS OF STRENGTH-TRAINED ATHLETES: NUTRITIONAL IMPLICATIONS

A. Weight Loss

Rapid weight loss among wrestlers and bodybuilders prior to competition in order to make their weight class is commonplace. Rapid weight loss, generally achieved by various methods of dehydration, may produce multiple problems for these athletes.[65,66] The short-term negative side effects include reduced muscular strength and endurance, increased fatigue, decreased plasma volume, which is associated with impaired cardiac function (i.e., higher heart rate, decreased stroke volume, and reduced cardiac output), decreased glomerular blood flow, and, consequently, reduced filtration rate, liver and muscle glycogen depletion, increased electrolyte losses, decreased oxygen consumption, and impaired thermoregulation. Heat exhaustion and heat stroke are possible outcomes, particularly when fluid loss exceeds 5% or more of total body water.

Weight losses during the competitive season compared to pretraining weights are typically 7 to 21 pounds or more, and represent a difference of about three weight classes.[65,66] Acute weight loss cycles may occur 15 to 30 times or more during the competitive season for wrestlers, and vary considerably among bodybuilders, depending upon the number of competitions and other training/competition factors. Lamar-Hildebrand et al.[13] reported that four female competitive bodybuilders gained 20 pounds while two others gained 10 pounds or less within a 4-week period following competition, suggesting that weight fluctuations in females approach those observed among male bodybuilders. Weight loss is generally achieved by restricting fluid and food intake, as well as other dehydrating practices, which include the use of saunas, sweat suits, laxatives, and diuretics, and even spitting.

Much of the research on the physiological effects of weight cycling has been conducted on obese subjects, especially females.[65] However, little work has been conducted in which the effects of weight cycling of athletes, in whom fluctuations in body weight largely reflect changes in body water and carbohydrate availability, are compared to the changes in body weight among obese subjects, in whom the fluctuations presumably reflect changes in adiposity. Additionally, it is not clear how differences in energy expenditure, and types of training (e.g., aerobic vs. strength) affect fluctuations in body weight/composition in comparison to the effects of adjusting energy intake, and the source of energy substrate (% of total kcal provided by fat, carbohydrate, and protein).

B. Considerations for Special Populations

Little attention has been given to the potential role of resistance strength training on weight loss of obese females. Ballor et al.[67] studied the effects of a 3-d per week resistance-training program on weight loss and the maintenance of LBM in obese women who averaged 35.9 ± 0.9% body fat. The 40 obese women were randomly assigned to one of four treatment groups: control, diet alone, exercise alone, or diet plus exercise. Significant increases in muscle area and strength were observed among the groups receiving the 8-week resistance training program. Weight training in combination with energy restriction was associated with the preservation of LBM in comparison to energy restriction alone. The investigators concluded that energy restriction and weight training acted independently on weight loss, since they did not observe any statistically significant interaction of diet and exercise. The energy intake of subjects was theoretically reduced by about 1000 kcal/d, although no data were reported to validate this assumption. Protein supplements were provided to ensure that protein intake was ≥1.0 g/d. Thus, it is not clear if protein supplementation had any potential role in maintaining LBM. It is also unclear if blood lipids and blood pressure were favorably affected among any of the treatment groups compared to the control group.

C. Blood Lipid Profiles

Since 1984, 12 investigations on the blood lipids of individuals engaged in some form of strength training have been published[6-9,10,12,68-73] (Table 3). All of these studies have been cross-sectional, except for the research by Kleiner et al.[9] and Peterson and Fahey.[70] Morgan et al.[12] studied females only, whereas Cohen et al.[68] and Bazzarre et al.[6,7] included both females and males in their surveys. All other studies were based on populations of males only. The sample size in most studies was relatively small, ranging from five males evaluated be Peterson and Fahey[70] to 76 South African male bodybuilders assessed by Faber et al., and 35 males in the longitudinal study of Kleiner et al.[9] Blood lipid profiles for all studies represent information obtained from a total of 40 females and 142 males (control subjects not included). The mean age of the populations surveyed ranged from 26 to 34 years for most studies.[6,7,9,10,68-71] The mean age of the Japanese weightlifters evaluated by Higuchi et al.[72] was only 19 years while the strength-trained females evaluated by Morgan et al.[12] had a mean age of 36 years.

Powerlifters were studied by Cohen et al.[68] and by Hurley et al.,[10] whereas bodybuilders were evaluated by other investigators.[6,10,69] The bodybuilders studied by Elliot et al.[69] were competitors in a regional competition of natural bodybuilders, whereas Bazzarre et al.[6,7] studied bodybuilders at national championships. The subjects in the other studies were generally classified as weightlifters or as individuals placed on a strength-training program.[12]

In most studies,[6-10,12,69,73] mean total cholesterol (TC) levels were generally below 200 mg%, however, TC values were consistently above 200 mg% in association with steroid use[9,68,70,71] (Table 3). Total cholesterol was 36 mg% higher among steroid-using (SU) body-builders compared to non-steroid users (NSU) studied by Kleiner et al.,[9] but only 14 mg% higher among SU vs. NSU strength-trained athletes evaluated by Costill et al.[71] TC declined from 223 to 200 mg% among five males studied by Peterson and Fahey.[70] TC levels for control subjects included in three investigations were within the same range as the strength-trained groups.[12,71,72]

Mean high-density lipoprotein (HDL) cholesterol (HDL-C) among males ranged from lows of 16 to 17 mg%, reported by Kleiner et al.,[9] Peterson and Fahey,[70] and Costill et al.,[71] among groups using steroids, to a high of 55 mg% among eight bodybuilders surveyed by Hurley et al.[10] (Table 3). Mean HDL-C was higher (NS) among bodybuilders with a high egg consumption (56 ± 13 mg%) compared to those with a low egg intake (50 ± 7 mg%).[8] Mean HDL-C ranged from 31 mg% among three female powerlifters[68] who used steroids to 56 mg% among two populations of female bodybuilders at the time of national competition.[6,7] Mean HDL2 cholesterol (HDL2-C) ranged from 0 among three female pow-erlifters who used steroids to 15–16 mg% among male bodybuilders.[7,9] HDL2-C values of 0 mg% observed among competitive bodybuilders and other strength-trained athletes ap-parently reflect the use of steroids. Mean HDL3 cholesterol (HDL3-C) ranged from 31 mg% among female powerlifters using steroids to 41 and 49 mg% among competitive female bodybuilders.[6,7] Mean HDL3-C among strength-trained males ranged from 22 mg%[68] to 32 mg%[9] among those who used steroids; and, from 41 mg%[7] to 49 mg%[6] among bodybuilders who reportedly did not use steroids.

Dietary intake was measured in only six of the studies that measured blood lipid profiles of strength-trained athletes[6-10,12] (Table 3). Food records were used to estimate nutrient intake in five of these studies.[6-9,12] Hurley et al.,[10] who used the 24-h recall and diet histories to evaluate nutrient intake, only reported the distribution of energy intake provided by protein, fat, and carbohydrate, while the other investigators provided more complete nutrient infor-mation. The nutrient content of these diets is summarized in an earlier section of this chapter. Kleiner et al.[9] and Bazzarre et al.[6,7] evaluated the relationships between dietary and anthro-pometric variables, and the lipid profiles of bodybuilders. None of the anthropometric or dietary variables were significantly associated with TC in the first study by Bazzarre et al.[7] However, percent body fat levels were positively and significantly associated with HDL-C ($r = .63; p = .04$) and HDL3-C ($r = .65; p = .03$). Saturated fat intake (which was quite low) was the only nutrient variable associated with any lipid variable, HDL2-C ($r = .60; p = 05$). Correlations reported by Kleiner et al.[9] were saturated fat intake with HDL3-C ($r = -.59; p = .05$); total fat intake and HDL3-C ($r = -.62; p = .04$); and, polyun-saturated fat intake with very low-density lipoprotein (VLDL)-C ($r = .69; p = .01$). The differences between the dietary and lipid correlations reported in these two studies may reflect large differences in energy and fat intakes between the two study populations, com-bined with large differences in body fat levels (6.0 vs. 13.5% between the groups; Table 3).

TABLE 3 Lipid Profiles, Energy Intake, and Anthropometric Data of Male and Female Bodybuilders and Weightlifters

Investigators	Study Design	Sample Size/Gender	Age of Subjects (years)	% Body Fat	Dietary Methods	Energy Intake (kcal)	TC (mg%)	HDL-C (mg%)	HDL2 (mg%)	HDL3 (mg%)	HDL-C/TC
Powerlifters											
Cohen et al., 1986[68]	Cross-sectional	3 female SU[a]	—	—	None	—	216	31	0	31	0.14
		9 male SU	—	—		—	291	24	2	22	0.08
Hurley et al., 1984[10]	Cross-sectional	8 males	31	14.0	24-h recall and diet history	NR	195	38	6	—	0.19
Bodybuilders											
Faber et al., 1986[8]	Cross-sectional	76 males	27 ± 6	15.4 ± 2.9	7-d food record	3187	176 ± 25	50 ± 7	—	—	0.28
						4143	189 ± 23	56 ± 13	—	—	0.30
Hurley et al., 1984[10]	Cross-sectional	8 males	29	12.0	24-hr recall and diet history	NR	172	55	12	—	0.32
Elliot et al., 1987[69]	Cross-sectional	16 males	25	7.2	None	—	158	45	—	—	0.28
		15 females	27	14.4		—	166	55	—	—	0.33
Kleiner et al., 1989[9]	Longitudinal	18 Male SU	30	13.1	3-d food record and food frequency	5739	214	16	2	17	0.07
		17 Male NSU[b]	26	13.8			178	46	16	32	0.26

Reference	Design	Subjects			Method						
Bazzarre et al., 1990[7]	Cross-sectional	19 males	28	6.0	7-d food records	2015	187	37	13	24	0.20
		8 females	28	9.8		2260	198	56	15	41	0.28
Bazzarre et al., 1992[6]	Cross-sectional	13 males	30	4.9	3-d food records	2620	154	48	4	45	0.31
		11 females	29	9.1		1597	145	56	7	49	0.39
Strength Training											
Peterson and Fahey, 1984[70]	Longitudinal	5 males	29	—	None	—	223	16	—	—	0.7
		On steroids					200	52	—	—	0.26
		Off steroids									
Costill et al., 1984[71]	Cross-sectional	9 SU	31	—	None	—	218	17	—	—	0.8
		13 NSU	32	—		—	204	45	—	—	0.22
		12 untrained	34	—		—	210	46	—	—	0.22
Morgan et al., 1986[12]	Cross-sectional	9 females Str Tx	36	BMI = 21.7	3-d weighed food records	1549	180	56	—	—	0.31
		9 female runners	27	BMI = 20.0		1888	182	72	—	—	0.39
		9 female controls	34	BMI = 24.3		2132	183	58	—	—	0.32
Higuchi et al., 1991[72]	Cross-sectional	15 male weight-lifters	19	BMI = 25.0	None	—	147	50	—	—	0.34
		13 untrained males	19	BMI = 22.0		—	146	61	—	—	0.42

a SU, Steroid users.
b NSU, Non-steroid users.

Although no significant correlations were observed between TC and any dietary variable in the former studies[7,9] Bazzarre et al.[6] more recently observed significant correlations between TC and dietary fat among competitive female, but not male, bodybuilders. The significant association in the more recent study may reflect the effect of gender. Dietary fiber intake was significantly associated with HDL-C in both competitive male and female bodybuilders, and with HDL3-C in competitive male, but not female, bodybuilders.[6] Vitamin C intake was significantly associated with HDL-C, HDL2-C, and HDL3-C in competitive male bodybuilders, and with HDL3-C in competitive female bodybuilders. Positive associations between dietary vitamin C intake and HDL-C have been reported in farmers and in other populations.[57]

Kohl et al.[73] evaluated the relationships between measures of musculoskeletal fitness and blood lipids in 5463 males 20 to 69 years of age attending a preventive medicine clinic between 1980 and 1987. On the basis of multiple regression analysis in which the effects of age and cardiorespiratory fitness were controlled, they found that HDL-C levels were significantly associated ($p < .0001$) with both the leg press and bench press. No significant associations were observed between TC and any of the four measures of musculoskeletal fitness.

VII. SUMMARY

Strength-trained athletes represent a wide variety of sports, and may engage in other forms of physical conditioning besides strength training. The evaluation of the nutritional status of any individual or group of athletes is based on a comprehensive evaluation of food intake, anthropometric measurements, laboratory tests, and an assessment of any signs and symptoms combined with the appropriate use of selected demographic and medical information. A wide range of specific methods are available for assessing each of the four components of nutritional assessment; and each method has certain advantages and limitations that tend to be characteristic of that method. Because of the homeostatic regulation of the constituents of the blood, serum and/or plasma values may not be indicative of nutritional problems until tissue stores are either depleted or saturated. Thus, special attention should be given to the potential development of nutrition problems associated with reliable and valid measures of food intake.

Coaches, trainers, health professionals, and athletes need to recognize the value of a complete nutritional assessment before using individual or group data as opposed to relying on the data obtained for a single component of the nutritional assessment process. The use of all four components of nutrition assessment increases the probability of detecting a nutrition problem when one usually does exist, and reduces the probability of assuming that an athlete has a nutrition problem when he or she really does not have one. Furthermore, the use of all four components of nutrition assessment may help to identify potential problems that would be considered marginal before a true deficiency state has a chance to develop. Dietary interventions to prevent deficient states are more likely to be successful if instituted early.

On the basis of the investigations published in the literature on strength-trained athletes, there clearly is considerable variability in the nutrient intakes among athletes. The individual variability reflects differences in gender, body mass, energy expenditure, and training status, as well as cultural differences and individual food preferences.

The few longitudinal studies that have been published on bodybuilders[9,13] consistently demonstrate dramatic changes in energy intake, and the distribution of energy substrates in the diet. Moderate increases in protein intake and dramatic decreases in dietary fat intake as a percentage of total calories suggest that bodybuilders develop dietary strategies which, combined with intensive, high-volume training, result in exquisitely low body fat levels in elite bodybuilders. Changes in food consumption patterns among bodybuilders reflect an avoidance of milk and other dairy products which results in marginal intakes of both calcium and vitamin D. No studies have been conducted to date that demonstrate an impact of these food preference cycles on reduced bone density in either female or male strength-trained athletes.

The composition of fat intake reported in the studies cited in the literature reflects a wide range of intakes regarding the polyunsaturated to saturated fat ratios in the diets of strength-trained athletes. Dietary cholesterol intake is above recommended levels for prevention of heart disease even when energy intakes have been curtailed in preparation for competition. Dietary cholesterol intake varies widely among bodybuilders, reflecting differences in the consumption of whole eggs vs. the consumption of egg whites. High intakes of tunafish and other seafood are common among bodybuilders, and may have some potential benefit on both lipid profiles as well as blood pressure. Dietary fiber has not been reported in most dietary studies, but appears to be well below guidelines associated with healthy diets.

Dietary vitamin and mineral intakes of both male and female strength-trained athletes tend to be at, or well above, recommended levels, with the exception of dietary zinc intake, which is marginal, and dietary copper intake for females. Biochemical measures of nutritional status for selected vitamins and minerals among athletes have not been commonly reported, but generally suggest a low prevalence of marginal or deficient levels. Problems of RBC hemolysis can dramatically elevate concentrations for some minerals, and special care should be taken to avoid the use of hemolyzed samples. The apparently widespread use of vitamin/ mineral supplements which have not been accounted for in most dietary studies of strength-trained athletes would theoretically increase the nutrient availability relative to the already adequate (or perhaps more than adequate) intakes among the individuals who use supplements (provided that the specific vitamin/mineral formulations represent the biologically active forms of each nutrient).

Functional improvements in body composition or other measures of strength performance as a consequence of dietary habits have not been impressive, although several studies on the protein requirements of strength-trained athletes have noted increased measures of lean body mass with increased dietary protein intakes.

Although older review articles on the protein needs of athletes have commonly reported no difference in protein requirements of athletes compared to ''general'' population, many of the studies suggest that the protein needs of highly trained athletes tend to fall within a range of 1.0 to 1.6 g/kg BW per day. At the lower limit, the differences in increased protein intake among athletes would represent an increase of at least 25% above the RDA, and perhaps as much as 200% above the RDA. Protein requirements of strength-trained athletes also appear to be less than that of endurance-trained athletes, but more research is needed.

The protein requirements of athletes should be met by the usual diets consumed by athletes. Thus, there is little need for alarm regarding the possibility of protein deficiency among athletes, and no convincing data that protein supplements are needed to meet requirements. The data do suggest that the level of protein adequacy is clearly dependent upon an adequate energy intake. Consequently, protein needs of strength-trained athletes and other highly trained athletes probably change during the course of the training, competitive, and recovery seasons. It is also important to recognize that given a sufficient period of time to allow for adaptation to training/competition stresses, most athletes should eventually achieve an equilibrium at which they will be in nitrogen balance. A positive energy balance associated with progressive increases in relative adiposity may also be associated with increased energy and protein efficiency, even among relatively lean athletes. Thus, energy intakes of about 3000 calories per day may be sufficient to achieve/maintain nitrogen balance in some athletes, provided they have adequate fat stores to meet the energy cost of training, while energy intakes of 5000 to 6000 calories may not be sufficient to maintain nitrogen balance if the athlete has reduced adipose tissue depots to levels below their usual body fat levels. The relationship of body fat levels to protein/energy needs of highly trained athletes is speculative at best, but future research on this issue may help explain some of the differences in protein needs of athletes (and body composition changes among athletes) as they physiologically adjust to different training demands. Until such data become available, it would be wise to obtain serial measurements of changes in body fat and lean body mass when evaluating the dietary adequacy of strength-trained athletes. A dramatic decrease in body fat levels, especially if combined with an absolute decrease in lean body mass, might be used as a guideline for caution in evaluating the adequacy of both energy and protein intakes. Based on personal diet counseling experiences, energy/food intakes of many athletes may be low because the athlete simply does not schedule time for eating.

The health status of strength-trained athletes is an important area of nutrition research. Weight loss practices in an effort to achieve competitive weight classes may place an athlete at risk of severe dehydration, electrolyte imbalances, thermoregulatory problems, and impaired kidney function, as well as a decline in performance associated with decreased strength and endurance.

The blood lipid profiles of strength-trained athletes reported in the literature have varied widely, ranging from values associated with an increased risk of cardiovascular heart disease to levels associated with good health. A wide range of values is present among athletes similar to the wide range observed for the population at large. While total cholesterol levels among highly trained competitive bodybuilders appear to be relatively low, HDL cholesterol levels tend to be lower than those reported for highly trained endurance athletes. HDL2 cholesterol levels appear also to be low and frequently are undetectable among steroid users. Steroid use has consistently been associated with elevated TC and extremely low HDL-C levels. The low body fat levels observed among highly trained competitive bodybuilders which also reflect training and dietary practices may account for the favorable lipid profiles observed among this group. Additionally, the intakes of vitamin C which tend to be about three to four times the RDA may also contribute to the HDL-C, HDL2-C, and HDL3-C observed among competitive bodybuilders.

REFERENCES

1. **Short, S.,** Dietary surveys and nutrition knowledge, in *Nutrition in Exercise and Sport,* Hickson, J. F. and Wolinsky, I., Eds., CRC Press, Boca Raton, FL, 1989, 309.
2. **Gibson, R.,** *Principles of Nutritional Assessment,* Oxford University Press, New York, 1990.
3. **Bazzarre, T. L. and Myers, M. P.,** The collection of food intake data in cancer epidemiology studies, *Nutr. Cancer,* 1, 22, 1979.
4. **Bazzarre, T. L. and Yuhas, J. A.,** Comparative evaluation of methods of collecting food intake data for cancer epidemiology studies, *Nutr. Cancer,* 5, 201, 1983.
5. **Short, S. and Short, W. R.,** Four-year study of university athletes' dietary intake, *J. Am. Diet. Assoc.,* 82, 632, 1983.
6. **Bazzarre, T. L., Kleiner, S. M., and Litchford, M. D.,** Nutrient intake, body fat and lipid profiles of competitive male and female bodybuilders, *J. Am. Coll. Nutr.,* 9, 136, 1990.
7. **Bazzarre, T. L., Kleiner, S. M., and Ainsworth, B. E.,** Vitamin C intake and lipid profiles of competitive male and female bodybuilders, *Int. J. Sport Nutr.,* 2, 260, 1992.
8. **Faber, M., Benade, A. J. S., and van Eck, M.,** Dietary intake, anthropometric measurements, and blood lipid values in weight training athletes, *Int. J. Sports Med.,* 7, 342, 1986.
9. **Kleiner, S. M., Calabrese, L. H., Fiedler, K. M., Naito, H. K., and Skibinski, C. I.,** Dietary influences on cardiovascular disease risk in anabolic steroid-using and non-using bodybuilders, *J. Am. Coll. Nutr.,* 8, 109, 1989.

10. **Hurley, B., Seals, D. R., Hagberg, J. M., Goldberg, A .C., Ostrove, S. M., Holloszy, J. O., Weist, W. G., and Goldberg, A. P.,** High-density lipoprotein cholesterol in bodybuilders vs. powerlifters, *JAMA,* 252, 507, 1984.

11. **Spitler, D., Diaz, F. J., Horvath, S. M., and Wright, J. E.,** Body composition and maximal aerobic capacity of bodybuilders, *J. Sports Med. Phys. Fitness,* 20, 181, 1980.

12. **Morgan, D. W., Cruise, R. J., Girardin, B. W., Lutz-Schneider, V., Morgan, D. H., and Qi, W. M.,** HDL-C concentrations in weight-trained, endurance-trained, and sedentary females, *Phys. Sportsmed.,* 14, 166, 1986.

13. **Lamar-Hildebrand, N., Saldanha, L., and Endres, J.,** Dietary and exercise practices of college-aged female bodybuilders, *J. Am. Diet. Assoc.,* 89, 1308, 1989.

14. **Fogleholm, G. M., Himberg, J.-J., Alopaeus, K., Gref, C.-G., Laadso, J. T., Lehto, J. J., and Mussalo-Rauhamaa, H.,** Dietary and biochemical indices of nutritional status in male athletes and controls, *J. Am. Coll. Nutr.,* 11, 181, 1992.

15. Food and Nutrition Board, National Academy of Sciences, *Recommended Dietary Allowances,* 10th ed., National Academy Press, Washington, D.C., 1989.

16. National Cholesterol Education Program, Report of the National Cholesterol Education Program Expert panel on Detection, Evaluation and Treatment of High Blood Cholesterol in Adults, *Arch. Intern. Med.,* 148, 36, 1988.

17. **Chen, J. D., Wang, J. F., Zhao, Y. W., Wang, S. W., Jiao, Y., and Hou, X. Y.,** Nutritional problems and measures in elite and amateur athletes, *Am. J. Clin. Nutr.,* 49, 1084, 1989.

18. **Heinemann, L. and Zerbes, H.,** Physical activity, fitness, and diet: behavior in the population compared with elite athletes in the GDR, *Am. J. Clin. Nutr.,* 49, 1007, 1989.

19. **Warren, B. J., Stone, M. H., Kearny, J. T., Fleck, S. J., Kraemer, W. J., and Johnson, R. L.,** The effect of amino acid supplementation on physiological and performance responses of elite junior weightlifters, *Med. Sci. Sports Exercise,* 23, S15, 1991.

20. **Hickson, J., Duke, M. A., Risser, W. L., Johnson, C. W., Palmer, R., and Stockton, J. E.,** Nutritional intake from food sources of high school football athletes, *J. Am. Diet. Assoc.,* 87, 1656, 1987.

21. **Hickson, J., Wolinsky, I., Pivarnik, J. M., Neuman, E. A., Itak, J. F., and Stockton, J. E.,** Nutritional profile of football athletes eating from a training table, *Nutr. Res.,* 7, 27, 1987.

22. **Bazzarre, T. L., Marquart, L. F., Izurieta, I. M., and Jones, A.,** Incidence of poor nutrition status among triathletes and control subjects, *Med. Sci. Sports Exercise,* 18, 590, 1986.

23. **Oddoye, E. B. and Margen, S.,** Nitrogen balance studies in humans: longterm effect of high nitrogen intake on accretion, *J. Nutr.,* 109, 363, 1979.

24. **Consalozio, C. F., Nelson, R. A., Matoush, L. O., Harding, R. S., and Canham, J. E.,** Nitrogen excretion in sweat and its relationship to nitrogen balance experiments, *J. Nutr.,* 79, 399, 1963.

25. **Dragan, G. I., Vasiliu, A., and Georgescu, E.,** Effects of increased supply of protein on elite weightlifters, in *Milk Proteins '84,* Galesloot, T. E. and Tinbergen, B. J., Eds., Pudoc, Wageningen, The Netherlands, 1985, 99.

26. **Frontera, W. R., Meredith, C. N., and Evans, W. J.,** Dietary effects on muscle strength gain and hypertrophy during heavy resistance training in older men, *Can. J. Sport Sci.,* 13, 13P, 1988.

27. **Lemon, P. W. R., MacDougall, J. D., Tarnopolsky, M. A., and Atkinson, S. A.,** Effect of dietary protein and body building exercise on muscle mass and strength gains, *Can. J. Sport Sci.,* 15, 14S, 1990.

28. **Tarnopolsky, M. A., Lemon, P. W. R., MacDougall, J. D., and Atkinson, S. A.,** Effect of body building exercise on protein requirements, *Can. J. Sports Sci.,* 15, 22S, 1990.

29. **Butterfield, G. and Calloway, D. J.,** Physical activity improves protein utilization in young men, *Br. J. Nutr.,* 51, 171, 1984.

30. **Celejowa, I. and Homa, M.,** Food intake, N and energy balance in Polish weightlifters during a training camp, *Nutr. Metab..,* 12, 259, 1970.

31. **Consolazio, C. F., Johnson, H. L., Nelson, R. A., Dramise, J. G., and Skala, J. H.,** Protein metabolism during intensive physical training in the young adult, *Am. J. Clin. Nutr.,* 28, 29, 1979.

32. **Decombaz, J., Reinhardt, R., Anantharaman, K., von Glutz, G., and Poortmans, J. R.,** Biochemical changes in a 100 km run: free amino acids, urea, and creatinine, *Eur. J. Appl. Physiol.,* 41, 61, 1979.

33. **Goranzon, H. and Forsum, E.,** Effect of reduced energy intake versus increased physical activity on the outcome of nitrogen balance experiments in man, *Am. J. Clin. Nutr.,* 41, 919, 1985.

34. **Gontzea, I. P., Sutzescu, P., and Dumitrache, S.,** The influence of muscular activity on nitrogen balance and on the need of man for proteins, *Nutr. Rep. Int.,* 10, 35, 1974.

35. **Gontzea, I. P., Sutzescu, P., and Dumitrache, S.,** The influence of adaptation to physical effort on nutrition balance in man, *Nutr. Rep. Int.,* 11, 231, 1975.

36. **Hickson, J. F., Wolinsky, I., Rodriguez, G. P., Pivarnik, J. M., Kent, M. C., and Shier, N. W.,** Failure of weight training to affect urinary indices of protein metabolism in men, *Med. Sci. Sports Exercise,* 18, 563, 1986.

37. **Kraut, H., Muller, E. A., and Muller-Wecker, H.,** Influence of the composition of dietary protein on nitrogen balance and muscle training, *Int. Z. Angew. Physiol. Einschl. Arbeitsphysiol.,* 17, 378, 1958.
38. **Laritcheva, K. A., Yalovaya, N. I., Shubin, V. I., and Smirnov, P. V.,** Study of energy expenditure and protein needs of top weight lifters, in *Nutrition, Physical Fitness, and Health,* Parizkova, J. and Rogozkin, V. A., Eds., University Park Press, Baltimore, 155, 1978.
39. **Lemon, P. W. R. and Mullin, J. P.,** Effect of initial muscle glycogen levels on protein catabolism during exercise, *J. Appl. Physiol. Respir. Environ. Exercise Physiol.,* 48, 624, 1980.
40. **Marable, N. L., Hickson, J. K., Korslund, M. K., Herbert, G., Desjardins, R. F., and Thye, F. W.,** Urinary nitrogen excretion as influenced by a muscle-building exercise program and protein variation, *Nutr. Rep. Int.,* 19, 795, 1979.
41. **Mole, P. and Johnson, R. E.,** Disclosure by dietary modification of an exercise-induced protein catabolism in man, *J. Appl. Physiol.,* 31, 185, 1971.
42. **Polykov, V. V.,** Nitrogen balance in man during reduced and increased energy expenditure, *Kosm. Biol. Aviakosm. Med.,* 8, 82, 1974.
43. **Refsum, H. E. and Stromme, S. B.,** Urea and creatinine production and excretion in urine during and after prolonged heavy exercise, *Scand. J. Clin. Lab. Invest.,* 33, 247, 1974.
44. **Tarnopolsky, M. A., MacDougall, J. D., and Atkinson, S. A.,** Influence of protein intake and training status on nitrogen balance and lean body mass, *J. Appl. Physiol.,* 64, 187, 1988.
45. **Todd, K. S., Butterfield, G., and Calloway, D. H.,** Nitrogen balance in men with adequate and deficient energy intake at three levels of work, *J. Nutr.,* 114, 2107, 1984.
46. **Walberg, J. L., Leddy, M. K., Sturgill, D. J., Hinkle, D. E., Ritchey, S. J., and Sebolt, D. R.,** Macronutrient content of a hypoenergy diet affects nitrogen retention and muscle function in weight lifters, *Int. J. Sports Med.,* 9, 261, 1988.
47. **Murdoch, S. D., Bazzarre, T. L., Wu, S. L., Herr, D., and Snider, I. P.,** Nitrogen balance in highly trained triathletes, *Med. Sci. Sports Exercise,* 24, S178, 1992.
48. **Liappes, N., Kelderbacher, S. D., Kesseler, K., and Bantzer, P.,** Quantitative study of free amino acids in human eccrine sweat excreted from the forearms of healthy trained and untrained men during exercise, *Eur. J. Appl. Physiol.,* 42, 227, 1979.
49. **Butterfield, G. E.,** Whole-body protein utilization in humans, *Med. Sci. Sports Exercise,* 19, S157, 1987.
50. **Dohm, G. L., Kasparek, G. J., Tapscott, E. B., and Barakat, H. A.,** Protein metabolism during endurance exercise, *Fed. Proc.,* 44, 348, 1985.
51. **Evans, W. J., Fisher, E. C., Hoerr, R. A., and Young, V. R.,** Protein metabolism and endurance exercise, *Phys. Sportsmed.,* 11, 63, 1983.
52. **Hagg, S. A., Morse, E. L., and Adibi, S. A.,** Effect of exercise on rate of oxidation, turnover, and plasma clearance of leucine in human subjects, *Am. J. Physiol. Endocrinol. Metab.,* 5, E407, 1982.
53. **Lemon, P. W. R.,** Protein and amino acid needs of the strength athlete, *Int. J. Sport Nutr.,* 1, 127, 1991.
54. **Young, V. R., Bier, D. M., and Pellet, P. L.,** A theoretical basis for increasing current estimates for the amino acid requirements in adult man with experimental support, *Am. J. Clin. Nutr.,* 50, 80, 1989.
55. **Bazzarre, T. L., Murdoch, S. D., Wu, S. L., and Snider, I. P.,** Amino acid response to two successive exhaustion trials and carbohydrate feeding, *J. Am. Coll. Nutr.,* 11, 501, 1992.
56. **Haralambie, G. and Berg, A.,** Serum urea and amino acid changes with exercise duration, *Eur. J. Appl. Physiol.,* 36, 39, 1976.
57. **Bazzarre, T. L., Wu, S. L., Murdoch, S. D., and Hopkins, R. G.,** Nutritional status, energy expenditure, body fat, stress and cardiovascular disease risk factors of North Carolina farm families, *Nutr. Res.,* 11, 1119, 1991.
58. **Bucci, L.,** Nutritional ergogenic aids, in *Nutrition in Exercise and Sport,* 1st ed., Hickson, J. F. and Wolinsky, I., Eds., CRC Press, Boca Raton, FL, 1989.
59. **Williams, M. H.,** Ergogenic aids, in *Sports Nutrition for the 90s: The Health Professionals Handbook,* Berning, J. R. and Steen, S. N., Eds., Aspen Publishers, Gaithersburg, MD, 1991.
60. **Chan, S. T. F., McLaughlin, S. J., Ponting, G. A., Biglin, J., and Dudley, H. A. F.,** Muscle power after glucose-potassium loading in undernourished patients, *Br. Med. J.,* 293, 1055, 1986.
61. **Hawkins, C. E., Walberg-Rankin, J., and Sebolt, D. R.,** Oral arginine does not affect body composition or muscle function in male weight lifters, *Med. Sci. Sports Exercise,* 23, S15, 1991.
62. **Howald, H., Segesser, B., and Korner, W. F.,** Ascorbic acid and athletic performance, *Ann. N.Y. Acad. Sci.,* 258, 458, 1975.
63. **Keith, R. E. and Merrill, E.,** The effects of vitamin C on maximum grip strength and muscular endurance, *J. Sports Med.,* 23, 145, 1980.
64. **Bramich, K. and McNaughton, L.,** The effects of two levels of ascorbic acid on muscular endurance, muscular strength and VO$_2$ max, *Int. Clin. Nutr. Rev.,* 7, 5, 1987.
65. **Saris, W. H. M.,** Physiological aspects of exercise in weight cycling, *Am. J. Clin. Nutr.,* 49, 1099, 1989.

66. **Freischlag, J.,** Weight loss, body composition, and health of high school wrestlers, *Phys. Sportsmed.,* 12, 121, 1984.
67. **Ballor, D. L., Katch, V. L., Becque, M. D., and Marks, C. R.,** Resistance weight training during caloric restriction enhances lean body weight maintenance, *Am. J. Clin. Nutr.,* 47, 19, 1988.
68. **Cohen, J. C., Faber, W. M., Benade, A. J. S., and Noakes, T. D.,** Altered serum lipoprotein profiles in male and female power lifters ingesting anabolic steroids, *Phys. Sportsmed.,* 14, 131, 1986.
69. **Elliot, D. L., Goldberg, L., Kuehl, K. S., and Catlin, D. H.,** Characteristics of anabolic-androgenic steroid-free male and female bodybuilders, *Phys. Sportsmed.,* 15, 169, 1987.
70. **Peterson, G. E. and Fahey, T. D.,** HDL-C in five elite athletes using anabolic-androgenic steroids, *Phys. Sportsmed.,* 12, 120, 1984.
71. **Costill, D. L., Pearson, D. R., and Fink, W. J.,** Anabolic steroid use among athletes: changes in HDL-C levels, *Phys. Sportsmed.,* 12, 113, 1984.
72. **Higuchi, M., Iwaoka, K., Ishii, K., and Kobayashi, S.,** Plasma lipoprotein and apolipoprotein in male weightlifters, *Med. Sci. Sports Exercise,* 23, S22, 1991.
73. **Kohl, H. W., Gordon, N. F., Vaandrager, H., and Blair, S. N.,** Musculoskeletal fitness and serum lipid levels in men, *Med. Sci. Sports Exercise,* 23, S22, 1991.
74. **Kleiner, S. M., Bazzarre, T. L., and Litchford, M. D.,** Metabolic profiles, diet and health practices of championship male and female bodybuilders, *J. Am. Diet. Assoc.,* 90, 962, 1990.

Chapter 18

OLYMPIC ATHLETES

Ann C. Grandjean
Jaime S. Ruud

CONTENTS

0-8493-7911-3/94/$0.00+$.50
© 1994 by CRC Press, Inc.

I. INTRODUCTION

It has been said that if one wants to win a gold medal, one has to select the right biological parents. No doubt genetics play a primary role in athletic ability. However, other factors can enhance or impede one's potential as an athlete.

A person's accomplishments in competitive sports are determined by a variety of behavioral, socioeconomic, cultural, and environmental factors. Nutrition is one of the environmental factors that can be controlled totally by the individual. Although good nutrition is important for normal growth and development and for maintaining health, for a world-class athlete, diet can make the difference in performance, assuming all other factors are equal.

What are the dietary habits of Olympic athletes? Are their nutritional needs different from nonelite athletes? Do they adhere to any special dietary regimens? What, if any, are the nutritional problems and dietary hurdles of these athletes? Given the limitations of the data, this chapter will attempt to answer these questions.

One of the difficulties in writing a chapter on "Olympic" athletes is distinguishing between Olympic, elite, and nonelite athletes. According to *The American Heritage Dictionary of the English Language, Olympic* has been defined as "of or belonging to the game...," whereas elite means "the best or most skilled." Olympic athletes, therefore, are rightfully considered elite. They are among the best. Butts[1] writes, "... one can find elite athletes at any and all levels of competition ...; however, most people think of the elite athlete as those individuals who are successful in national or international competition, such as the Olympics."

There are certain characteristics that exemplify the subpopulation of athletes referred to as Olympians. For one, they are more heterogenous than other groups of athletes. They may attend high school or college, or be a high school dropout, or hold an advanced degree. They may be in the armed forces. They may live with their immediate family, a spouse, other roommates, or alone. They may be adolescents or parents of adolescents. Olympic sports cover a wider variety of sports than seen in professional, college, or high school athletics. For example, while swimming, basketball and wrestling are common at all levels, sports such as orienteering, team handball, luge, speed skiing, and table tennis are not.

Olympians represent a group of very dedicated and hard-working athletes who are training at the limit of their physical capacity,[2] which sets them apart from their less successful counterparts. Even though the "experienced" marathon runner may average 46 km per week,[3] the elite runner is training between 90 amd 150 km per week.[2] Road cyclists may ride 400 to 600 miles during a training week.

Winning a gold medal in international competition, such as the Winter or Summer Olympics, is a common goal for these athletes. They travel to numerous countries to train and compete. For example, members of the U.S. Luge Team train in Eastern European countries for several months, attend college in the U.S., and train at Lake Placid, New York, for a portion of the year. Bonnie Blair, U.S. Olympic speedskater, skates from October to March and then trains in other ways from May to October.[4]

Olympic athletes, among other attributes, possess a positive self-concept, function with a strong sense of personal autonomy, and have a high expectancy of success.[5] Ewing and co-workers[6] assessed the psychological characteristics of male elite hockey players across the country and found the athletes identified "the desire to go to a higher level" as the most important reason for participating in hockey.

II. NUTRITIONAL PROFILE

Olympic athletes are thought by many to be the epitome of physical health and thus their nutritional status is presumed to be superior to that of other athletes as well as nonathletes. Surveys have shown the eating habits of elite athletes closely resemble those of nonathletes, with the exception of total calories. Grandjean[7] reported higher mean energy intakes for athletes than the general U.S. population, but the percentage of calories from carbohydrates, protein, and fat was similar between the two groups.

Data[8] have been collected on 357 elite athletes, including 103 Olympians (Table 1). Daily energy intakes ranged from 1712 to 6065 calories per day for the male Olympians and from 1235 to 4854 for female Olympians. Considering the majority of these athletes train heavily on a daily basis, group mean carbohydrate intakes could be considered low, ranging from 4.2 to 6.5 g/kg body weight for men and 4.4 to 7.1 g/kg body weight for women. Mean protein intakes for male groups ranged from 1.5 to 2.2 g/kg body weight, supplying 14 to 19% of energy, and 1.0 to 1.7 g/kg body weight for female athletes, supplying 12 to 15% of energy. Fat intakes ranged from means of 29 to 41% for the men and 29 to 34% for the women.

Mean intakes of vitamins and minerals for all male elite athletes studied by Grandjean[8] met or exceeded the Recommended Dietary Allowance (RDA). Elite female athletes, on the other hand, consumed less than 100% of the RDA for iron, calcium, zinc, and vitamin B_6. Vitamin C intakes from food alone were high in male and female cyclists, representing 586% and 425% of the RDA, respectively. Vitamin B_{12} intakes were also high (499% of the RDA) for the group of weightlifters.

Food intake data have also been reported on 419 athletes competing primarily on an international level, including several European, world, and Olympic medal winners.[9] Eating habits varied greatly with gender and sport. As was also true of athletes in Grandjean's study, energy intakes were highest in male endurance sports and the lowest in female athletes where body composition is a major concern. Only five sport groups reached the level of 55% of total calories from carbohydrates. Extremely low fat intakes (<25%) were reported for Tour de France and Tour de l'Avenir athletes.

In general, vitamin intakes for the total group studied by van Erp-Baart and colleagues[10] were adequate, with the exception of low vitamin B_6 and B_1 intakes in professional cyclists. The authors attributed this to high intake of refined foods, such as sweet cakes or soft drinks. With respect to mineral intake, the authors concluded that calcium and iron may be problematic for young female athletes who are dieting. The major differences in food choices between the sport groups were in meat intake; endurance athletes tended toward a vegetarian diet.

III. DIETARY SUPPLEMENTS

Elite athletes are more inclined to read about nutrition and its effect on performance. Therefore, the amount of information as well as misinformation they possess is generally greater than for other athletes. Despite the scientific data disproving the ergogenic effects of dietary supplements, many Olympians and Olympic hopefuls take a variety of nutrient and non-nutrient supplements. Of the aforementioned Olympians, 52% reported routine use of dietary supplements.[8] Patterns emerge when the data are analyzed by sport (Table 2), with male and female cyclists being the largest consumers of nutritional supplements. Similar results were reported by van Erp-Baart et al.,[10] who found a high supplement use by professional cyclists and body builders. Tour de France cyclists studied by Saris et al.[11] took several concentrated vitamin/mineral supplements, particularly iron and vitamin B_{12}.

Although little is known about the rationale for supplement use by Olympic athletes, one would assume it is to improve performance, to gain a competitive edge, and to be the best. Burke and Read,[12] who studied the eating habits of elite Australian football players, found the most frequently reported reasons for taking vitamins were to compensate for poor nutrition and lifestyle or in response to respiratory infections and excess alcohol consumption. Some players also felt dietary supplements would compensate for tiredness and loss of appetite due to heavy training.

TABLE 1 Nutrient Intake of 103 Olympic Athletes

	n	kcal/d	kcal/kg	Protein			Carbohydrate			Fat		
				Per day (g/d)	Per weight (g/kg)	% of total energy	Per day (g/d)	Per weight (g/kg)	% of total energy	Per day (g/d)	Per weight (g/kg)	% of total energy
Males												
Cycling	9	4269	59	160	2.2	15	471	6.5	43	196	2.7	41
Distance running	11	3107	45	124	1.8	16	420	6.1	53	106	1.5	29
Figure skating	7	2533	43	103	1.8	16	336	5.8	52	88	1.5	31
Hockey	8	3468	43	156	1.9	18	343	4.2	39	155	1.9	39
Judo	7	3159	42	114	1.5	14	358	4.9	45	127	1.7	36
Weightlifting	21	3758	41	178	1.9	19	372	4.2	39	165	1.8	38
Females												
Cycling	10	3009	52	100	1.7	13	409	7.1	53	111	1.9	31
Distance running	9	2142	42	82	1.6	15	275	5.4	50	74	1.4	30
Figure skating	8	1866	40	66	1.4	14	248	5.3	52	69	1.5	33
Judo	4	1966	32	62	1.0	12	264	4.4	53	77	1.2	34
Tennis	9	2040	35	80	1.4	15	279	4.8	54	68	1.2	29

**TABLE 2 Percent of Athletes
Reporting Routine Use of
Supplements by Sport**

Sport	Percent
Males	
Cycling	66
Distance running	54
Weightlifting	47
Judo	42
Hockey	37
Figure skating	14
Females	
Cycling	100
Distance running	66
Tennis	55
Figure skating	37

IV. DIETARY CONCERNS

The Olympic athlete's nutritional program is comprised of four phases: training, precompetition, during competition, and postcompetition. The importance of each of these phases and the specific dietary recommendations vary with the individual and the sport. For example, during competition, nutrition for a marathon runner or road cyclist is much different than for the gymnast or figure skater. The energy expenditure of Tour de France cyclists is the highest recorded for an athletic event. To maintain body weight, these athletes have to eat more than 6000 calories a day during competition.[13] Kirsch and von Ameln[14] studied distance runners, cyclists, and sedentary men, and found that cyclists and runners "nibbled," which was characterized by frequent small meals and drinks. The eating frequency was at least four to six times and often more, and the intervals between the meals and drinks were short. The 357 athletes studied by Grandjean averaged 2.7 ± .4 meals per day plus 1.6 ± 1.0 snacks per day.

Often, the stress of hard training can suppress appetite, making it increasingly difficult for the athlete to consume adequate calories and carbohydrate on a regular basis. In fact, many Olympic athletes are unable to maintain a regular meal schedule. Training for several hours a day leaves little time for preparing and ingesting meals, a dilemma shared by professional dancers. Cohen et al.[15] reported during the dance season, members of the American Ballet Theatre danced from 10:30 A.M. until 11:00 P.M. daily. No special time was set aside for lunch, and half of the dancers waited until after the final performance to consume the major meal of the day. As a result, the dancers' diets were often monotonous and unbalanced, particularly those of the women, who selected basically the same foods every day.

In addition to long training hours, travel is another disruption for athletes who compete on an international level. Food intake often depends on local restaurant facilities, and, thus, access to familiar foods may be limited. This can become a problem, especially for athletes with high calorie requirements. Additionally, eating atypical foods for long periods of time can have negative emotional and psychological effects.

Most Olympians have devoted the better part of their lives to intense training in hopes of being the best in the world. And for many, there is only one moment in time to achieve their ultimate dream. One of an Olympian's greatest fears is to become sick or sustain an injury just prior to, or during, the Olympic Games. As exemplified in the 1992 Winter Games, food-borne illness and gastrointestinal distresses of other etiology can prohibit competing or diminish performance; thus, a safe food supply at the Games is a major concern of all host countries and one of many reasons why years of planning and training food service employees precede the Games.

The challege for food service at the Olympic games, in addition to a safe food supply, is to satisfy the desires and preferences of a diverse group of athletes. Host countries do an excellent job of meeting these needs by providing a wide variety of foods in a buffet setting and the use of box lunches for athletes whose competition venues are away from the Village.

V. DIETARY RECOMMENDATIONS

The relationships of various nutrients to athletic performance have been studied, and dietary recommendations have been made.[16-18] This section provides a brief overview of some current recommendations. Other chapters in this volume provide a more comprehensive discussion of specific nutrients.

A. Carbohydrate

Because dietary carbohydrate contributes directly to maintenance of body carbohydrate stores,[19] athletes participating in strenuous, long-term exercise have been advised to consume a diet containing 60 to 70% of total calories from carbohydrate.[20] While recommendations for dietary carbohydrate intake have traditionally been made on a percentage basis,[21] a recommendation for carbohydrate intake relative to body weight is more operative.[7,16,22-24] A diet containing 8 to 10 g of carbohydrate/kg body weight per day should prevent glycogen depletion during heavy training.[16] However, it is unknown whether athletes consuming less than this amount will have impaired performance. Studies are warranted to evaluate the effects of different types and amounts of dietary carbohydrate on training and performance capabilities, and there is need for research on carbohydrate requirements of athletes participating in short-term muscular exercise.

B. Protein

The available research on protein requirements suggests that some athletes may need more than the current RDA of 0.8 g/kg body weight per day.[25] Nitrogen balance studies in endurance athletes show the requirement for protein may be between 0.94 and 1.8 g/kg body weight per day.[26-29] Strength athletes may need slightly more.[17] In most cases, the additional amount of protein can be obtained easily by a normal mixed diet, as long as adequate amounts of food are consumed. Energy intake is a primary consideration, as protein requirement increases as energy intake decreases.[30] Thus, weight-conscious athletes may require a more protein-dense diet to cover needs.

C. Vitamins and Minerals

The RDA is the standard currently used in the U.S. for evaluating the adequacy of nutrient intakes of groups of people. It represents a level of intake sufficient to meet the nutrient needs of most healthy people. While intakes less than the RDA are not necessarily considered inadequate, the more a mean intake falls below this standard, the greater is the number of people for which it is potentially inadequate.[31]

A balanced diet sufficient in calories should provide adequate levels of vitamins and minerals, and there are few data showing that vitamin and/or mineral supplementation beyond 100% of the RDA will enhance performance.[25] Taken in excess, vitamins and minerals provide no advantage, can be toxic, and may interfere with the absorption and metabolism of other nutrients. On the other hand, minerals that affect peak bone mass and exercise endurance, such as calcium and iron, may require special attention among athletes who are low energy consumers, e.g., figure skaters and gymnasts.

VI. CONCLUSION

Olympic athletes are a very dedicated group of individuals with a high expectancy of success. Although the available research indicates that their eating habits are not unique compared to other groups of athletes, they are high supplement users and their dietary concerns are performance-related. Two factors that interfere with adequate food consumption in these athletes are long training hours and travel.

Although the relationship between nutrition and performance has been studied for several years, methodologies are not always consistent; sample sizes are often small; level of accomplishment, type of sport, and training season vary from study to study; and data are not collected, analyzed, and reported in a consistent manner. Only when a substantial pool of data accumulates will more accurate profiles emerge and allow for more specific recommendations to be made.

REFERENCES

1. **Butts, N. K.**, Profiles of elite athletes: physical and physiological characteristics, in *The Elite Athlete*, Butts, N. K., Gushiken, T. T., and Zarins, B., Eds., Spectrum Publications, Jamaica, NY, 1985, 183.
2. **Holmich, P., Darre, E., Jahnsen, F., and Hartvig-Jensen, T.**, The elite marathon runner: problems during and after competition, *Br. J. Sports Med.*, 22, 19, 1988.
3. **Nieman, D. C., Butler, J. V., Pollett, L. M., Dietrich, S. J., and Lutz, R. D.**, Nutrient intake of marathon runners, *J. Am. Diet. Assoc.*, 89, 1273, 1989.
4. **Bakoulis, G. and Fox, M.**, The Olympic edge, *Health*, February, 1988, p. 65.
5. **Parsons, T. W., Bowden, D., Garrett, M., McDonald, J., Schrock, M., Tesnow, D., and Wright, R.**, Profile of the elite athlete, *Coaching Rev.*, 9, 62, 1986.
6. **Ewing, M. E., Feltz, D. L., Schultz, T. D., and Albrecht, R. R.**, Psychological characteristics of competitive young hockey players, in *Competitive Sports for Children and Youth*, Brown, E. W. and Branta, C. F., Eds., Human Kinetics, Champaign, IL, 1988, 49.
7. **Grandjean, A. C.**, Macronutrient intake of US athletes compared with the general population and recommendations made for athletes, *Am. J. Clin. Nutr.*, 49, 1070, 1989.
8. **Grandjean, A. C.**, in preparation.
9. **van Erp-Baart, A. M. J., Saris, W. H. M., Binkhorst, R. A., Vos, J. A., and Elvers, J. W. H.**, Nationwide survey on nutritional habits in elite athletes. I. Energy, carbohydrate, protein, and fat intake, *Int. J. Sports Med.*, 10 S3, 1989.
10. **van Erp-Baart, A. M. J., Saris, W. H. M., Binkhorst, R. A., Vos, J. A., and Elvers, J. W. H.**, Nationwide survey on nutritional habits in elite athletes. II. Mineral and vitamin intake, *Int. J. Sports Med.*, 10, S11, 1989.
11. **Saris, W. H. M., Schrijver, J., van Erp-Baart, M. A., and Brouns, F.**, Adequacy of vitamin supply under maximal sustained workloads: the Tour de France, *Int. J. Vitam. Nutr. Res. Suppl.*, 30, 205, 1989.
12. **Burke, L. M. and Read, R. S. D.**, A study of dietary patterns of elite Australian football players, *Can. J. Sport Sci.*, 13, 15, 1988.
13. **Saris, W. H. M., van Erp-Baart, M. A., Brouns, F., Westerterp, K. R., and ten Hoor, F.**, Study on food intake and energy expenditure during extreme sustained exercise: the Tour de France, *Int. J. Sports Med.*, 10, S26, 1989.
14. **Kirsch, K. A. and Von Ameln, H.**, Feeding patterns of endurance athletes, *Eur. J. Appl. Physiol.*, 47, 197, 1981.
15. **Cohen, J. L., Potosnak, L., Frank, O., and Baker, H.**, A nutritional and hematologic assessment of elite ballet dancers, *Phys. Sportsmed.*, 13, 43, 1985.
16. **Sherman, W. M. and Wimer, G. S.**, Insufficient dietary carbohydrate during training: does it impair athletic performance?, *Int. J. Sport Nutr.*, 1, 28, 1991.
17. **Lemon, P. W. R.**, Protein and amino acid needs of the strength athlete, *Int. J. Sport Nutr.*, 1, 127, 1991.
18. **Leaf, A. and Frisa, K. B.**, Eating for health or for athletic performance?, *Am. J. Clin. Nutr.*, 49, 1066, 1989.
19. **Christensen, E. H. and Hansen, O.**, Arbeitsfahigkeit und Ernahrung, *Skand. Arch. Physiol.*, 81, 160, 1939.

20. **Costill, D. L., Sherman, W. M., Fink, W. J., Maresh, C., Witten, M., and Miller, J. M.,** The role of dietary carbohydrate in muscle glycogen resynthesis after strenuous running, *Am. J. Clin. Nutr.,* 34, 1831, 1981.

21. **Sherman, W. M.,** Carbohydrates, muscle glycogen and muscle glycogen supercompensation, in *Ergogenic Aids in Sport,* Williams, M. H., Ed., Human Kinetics, Champaign, IL, 1983, 3.

22. **Sherman, W. M., Brodowicz, G., Wright, D. A., Allen, W. K., Simonsen, J., and Dernbach, A.,** Effects of 4 h preexercise carbohydrate feedings on cycling performance, *Med. Sci. Sports Exercise,* 21, 598, 1989.

23. **Sherman, W. M.,** Carbohydrate feedings before and after exercise, in *Perspectives in Exercise Science and Sports Medicine,* Vol. 4, *Ergogenics — Enhancement of Performance in Exercise and Sport,* Lamb, D. R., and Williams, M. H., Eds., Brown & Benchmark, 1992, 1.

24. **Lamb, D. R., Rinehardt, K. F., Bartels, R. L., Sherman, W. M., and Snook, J. T.,** Dietary carbohydrate and intensity of interval swim training, *Am. J. Clin. Nutr.,* 52, 1058, 1990.

25. Food and Nutrition Board, National Academy of Sciences, *Recommended Dietary Allowances,* 10th rev. ed., National Academy Press, Washington, D.C., 1989.

26. **Meredith, C. N., Zackin, M. J., Frontera, W. R., and Evans, W. J.,** Dietary protein requirements and body protein metabolism in endurance trained men, *Appl. Physiol.,* 66, 2850, 1989.

27. **Friedman, J. E. and Lemon, P. W. R.,** Chronic endurance exercise on retention of dietary protein, *Int. J. Sports Med.,* 10, 118, 1989.

28. **Tarnopolsky, M. A., MacDougall, J. D., and Atkinson, S. A.,** Influence of protein intake and training status on nitrogen balance and lean body mass, *J. Appl. Physiol.,* 64, 187, 1988.

29. **Brouns, F., Saris, W. H. M., Stroecken, J., Beckers, E., Thijssen, R., Rehrer, N. J., and ten Hoor, F.,** The effect of diet manipulation and repeated sustained exercise on nitrogen balance, a controlled Tour de France simulation study, part 3, in *Food and Fluid Related Aspects in Highly Trained Athletes,* Brouns, F., Ed., De Vrieseborch, Haarlem, The Netherlands, 1988, 73.

30. **Ivengar, A. and Narasinga Rao, R. S.,** Effect of varying energy and protein intake on nitrogen balance in adults engaged in heavy manual labour, *Br. J. Nutr.,* 41, 19, 1979.

31. **Guthrie, H. A.,** Interpretation of data on dietary intake, *Nutr. Rev.,* 47, 33, 1989.

Chapter 19

NUTRITION AND PERFORMANCE AT ENVIRONMENTAL EXTREMES*

Eldon W. Askew

CONTENTS

---

* The views, opinions, and/or findings contained in this report are those of the author and should not be construed as an official Department of the Army position, policy, or decision, unless so designated by other official documentation.

I. INTRODUCTION

Humans are remarkably adaptive animals, having learned to survive and even thrive in environments outside their normal "comfort" zone. Man accomplishes these adaptations through metabolic and behavioral changes. Environments that threaten to overwhelm the ability of man to adjust his metabolism and/or change behavioral strategies have been referred to as "hostile" environments.[1] This terminology is a misnomer, since man can function safely and effectively in extremes of environments, provided adequate behavioral precautions (e.g., clothing, shelter, food, water) are taken. The environment becomes "hostile" only when man has entered it unprepared or the environment is so severe that it threatens to surpass man's ability to adapt or respond appropriately to its challenges.

Although man is a remarkably adaptive animal, he has limitations. One of these limitations is homeothermy. Shephard[2] described mankind as being "... metabolic hostages of the homeothermic condition." This means regardless of the environmental temperatures, man must defend the normal body temperature of 37°C (98.5°F) within a relative narrow range of temperatures. We have several physiologic defense mechanisms at our disposal (e.g., shivering, sweating, vasodilation, or vasoconstriction) to help maintain homeothermy. When the capability of these defense mechanisms is exceeded and body core temperature drops below 35°C (95°F) or rises above 41°C (106°F), the human body functions at such reduced efficiency that both physical and mental performance deteriorates rapidly.[2,3] Left unchecked, hypothermia and hyperthermia can be life threatening. Hypoxia associated with high-altitude environments can also impose severe restrictions on physical performance and jeopardize survival.[4] High altitudes are usually accompanied by cold temperatures, compounding environmental stress and metabolic challenge.

The body's metabolic response to heat, cold, and hypoxia can also be impaired by inadequate nutrition. This is depicted schematically in Figure 1. Appetite and thirst responses are frequently inappropriate in these environmental extremes, leading to inadequate calorie or fluid intakes. The availability of water and food is often limited due to logistical constraints. Backpackers, mountaineers, and explorers are usually limited to the food they can carry with them in their packs. The weight of these packs is critical; often food and water are sacrificed to make room for essential equipment, clothing, and gear. Inadequate dietary energy (particularly carbohydrate and protein) can result in glycogen depletion and loss of lean body mass. This, in turn can result in impaired thermoregulation and impaired muscle strength, coordination, and endurance. Inadequate fluid intakes coupled with increased sweating, loss of lung-humidified air to an arid environment or altitude, or cold-induced diuresis can lead to dehydration and compromised thermoregulation and endurance. The usual increased energy and fluid demands for work in environmental extremes can be exacerbated by anorexia (hypophagia) and inappropriate thirst response (hypodipsia). The effects of hypophagia and hypodipsia can be further complicated by the general lack of food and water in cold, desert, or high-altitude settings. Negative energy and fluid balances can combine to cause substantial decreases in physical performance capacities.[5-9]

Expeditionary or recreational outdoor activities are frequently conducted in hot, cold, high-altitude, or rugged-terrain environments. Mountaineering, cross-country skiing, snowshoeing, sledging, and backpacking can be as physically demanding as more conventional sporting events, plus there is an added element of danger. The wilderness is much less forgiving of mistakes than a more "civilized" environment where medical care is just minutes away. A miscalculation of physical ability or inadequate preparation can be life threatening in environmental extremes. Proper education, planning, preparation, equipment, and training are essential for work in the heat, cold, and high altitudes.

Proper nutrition is an often-overlooked but critical component of effective work under these conditions. The information in this chapter may be useful to individuals planning

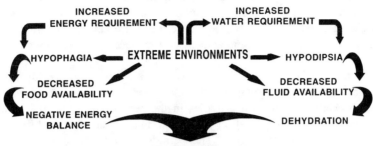

CASCADE EFFECT OF ENVIRONMENTAL EXTREMES
ON WORK PERFORMANCE

INCREASED
ENERGY REQUIREMENT

INCREASED
WATER REQUIREMENT

HYPOPHAGIA ← EXTREME ENVIRONMENTS → HYPODIPSIA

DECREASED
FOOD AVAILABILITY

DECREASED
FLUID AVAILABILITY

NEGATIVE ENERGY
BALANCE

DEHYDRATION

CONSEQUENCES
* IMPAIRED THERMOREGULATION
* KETOSIS
* PERTURBED ACID-BASE BALANCE
* DEPLETED MUSCLE GLYCOGEN
* DETERIORATION OF FINE MOTOR COORDINATION
* DIMINISHED WORK CAPACITY

FIGURE 1. Schematic representation of the influence of extreme environments upon energy balance, hydration status, and resultant consequences. This generalized diagram illustrates the influence of heat, cold, and/or high altitude on the cascade of events that can lead to physiological consequences and impaired performance.

TABLE 1 Energy Requirements for Physical Activity in Temperate, Cold, and Hot Environments

	Environment		
Physical activity	**Temperate[a]**	**Cold (kcal/kg BW)**	**Hot**
Light	32–44	35–46	40–54
Moderate	45–52	47–55	55–61
Heavy	53–63	56–68	62–75

[a] Altitude energy requirements are similar to temperate.

From Consolazio, C. F., *Army Research and Development Newsmagazine*, November 1966, p. 24. With permission.

nutritional support for work in hot (greater than 30°C/86°F), cold (less than 0°C/32°F), or at high-altitude (greater than 3050 m/10,000 ft elevation) environments.

II. ENVIRONMENT, METABOLISM, AND NUTRIENT REQUIREMENTS

Extremes in the external environment can influence the requirements for certain nutrients,[10-13] and may have implications for people who live or recreate, and athletes who train or compete, under these conditions.[14,15] The need for additional vitamins and minerals may be influenced by certain environments, but the two nutrients most often in short supply are energy (more specifically carbohydrate) and water. Achieving energy balance is often difficult, for the reasons illustrated in Figure 1. Consolazio[16] estimated energy requirements for work in temperate, hot, cold, and high-altitude environments. These guidelines are shown Table 1.

Athletes can sustain a high-level work output only when they manage to maintain energy balance.[17] Work is not necessarily severely impaired following hypocaloric diets.[8] More commonly, the upper limit of power output during endurance exercise with intensity greater than 60% $\dot{V}O_2$ max is limited[17] during energy deficiency and the ability of muscles to resist fatigue may be reduced.[18,19] Energy (more specifically carbohydrate) deficiency results in reduced muscle glycogen stores[15] and an increased reliance upon body fat stores to support work output.[5]

Trekkers often take along high-fat foods to increase the energy density of their diets. Under most circumstances, relying upon dietary or body fat stores to meet energy requirements in high energy expenditure activities in the heat, cold, or at high altitude is not advisable. Given a sufficient period for adaptation, muscles are able to shift their substrate utilization from carbohydrate to lipid.[20] This permits maintenance of only a relatively low-intensity work load. High-fat diets are not generally recommended for environmental extremes where high power outputs are necessary (due to the requirement of carbohydrate by muscles for maximum power output).[17] High-fat diets may not be well tolerated (reduced appetite appeal or digestibility) in hot or high-altitude settings; however, they seem to be tolerated relatively well in cold environments close to sea level.

Exposures to extreme heat, cold, or high altitude alters muscle metabolism by a variety of factors, including muscle temperature, pH, O_2 tension, as well as cofactor and substrate availability.[21] As an example, unacclimatized individuals generally exhibit greater muscle glycogen breakdown, glycolytic flux, and lactate accumulation in extreme environments compared to temperate conditions at sea level.[21] (The "lactate paradox" of diminished blood lactate following *maximal* exercise at altitude compared to sea level is an exception to this generalization.[22])

III. NUTRIENT REQUIREMENTS FOR WORK IN HOT ENVIRONMENTS

Adequate fluid replacement overshadows all other considerations of nutrient requirements for work in a hot environment. Drinking adequate water for work in the heat prevents dehydration, heat illness, and reduced performance.[6,23] Heat acclimation can reduce sodium requirements for work in the heat[7] but water requirements remain relatively unaffected.[6,24] Thirst is a poor indicator of hydration status.[23] Intense thirst is usually noticed at 5 to 6% body weight loss due to dehydration. By this time physical performance is compromised. Vague discomfort, lethargy, weariness, sleepiness, and apathy, as well as elevated body core temperature, heart rate, and muscular fatigue are noted as body water loss reaches the 3 to 5% level. The magnitude of the increase in body core temperature and heart rate elicited by dehydrating exercise is linearly related to the level of body water deficit.[25]

Severe hypohydration can lead to decreased blood volume and increased plasma osmolality, which can decrease sweating and heat dissipation.[25,26] Eighty percent of the energy metabolized during exercise in a hot environment is liberated as heat (20% is utilized for mechanical work) and 80 to 90% of heat dissipation during exercise in a hot-dry environment is accomplished by the evaporation of sweat.[27,28] Water consumed during exercise in the heat can move to the sweat glands within 9 to 18 min of ingestion, where it is available for cooling the body.[27] Each milliliter of sweat evaporated from the skin will lead to a heat loss or dissipation of approximately 0.6 kcal.[28] Sweat rates are highly variable between individuals, but can reach 2 l/h for prolonged time periods.[29] Dehydration depends in large part upon sweat loss, which is in turn determined by exercise intensity and duration, as well as environmental factors such as temperature, solar load, wind speed, and relative humidity and clothing. The influence of these factors on water requirements for work in the heat is illustrated in Table 2.[30,31]

It is important to note under certain environmental conditions a 10°F increase in temperature can cause a 50 to 60% increase in water requirements at *rest*. Superimposing an increased

TABLE 2 Water Requirements (l/h) for Rest and Work in the Heat as Influenced by Solar Load and Temperature

Temperature and relative humidity (°F @ % rh)	Indoors (no solar load)				Outdoors (clear sky)			
	Rest	Light	Medium	Heavy	Rest	Light	Medium	Heavy
85 @ 50	0.2	0.5	1.0	1.5	0.5	0.9	1.3	1.8
96 @ 50	0.3	0.9	1.3	1.9	0.8	1.2	1.7	2.0
105 @ 30	0.6	1.0	1.5	2.0	0.9	1.3	1.9	2.0
115 @ 20	0.8	1.2	1.7	2.0	1.1	1.5	2.0	2.0
120 @ 20	0.9	1.3	1.9	2.0	1.3	1.7	2.0	2.0

Note: The values for water requirements in l/h were calculated according to the prediction model of Shapiro et al.[30] by L. A. Stroschein, Biophysics and Biomedical Modeling Division, U.S. Army Research Institute of Environmental Medicine, Natick, MA. The following conditions were assumed in these calculations: clothing, tropical fatigues; heat-acclimatized subjects; wind speed 2 m/s.

work load at high temperatures greatly increases fluid requirements. The solar load, relative humidity, clothing, wind speed, and prior acclimation to heat all interact in determining sweat rates, insensible water loss, and water requirements at any given workload.[31] Consolazio[16] recommended up to 12 l of water per day for soldiers engaged in heavy physical activity in 100°F weather. While this level of water intake may be necessary to replenish fluid losses in a hot environment, it may be difficult to ingest such a large volume. As an example, it would be necessary to consume 1 l of water upon arising in the morning, 1 l with each of three meals and 1 l for each hour during an 8-h work day to achieve a daily intake of 12 l. This rate of fluid consumption is possible, but requires conscious effort. The U.S. military refers to planned or programmed water drinking as "water discipline"[32] and credits this doctrine for the relatively low incidence of U.S. heat casualties in the 1990–1991 Desert War in Iraq and Kuwait.

As a general rule, salt supplements are not necessary for work in the heat unless water is available but food is not.[33] Since the typical daily American diet contains 6 to 18 g of NaCl,[34] replacement of sodium lost during exercise in the heat can usually be met by consuming normally salted food in proportion to caloric requirements.[16,33] This is usually an adequate amount of sodium to replace that lost in sweat in a hot environment. Armstrong et al.[35] demonstrated that humans could successfully acclimate to work in the heat on as little as 6 g of NaCl/d although higher levels of sodium intake (8 g) reduced some of the adverse symptoms asssociated with this period of heat acclimation.

Sodium losses can, however, be quite high at sustained moderate work rates in a hot environment. Sweat losses amounting to 12 l/24 h can result in the loss of 11,000 to 16,500 mg of Na$^+$ per day.[36] Under these conditions sodium replacement will require liberal salting of food, drinking water that contains 1.0 g of NaCl/l[16] (390 mg Na$^+$), or consuming sodium-containing "sports" beverages in place of a portion of the 12 l/d water requirement. Sodium supplementation should be given consideration only when fluid replacement is adequate. Barr et al.[37] found that sodium replacement during exercise in the heat does not appear necessary for moderate-intensity work up to 6 h duration. Excess salt consumption can place an added burden on water requirements in all environments (Figure 2).[38] In addition to increasing water requirements, high salt intake (without adequate water intake) can elevate plasma osmolality, which can lead to decreased sweating and as a result, increase thermal strain during work.[24]

Although water and sodium replenishment are the primary nutrients of concern in a hot environment, consideration should also be given to providing adequate energy. Food and

Influence of salt intake on water requirements

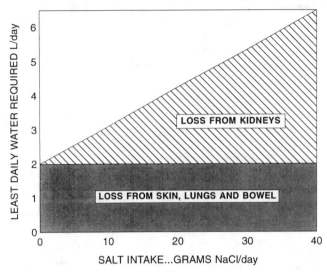

FIGURE 2. Estimated minimum daily water requirement of a sedentary man weighing 70 kg at an ambient temperature of 75°F, relative humidity of 19%, consuming 0 to 30 g of NaCl/day. (From Baker, E. M., Plough, I. C., and Allen, T. H., *Am. J. Clin. Nutr.*, 12, 394, 1963. With permission.)

water intakes are closely related; food intake is reduced during water deprivation and water intake is reduced during starvation.[39] Energy requirements for work in the heat may be elevated 0.5% for each 1°F increase as the ambient temperature increases from 86 to 104°F.[16] Below temperatures of 86°F (30°C) temperature has little influence on energy requirements until cold temperatures (requiring additional clothing to prevent excessive heat loss) are reached. The relatively small increase in energy requirements for work at high temperatures is believed to be attributable to increased cardiovascular work needed to dissipate heat, increased sweat gland activity, and metabolic rate. Consolazio et al.[40] found approximately a 10% increase in metabolic cost for work at 100°F compared to work at 70°F. Sawka et al.[41] subsequently demonstrated that heat acclimation can lower the rate of metabolism during exercise in the heat by as much as 3%, indicating that the actual increase in energy requirements for work at high ambient temperatures may vary with the degree of heat acclimation of the individual.

Work in the heat has implications with regard to muscle glycogen synthesis and utilization.[15] Fink et al.[42] found that exercise in the heat increased muscle glycogen utilization, although this has not been observed in all studies.[26,43] Hargreaves[15] speculated that a reduction in muscle blood flow, increased muscle temperature, and elevated catecholamines may contribute to stimulation of muscle glycogenolysis during exercise in the heat. Surprisingly, hypohydration comprising up to 5% body weight loss does not seem to impair muscle glycogen synthesis after exercise.[44] These observations indicate that exercise in the heat may increase glycogen utilization.

Sustained heavy sweat rates increase the loss of sodium and a number of other nutrients, including chloride, potassium, calcium, magnesium, iron, and nitrogen.[36] There is little evidence to suggest these nutrients cannot be replaced adequately by a normal diet.[29] Vitamin supplementation for work in the heat is also unnecessary, with two possible exceptions.[14] Vitamin C has been reported to facilitate heat acclimation,[11] and multiple B vitamins have been reported to lessen fatigue during work in the heat.[12] Generally speaking, vitamin and mineral supplements will be advantageous only for those with extremely poor dietary habits. Water supplementation during work in the heat is more critical than carbohydrate supplementation,[29] since performance will be impacted sooner by heat and dehydration than muscle glycogen supply. Hence, the provision of water should take precedence over carbohydrate and electrolytes during exercise in the heat,[29] although carbohydrate-containing beverages may be more effective than plain water in the support of continuous exercise lasting longer than 50 min.[27] The key to carbohydrate and water provision during work in the heat is to administer them simultaneously (commercial carbohydrate/electrolyte or ''sports'' drinks containing 5 to 10% carbohydrate are appropriate). These sports drinks typically contain ~20 meq Na^+/l to promote glucose and water absorption from the gut. If it is not feasible to use a carbohydrate/electrolyte drink, concentrate on rehydration with plain water accompanied by adequate food salted a bit more than normal.

Hydration with solutions containing 1 g of glycerol/kg body weight prior to work in the heat may help maintain a better hydration status than plain water alone.[45] This effect is believed to be due to glycerol's hyperhydrating properties. Glycerol seems to provide a fluid reservoir in the interstitial spaces with body tissues. The ingestion of a glycerol solution and water compared to water alone results in decreased urine output, decreased body temperature, increased sweat rate, and lower heart rate during moderate work in the heat.[45] Glycerol-induced hyperhydration appears to be a promising method of reducing the thermal burden during moderate exercise in the heat.

IV. NUTRIENT REQUIREMENTS FOR WORK IN COLD ENVIRONMENTS

Energy requirements are the major consideration for providing nutritional support in a cold environment.[46] Energy expenditure in hot and high-altitude environments is usually limited by the rate of heat buildup and hypoxia, respectively, whereas in a cold environment the rate of energy expenditure is usually not restricted by the heat burden or hypoxia. In addition, high rates of energy expenditure in the cold (~7000 kcal/d) have been attributed to the high degree of motivation of cold-weather expedition team members.[47] Energy requirements in a cold environment are influenced by the intensity of the cold, windspeed, physical difficulties associated with working under winter conditions (preparing shelters, melting snow, locomotion on icy or snow-covered surfaces, etc.) and the light–dark cycle in arctic areas.[48,49] At the same time that energy requirements are high, energy intakes may be reduced by such factors as monotony of the diet and the difficulty of preparing food for consumption under adverse conditions.

Cold exposure increases energy requirements. Most investigators would agree with this statement, but there are several caveats. Johnson and Kark[50] reported that people in a cold climate normally eat more than those in a warm climate. Gray et al.[51] suggested that increased energy requirements were primarily due to a ''hobbling'' effect of the weight of the clothing and associated inefficiencies of locomotion. Teitlebaum and Goldman[52] subsequently demonstrated that the energy expenditure increase attributable to the weight of arctic clothing (24.6 lbs) was greater than that which could be accounted for by the weight of the clothing alone and attributed it to ''friction drag'' between the multiple layers of arctic clothing. The weight of cold-weather clothing has decreased as technology has improved; however, clothing is still a considerable burden.

Properly outfitted, modern cold-weather clothing ensembles now weigh 15 to 20 lbs and still account for the major part of the additional energy expenditure in cold not attributed to discernable work such as skiing, snowshoeing, sledging, etc. Mechanical inefficiencies associated with ''clothing friction'' and ''hobbling'' combine with small energy requirements to heat and humidify inspired air and air ''pumped'' into and out of clothing sleeves and seams. These factors contribute to a 10 to 15% increase in the metabolic cost of working in the cold.[40,52,53]

Energy requirements for activities in a cold environment are considerably higher when accompanied by heavy work. However, provided that adequate clothing is worn and allowances are made for the increased weight of the clothing, increases in energy requirements are usually comparable to those for similar activities in a temperate environment.[54,55] (However, energy requirements for an activity may be higher in certain cold environments if the terrain is inefficient for locomotion due to ice or snow.) Cold-weather energy expenditures can range from approximately 3200 kcal/d in low-activity situations to 5000 kcal/d during sledging and manhauling activities.[1] Although considerably higher rates of energy expenditure have been reported,[47] 4500 kcal/d is a reasonable target figure for planning purposes. Recent measurements of U.S. Military cold-weather energy expenditure utilizing the doubly labeled water technique ($D_2{}^{18}O$) confirmed that 4000 to 5000 kcal/d will usually meet cold-weather energy requirements.[56]

The dietary patterns of natives of arctic and subarctic regions and their obvious success in coping with harsh environments have influenced arctic explorers to embrace diets high in fat and led to the general belief that diets high in fat impart a special advantage for work in the cold. Such information is largely anecdotal and probably relates more to the availability of local foods (seal, fish, whale, caribou) and the familiarity of Eskimos with these foods than any real nutritional advantage. Indeed, many Alaskan natives (Eskimos, Indians, and Aleuts) currently consume diets containing 38% of the energy from fat, which is similar to that of the general U.S. population (37%).[57] This change toward lower-fat diets probably reflects the availability of a changing supply of local foods rather than any conscious or unconscious choice influenced by cold weather. Swain et al.[58] reported the caloric consumption distribution pattern of military troops stationed in cold, temperate, and tropical areas was similar across these environments.

Few studies in the literature deal specifically with nutrient requirements in the cold. These limited studies support the concept that cold does not cause a greater demand for any nutrients other than calories.[50,59,60] Anecdotal reports of "craving" classes of food such as fat or carbohydrate have not been substantiated,[59] yet the idea persists that high-fat diets are especially appopriate for cold-weather operations.

Humans can adapt over a period of time to a high-fat diet[20,61] and much of the submaximal endurance type of work in the cold such as cross-country skiing, snowshoeing, and sledging can be supported by $\dot{V}O_2$ max efforts of less than 60%. These moderate sustained power outputs can be supported relatively well by high levels of lipid oxidation.[17,61]

The question next arises: "Does the consumption of a high-fat diet in the cold increase cardiovascular health risk?" It would be irresponsible to recommend a chronically high-fat diet; however, it appears that cardiovascular risk is minimized by the high rate of caloric expenditure associated with work in the cold. An example of this can be seen in the data of Ekstedt et al.[62] (Table 3). Despite consuming a diet containing twice the fat and cholesterol of the low-fat group, cross-country skiers fed the high-fat diet decreased their cholesterol, very-low-density lipoproteins (VLDL), and triglycerides over an 8-d period of cross-country skiing in the cold. The observed decreases were similar to those of the low-fat group and suggests that, in the short run, at least, hard physical work can lessen the normally adverse effect of a high-fat diet on blood lipids.

In addition to the anecdotal, historical, and scientific evidence that high-fat diets are well tolerated in the cold, there is also evidence to suggest that high-fat diets may improve cold tolerance provided that meals are fed at regular intervals during cold exposure[63] (Figure 3).

Despite the arguments that can be made for high-fat diets in the cold, there is evidence suggesting that carbohydrates are more important than fat in fueling metabolic heat production during cold exposure.[21,64] An illustration of this can be seen in Figure 4. Vallerand and Jacobs[64] studied the contribution of protein, carbohydrate, and fat to energy expenditure

TABLE 3 Effect of Low- or High-Fat Diets on Percent Change of Serum Lipids During Eight Days Cross-Country Ski Exercise

	Diets[a]	
	Low Fat	High fat
Total cholesterol	-26.4 ± 4.3	-19.9 ± 2.9
VLDL-LDL cholesterol	-38.1 ± 3.0	-41.1 ± 5.7
HDL cholesterol	$+5.9 \pm 2.3$	$+19.0 \pm 3.8$
Triglycerides	-30.6 ± 6.8	-32.6 ± 8.0
Body weight, kg	-0.2 ± 0.5	-0.9 ± 0.4

Note: Data from Ekstedt et al.[62] $N = 7$, 8-d cross country ski trip with backpack weighing 30 kg, total distance covered 160 km.

[a] Low-fat diet, 3800 kcal/d, 26% fat, 260 mg cholesterol per day; high-fat diet, 3800 kcal/d, 52% fat, 480 mg cholesterol/day. Values shown are mean ± SD of percent differences before and after ski trip.

EFFECT OF DIET COMPOSITION AND FREQUENCY OF EATING ON COLD TOLERANCE

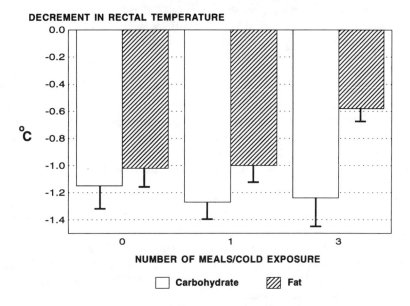

FIGURE 3. The effect of high-carbohydrate (66% of the kcal) or high-fat (73% of the kcal) diets on cold tolerance (decrease in rectal temperature) during clothed cold exposure at −20°F. The data for 0 meals was for 6 h of cold exposure; the date for 1 or 3 meals (600 kcal/meal) was for 8 h of cold exposure. The differences between 0 or 1 meal were not significant. The differences between carbohydrate and fat for 3 meals was significant ($p < .0001$). (Adapted from Mitchell, H. H. et al., *Am. J. Physiol.*, 146, 84, 1946. With permission.)

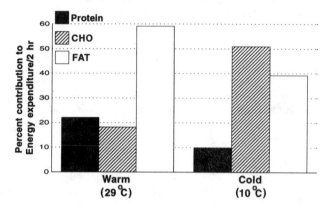

**Influence of cold exposure on
calorie source for resting energy expenditure**

FIGURE 4. Influence of cold exposure on the calorie source for energy expenditure in resting male subjects. Seven subjects were exposed to both warm (29°C) and cold (10°C) conditions for 2 h while they rested (clothed in shorts). Cold exposure induced a body heat debt of 825.9 ± 63.3 kJ, whereas warm exposure produced a heat gain of 92.4 ± 19.2 kJ. Energy expenditure in the cold was 1519.4 ± 150.6 kJ, whereas in the warm it was 617.8 ± 28 kJ. (Data from Vallerand, A. L. and Jacobs, I., *Eur. J. Appl. Physiol.*, 58, 873, 1989. With permission.)

during 2-h exposures of semi-nude men to warm (29°C) or cold (2°C) environments. Cold exposure elevated energy expenditure almost 2.5 times over that observed for subjects in the warm environment. This increase in energy expenditure resulted in an increase in carbohydrate oxidation of 588% and a 63% increase in fat oxidation. Protein oxidation was unaffected. These results demonstrate that cold exposure causes a much greater increase in carbohydrate utilization than lipid. They also suggest that both fat and carbohydrate fuel the shivering response in humans, with carbohydrate (presumably glycogen) being the more important of the two fuel sources. Shivering is impaired by fasting and hypoglycemia.[65,66] Light exercise in the cold results in lower muscle glycogen levels than similar exercise at normal temperature.[67] These observations, coupled with the observation that low muscle glycogen levels are associated with a more rapid body cooling during cold exposure,[68] suggests that muscle glycogen and blood glucose are important, if not critical, fuels for thermogenesis from shivering.[69] Fat can potentially contribute to thermogenesis by fueling the shivering response and/or through triglyceride–fatty acid cycling.[70] The relative importance of these two cycles in humans is not known.[71] Young et al.[71] have reported that metabolic heat production was not significantly affected by dietary lowering of muscle glycogen stores prior to cold exposure, indicating either that fat can adequately fuel cold-induced thermogenesis under reduced muscle glycogen concentrations or that a critical level of muscle glycogen depletion had not been reached. Martineau and Jacobs[72] were unable to alter the thermal responses to cold exposure by simultaneously lowering muscle glycogen and plasma free fatty acids, leading them to suggest that thermal and metabolic responses in the cold can rapidly adjust to compensatory utilization of alternative fuels. Although the lowering of carbohydrate stores does not necessarily result in reduced heat production,[71,72] there is evidence to suggest that a stimulation of carbohydrate oxidation by the ingestion of an ephedrine–caffeine mixture can improve cold tolerance in humans.[73]

Water requirements for work in cold environments are similar to those for temperate environments.[74] Roberts et al.[75] suggested that it is possible to remain adequately hydrated in the cold (at low activity levels) on a minimum of 3 l of water per day. A more generous allowance of 4 to 6 l/d will cover increased fluid requirements for humidifying inspired air and a certain degree of sweating that may accompany moderate to heavy work levels. Jones[76] reported D_2O-measured turnover rates of 3 to $4\frac{1}{2}$ l/d for U.S. Marines conducting cold-weather training and Edwards et al.[77,78] and King et al.[79] reported water consumption rates of 3.5 to 5 l/d for U.S. Army solders engaged in arctic cold-weather training. Although water requirements are not high in the cold, the consequences of dehydration are still important. Exposure to cold can cause a reduction in the sense of thirst and consequently reduced water consumption.[77,80] This relationship was observed by Edwards and Roberts,[77] who noted that elevated urine specific gravities (>1.030) were associated with the consumption of less than 2 l of water per day by soldiers working in the cold. When forced drinking was initiated, water consumption in these soldiers doubled and urine specific gravities rapidly decreased to the normal range of 1.020. They also found that water consumption and food intake were strongly correlated ($r = .76$).[77] Dann et al.[80] observed marked voluntary dehydration in a control group during a 4.5-h, 1700-m, cold-weather (0°C) march. The control group exhibited evidence of dehydration, decreased glomerular filtration rate, osmotic clearance, and urine volume compared to the imposed drinking discipline group. Dann et al.[80] calculated that a fluid intake of 150 ml/h during exercise in the cold would be required to maintain a urinary flow rate of about 1 ml/kg/h necessary for a good state of hydration.

Hypohydration in the cold can reduce food consumption, efficiency of physical and mental performance and resistance to cold exposure.[81] While adequate fluid intake is paramount in preventing hypohydration in the cold, it is also prudent to consider the temperature of fluid and food provided for work in the cold. Warm fluids and heated foods are generally recommended in the cold, whenever possible, to impart a feeling of warmth and well-being.[81] The warming effect of a hot beverage in the cold is probably related to its effect upon subsequent vasodilation and increased blood flow to cold extremities rather than to the actual quantity of heat contained in the ingested fluid. Wilson and Culik[82] have provided the thought-provoking suggestion that the real advantage to providing warm food in the cold is the net heat savings that results to the body compared to ingesting ambient temperature (cold) food. Their calorimetric calculations based upon observations conducted with penguins fed warm or cold krill (fish) suggest that up to 13% of the daily energy expenditure of the penguin may be devoted to heating cold ingested food to body temperature. The lesson for human sojourners in the cold is apparent and can probably be taken to heart even in the absence of similar human studies.

It is clear that in a cold environment, man must adapt his behavior to minimize cold exposure and achieve homeothermy; failure to do so will result in rapid performance decrements and even death. The energy costs of performing any task under extreme cold conditions is higher than performing the same task under temperate conditions because of the difficulties in working in heavy clothing and traveling in snow. Working in cold environments does not lead to an increased requirement for any nutrient other than energy. Carbohydrate intake may be of concern if high power output (>50% $\dot{V}O_2$ max) is required for extended periods of time. Replenishment of muscle glycogen stores will assure the availability of this fuel during exercise and shivering to support thermogenesis and aid the body in fighting hypothermia. Caloric demands for moderate to high activity levels in arctic and subarctic areas are usually adequately supported by 4000 to 5000 kcal/d.

Weight loss is common during cold-weather field expeditions, often due to the monotony of the diet and difficulty in preparing food, coupled with increased energy expenditures. Water requirements are not increased in cold-weather operations, but intakes may be decreased due to the difficulty of melting snow and ice and the tendency of cold weather travelers to utilize dry foods that will not freeze and can be eaten without thawing. Inadequate hydration may decrease the body's ability to adjust to cold stress.

V. NUTRIENT REQUIREMENTS FOR WORK AT HIGH ALTITUDE

Abrupt exposure to altitudes greater than 10,000 ft (3050 m) elevation is frequently associated with symptoms of altitude sickness.[83] Altitude sickness is a generalized term referring to a combination of symptoms, including headaches, anorexia, nausea, vomiting, and malaise. The experienced mountaineer knows that gradual acclimation to progressively higher altitude exposure is the best preventive medicine for high-altitude sickness.[84,85] Gradual ascent over a period of days from sea level to high altitude is accompanied by a number of simultaneous physiologic adaptations that permit the accomplishment of significant work with minimal physical symptoms other than an increased perceived exertion. Unfortunately, it is not always practical or possible to delay ascent to altitude. Soldiers and rescue workers frequently must travel abruptly to high altitudes to perform critical missions. Prior acclimation is not possible. Abrupt transportation from sea level to high altitude is usually accompanied by debilitating altitude sickness influencing symptoms, mood, and performance.[85,86] These uncomfortable symptoms usually increase in intensity for periods of up to 48 h after altitude exposure and then gradually lessen.[87] Unfortunately, it is usually during the first 48 h at altitude that critical work must be accomplished. Although there is some debate as to whether altitude exposure causes an absolute increase in energy requirements above that of similar work performed at sea level,[55,88] the usual activities associated with missions at altitude and the lack of adequate food intakes almost invariably result in an initially negative energy balance.[89-91] Altitude exposure (and the accompanying hypoxia) is associated with a 17 to 27% increase in basal metabolic rate which raises energy requirements above sea level.[92] However, altitude exposure is often accompanied by a decrease in voluntary energy expenditure which may cancel the new effect of an increase in basal metabolic rate.[92] Energy expenditures in experienced and motivated climbers can be quite high[90] and depend upon the activity level.

Rose et al.[93] observed depressed food intakes and weight loss at altitude even under the chamber conditions of Operation Everest II. In this study, work requirements were relatively low and a thermoneutral hypobaric environment with an adequate quantity and variety of palatable food was provided. Reduced food intake under these conditions indicated that hypoxia by itself was a major factor reducing appetite and food intake. Adequate food intake can be achieved at altitude but it requires a concerted conscious effort of dietary management and forced eating.[92] The usual combination of anorexia and reduced food intake can potentially exert a negative effect on work performance at even moderate altitude.[55] Food intakes are usually reduced 10 to 50% during acute altitude exposure.

Numerous pharmacological attempts to reduce acute mountain sickness have been investigated, with limited success. High-carbohydrate diets have been recommended as a "nonpharmacological" method to reduce the symptoms associated with acute mountain sickness.[1] To be effective, these diets should be fed prior to and during the initial 3- to 4-d critical period of acute altitude exposure. It should be noted that only a limited number of investigators have studied high-carbohydrate diets or carbohydrate supplements for the relief of acute mountain sickness and performance enhancement. Most, but not all, have reported some beneficial effects upon symptoms, mood, and performance. Consolazio et al.[94] conducted a study at 14,000 ft elevation with two groups of young sea level natives transported abruptly to altitude. One group consumed a normal diet containing 35% of the calories in the form of carbohydrate. The second group consumed a diet containing approximately 70% of the calories from carbohydrate. The normal carbohydrate group was more nauseated, less energetic, and more depressed than the group consuming the high-carbohydrate diet. The normal carbohydrate group also experienced greater heart pounding, was more irritable, more tired, and less happy than the high carbohydrate group. They also felt less lively and experienced greater shortness of breath. Both groups experienced dizziness, cramping, headaches, and trouble sleeping to approximately the same degree. Work performance was compared in a relatively high-exertion, short-duration protocol consisting of walking on a treadmill at 3.5 mph on an 8% grade carrying a 20-kg pack. During the sea level control period all men completed the 15-min walk but at altitude, the normal carbohydrate group averaged only 4.5 min, while the high-carbohydrate group averaged 9.8 min until exhaustion. Askew et al.[89] studied exercise at high altitude under conditions designed to stress muscle glycogen stores. They abruptly transported three groups of soldiers from sea level to 4100 m (13,500 ft) elevation (summit of Mauna Kea, Hawaii). One group of solders remained sedentary and consumed a normal military field ration (45% carbohydrate) during 4 d at this elevation. The other two groups were paired according to their $\dot{V}O_2$ max determined at sea level and exercised for 2 h/d at altitude by running on a cross-country course at an exertion level of 70% of their maximum heart rate. One of the exercise groups consumed the same 45% carbohydrate ration as the sedentary group. The other exercise group consumed the same basal diet as the other two groups but received approximately 200 g of carbohydrate supplement per day through glucose polymer-supplemented beverages (approximately 40 g of carbohydrate per 8-oz beverage). The nonsupplemented groups consumed similar beverages sweetened with a non-nutritive sweetener. All beverages were provided *ad libitum*. The nonsupplemented group consumed an average of 190 g of carbohydrate per day, whereas the group receiving the carbohydrate supplement consumed an average of 400 g of carbohydrate per day during the 4 d at altitude. Total voluntary mileage covered during the 2 h/d running period was recorded daily. The carbohydrate-supplemented group logged a significantly greater ($p < .05$) 12% total miles covered over the course of this 4-d study. In addition to improving energy balance, carbohydrate supplementation also improved nitrogen balance in the initial phase of acute altitude exposure. Butterfield et al.[92] have confirmed that the negative nitrogen balances encountered at altitude is not due to any decrease in protein digestibility or absorption, but primarily due to negative energy balances.

The exact mechanism by which carbohydrate exerts a beneficial effect on relieving symptoms of altitude sickness and prolongs endurance at altitude is not known. Hansen et al.[95] showed that blood oxygen tension is increased by a high-carbohydrate diet and Dramise et al.[96] reported that carbohydrate can increase lung pulmonary diffusion capacity at altitude. The energy production per liter of oxygen uptake is greater when carbohydrate is the energy source compared to fat (carbohydrate, 5.05 kcal/l O_2; fat, 4.69 kcal/l O_2) regardless of the oxygen tension in the inspired air.[97] Taken together, these different lines of evidence suggest that carbohydrate is a more efficient energy source for work at reduced oxygen tension.[98] The beneficial effect of high-carbohydrate diets on physical performance at sea level is well known.[9] Carbohydrate can prolong endurance by its effect on muscle glycogen stores which are in turn closely related to endurance. It is unlikely that the ergogenic effect of the high-carbohydrate diets at altitude reported by Consolazio et al.[94] was related to a specific muscle glycogen effect, since the short exercise time periods (<10 min) should not have been limited by glycogen stores, but may have been related to the provision of blood glucose to the working hypoxic muscles. Caffeine has also been reported to enhance relatively short-term, high-intensity work at simulated high altitude,[99] perhaps via a similar influence upon blood glucose availability.

There is little evidence that chronic or acute altitude exposure increases the requirement for any specific nutrient[100] other than possibly vitamin E[10] and iron.[13] Some workers have noted that supplementation of vitamins having an antioxidant function may be desirable at high altitude.[10,14,101] Simon-Schnass[10] reported that supplemental vitamin E (2 × 200 mg daily) during a prolonged stay at high altitude prevented a "deterioration" of blood flow and a decrease in physical performance associated with free radical damage to cellular antioxidant defense systems. Simon-Schnass[10] theorized that the "oxidative stress" during

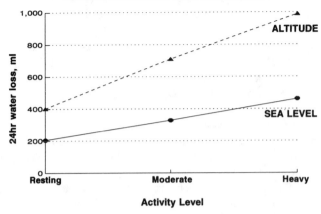

**Calculated 24 hour water respiratory loss during
rest and work at sea level and altitude**

FIGURE 5.   Calculation of 24-h respiratory water loss at three activity levels at sea level and at altitude. Resting and moderate estimations are at sea level and 5570 m. The estimation for heavy activity is at sea level (hill walking) and ~8000 m (climbing). Detailed information on the equations and assumptions involved in the calculation of these values can be found in Milledge, J., *Newsletter of the International Society for Mountain Medicine,* 2, 5, 1992. (After Milledge,[103] with permission.)

hypoxia is a consequence of alterations in the oxidation–reduction potential leading to lipid peroxidation and free radical production and subsequent oxidative injury to tissue and blood.

The suggestion that supplementary dietary iron may be beneficial at altitude stems from the observation that there is an increased erythropoietic response to altitude exposure as the oxygen delivery system of the blood attempts to support increased hemoglobin synthesis at high altitude.[83] Although Hornbein[102] concluded that normal dietary iron intakes are adequate to support increased hemoglobin synthesis for males at high altitude, Hannon[13] suggested that females exposed to high altitude may benefit from a dietary iron supplement.

Water requirements at altitude may be greater than those at sea level, due to the low humidity of the atmosphere at altitude and hyperventilation associated with altitude exposure.[13,55,98] Normal water consumption and normal to slightly reduced urine outputs at altitude (compared to sea level) can still lead to dehydration when accompanied by an increased rate of insensible water loss. The risk of dehydration is high at altitude due to water loss in breath and sweat coupled with the difficulty of obtaining adequate water.[103] Based upon the equations and assumptions of Ferrus et al.,[104] Milledge[103] has estimated that the rate of respiratory water loss is probably less than 1 l/d. This is still about twice the rate of respiratory water loss for an equivalent activity at sea level. Milledge[103] has calculated theoretical 24-h respiratory water loss at rest and at work at sea level and at high altitude. These predictions are shown in Figure 5.

An inappropriate thirst response coupled with an increase in insensible water loss and a transient diuresis during the initial hours of altitude exposure, can result in rapid dehydration if adequate fluid is either unavailable or neglected.[105]

High altitude and cold environments are often similar with respect to the thermal challenge, tempting one to categorize work in snow and cold at sea level with work under similar conditions at altitude. There are some distinct differences which should be considered when planning nutritional support at high altitude. Fat, while tolerated relatively well in the cold at sea level, may not be as well tolerated in diets at high altitude. The symptoms of acute altitude exposure may worsen, especially if fat displaces carbohydrate from the diet. Although high-fat foods are energy dense and reduce the weight/calorie aspect of food carried on

TABLE 4 Generalized Influence of Environment upon Nutrient Utilization

	Environment		
Utilization	Heat	Cold	Altitude
Dietary tolerance			
Carbohydrate	+	0	+
Fat	−	+	−
Protein	−	0	0
Metabolism			
Carbohydrate	+	+	+
Fat	0	+	−
Protein	0	0	0
Performance			
Carbohydrate	+[a]	+	+
Fat	−	0, +	−
Protein	−	0	0

Note: These generalizations are qualitative in nature and are drawn from the literature reviewed in this chapter. As with all generalizations, there are exceptions. A (+) indicates an augmentation, (−) a diminishment, and (0) is no change.

[a] The enhancement of performance by carbohydrate in the heat assumes adequate water.

climbs, fat requires more oxygen for metabolism than carbohydrate and will place a small, but added, burden upon the already overtaxed oxygen economy of the climber. Fat absorption may also be reduced as the climber exceeds elevations above 6300 m;[106] however, elevations commonly reached by recreational skiers, snowshoers, and backpackers are usually not associated with impaired fat absorption.[92] One other difference between cold exposure at sea level and high altitude is the calorigenic response to cold. Cold exposure during hypoxia results in an increased reliance upon shivering for thermogenesis due to a reduction in nonshivering thermogenesis at altitude.[107,108] Robinson and Haymes[108] suggested that this is due to a reduction in aerobic catabolism of free fatty acids during hypoxia.

Inappropriate thirst and appetite responses, together with increased insensible water loss, transient diuresis, and increased energy expenditures, can lead to rapid dehydration and glycogen depletion if adequate food and fluid is neglected. Dehydration may intensify the symptoms of altitude sickness and result in even lower food intakes. One of the most effective and practical performance-sustaining measures that can be adopted upon arrival at high altitude is to consume a minimum of 3 to 4 l of fluid per day containing 200 to 300 g of carbohydrate in addition to that contained in the diet. This should prevent dehydration, improve energy balance, improve the oxygen delivery capability of the circulatory system, replenish muscle glycogen, and conserve body protein levels.

VI. SUMMARY

A generalized summary of the influence of environment upon nutrient utilization is depicted in Table 4. The challenge of providing adequate nutrition in environmental extremes is one of furnishing a palatable diet generally high in carbohydrate to meet high energy demands. Adequate fluid replacement is critical in any environment. Dehydration can reduce appetite and compromise thermoregulation. Practical dietary recommendations can be made

TABLE 5 Do's and Don'ts for Recreational and Expedition Meal Planning

DO provide group/hot meals whenever possible. People will generally eat more when warm meals are consumed "socially".

DON'T assume that everyone is eating adequately in group feeding situations. A meal prepared is not necessarily a meal eaten.

DO schedule breaks for meals and snacks even when individual food will be consumed for the meal or snack. Left to their own initiative people will frequently skip or shorten meals to accomplish tasks they feel are more "important".

DON'T allow snack food to substitute for meals. Snacks should augment or supplement daily meals, primarily as a means to increase total daily energy or carbohydrate intake. Snacks should be a morale and performance booster, not an obsession.

DO observe what food items are being consumed. Picky dietary habits can lead to imbalances of vitamins, minerals, or energy. Vitamin and mineral supplements are usually not needed; a multivitamin supplement can provide some "insurance" for finicky eaters.

DON'T permit individuals to use the expedition as a "crash" weight loss program. Dehydrated, ketotic, and weak team members jeopardize the safety of others as well as themselves.

DO encourage water consumption with meals. Meal time is often a major fluid consumption point due to the opportunity to prepare beverages, soups, and other water-containing food items.

DON'T permit food and personal hygiene to slip just because you are in the field. Clean hands, clean utensils, and disinfected water are requisite for safe food preparation.

to optimize performance in environmental extremes. Some practical guidelines for recreational or expedition meal planning in environmental extremes are shown in Table 5. Proper nutrition can prevent or minimize performance decrements that often accompany environmental stress and help to make a "hostile" environment a bit less "hostile".

ACKNOWLEDGMENTS

The assistance of Sharon L. Askew and Deborah Jezior in the preparation of this manuscript is gratefully acknowledged.

REFERENCES

1. **Askew, E. W.,** Nutrition and performance under adverse environmental conditions, in *Nutrition in Exercise and Sport,* Hickson, J. F., Jr. and Wolinsky, I., Eds., CRC Press, Boca Raton, FL, 1989, 367.
2. **Shepherd, R. J.,** Adaptation to exercise in the cold, *Sports Med.,* 2, 59, 1985.
3. **Knochel, J. P.,** Environmental heat illness, *Arch. Intern. Med.,* 133, 841, 1974.
4. **Buskirk, E. R.,** Decrease in physical working capacity at high altitude, in *Biomedicine of High Terrestrial Elevations,* Hegnauer, A. H., Ed., Technical Report No. 68-50, U.S. Army Research Institute of Environmental Medicine, Natick, MA, January, 1969, p. 204.
5. **Moore, R. J., Friedl, K. E., Kramer, T. R., Martinez-Lopez, L. E., Hoyt, R. W., Tulley, R. E., Delany, J. P., Askew, E. W., and Vogel, J. A.,** *Changes in Soldier Nutritional Status and Immune Function During the Ranger Training Course,* Technical Report No. T13-92, U.S. Army Research Institute of Environmental Medicine, Natick, MA, September, 1992.
6. **Gisolfi, C. V.,** Impact of limited fluid intake on performance, in *Predicting Decrements in Military Performance Due to Inadequate Nutrition,* National Academy Press, Washington, D.C., 1986, 17.
7. **Hubbard, R. W., Armstrong, L. E., Evans, P. K., and DeLuca, J. P.,** Long-term water and salt deficits — a military perspective, in *Predicting Decrements in Military Performance Due to Inadequate Nutrition,* National Academy Press, Washington, D.C., 1986, 29.
8. **Johnson, H. L.,** Practical military implications of fluid and nutritional imbalances for performances, in *Predicting Decrements in Military Performance Due to Inadequate Nutrition,* National Academy Press, Washington, D.C., 1986, 55.

9. **Askew, E. W.,** Effect of protein, fat and carbohydrate deficiencies on performance, in *Predicting Decrements in Military Performance Due to Inadequate Nutrition,* National Academy Press, Washington, D.C., 1986, 189.

10. **Simon-Schnass, I. M.,** Nutrition at high altitude, *J. Nutr.,* 122, 778, 1992.

11. **Strydhom, N. B., Kotze, M. E., van der Walt, W. H., and Rogers, G. G.,** Effect of ascorbic acid on rate of heat acclimation, *J. Appl. Physiol.,* 41, 202, 1976.

12. **Early, R. G. and Carlson, B. R.,** Water-soluble vitamin therapy in the delay of fatigue from physical activity in hot climatic conditions, *Int. Z. Angew. Physiol.,* 27, 43, 1969.

13. **Hannon, J. P.,** Nutrition at high altitude, in *Environment Physiology: Aging, Heat and Attitude,* Horvath, S. M. and Yousef, M. K., Eds., Elsevier, Amsterdam, 1980, 309.

14. **van der Beek, E. J.,** Vitamin supplementation and physical exercise performance, *J. Sports Sci.,* 9, 77, 1991.

15. **Hargreaves, M.,** Carbohydrates and exercise, *J. Sports Sci.,* 9, 17, 1991.

16. **Consolazio, C. F.,** Nutrient requirements of troops in extreme environments, *Army Research and Development Newsmagazine,* November 1966, p. 24.

17. **Westerterp, K. R. and Saris, W. H. M.,** Limits of energy turnover in relation to physical performance, achievement of energy balance on a daily basis, *J. Sports Sci.,* 9, 1, 1991.

18. **Barclay, C. J. and Loiselle, D. S.,** Dependence of muscle fatigue on stimulation protocol: effect of hypocaloric diet, *J. Appl. Physiol.,* 72, 2278, 1992.

19. **Askew, E. W., Munro, I., Sharp, M. A., Siegel, S., Popper, R., Rose, M. S., Hoyt, R. W., Martin, J. W., Reynolds, K., Lieberman, H. R., Engell, D., and Shaw, C. P.,** Nutritional Status and Physical and Mental Performance of Special Operations Soldiers Consuming the Ration, Lightweight, or the Meal, Ready-to-Eat Military Field Ratio During a 30-Day Field Training Field Training Exercise, Technical Report No. T7-87, U.S. Army Research Institute of Environmental Medicine, Natick, MA, March, 1987.

20. **Phinney, S. D., Bistrian, B. R., Evans, W. J., Gervino, E., and Blackburn, G. L.,** The human metabolic response to chronic ketosis without caloric restriction: preservation of submaximal exercise capability with reduced carbohydrate oxidation, *Metabolism,* 32, 769, 1983.

21. **Young, A. J.,** Energy substrate utilization during exercise in extreme environments, in *Exercise and Sport Sciences Reviews,* Vol. 18, Pandolf, K. B., Ed., Williams & Wilkins, Baltimore, 1990, 65.

22. **Brooks, G. A., Wolfel, E. E., Groves, B. M., Bender, P. R., Butterfield, G. E., Cymerman, A., Mazzeo, R. S., Sutton, J. R., Wolfe, R. R., and Reeves, J. T.,** Muscle accounts for glucose disposal but not blood lactate appearance during exercise after acclimatization to 4,300 m, *J. Appl. Physiol.,* 72, 2435, 1992.

23. **Sawka, M. N. and Neufer, P. D.,** Interaction of water bioavailability, thermoregulation and exercise performance, in *Fluid Replacement and Heat Stress,* Marriott, B. M., and Rosemont C., Eds., National Academy Press, Washington, D.C., 1989, VII-1.

24. **Sawka, M. N., Francesconi, R. P., Young, A. J., and Pandolf, K. B.,** Influence of hydration level and body fluids on exercise performance in heat, *JAMA,* 252, 1165, 1984.

25. **Sawka, M. N., Young, A. J., Francesconi, R. P., Muza, S. R., and Pandolf, K. B.,** Thermoregulatory and blood response during exercise at graded hypohydration levels, *J. Appl. Physiol.,* 59, 1394, 1985.

26. **Young, A. J., Sawka, M. N., Levine, L., Cadarette, B. S., and Pandolf, K. B.,** Skeletal muscle metabolism during exercise is influenced by heat acclimation, *J. Appl. Physiol.,* 59, 1929, 1985.

27. **Armstrong, L. E.,** Is fluid intake important in the control of body temperature? If yes, which fluid is best in a hot environment?, *Nat. Strength Conditioning Assoc. J.,* 13, 68, 1991.

28. **Brouns, F.,** Heat-sweat-dehydration-rehydration: a praxis oriented approach, *J. Sports Sci.,* 9, 143, 1991.

29. **Maughan, R. J.,** Fluid and electrolyte loss and replacement in exercise, *J. Sports Sci.,* 9, 117, 1991.

30. **Shapiro, Y., Pandolf, K. B., and Goldman, R. F.,** Predicting sweat loss response to exercise, environment and clothing, *Eur. J. Appl. Physiol.,* 48, 83, 1982.

31. **Pandolf, K. B., Stroschein, L. A., Drolet, L. L., Gonzalez, R. R., and Sawka, M. N.,** Prediction modeling of physiological responses and human performance in the heat, *Comput. Biol. Med.,* 16, 319, 1986.

32. **Glenn, J. F., Burr, R. E., Hubbard, R. E., Mays, M. Z., Moore, R. J., Jones, B. H., and Krueger, G. P.,** Sustaining Health and Performance in the Desert: Environmental Medicine Guidance for Operations in Southwest Asia, Technical Note No. 91-1, U.S. Army Research Institute of Environmental Medicine, Natick, MA, December, 1990.

33. **Hubbard, R. W., Mager, M., and Kerstein, M.,** Water as a tactical weapon: a doctrine for preventing heat casualties, *Proc. Army Sci. Conf.,* 2, 125, 1982.

34. **Beauchamp, G. K.,** The human preference for excess salt., *Am. Sci.,* 75, 27, 1987.

35. **Armstrong, L. E., Hubbard, R. W., Askew, E. W., DeLuca, J. P., O'Brian, C., Pasqualicchio, A., and Francesconi, R. P.,** Response to moderate and low sodium diets during exercise-heat acclimation, *Int. J. Sports Nutr.,* in press.

36. **Costill, D. L.,** Sweating: its composition and effects on body fluids, in *The Marathon: Physiological, Medical, Epidemiological and Psychological Studies,* Milvy, P., Ed., New York Academy of Sciences, New York, 1977, 160.

37. **Barr, S. I., Costill, D. L., and Fink, W. J.,** Fluid replacement during prolonged exercise: effects of water, saline, or no fluid, *Med. Sci. Sports Exercise,* 23, 811, 1991.

38. **Baker, E. M., Plough, I. C., and Allen, T. H.,** Water requirements of men as related to salt intake, *Am. J. Clin. Nutr.,* 12, 394, 1963.

39. **Greenleaf, J. E.,** Environmental issues that influence intake of replacement beverages, in *Fluid Replacement and Heat Stress,* Marriott, B. M., and Rosemont, C., Eds., National Academy Press, Washington, D.C., 1989, 15.

40. **Consolazio, C. F., Matoush, L. O., Nelson, R. A., Torres, J. B., and Isaac, G. J.,** Environmental temperature and energy expenditures, *J. Appl. Physiol.,* 18, 65, 1963.

41. **Sawka, M. N., Pandolf, K. B., Avellini, B. A., and Shapiro, Y.,** Does heat acclimation lower the rate of metabolism elicited by muscular exercise?, *Aviat. Space Environ. Med.,* 54, 27, 1983.

42. **Fink, W. J., Costill, D. L., and van Handel, P. J.,** Leg muscle metabolism during exercise in the heat and cold, *Eur. J. Appl. Physiol.,* 34, 183, 1975.

43. **Nielsen, B., Savard, G., Richter, E. A., Hargreaves, M., and Saltin, B.,** Muscle blood flow and muscle metabolism during exercise and heat stress, *J. Appl. Physiol.,* 69, 1040, 1990.

44. **Neufer, P. D., Sawka, M. N., Young, A. J., Quigley, M. D., Latzka, W. A., and Levine, L.,** Hypohydration does not impair skeletal muscle glycogen resynthesis after exercise, *J. Appl. Physiol.,* 70, 1490, 1991.

45. **Lyons, T. P., Riedesel, M. L., Meuli, L. E., and Chick, T. W.,** Effects of glycerol-induced hyperhydration prior to exercise in the heat on sweating and core temperature, *Med. Sci. Sports Exercise,* 22, 477, 1990.

46. **Askew, E. W.,** Nutrition for a cold environment, *Physician Sportsmed.,* 17, 77, 1989.

47. **Stroud, M. A.,** Effects on energy expenditure of facial cooling during exercise, *Eur. J. Appl. Physiol.,* 63, 376, 1991.

48. **Henschell, A.,** Energy balance in cold environments, in *Cold Injury,* Horvath, S. M., Ed., Josiah Macy Foundation, New York, 1960, 303.

49. **Campbell, I. T.,** Nutrition in adverse environments. II. Energy balance under polar conditions, *Hum. Nutr. Appl. Nutr.,* 36A, 165, 1982.

50. **Johnson, R. E. and Kark, R. M.,** Environment and food intake in man, *Science,* 105, 378, 1947.

51. **Gray, E. L., Consolazio, C. F., and Kark, R. M.,** Nutritional requirements for men at work in cold, temperature and hot environments, *J. Appl. Physiol.,* 4, 270, 1951.

52. **Teitlebaum, A. and Goldman, R. F.,** Increased energy cost with multiple clothing layers, *J. Appl. Physiol.,* 32, 743, 1972.

53. **Romet, T. T., Shephard, R. J., Frim, J., and Goode, R. C.,** The metabolic cost of exercising in cold air ($-20°C$), *Arctic Med. Res.,* 47 (Suppl. 1), 280, 1988.

54. **Consolazio, C. F.,** Energy metabolism and extreme environments (heat, cold, high altitude), *Proc. 8th Int. Cong. Nutr.,* Excerpta Medica Int. Cong. Ser. Amsterdam, No. 213, 1969.

55. **Buskirk, E. R. and Mendez, J.,** Nutrition, environment and work performance with special reference to altitude, *Fed. Proc.,* 26, 1760, 1967.

56. **Delany, J. P., Moore, R. J., and Hoyt, R. W.,** Use of doubly labeled water for energy expenditure of soldiers during training exercises in a cold environment, *Int. J. Obesity,* 15, 48, 1991.

57. **Nobmann, E. D., Byers, T., Lanier, A. P., Hankin, J. H., and Jackson, M. Y.,** The diet of Alaska native adults: 1987–1988, *Am. J. Clin. Nutr.,* 55, 1024, 1992.

58. **Swain, H. L., Toth, F. M., Consolazio, C. F., Fitzpatrick, W. H., Allen, D. J., and Koehn, C. J.,** Food consumption of soldiers in a subarctive climate (Fort Churchill, Manitoba, Canada, 1947–1948), *J. Nutr.,* 38, 63, 1949.

59. **Rodahl, K.,** Nutritional requirements in cold climates, *J. Nutr.,* 53, 575, 1954.

60. **Rodahl, K., Horvath, S. M., Birkhead, N. C., and Issekutz, B., Jr.,** Effects of dietary protein on physical work capacity during severe cold stress, *J. Appl. Physiol.,* 17, 763, 1962.

61. **Bjorntorp, P.,** Importance of fat as a support nutrient for energy: metabolism of athletes, *J. Sports Sci.,* 9, 71, 1991.

62. **Ekstedt, B., Jonsson, E., and Johnson, O.,** Influence of dietary fat, cholesterol and energy on serum lipids at vigorous physical exercise, *Scand. J. Clin. Lab. Invest.,* 51, 437, 1991.

63. **Mitchell, H. H., Glickman, N., Lambert, E. H., Keeton, R. W., and Fahnestock, M. K.,** The tolerance of man to cold as affected by dietary modification: carbohydrate versus fat and the effect of the frequency of meals, *Am. J. Physiol.,* 146, 84, 1946.

64. **Vallerand, A. L. and Jacobs, I.,** Rates of energy substrates utilization during human cold exposure, *Eur. J. Appl. Physiol.,* 58, 873, 1989.

65. **Haight, J. S. J. and Keating, W. R.,** Failure of thermoregulation induced by exercise and ethanol, *J. Physiol.,* 229, 87, 1973.

66. **MacDonald, I. A., Bennett, T., and Sainsburg, R.,** The effect of a 48 hour fast on the thermoregulatory responses to graded cooling in man, *Clin. Sci.,* 67, 445, 1984.

67. **Jacobs, I., Romet, T. T., and Kerrigan-Brown, D.,** Muscle glycogen depletion during exercise at 9°C and 21°C, *Eur. J. Appl. Physiol.,* 54, 35, 1985.

68. **Martineau, L. and Jacobs, I.,** Muscle glycogen availability and temperature regulation in humans, *J. Appl. Physiol.,* 66, 72, 1989.

69. **Martineau, L. and Jacobs, I.,** Muscle glycogen utilization during shivering thermogenesis in humans, *J. Appl. Physiol.,* 65, 2046, 1988.

70. **Wolfe, R. R., Klein, S., Carraro, F., and Weber, J. M.,** Role of triglyceride-fatty acid cycle in controlling fat metabolism in humans during and after exercise, *Am. J. Physiol.,* 258, E382, 1990.

71. **Young, A. J., Sawka, M. N., Neufer, P. D., Muza, S. R., Askew, E. W., and Pandolf, K. B.,** Thermoregulation during cold water immersion is unimpaired by low muscle glycogen levels, *J. Appl. Physiol.,* 66, 1809, 1989.

72. **Martineau, L. and Jacobs, I.,** Effects of muscle glycogen and plasma FFA availability on human metabolic responses in cold water, *J. Appl. Physiol.,* 71, 1331, 1991.

73. **Vallerand, A. L., Jacobs, I., and Kavanagh, M. F.,** Mechanism of enhanced cold tolerance by an ephedrine-caffeine mixture in humans, *J. Appl. Physiol.,* 67, 438, 1989.

74. **Welch, B. E., Buskirk, E. R., and Iampietro, P. F.,** Relation of climate and temperature to food and water intake in man, *Metabolism,* 7, 141, 1958.

75. **Roberts, D. E., Patton, J. F., Pennycook, J. W., Jacey, M. J., Tappan, D. V., Gray, P., and Heyder, E.,** Effects of Restricted Water Intake on Performance in a Cold Environment, Technical Report, No. T2/84, U.S. Army Research Institute of Environmental Medicine, Natick, MA, 1984.

76. **Jones, T. E.,** unpublished observations, U.S. Army Research Institute of Environmental Medicine, Natick, MA, 1993.

77. **Edwards, J. S. A. and Roberts, D. E.,** The influence of a calorie supplement on the consumption of the meal, ready-to-eat in a cold environment, *Milit. Med.,* 156, 466, 1991.

78. **Edwards, J. S. A., Roberts, D. E., and Mutter, S. H.,** Rations for use in a cold environment, *J. Wilderness Med.,* 3, 27, 1992.

79. **King, N., Mutter, S. H., Roberts, D. E., Sutherland, M. R., and Askew, E. W.,** Field feeding the army in Alaska during a cold weather field training exercise: evaluation of the 18-man arctic tray pack ratio module, the Meal, Ready-to-Eat and the Long Life Ration Packet, *Milit. Med.,* 158(7), July 1993, in press.

80. **Dann, E. J., Gillis, S., and Burstein, R.,** Effect of fluid intake on renal function during exercise in the cold, *Eur. J. Appl. Physiol.,* 61, 133, 1990.

81. **Young, A. J., Roberts, D. E., Scott, D. P., Cook, J. E., Mays, M. Z., and Askew, E. W.,** Sustaining Health and Performance in the Cold: Environmental Medicine Guidance for Cold-Weather Operations, Technical Note No. 92-2, U.S. Army Research Institute of Environmental Medicine, Natick, MA, 1992.

82. **Wilson, R. P. and Culik, B. M.,** The cost of a hot meal: facultative specific dynamic action may ensure temperature homeostasis in post-ingestive endotherms, *Comp. Biochem. Physiol.,* 100A, 151, 1991.

83. **Haymes, E. M. and Wells, C. L.,** Altitude and Performance, in *Environment and Human Performance,* Human Kinetics Publishers, Champaign, IL, 1986, 69.

84. **Evans, W. O., Robinson, S. M., Horstman, D. H., Jackson, R. E., and Weiskopf, R. B.,** Amelioration of the symptoms of acute mountain sickness by staging and acetazolamide, *Aviat. Space Environ. Med.,* 47, 512, 1976.

85. **Hansen, J. E., Harris, C. W., and Evans, W. O.,** Influence of elevation of origin, rate of ascent and a physical conditioning program on symptoms of acute mountain sickness, *Milit. Med.,* 132, 585, 1967.

86. **Shukitt-Hale, B., Banderet, L. E., and Lieberman, H. R.,** Relationships between symptoms, moods, performance, and acute mountain sickness at 4700 meters, *Aviat. Space Environ. Med.,* 62, 865, 1991.

87. **Carson, R. P., Evans, W. O., Shields, J. L., and Hannon, J. P.,** Symptomatology, pathophysiology, and treatment of acute mountain sickness, *Fed. Proc.,* 28, 1085, 1969.

88. **Johnson, H. L., Consolazio, C. F., Krzywicki, H. J., and Isaac, G. J.,** Increased energy requirements of man after abrupt altitude exposure, *Nutr. Rep. Int.,* 4, 77, 1971.

89. **Askew, E. W., Claybaugh, J. R., Hashiro, G. M., Stokes, W. S., Sato, A., and Cucinell, S. A.,** Mauna Kea. III. Metabolic Effects of Dietary Carbohydrate Supplementation During Exercise at 4100 m Altitude, Technical Report No. T12-87, U.S. Army Research Institute of Environmental Medicine, Natick, MA, May 1987.

90. **Reynolds, R. D., Howard, M. P., Deuster, P., Lickteig, J. A., Conway, J., Rumpler, W., and Seale, J.,** Energy intakes and expenditures on Mt. Everest, *FASEB J.,* 6, A1084, 1992.

91. **Edwards, J. S. A., Askew, E. W., King, N., Fulco, C. S., Hoyt, R. W., and DeLany, J. P.,** An Assessment of the Nutritional Intake and Energy Expenditure of Unacclimatized U.S. Army Soldiers Living and Working at High Altitude, Technical Report No. T/10-91, U.S. Army Research Institute of Environmental Medicine, Natick, MA, June 1991.

92. **Butterfield, G. E., Gates, J., Fleming, S., Brooks, G. A., Sutton, J. R., and Reeves, J. T.,** Increased energy intake minimizes weight loss in men at high altitude, *J. Appl. Physiol.,* 72, 1741, 1992.

93. **Rose, M. S., Houston, C. S., Fulco, C. S., Coates, G., Sutton, J. R., and Cymerman, A.,** Operation Everest. II. Nutrition and body composition, *J. Appl. Physiol.,* 65, 2545, 1988.

94. **Consolazio, C. F., Matoush, L. O., Johnson, H. L., Krzywicki, H. J., Daws, T. A., and Isaac, G. J.,** Effects of high-carbohydrate diets on performance and clinical symptomatology after rapid ascent to high altitude, *Fed. Proc.,* 28, 937, 1969.

95. **Hansen, J. E., Hartley, L. H., and Hogan, R. P.,** Arterial oxygen increase by high-carbohydrate diet at altitude, *J. Appl. Physiol.,* 33, 441, 1972.

96. **Dramise, J. G., Inouye, C. M., Christensen, B. M., Fults, R. D., Canham, J. E., and Consolazio, C. F.,** Effects of a glucose meal on human pulmonary function at 1600 m and 4300 m altitudes, *Aviat. Space Environ. Med.,* 46, 365, 1975.

97. **Durnin, J. V. G. A. and Passmore, R., Eds.,** *Energy, Work and Leisure,* Heinemann, London, 1967, 16.

98. **Maher, J. T.,** Nutrition and altitude acclimatization, in *Handbook of Nutritional Requirements in a Functional Context,* Volume 2, Rechcigl, M. R., Jr., Ed., CRC Press, Boca Raton, FL, 1981, 549.

99. **Fulco, C. S., Rock, P. B., Trad, L. A., Rose, M. S., Forte, V. A., Young, P. M., and Cymerman, A.,** The Effect of Caffeine on Endurance Time to Exhaustion at High Altitude, Technical Report No. T17-89, U.S. Army Research Institute of Environmental Medicine, Natick, MA, 1989.

100. **Agnew, J.,** A review of the effects of high altitude on nutrition in man, *Nutr. Rep. Int.,* 32, 187, 1985.

101. **Aldashev, A. A.,** Metabolic basis for dietary recommendations under alpine conditions, *Alma-Ata Zdravookhraneiye Kazakhstana,* (No. 7) July, 1985, p. 35.

102. **Hornbein, T. F.,** Evaluation of iron stores as limiting high-altitude polycythemia, *J. Appl. Physiol.,* 17, 243, 1962.

103. **Milledge, J.,** Respiratory water loss at altitude, *Newsletter Int. Soc. Mountain Med.,* 2 (No. 3), 5, 1992.

104. **Ferrus, L., Commenges, D., Gire, J., and Varene, P.,** Respiratory water loss as a function of ventilatory or environmental factors, *Res. Physiol.,* 56, 11, 1984.

105. **Krzywicki, H. J., Consolazio, C. F., Johnson, H. L., Nielsen, W. C., and Barnhart, R. A.,** Water metabolism in humans during acute high-altitude exposure, *J. Appl. Physiol.,* 30, 806, 1971.

106. **Boyer, S. J. and Blume, F. D.,** Weight loss and changes in body composition at high altitude, *J. Appl. Physiol.,* 57, 1580, 1984.

107. **Blatteis, C. M. and Lutherer, L. O.,** Effect of altitude exposure on thermoregulatory response of man to cold, *J. Appl. Physiol.,* 41, 848, 1976.

108. **Robinson, K. A. and Haymes, E. M.,** Metabolic effects of exposure to hypoxia plus cold at rest and during exercise in humans, *J. Appl. Physiol.,* 68, 720, 1990.

Chapter 20

IMMUNE FUNCTION IN EXERCISE, SPORT, AND INACTIVITY

Laurie Hoffman-Goetz
Ronald Ross Watson

CONTENTS

0-8493-7911-3/94/$0.00+$.50
© 1994 by CRC Press, Inc.

I. INTRODUCTION

The concept that exercise modulates immunological responses derives primarily from three types of observations:

1. Acute physical stress (e.g., rotational, restraint, handling, surgical) influences a variety of immune parameters.
2. Many of the neuroendocrine changes elicited by acute physical and psychological stress, such as increased sympathetic activity and elevated epinephrine and cortisol levels, also occur during intense exercise.
3. Increased episodes of infectious disease, especially of the upper respiratory tract, have been reported to occur (although mainly anecdotal) in athletes during periods of intense training.

In addition, psychologically stressful events have been correlated with an increased incidence of various infections;[1,2] competitive exercise also involves a measure of psychological stress. In contrast, the biological rationale for linking exercise conditioning and fitness with persistent changes in immune function stems, in part, from several reports of reduced growth of experimental tumors in animals given long-term exercise training.[3-6] Although spontaneously arising cancers in humans are largely nonimmunogenic, several natural immune mechanisms, including macrophage and natural killer (NK)-cell-mediated cytotoxicity, are thought to serve as a first line of defense; it is, therefore, tempting to speculate that if training results in persistent changes in natural immunity, then this should be reflected in some alteration in the growth of tumors.

This review focuses on the effects of physical conditioning, exercise, and inactivity on the immune system, and in particular on cellular and natural immune mechanisms. The term *cellular immunity* refers to immunological effects mediated by specifically sensitized lymphocytes. *Natural immunity* involves that aspect of host defense that does not display specificity to antigen (or only partial specificity) and includes NK cells, macrophages, and other phagocytic cells.

Whenever possible, the immunological changes in humans undergoing exercise is described. However, since much of the recent work on exercise and immune functions has been done in animal models, examples of these are given with a view of what might occur in humans. In addition, the clinical relevance of exercise-mediated changes in immune functions will be considered. If exercise significantly changes immune functions or if immune parameters change during prolonged inactivity, this is potentially of critical importance for overall health. The nutritionist who is monitoring changes in dietary consumption during inactivity or activity and evaluating health risks needs this relationship defined. Therefore, it is appropriate to review various areas of the research literature that relate to physical fitness and immune function. These range from the effects of weightlessness and inactivity in astronauts, to the effects of short bouts of intense exercise by athletes, to the effects of moderate-intensity training programs by average, healthy individuals. Recent reviews on general aspects of exercise and immunity,[7,8] exercise and immunoglobulins,[9] and exercise, immunity, and cancer[10] are available.

II. ACUTE EXERCISE AND IMMUNE FUNCTIONS

Perhaps the most widely utilized paradigm to assess the impact of exercise on immunity has been that of a single aerobic exercise session. Despite variations in the type, duration, and intensity of the work, the timing of the immune assessments, and differences in initial fitness levels of the subjects, several consistent patterns emerge regarding leukocyte and lymphocyte numbers. First, physical exercise results in a transient leukocytosis which quickly returns to preexercise values.[11-22] Most studies suggest that the basal number of leukocytes and the leukocytosis following acute exercise are not changed by exercise training.[15,16,23]

An exception to this is a recent study[17] in which the absolute number of leukocytes (neutrophils) obtained from subjects at rest was smaller after than before training. Second, the transient increase in leukocyte number includes a striking lymphocytosis with a portion of the lymphocytosis due to an increase in the absolute or relative numbers of NK cells.[17,18,20,24-26] The absolute or relative numbers of T-lymphocyte subsets, defined by monoclonal antibodies, is more variable, with some studies reporting an increase in cytotoxic/suppressor (CD8 +) phenotypes[17,18] and others reporting no changes in the cytotoxic/suppressor population after exercise.[20,24,27,28] Field et al.[20] suggest that the differences observed in the proportion of cytotoxic/suppressor lymphocytes after exercise may reflect changes in cell density and subsequent recovery in density gradients and/or contamination by a subset of NK cells that expresses low levels of the CD8 + antigen. Alternatively, this difference in reports of the CD8 + subset of lymphocytes after exercise may reflect sampling times; a recent study[29] demonstrated that the total number of CD8 + cells increased overproportionately immediately after cessation of intensive exercise to exhaustion (0 and 5 min postexercise) followed by a rapid drop below preexercise values at +30 and +60 min. The phenomenon of exercise-mediated leukocytosis and lymphocytosis appears to characterize pathophysiological as well as normal physiological conditions. For example, in a clinical case report of a patient with leukemia, strenuous exercise was associated with a striking leukocytosis, lymphocytosis, and an increase in CD8 + lymphocytes and large granular lymphocytes.[30]

The physiological mechanisms accounting for the leukocytosis/lymphocytosis of exercise have been suggested to include the effects of catecholamines and corticosteroids on leukocyte mobilization, interaction between leukocytes and endothelial cells in terms of adhesion, differences in the density of β-adrenergic receptors on the various leukocyte populations, and differential involvement of leukocytes in extravascular tissues.[17,31-34] However, in one recent study[35] neither the initial increase nor the subsequent decrease in plasma cortisol concentration after maximal exercise was essential for the magnitude of the delayed leukocytosis. Furthermore, although the number of β-adrenergic receptors varies among T-lymphocyte subsets, only natural killer cells show an increase in the number of receptors *in vivo* with dynamic exercise.[36]

The *in vitro* proliferative response of lymphocytes to mitogenic stimuli is a commonly used method to characterize functional status. A limited number of studies have assessed the proliferative responses of human and rodent lymphocytes isolated after exercise. The majority of reports indicate that lymphocyte responses to T-cell mitogens are reduced after a single episode of exercise.[20,28,37-41] In contrast, a brisk 45-min walking bout was reported not to affect lymphocyte mitogenic responses to Concanavalin A.[42] The direction of the effect of acute exercise on B-lymphocyte proliferative responses tends to suggest a similar immunosuppression after exercise; reductions were observed in the numbers of IgG, IgM, and IgA-secreting B cells after stimulation with pokeweed mitogen[43] and in mouse splenic-lymphocyte proliferation to lipopolysaccharide in trained animals immediately after an exhaustive exercise.[44]

Delineation of the biological mechanisms involved in the acute exercise-mediated suppression in lymphocyte mitogenesis is fundamental to understanding the potential health impact of this phenomenon. Several factors appear to be potentially involved:

1. Exercise-associated increases in endogenous opioids may contribute to the immunosuppression since subcutaneous injection of naltrexone before an acute swimming session in rats blocks the expected immunosuppression to mitogen.[45]
2. Acute exercise is associated with increased *in vitro* monocyte/macrophage production of prostaglandin E (PGE) during and for 2 h after an exercise session.[46] PGE is thought to have down-regulatory effects on various functions of macrophages, including IL-1β release,[47] and it is possible that a reduction in IL-1 release could attenuate the early signaling events in T-helper lymphocytes.

Indeed, there is evidence to suggest that the functional balance between IL-1 and PGE production by monocytes determines whether suppression or augmentation is observed.[47] Nevertheless, the PGE/IL-1 hypothesis has been difficult to reconcile with the observed data on IL-1 levels after exercise; the production of this cytokine has been reported to increase after exercise when measured by the thymocyte proliferation assay or bioassay.[48,49] Moreover, membrane-bound and perivascular IL-1β has been demonstrated in skeletal muscle after strenuous, eccentric exercise.[50] These observations notwithstanding, it is likely that the increase in IL-1 levels reflects the specific sampling time, the plasma volume changes concomitant with exercise, and the extent of skeletal muscle damage with exercise (e.g., eccentric exercise). A recent study which utilized a specific RIA to assay plasma IL-1 concentration and which presented concentrations corrected for plasma volume shifts found that IL-1 levels were unchanged 2 h after cycle ergometry (concentric) exercise relative to preexercise levels.[51]

3. It is possible that the exercise-associated reduction in mitogenesis reflects differential responsiveness to mitogens of specific subpopulations of T cells from exercised vs. nonexercised subjects. In this regard, Randall Simpson et al.[52] found an increased percentage of cytotoxic/suppressor mouse splenic lymphocytes (Lyt-2+ cells) in culture from animals given exhaustive exercise relative to controls.

The effects of acute exercise on the production of other immunoregulatory cytokines have been investigated only to a limited extent, and often the direction of the exercise effects is confusing. For example, IL-2 production from mitogen-stimulated lymphocytes is reduced[28] or increased[53] after exercise. One study reported both a decrease and an increase in plasma IL-2 levels after exercise depending upon sampling time: reductions for up to 2 h with an increase above resting values by 24 h after exercise.[54] Tumor necrosis factor (TNF) α was significantly increased after a 5-km race[54] or 2.5 h of running.[55] The physiological significance of an increase in TNF molecules after exercise is not known. However, recent evidence shows that not only are TNFs able to kill certain target cells, TNFα has the capacity to alter the susceptibility of cells to reactive oxygen species;[56] this observation is especially noteworthy given that blood antioxidant enzymes, glutathione peroxidase and catalase, increase in response to endurance training[57] or to the related lifestyle, such as increased intake of vitamin E and ascorbic acid. To date, there is only one report of exercise increasing the plasma levels of interferon-α.[58]

Short, vigorous exercise is likely to enhance several aspects of neutrophil and macrophage phagocytic capacity. Neutrophil activation, as measured by myeloperoxidase concentration (a neutrophil enzyme involved in oxygen-dependent killing of phagocytosed particles), was increased after extremely short (<10 min), vigorous ergometry exercise.[59] Neutrophil H_2O_2 production, as an indicator of microbicidal activity, was elevated after 1 h of aerobic exercise at 60% of $\dot{V}O_2$ max,[60] but was depressed in another study in which subjects were exercised at a comparable workload and in which neutrophils were stimulated with phorbol myristate acetate to generate hydrogen peroxide.[61] Dziedziak[62] found that granulocyte chemiluminescence (a measure of metabolic activity) increased after light cycling exercise (50% of $\dot{V}O_2$ max) and decreased after intense exercise (80% of $\dot{V}O_2$ max). In another measure of neutrophil function, Rodriguez et al.[63] reported that opsonization of *Candida albicans* and candidicide capacity increased significantly after exercise. Macrophage phagocytic functions (apart from the role that macrophages play in IL-1 and PGE generation) were increased after a single exhaustive 15-km run in humans[64] and after swimming to exhaustion in rats.[65] Interestingly, Voronina and Mayanskii[66] found that in mice and rats, exercise reduced the number of blood monocytes and peritoneal macrophages while the number of alveolar macrophages was increased. Tissue-specific changes have also been reported for lymphocyte subsets after exercise.[67] Whether exercise influences the activation state and phagocytic capacity of macrophages differentially by tissue compartment has not been tested. Finally, mouse peritoneal macrophages obtained after exhaustive exercise were better able to retard the growth of cultured sarcoma cells compared to the cytostatic capacity of macrophages obtained from nonexercised animals.[68] Since neutrophils and macrophages are fundamental to immune and inflammatory responses, results indicating that exercise may enhance some aspects of phagocytic function warrant further investigation.

Because NK cells play an important role in host-nonspecific defense responses in viral infections and cancer,[69,70] the impact of acute exercise on this immune cell has been the topic of numerous reports. Several studies document that the frequency of human blood lymphocytes positive for monoclonal antibodies against various NK-cell surface markers increases after exercise.[27,71-73] The source of these NK cells is unknown, but animal studies suggest that the increase in NK numbers in blood is due to a concurrent demargination from other tissue compartments, such as the spleen,[74] and entry into the circulating pool. The increase in the proportion of blood NK cells after exercise also appears to characterize individuals across several fitness groups and in response to acute exercise of varying intensities and durations.[24] Interestingly, the increase in NK-cell number and percentage was shown to be consistent when subjects performed the exercise repeatedly over 5 d.[25] NK-cell activity increases after acute exercise, followed by a reduction in cytotoxic activity which is typically present several hours after exercise.[27,46,71,75] The increase in NK activity at the end of exercise is likely due to the increase in NK-cell numbers postexercise. However, the delayed reduction in NK cytolytic activity after exercise cannot be easily explained by changes in NK-cell numbers since, typically, this latter parameter has returned to baseline. The delayed, reduced cytotoxicity may well reflect fluctuations in neuroendocrine factors during the exercise session. For example, Kappel et al.[76] found the increase and subsequent decrease in NK cytolytic function in response to physical exercise also occurred following an infusion of epinephrine, and it has been well documented that NK cells have receptors for a variety of neuroendocrine factors including epinephrine.[77,78] Indeed, β-adrenergic stimulation of NK cells *in vitro* inhibits cytotoxicity;[79] nevertheless, whether exercise-induced elevations in blood epinephrine levels explain the delayed suppression in NK activity remains to be empirically tested.

III. EXERCISE TRAINING, FITNESS, AND IMMUNE RESPONSES

In contrast to the evidence that an acute exercise bout (of either maximal or submaximal intensity) modulates immune function, less is known about the impact of chronic exercise, exercise training, or physical conditioning on immune parameters. The impact of chronic exercise and training on leukocyte and lymphocyte numbers is inconsistent. For example, an older study[80] reported the absolute numbers of blood leukocytes and lymphocytes obtained at rest to be low among some marathon runners. Papa et al.[81] also reported the absolute number of lymphocytes and the percentage of T lymphocytes to be lower in water-polo players relative to untrained controls in blood samples obtained at rest. In contrast, body builders and trained swimmers did not differ in baseline numbers of leukocytes, lymphocytes, or neutrophils relative to sedentary controls;[21] no difference in the absolute number of neutrophils or monocytes was observed in conditioned cyclists relative to untrained controls sampled at rest.[82] Healthy, previously inactive men who trained aerobically (40 to 50 min/d, 5 d/week for 15 weeks) did not have a significant change in the percentage of total lymphocytes as a consequence of training although the number of T lymphocytes (measured by the E-rosetting technique) was increased.[83] At rest, the percentage of T lymphocytes (also determined by the E-rosetting technique) was lower among ballet students than controls.[84] Finally, a recent study found that in women assigned to a walking training program for 15 weeks, the total number of lymphocytes and T cells was reduced at 6 weeks but not at 15 weeks relative to pretraining levels.[85] This apparent inconsistency in the reported effects of exercise training on baseline leukocyte numbers may well be due to the timing of blood sample collections in relation to the last exercise session and training protocol.

There are relatively few studies in humans on the effects of long-term exercise conditioning on lymphocyte function either at rest or in response to an acute exercise session. In response to intense exercise, elite marathoners[37] and kayakists[39] had reductions in blood-lymphocyte response to mitogens; MacNeil et al.[38] also found reduced lymphocyte blastogenesis in response to mitogen stimulation after cycle-ergometry exercise undertaken at intensities up to 75% of maximum oxygen consumption regardless of exercise duration in highly fit subjects. In contrast, spontaneous blastogenesis (i.e., without mitogenic stimulation) was increased in marathoners following a 3-h run to exhaustion.[19] In general, though, the results of human studies indicate that highly conditioned subjects experience a suppression in lymphocyte function following acute exercise, which is qualitatively similar to the responses observed in untrained subjects after acute exercise. Although it is possible that training may blunt the magnitude of the lymphocyte immunosuppression, it is not surprising that the stability of this exercise-stress effect holds across fitness groups. In response to acute exhaustive exercise, swim-trained rats[41] and treadmill-trained mice[86] had suppressed splenic-lymphocyte proliferation responses to mitogens. Exercise training, apart from the immediate effects of exercise, appears to augment splenic-lymphocyte response to mitogens in rodents in some studies[45,87] but not in others.[86]

Exercise training enhances NK-cell activity, although this effect has not always been consistent. Elderly women who underwent a 16-week aerobic exercise program (three times per week) had an elevated baseline NK activity relative to undertrained women[88] as well as an increase in NK activity immediately after acute treadmill exercise. In another longitudinal training study, elderly women enroled in a brisk walking program for 15 weeks showed an increase in NK activity at 6 weeks relative to controls;[89] however, the interpretation of this finding is open, since at 15 weeks there was no further increase in NK activity and at this time the controls also showed an increase in NK activity. Baseline NK-cell cytolytic activity against tumor targets *in vitro* was higher in trained racing cyclists than in untrained subjects.[90] In contrast, the lysis of target cell by NK cells was decreased significantly after physical training.[83] Experimental work in animals supports the hypothesis that exercise conditioning enhances NK activity with increases in both total splenic-NK activity[91] and NK activity expressed relative to the number of NK cells.[74] In a very interesting study of an aerobic-exercise training program for individuals seropositive for HIV-1, seropositive men who received exercise training had less of a drop in NK numbers after notification of HIV status than seropositive individuals who did not exercise;[92] no differences were reported between the exercise and nonexercise groups for *in vitro* NK-cell cytolytic activity.

In sum, while there is experimental evidence to support a training-mediated enhancement of NK-cell function, the strength of this effect is relatively weak due to the limited number of studies and the occasional discrepancy in the direction of the effects. Further, even if there is an augmentation of NK activity, the physiological mechanisms have not been studied. Such enhanced function can be due to multiple factors including increased numbers of NK cells, differences in the responsiveness of NK cells to cytokine signals leading to more effective killers (interferon-γ and interleukin-2-stimulated LAK cells), or other fundamental changes in NK cells (e.g., increased protein synthesis of hydrolytic enzymes such as perforin).

IV. IMMUNOMODULATION BY INACTIVITY AND WEIGHTLESSNESS

In parallel with the literature on exercise and immune modulation are studies which try to evaluate the impact of inactivity and deconditioning on the immune system. The strategy for assessing the impact of inactivity and deconditioning on immunity includes the role of prolonged bedrest due to disease, reduced mobility due to aging, inactivity due to spinal-cord injury, and reduced activity during space flight. Each of these conditions includes other physiologic and pathophysiologic variables in addition to inactivity which limits the interpretation of immune changes. To illustrate the methodological problems of trying to assess inactivity, deconditioning, and immune function, we will consider evidence on the impact of space flight on the immune system.

Space flight has profound physiological effects including cardiovascular deconditioning[93] and reduced tolerance to exercise upon return to Earth's gravity.[94,95] However, space flight also involves the individual and interactive effects of reduced exercise, weightlessness, possible radiation exposure (especially on long-term manned space missions), and psychological stress. Partitioning the impact of each of these factors on immune parameters during space flight has proven to be challenging. Several brief reviews of the immune response to space flight, weightlessness, and hypergravity highlight many of the issues in this area.[96-98]

Data from early space flights suggested changes in leukocyte number indicative of a stress response. Both animal and human subjects demonstrated postflight neutrophilia and lymphopenia. Transient neutrophilia, reversible by the second postflight day, was observed in the Apollo astronauts, perhaps due to increased blood epinephrine and steroid levels associated with stress;[93] this neutrophilia following space flight has been confirmed in other studies.[99] The underlying mechanism for the neutrophilia is unclear but may reflect stress-induced increases in epinephrine and/or cortisol. Whether neutrophils function normally after space flight is untested in the laboratory. Since acute exercise stress (rather than lack of exercise) also evokes a corticoid-mediated neutrophilia,[100] it is likely that the neutrophilia associated with short space flight reflects general responses to stress rather than reduced exercise activity.

Probably the greatest amount of published data on immune responses during space flight has focused on T-lymphocyte function. The early reports of U.S. Apollo astronauts and Soviet Soyuz cosmonauts gave inconsistent results;[101,102] while the accounts are historically interesting, lack of procedural details and limitations of the methodology used to assess T-lymphocyte function make the interpretation of results difficult. Most, but not all,[103] later reports suggest that *in vitro* T-lymphocyte responsiveness to mitogens is suppressed during space flight.[104,105] In one study, human lymphocytes obtained before flight and exposed to the T-cell mitogen concanavalin A (Con A) during a U.S. Spacelab mission had less than 3% of the mitogenic activity of control (ground-based) cultures.[106] Bechler et al.[107] reported that T lymphocytes, obtained from astronauts during space flight and stimulated with Con A, showed a 90% reduction in mitogenesis relative to responses obtained at preflight. The similarity in the pattern of this response to the reduced lymphocyte mitogenesis after acute exercise is striking and would indicate, at least conceptually, that similar neuroendocrine stress mediates immune changes in both acute exercise and spaceflight. Indeed, Gmünder et al.[108] have suggested that the immunological profile to exercise is similar to that occurring following space flight. However, delineation and comparison of common neuroendocrine mechanisms in response to space flight and exercise have not been pursued clinically or experimentally. Moreover, it should be noted that although these limited studies of T-lymphocyte responsiveness during space flight suggest a suppression in function, there are no reports of clinically significant disease in space resulting from depressed cellular immunity. It is unknown whether this reflects a true lack of association between the suppression of lymphocyte function and health status or a bias in reporting of some illnesses due to negative publicity.[98]

Recent medical reports of the Soviet Mir and Salyut missions indicate that the suppression in lymphocyte function observed during space flight may also relate to the duration of exposure to reduced gravity.[109] Konstantinova and colleagues[110] described marked suppression in PHA responsiveness of T lymphocytes, as well as in T-helper-cell functional activity, from cosmonauts who had lived in orbital stations from 112 to 366 d; short-term space flight was not associated with suppression of PHA-induced mitogenesis, and with relatively minor changes in T-helper lymphocyte function, compared with preflight levels. Significant reductions in the capacity of blood NK cells to bind K-562 tumor target cells *in vitro* was also observed in cosmonauts after 1 d of recovery following long-duration space flights. Concurrent changes in the redistribution of lymphocytes from blood to bone marrow[110] may account for the immune suppression observed after long-duration space flight.

Alternatively, changes in the activity, secretion, or signal transduction of immunoregulatory cytokines, such as interleukin-2 (IL-2) or the interferons, may be involved. IL-2 activity fell significantly in cosmonauts after long-duration space flight.[110] IL-2 receptor expression was also depressed in postflight samples taken from those cosmonauts required to perform extravehicular activities during flight; the defect in IL-2 receptor expression was normalized following stimulation with phorbol myristate acetate (PMA) which directly activates protein kinase C in lymphocytes.[111] Interestingly, the ability to produce IL-2 was enhanced in two out of three individuals after space flight.[111] These findings suggest that one potential mechanism involved in the suppression of T-lymphocyte proliferation observed with space flight relates to changes in signal transmission from lymphocyte membranes to the nucleus. Information about the regulation of other cytokines during space flight is more limited. There is some evidence that the secretion of interferons is depressed by space flight. In mice and rats maintained in an antiorthostatic position to simulate some aspects of weightlessness, interferon-α/β production was inhibited.[112,113] Interferon-γ production by splenocytes of rats flown in the Space Shuttle SL-3 for 1 week was undetectable relative to ground-based controls.[114] Human IL-1[111] and rat IL-3[114] production are apparently unaffected by space flight. Despite the biological attractiveness of the altered-cytokine hypothesis to explain the suppression in lymphocyte mitogenesis with prolonged weightlessness, several cautionary notes are warranted. First, since most alterations in immune measures are observed postflight, it is possible that these reflect the immediate psychological and hormonal impact of reentry stress rather than the effects of prolonged weightlessness and physical inactivity. Second, the results on human subjects are obtained on a very small number of cases for any given space mission, which limits the statistical confidence in the data. Third, results of space-flight studies are always complicated by changes in atmosphere, the fact that subjects are exposed to both hypergravity and hypogravity, and the varying duration of exposure to weightlessness.

Studies which partition the role of individual components of space flight (physical inactivity, radiation exposure, weightlessness, psychological stress) on immune suppression are limited. Evidence that reduced physical activity is involved in immune alterations during space flight is circumstantial at best. Apollo astronauts had increased concentrations of acute-phase reactant proteins (e.g., ceruloplasmin, α_2-macroglobulin), whereas these proteins remained unchanged in later Skylab astronauts; the difference in acute-phase reactant responses between the two programs has been suggested to reflect an increase in the amount of physical exercise during the Skylab mission.[97,115] Moreover, there is little indication that spacecraft in orbit are exposed to excessive radiation given the protection by the Earth's magnetic fields forming the Van Allen belts. Indeed, as noted by Fowler,[98] on a 90-d Skylab mission, the average maximum radiation dose was 7.7 rad, which is well within the safe range for humans.[116] In contrast, the effects of hypogravity, hypergravity, and weightlessness on immune functions have been studied in a variety of experimental models. Some of these experiments used clinostats (which rotate cells in various directions), water immersion, bedrest, or tail suspension with or without head-down tilt (antiorthostatic position).[96] Early reports indicated that hypogravity depresses, whereas hypergravity enhances, some aspects of lymphocyte mitogenic responses.[117] These findings were confirmed by Guanghua and colleagues.[118] Rats exposed to whole-body suspension for 3 weeks had significantly lower splenic-lymphocyte counts, spleen and thymic weights, and serum-lysozyme concentration relative to controls; hypergravity tended to be associated with higher splenic-lymphocyte numbers. Again, the mechanism accounting for these immunological changes was suggested to be stress-related, although the dichotomy of stress effects (hypo- vs. hypergravity) was not addressed. In a 56-d ground simulation of space life without radiation or weightlessness, there was no change in lymphocyte reactivity in the few measures done.[119] Using only three subjects who were given daily exercise and exposed to transverse acceleration on a centrifuge for 62 d, there was a decline in phagocytosis of monocytes in the nonexercising men.[120] A recent study[121] raises the possibility that the immunological changes observed with weightlessness are due, at least in part, to changes in lymphocyte adhesion rather than black-box "stress" effects. Human lymphocytes grown on a hydrophobic polymer that prevents cells from anchoring to and spreading on the coated surface had reduced mitogenesis in response to Con A and lower interferon-γ production.

There is clearly a very limited amount of information on the totality of the effects of space flight, including changes in physical activity and fitness on the immune system. This is due to the limited number of modern assays performed on immune cells and products from individuals living and working in space. Most studies have focused on T-lymphocyte function upon reentry from space flight relative to either preflight values or unstressed controls. The majority of these report indicate abnormal T-lymphocyte mitogenesis, which may be due to poor production of immunoregulatory signal proteins. Changes in signal proteins may occur at the level of lymphocyte–lymphocyte interactions (e.g., IL-2) or in the differentiation of lymphoid progenitor cells. In this later regard, progenitors of rat fibroblasts in bone marrow (CFU_f) are depressed after 2 weeks in space.[122] and this raises the possibility of concomitant changes in (fibroblastogenic) colony-stimulating growth factors. The response of rat bone-marrow cells to CSF_m (monocyte-macrophage) was impaired after 12.5 d of space flight, although unintentional confounding by a 42-h fast may have contributed to this effect.[123] Changes in the levels of hormones, such as corticosteroids, and in cell-to-cell and cell-to-matrix adhesion properties may also contribute to the alterations in immune responses observed during space flight. Finally, whether such changes in immunoregulatory molecules and lymphocyte-adhesion properties have a component of changed fitness due to inactivity, or reduced demands on muscles due to lack of gravity, is possible but essentially untested.

V. ENDOCRINE MEDIATORS OF IMMUNOMODULATION

The general and specific hormonal responses to exercise have been the subject of numerous reviews.[124-126] In this section, some of the major findings for glucocorticoids, catecholamines, and endorphins are summarized with respect to the implications for modulation of immune functions. Recent reviews and books dealing with neuroendocrine–immune interactions in general and specifically in response to stress are available.[127,128] One of the classic hormonal changes with many acute-stress situations is the increase in glucocorticoid secretion by the adrenal cortex in response to signals from adrenocorticotrophin hormone (ACTH) produced by the anterior pituitary. Exercise-induced stress results in increased glucocorticoid production in subjects classified as having a sedentary physical status.[129] Subjects classified as active do not exhibit an exercise-related increase in glucocorticoid production unless given higher work loads.[129] Increases in plasma levels of cortisol, the primary glucocorticoid in humans, are dependent upon relative workloads of 60% of $\dot{V}O_2$ max or greater.[130] It has been suggested that an increase in plasma cortisol levels over time may contribute to some of the physiological adaptations to training.[124] Not unexpectedly, ACTH concentrations also increase with exercise.[125,131]

For many years, it has been noted that elevated glucocorticoids produce a lymphocytopenia and have marked effects of the migration and distribution patterns of leukocytes.[132] In general, lymphocyte proliferation responses to mitogens are reduced by the addition of glucocorticoids *in vitro*.[133,134] Glucocorticoids also inhibit a variety of hormones and neuropeptides (insulin, ACTH, CRF, β-endorphin, ADH), lymphokines and monokines (IL-1, TNF, IFN-γ), and inflammatory agents (histamine, eicosanoids, elastase).[135,136] These observations present a more complex role for endogenous glucocorticoids in modulating immune functions and have implications for overall metabolism and homeostasis.

ACTH has immunomodulatory effects independent of the actions of glucocorticoids.[127] For example, ACTH, per se, suppresses the *in vitro* production of interferon-γ by T lymphocytes.[137] ACTH blocks the ability of preformed interferon to activate macrophages to a tumoricidal state.[138] Interestingly, human and mouse lymphocytes express immunoreactive ACTH after viral infection, interaction with tumor cells, or after exposure to bacterial lipopolysaccharide.[127,139,140] Constitutive production of ACTH by a subset of mouse splenic macrophages has also been observed,[141] and IL-1 can stimulate ACTH and corticosterone production in mice and rats.[142] These observations support the argument in favor of bidirectional interactions between the immune and central nervous systems[127] and raise several questions with respect to exercise. First, there is the possibility that traumatic exercise, involving muscle damage and infiltration by immune cells, could lead to *de novo* production of ACTH by macrophages and lymphocytes with subsequent immune suppression. Second, the elevation in IL-1 levels observed after acute, eccentric exercise[48] may stimulate central ACTH production, also leading to an eventual down-regulation in immune function. In experimental animals, plasma glucocorticoids, chiefly corticosterone, are elevated soon after stress induction, followed by a gradual recovery to basal levels.[136] The number of circulating lymphocytes inversely parallels the stress-related increases in plasma corticosterone, followed by a recovery to normal levels. However, while exercise stress increases ACTH and glucocorticoids in humans, simple correlations between exercise-induced changes in these hormones and immune alterations have not been found. Part of the difficulty in linking exercise-mediated changes in ACTH and corticoids with immune changes may relate to dissociation between the timing of sampling for peak hormone levels and later steroid hormone effects, the use of *in vivo* vs. *in vitro* analysis of corticoid effects on immune function, and the growing complexity of interactions between "classic" stress hormones and immunoregulatory cytokines.

One of the most consistent and important effects of physical exercise is the increase in sympathoadrenal activity, with a consequent increase in the plasma levels of the catecholamine hormones, epinephrine and norepinephrine. Epinephrine and norepinephrine have well-documented effects on heart rate, vasomotor activity, metabolic rates of skeletal muscle, and substrate utilization.[124,125] Increases in catecholamine concentrations have been shown to be related to the intensity of exercise as a percentage of $\dot{V}O_2$ max.[124,143,144] At the same relative intensities of physical work, endurance-trained athletes have higher plasma-epinephrine concentrations[145] and an increased capacity to secrete epinephrine[146] compared to untrained individuals.

Epinephrine has potent effects on cells of the immune system. For example, *in vivo* infusion of epinephrine results in leukocytosis including lymphocytosis and neutrophilia.[33] Addition of epinephrine to lymphocyte cultures is associated with reduced blastogenic responses to mitogens;[147-149] this effect is partly dependent upon the concentration of the hormone in culture.[150] Pretreatment of lymphocytes with low concentrations of epinephrine followed by removal of the drug increased NK-cell cytolytic activity, whereas direct addition of epinephrine to NK-cell–target-cell cultures inhibits cytolysis.[151] More recently it has been shown that IL-2-stimulated proliferative responses to T lymphocytes are inhibited by activation of β-adrenoceptors.[152] From this type of study, the view has emerged that β-adrenergic stimulation of intracellular cAMP leads to inhibiton of lymphocyte proliferation and effector functions.

The potential role of epinephrine in mediating exercise-stress-related immune changes has been described by Kappel et al.[76] Intravenous infusion of epinephrine into eight healthy untrained subjects — at concentrations comparable to those observed with exercise at 75% of $\dot{V}O_2$ max for 1 h — leads to an increase in NK-cell activity (lysis per fixed number of cells) followed by a drop in NK activity 2 h later. Because epinephrine infusion also results in an increase in the percentage of NK cells,[33,153] the immediate postexercise increase in NK activity probably reflects changes in the size of the NK-cell pool. Again, as described earlier, the reduction in NK activity 2 h after exercise is thought to be due to an epinephrine-mediated increase in monocytes expressing PGE_2 and down-regulation of NK-cell activity.[46,76]

Much less is known about the impact of the endogenous opioid peptides and other neuropeptides on the behavior of immune cells during exercise stress. The evidence that changes in immune function with exercise are due to endogenous opioids is largely based on studies linking stress (especially tail-shock stress in rodents) to increased opioid secretion and subsequent immunoregulation[154-156] and the documentation that β-endorphin levels are elevated following exercise.[157-160] Whether the increase in blood β-endorphin concentrations are related to the intensity and duration of physical work is ambiguous, with reports indicating a curvilinear relationship[158] or no relationship between intensity of exercise and β-endorphin levels.[157] Endogenous opioids have multiple effects on immune cells depending upon the specific opioid peptide, which opioid receptor is activated, and the concentration of the opioid peptide.[161] For example, Johnson and associates[137] reported decreased numbers of mouse splenocytes producing antibody in a plaque-forming assay when α-endorphin, met-enkephalin, and leu-enkephalin where used, but no effect was observed using β-endorphin. NK-cell cytotoxicity was enhanced by low (10 f*M*) concentrations of β-endorphin and higher concentrations of met-enkephalin, but not by leu-enkephalin or α-endorphin.[162] A relatively recent study on exercise and endogenous opioids suggests that the increase in NK-cell cytotoxicity immediately after exercise may be partly due to the actions of β-endorphin. Fiatarone et al.[72] showed that administration of naloxone (an opioid antagonist) prior to maximal cycle-ergometry exercise blocked the expected immediate postexercise increase in NK-cell cytolytic activity seen in placebo controls; the increase in the percentage of blood NK cells (Leu 11a and Leu 19) observed postexercise was not significantly affected by prior treatment with naloxone. Finally, in a study of Norwegian military cadets, inhibition of monocyte function *in vitro* was observed following vasoactive intestinal peptide (VIP) administration in subjects who were given 3 d of continuous physical activity at 35% of $\dot{V}O_2$ max; inhibition was greater than on the control day.[163] The significance of this finding is unclear given the absence of published data on the levels of VIP or the expression of VIP receptors on lymphocytes and monocytes in response to exercise stress.

VI. EXERCISE, INACTIVITY, AND DISEASE

Despite the growing evidence that exercise and fitness modify immune functions, the clinical relevance of these changes is largely speculative. Part of the difficulty in evaluating the causal nature of exercise-induced changes in immune parameters in humans to disease risk is due to methodological concerns in measuring physical activity and fitness in large populations, the factor of positive health behaviors being associated (such as absence of smoking with exercise conditioning), and the multifactorial etiology of chronic diseases including those with an immunological component. Even with respect to infectious diseases, there is no clear consensus as to whether exercise-mediated immune changes are protective, detrimental, or of little consequence for occurrence of disease episodes.

Hoffman-Goetz and MacNeil[10] reviewed the evidence linking exercise with natural immunity and cancer. Numerous epidemiological[164-169] and experimental[3,4,170,171] studies suggest that regular physical activity in humans reduces the risk for some cancers — cancers of the colon, breast and reproductive tract — and reduces the occurrence of chemically induced or transplanted tumors in animals. Inactivity or sedentariness, as measured by occupational physical activity, is positively associated with increased relative risk for cancers of the colon.[172,173] However, the possibility of exercise-mediated immunological changes as underlying mechanisms in cancer risk was not addressed in these studies. A recent report[174] showed that in mice given moderate-intensity treadmill exercise for 12 weeks and injected with an experimental fibrosarcoma 3 weeks prior to cessation of training, *in vitro* splenic NK-cell activity was higher in exercised animals who did not have successful tumor take than in sedentary controls; *in vitro* NK-cytolytic activity was not different between exercised and sedentary animals with successful tumor implants. *In vivo* retention in the lungs of radiolabeled tumor cells was lower in mice given voluntary physical activity through in-cage running wheels for 9 weeks than in sedentary controls;[131] administration of an antibody which blocked natural immune responses prior to injection of the labeled tumor cells increased retention of radioactivity in the lungs of exercised animals. These data suggest, then, that exercise-mediated augmentation of natural immune functions modifies the growth of experimental tumors in the lungs, though likely at the early stages of initial implantation. This fits with the observation that NK cells constitute an important defense mechanism in the circulation rather than in alveolar space or lung parenchyma.[175] Whether exercise-mediated increases in NK-cell activity affects the development of spontaneous tumors has not been investigated.

Under selected conditions, exercise may alter immune function or cell location resulting in increased death or damage.[176] For example, during coxsackie B3 infection in mice, T cells migrate to the heart accompanied by myocardial calcification. Mice infected with the virus and forced to swim had four times the number of T cells, sensitized to the virus, which were redirected to the heart from other parts of the body. More severe myocardial calcification occurred. A recent report[177] indicates that the increased inflammatory and necrotic lesions seen in exercised mice with coxsackie B viral myocarditis is associated with decreased mobilization of macrophages, followed by an increased tissue destruction possibly mediated by cytotoxic T lymphocytes.

Scientific opinions vary regarding the susceptibility of trained subjects to upper respiratory tract infections (URI) and the relationship to immune parameters.[178] Acute exercise to exhaustion may increase susceptibility to infections among elite athletes.[179] URI were the primary medical reason for absence from training among elite Nordic skiers.[180] In women given a 15-week exercise-training program, elevated NK-cell activity was observed at 6 weeks but not at 15 weeks, and the trained women had reduced URI symptomatology compared to sedentary controls; no significant correlations were found for changes in NK-cell activitiy and symptomatology at 6 or 15 weeks.[89] Again, while it is tempting to speculate that training-associated enhancement in immune functions, including innate immunity, protects against infectious disease, direct clinical observations are lacking.

VII. SUMMARY

On the basis of experimental studies involving humans and animals, the tentative conclusion that acute, intense exercise depresses and that regular, moderate exercise enhances immune functions is put forward. Conversely — and largely by extrapolation — long-term inactivity, such as that experienced during space travel, could be potentially immunosuppressive. Biologically credible and parsimonious mechanisms to account for the immunomodulatory effects of exercise have not been well described. Neuroendocrine explanations, based upon analogy with other stress paradigms, have been suggested to underlie the acute-exercise effects. Hormonal mediation of long-term adaptations in the immune system with regular physical activity and fitness is theoretically possible but essentially unproven. Moreover, the clinical relevance of such immunomodulation remains open. Despite these caveats, to the extent that regular physical activity is an important component of public health-promotion strategies, research aimed at systemically identifying immunological changes with exercise and the health implications of these changes are both timely and necessary.

ACKNOWLEDGMENT

This work was supported by funding from the Natural Sciences and Engineering Research Council of Canada and from the Canadian Fitness and Lifestyle Research Institute.

REFERENCES

1. **Kemeny, M., Zegans, L., and Cohen, F.,** Stress, mood, immunity, and recurrence of genital herpes, *Ann. N.Y. Acad. Sci.,* 494, 735, 1987.
2. **Zarski, J.,** Hassles and health: a replication, *Health Psychol.,* 3, 243, 1984.
3. **Baracos, V. E.,** Exercise inhibits progressive growth of the Morris hepatoma 7777 in male and female rats, *Can. J. Physiol. Pharmacol.,* 67, 864, 1988.
4. **Cohen, L. A., Choi, K., and Wang, C.-X.,** Influence of dietary fat, caloric restriction, and voluntary exercise on *N*-nitrosomethylurea-induced mammary tumorigenesis in rats, *Cancer Res.,* 48, 4276, 1988.
5. **Kritchevsky, D.,** Influence of caloric restriction and exercise on tumorigenesis in rats, *Proc. Soc. Exp. Biol. Med.,* 193, 35, 1990.
6. **Rusch, H. P. and Kline, B. E.,** The effect of exercise on the growth of a mouse tumor, *Cancer Res.,* 4, 116, 1944.
7. **Keast, D., Cameron, K., and Morton, A. R.,** Exercise and the immune response, *Sports Med.,* 5, 248, 1988.
8. **Hoffman-Goetz, L.,** Exercise and the immune response, in *Encyclopedia of Immunology,* Roitt, I. M. and Delves, P. J., Eds., W. B. Saunders, London, 1992, 528.
9. **Nieman, D. C. and Nehlsen-Cannarella, S. L.,** The effects of acute and chronic exercise on immunoglobulins, *Sports Med.,* 11, 183, 1991.
10. **Hoffman-Goetz, L. and MacNeil, B.,** Exercise, natural immunity, and cancer: causation, correlation, or conundrum, in *Exercise and Disease,* Watson, R. R. and Eisinger, M., Eds., CRC Press, Boca Raton, FL, 1992, 37.
11. **Andersen, K. L.,** Leukocyte response to brief, severe exercise, *J. Appl. Physiol.,* 7, 671, 1955.
12. **McCarthy, D. A. and Dale, M. M.,** The leukocytosis of exercise: a review and a model, *Sports Med.,* 6, 333, 1988.
13. **Galun, E., Burstein, R., Assia, E., Tur-Kaspa, I., Rosenblum, J., and Epstein, Y.,** Changes of white blood cell count during prolonged exercise, *Int. J. Sports Med.,* 8, 253, 1987.
14. **Gimenez, M., Mohan-Kumar, T., Humbert, J. C., DeTalance, N., and Buisine, J.,** Leukocyte, lymphocyte and platelet response to dynamic exercise, *Eur. J. Appl. Physiol.,* 55, 465, 1986.
15. **Gimenez, M., Mohan-Kumar, T., Humbert, J. C., DeTalance, N., Teboul, M., and Belenguer, F. J. A.,** Training and leukocyte, lymphocyte and platelet response to dynamic exercise, *Int. J. Sports Med.,* 27, 172, 1987.
16. **Oshida, Y., Yamanouchi, Y., Hayamizu, S., and Sato, Y.,** Effects of acute physical exercise on lymphocyte subpopulations in trained and untrained subjects, *Int. J. Sports Med.,* 9, 137, 1988.
17. **Ferry, A., Picard, F., Duvallet, A., Weill, B., and Rieu, M.,** Changes in blood leukocyte populations induced by acute maximal and chronic submaximal exercise, *Eur. J. Appl. Physiol.,* 59, 435, 1990.
18. **Nieman, D. C., Nehlsen-Cannarella, S. L., Donohue, K. M., Chritton, D. B. W., Haddock, B. L., Stout, R. W., and Lee, J. W.,** The effects of acute moderate exercise on leukocyte and lymphocyte subpopulations, *Med. Sci. Sports Exerc.,* 23, 578, 1991.

19. Nieman, D. C., Berk, L. S., Simpson-Westerberg, M., Arabatzis, K., Youngberg, S., Tan, S. A., Lee, J. W., and Eby, W. C., Effects of long-endurance running on immune system parameters and lymphocyte function in experienced marathoners, *Int. J. Sports Med.*, 10, 317, 1989.

20. Field, C. J., Gougeon, R., and Marliss, E. B., Circulating mononuclear cell numbers and function during intense exercise and recovery, *J. Appl. Physiol.*, 71, 1089, 1991.

21. Ciusani, E., Grazzi, L., Salmaggi, A., Eoli, M., Ariano, C., Vescovi, A., Parati, E., and Nespolo, A., Role of physical training on immune function: preliminary data, *Intern. J. Neurosci.*, 51, 249, 1990.

22. Martina, B., Schreck, M., Droste, C., Roskamm, H., Tichelli, A., and Speck, B., Physiologic exercise-induced lymphocytosis, *Blut*, 60, 255, 1990.

23. Soppi, E., Varjo, P., Eskola, J., and Laitinen, L. A., Effect of strenuous physical stress on circulating lymphocyte number and function before and after training, *J. Clin. Lab. Immunol.*, 8, 43, 1982.

24. Kendall, A., Hoffman-Goetz, L., Houston, M., MacNeil, B., and Arumugam, Y., Exercise and blood lymphocyte subset responses: intensity, duration and subject fitness effects, *J. Appl. Physiol.*, 69, 251, 1990.

25. Hoffman-Goetz, L., Randall Simpson, J., Cipp, N., Arumugam, Y., and Houston, M., Lymphocyte subset responses to repeated submaximal exercise in men, *J. Appl. Physiol.*, 68, 1069, 1990.

26. Deuster, P. A., Curiale, A. M., Cowan, M. L., and Finkelman, F. D., Exercise-induced changes in populations of peripheral blood mononuclear cells, *Med. Sci. Sports Exerc.*, 20, 276, 1988.

27. Pedersen, B. K., Tvede, N., Hansen, F. R., Andersen, V., Bendix, T., Bendixen, G., Galbo, H., Haahr, P. M., Klarlund, K., Sylvest, J., Thomsen, B. S., and Halkjær-Kristensen, J., Modulation of natural killer cell activity in peripheral blood by physical exercise, *Scand. J. Immunol.*, 27, 673, 1988.

28. Tvede, N., Pedersen, B. K., Hansen, F. R., Bendix, T., Christensen, L. D., Galbo, H., and Halkjær-Kristensen, J., Effect of physical exercise on blood mononuclear cell subpopulations and *in vitro* proliferative responses, *Scand. J. Immunol.*, 29, 383, 1989.

29. Gabriel, H., Urhausen, A., and Kindermann, W., Circulating leucocyte and lymphocyte subpopulations before and after intensive endurance exercise to exhaustion, *Eur. J. Appl. Physiol.*, 63, 449, 1991.

30. Mulligan, S. P., Wills, E. J., and Young, G. A. R., Exercise-induced CD8 lymphocytosis: a phenomenon associated with large granular lymphocyte leukaemia, *Brit. J. Haematol.*, 75, 175, 1990.

31. Frey, M. J., Mancini, D., Fischberg, D., Wilson, J. R., and Molinoff, P. B., Effect of exercise duration on density and coupling of beta-adrenergic receptors on human mononuclear cells, *J. Appl. Physiol.*, 66, 1495, 1989.

32. Foster, N. K., Martyn, J. B., Rangno, R. E., Hogg, J. C., and Pardy, R. L., Leukocytosis of exercise: role of cardiac output and catecholamines, *J. Appl. Physiol.*, 61, 2218, 1986.

33. Crary, B., Hauser, S. L., Borysenko, M., Kutz, I., Hoban, C., Ault, K. A., Weiner, H. L., and Benson, H., Epinephrine-induced changes in the distribution of lymphocyte subsets in peripheral blood of humans, *J. Immunol.*, 131, 1178, 1983.

34. Katz, P., Zaytoun, A. M., and Lee, J. H., The effects of *in vivo* hydrocortisone on lymphocyte-mediated cytotoxicity, *Arthritis Rheum.*, 27, 72, 1984.

35. Hansen, J.-B., Wilsgard, L., and Osterud, B., Biphasic changes in leukocytes induced by strenuous exercise, *Eur. J. Appl. Physiol.*, 62, 157, 1991.

36. Maisel, A. S., Harris, T., Rearden, C. A., and Michel, M. C., β-Adrenergic receptors in lymphocyte subsets after exercise. Alterations in normal individuals and patients with congestive heart failure, *Circulation*, 82, 2003, 1990.

37. Eskola, J., Russkanen, O., Soppi, E., Viljanen, M., Jarvinen, M., and Toivonen, H., Effect of sport stress on lymphocyte transformation and antibody formation, *Clin. Exp. Immunol.*, 32, 339, 1978.

38. MacNeil, B., Hoffman-Goetz, L., Kendall, A., Houston, M., and Arumugam, Y., Lymphocyte proliferation responses after exercise in men: fitness, intensity, and duration effects, *J. Appl. Physiol.*, 70, 179, 1991.

39. Fry, R. W., Morton, A. R., and Keast, D., Acute intense interval training and T-lymphocyte function, *Med. Sci. Sports Exerc.*, 24, 339, 1992.

40. Ferry, A., Rieu, P., Laziri, F., Guezennec, C. Y., El Habazi, A., Le Page, C., and Rieu, M., Immunomodulation of thymocytes and splenocytes in trained rats, *J. Appl. Physiol.*, 71, 815, 1991.

41. Mahan, M. P. and Young, M. R., Immune parameters of untrained or exercise-trained rats after exhaustive exercise, *J. Appl. Physiol.*, 66, 282, 1989.

42. Nehlsen-Cannarella, S. L., Nieman, D. C., Jessen, J., Chang, L., Gusewitch, G., Blix, G. G., and Ashley, E., The effects of acute moderate exercise on lymphocyte function and serum immunoglobulin levels, *Int. J. Sports Med.*, 12, 391, 1991.

43. Tvede, N., Heilmann, C., Halkjær-Kristensen, J., and Pedersen, B. K., Mechanisms of B-lymphocyte suppression induced by acute physical exercise, *J. Clin. Lab. Immunol.*, 30, 169, 1989.

44. Hoffman-Goetz, L., Thorne, R. J., and Houston, M. E., Splenic immune responses following treadmill exercise in mice, *Can. J. Physiol. Pharmacol.*, 66, 1415, 1988.

45. **Ferry, A., Weill, B., Amiridis, I., Laziry, F., and Rieu, M.,** Splenic immunomodulation with swimming-induced stress in rats, *Immunol. Lett.,* 29, 261, 1991.

46. **Pedersen, B. K., Tvede, N., Klarlund, K., Christensen, L. D., Hansen, F. R., Galbo, H., Kharazmi, A., and Halkjær-Kristensen, J.,** Indomethacin *in vitro* and *in vivo* abolishes post-exercise suppression of natural killer cell activity in peripheral blood, *Int. J. Sports Med.,* 11, 127, 1990.

47. **Bloom, E. T. and Babbitt, J. T.,** Prostaglandin E2, monocytes adherence and interleukin-1 in the regulation of human natural killer cell activity by monocytes, *Nat. Immun. Cell. Growth Regul.,* 9, 36, 1990.

48. **Cannon, J. G., Evans, W. J., Hughes, V. A., Meredith, C. N., and Dinarello, C. A.,** Physiological mechanisms contributing to increased interleukin-1 secretion, *J. Appl. Physiol.,* 61, 1869, 1986.

49. **Lewicki, R., Tchórzewski, H., Majewska, E., Nowak, Z., and Baj, Z.,** Effect of maximal physical exercise on T-lymphocyte subpopulations and on interleukin 1 (IL 1) and interleukin 2 (IL 2) production *in vitro*, *Int. J. Sports Med.,* 9, 114, 1988.

50. **Cannon, J. G., Fielding, R. A., Fiatarone, M. A., Orencole, S. F., Dinarello, C. A., and Evans, W. J.,** Increased interleukin 1β in human skeletal muscle after exercise, *Am. J. Physiol.,* 257, R451, 1989.

51. **Randall Simpson, J. and Hoffman-Goetz, L.,** Exercise, serum zinc, and interleukin-1 concentrations in man: some methodological considerations, *Nutr. Res.,* 11, 309, 1991.

52. **Randall Simpson, J. A., Hoffman-Goetz, L., Thorne, R., and Arumugam, Y.,** Exercise stress alters the percentage of splenic lymphocyte subsets in response to mitogen but not in response to interleukin-1, *Brain Behav. Immun.,* 3, 119, 1989.

53. **Shechtman, O., Elizondo, R., and Taylor, M.,** Exercise augments interleukin-2 induction, *Med. Sci. Sports Exerc.* (abstract), 20, S18, 1988.

54. **Espersen, G. T., Elbæk, A., Ernst, E., Toft, E., Kaalund, S., Jersild, C., and Grunnet, N.,** Effect of physical exercise on cytokines and lymphocyte subpopulations in human peripheral blood, *APMIS,* 98, 395, 1990.

55. **Dufaux, B. and Order, U.,** Plasma elastase-α1-antitrypsin, neopterin, tumor necrosis factor, and a soluble interleukin-2 receptor after prolonged exercise, *Int. J. Sports Med.,* 10, 434, 1989.

56. **Pogrebniak, H. W., Prewitt, T. W., Matthews, W. A., and Pass, H. I.,** Tumor necrosis factor-α alters response of lung cancer cells to oxidative stress, *J. Thorac Cardiovasc. Surg.,* 102, 904, 1991.

57. **Robertson, J. D., Maughan, R. J., Duthie, G. G., and Morrice, P. C.,** Increased blood antioxidant systems of runners in response to training load, *Clin. Sci.,* 80, 611, 1991.

58. **Viti, A., Muscettla, M., Pauiesi, L., Bocci, V., and Almi, A.,** Effect of exercise on plasma interferon levels, *J. Appl. Physiol.,* 59, 426, 1985.

59. **Pincemail, J., Camus, G., Roesgen, A., Dreezen, E., Bertrand, Y., Lismonde, M., Deby-Dupont, G., and Deby, C.,** Exercise induces pentane production and neutrophil activation in humans. Effect of propranolol, *Eur. J. Appl. Physiol.,* 61, 319, 1990.

60. **Smith, J. A., Telford, R. D., Mason, I. B., and Weidemann, M. J.,** Exercise, training and neutrophil microbicidal activity, *Int. J. Sports Med.,* 11, 179, 1990.

61. **Macha, M., Shlafer, M., and Kluger, M. J.,** Human neutrophil hydrogen peroxide generation following physical exercise, *J. Sports Med. Phys. Fitness,* 30, 412, 1990.

62. **Dziedziak, W.,** The effect of incremental cycling on physiological functions of peripheral blood granulocytes, *Biol. Sport,* 7, 239, 1990.

63. **Rodriguez, A. B., Barriga, C., and De La Fuente, M.,** Phagocytic function of blood neutrophils in sedentary young people after physical exercise, *Int. J. Sports Med.,* 12, 276, 1991.

64. **Fehr, H.-G., Lötzerich, H., and Michna, H.,** The influence of physical activity on peritoneal macrophage function: histochemical and phagocytic studies, *Int. J. Sports Med.,* 9, 77, 1988.

65. **De La Fuente, M., Martin, M. I., and Ortega, E.,** Changes in the phagocytic function of peritoneal macrophages from old mice after strenuous physical exercise, *Comp. Immunol. Microbiol. Infect. Dis.,* 13, 189, 1990.

66. **Voronina, N. P. and Mayanskii, D. N.,** Effect of intensive physical exercise on macrophage functions, *Bull. Exp. Med. Biol.,* 104, 1120, 1987.

67. **Hoffman-Goetz, L., Thorne, R., Randall Simpson, J., and Arumugam, Y.,** Exercise stress alters murine lymphocyte subset distribution in spleen, lymph nodes and thymus, *Clin. Exp. Immunol.,* 76, 307, 1989.

68. **Lötzerich, H., Fehr, H.-G., and Appell, H.-J.,** Potentiation of cytostatic but not cytolytic activity of murine macrophages after running stress, *Int. J. Sports Med.,* 11, 61, 1990.

69. **Herberman, R. B. and Ortaldo, J. R.,** Natural killer cells: their role in defense against disease, *Science,* 214, 24, 1981.

70. **Levy, S. M., Herberman, R. B., Lee, J., Whiteside, T., Beadle, M., Heiden, L., and Simons, A.,** Persistently low natural killer cell activity, age, and environmental stress as predictors of infectious morbidity, *Nat. Immun. Cell Growth Regul.,* 10, 289, 1991.

71. **Brahmi, Z., Thomas, J. E., Park, M., and Dowdeswell, I. R. G.,** The effect of acute exercise on natural killer cell activity of trained and sedentary human subjects, *J. Clin. Immunol.,* 5, 321, 1985.

72. **Fiatarone, M. A., Morley, J. E., Bloom, E. T., Benton, D., Makinodan, T., and Solomon, G. F.,** Endogenous opioids and the exercise-induced augmentation of natural killer cell activity, *J. Lab. Clin. Med.,* 112, 544, 1988.

73. **Kotani, T., Aratake, Y., Ishiguro, R., Yamamoto, I., Uemura, Y., Tamura, K., and Ohtaki, S.,** Influence of physical exercise on large granular lymphocytes, leu-7 bearing mononuclear cells and natural killer activity in peripheral blood-NK-cells and NK-activity after physical exercise, *Acta Haematol. Jap.,* 50, 1210, 1987.

74. **Randall Simpson, J. and Hoffman-Goetz, L.,** Exercise stress and murine natural killer cell function, *Proc. Soc. Exp. Biol. Med.,* 195, 129, 1990.

75. **Fiatarone, M. A., Morley, J. E., Bloom, E. T., Benton, D., Solomon, G. F., and Makinodan, T.,** The effect of exercise on natural killer cell activity in young and old subjects, *J. Gerontol.,* 44, M37, 1989.

76. **Kappel, M., Tvede, N., Galbo, H., Haahr, P. M., Kjær, M., Linstow, M., Klarlund, K., and Pedersen, B. K.,** Evidence that the effect of physical exercise on NK cell activity is mediated by epinephrine, *J. Appl. Physiol.,* 70, 2530, 1991.

77. **Plaut, M.,** Lymphocyte hormone receptors, *Ann. Rev. Immunol.,* 5, 621, 1987.

78. **Rabin, B. S., Cohen, S., Ganguli, R., Lysle, D. T., and Cunnick, J. E.,** Bidirectional interaction between the central nervous system and the immune system, *Crit. Rev. Immunol.,* 9, 279, 1989.

79. **Katz, P., Zaytoun, A. M., and Fauci, A. S.,** Mechanisms of human cell-mediated cytotoxicity. I. Modulation of natural killer cell activity by cyclic nucleotides, *J. Immunol.,* 129, 287, 1982.

80. **Green, R. L., Kaplan, S. S., Rabin, B. S., Stanitski, C. L., and Zdziarski, U.,** Immune function in marathon runners, *Ann. Allergy,* 47, 73, 1981.

81. **Papa, S., Vitale, M., Mazzotti, G., Neri, L. M., Monti, G., and Manzoli, F. A.,** Impaired lymphocyte stimulation induced by long-term training, *Immunol. Lett.,* 22, 29, 1989.

82. **Lewicki, R., Tchorzewski, H., Denys, A., Kowalska, M., and Golinska, A.,** Effect of physical exercise on some parameters of immunity in conditioned sportsmen, *Int. J. Sports Med.,* 8, 309, 1987.

83. **Watson, R. R., Moriguchi, S., Jackson, J. C., Werner, L., Wilmore, J. H., and Freund, B. J.,** Modification of cellular immune functions in humans by endurance exercise training during β-adrenergic blockade with atenolol or propranolol, *Med. Sci. Sports Exerc.,* 18, 95, 1986.

84. **Xusheng, S., Yugi, X., Yongguang, Z., and Li, S.,** Effect of ballet on immunity in young people, *J. Sports Med. Phys. Fitness,* 30, 397, 1992.

85. **Nehlsen-Cannarella, S. L., Nieman, D. C., Balk-Lamberton, A. J., Markoff, P. A., Chritton, D. B. W., Gusewitch, G., and Lee, J. W.,** The effects of moderate exercise training on immune response, *Med. Sci. Sports Exerc.,* 23, 64, 1991.

86. **Hoffman-Goetz, L., Keir, R., Thorne, R., Houston, M., and Young, C.,** Chronic exercise stress in mice depresses splenic T lymphocyte mitogenesis *in vitro, Clin. Exp. Immunol.,* 66, 551, 1986.

87. **Tharp, G. D. and Preuss, T. L.,** Mitogenic responses of T-lymphocytes to exercise training and stress, *J. Appl. Physiol.,* 70, 2535, 1991.

88. **Crist, D. M., Mackinnon, L. T., Thompson, R. F., Atterborn, H. A., and Egan, P. A.,** Physical exercise increases natural cellular-mediated tumor cytotoxicity in elderly women, *Gerontol.,* 35, 66, 1989.

89. **Nieman, D. C., Nehlsen-Cannarella, S. L., Markoff, P. A., Balk-Lamberton, A. J., Yang, H., Chritton, D. B. W., Lee, J. W., and Arabatzis, K.,** The effects of moderate exercise training on natural killer cells and acute upper respiratory tract infections, *Int. J. Sports Med.,* 11, 467, 1990.

90. **Pedersen, B. K., Tvede, N., Christensen, L. D., Klarlund, K., Kragbak, S., and Halkjær-Kristensen, J.,** Natural killer cell activity in peripheral blood of highly trained and untrained persons, *Int. J. Sports Med.,* 10, 129, 1989.

91. **Ndon, J. A., Snyder, A. C., Foster, C., and Wehrenberg, W. B.,** Effects of chronic intense exercise training on the leukocyte responses to acute exercise, *Int. J. Sports Med.,* 13, 176, 1992.

92. **LaPerriere, A. R., Antoni, M. H., Schneiderman, N., Ironson, G., Klimas, N., Caralis, P., and Fletcher, M. A.,** Exercise intervention attenuates emotional distress and natural killer cell decrements following notification of positive serologic status for HIV-1, *Biofeedback Self Regul.,* 15, 229, 1990.

93. **Berry, C. A.,** Medical legacy of Apollo, *Aerospace Med.,* 45, 1046, 1974.

94. **Merz, B.,** The body pays a penalty for defying the law of gravity, *JAMA,* 256, 2040, 1986.

95. **Vasquez, T. E., Pretorius, H. T., and Rimkus, D. S.,** Space medicine: A review of current concepts, *West J. Med.,* 147, 292, 1987.

96. **Barone, R. P. and Caren, L. D.,** The immune system: effects of hypergravity and hypogravity, *Aviat. Space Environ. Med.,* 55, 1063, 1984.

97. **Criswell-Hudak, B.,** Immune response during space flight, *Exp. Gerontol.,* 26, 289, 1991.

98. **Fowler, J. F., Jr.,** Dermatology in space: the final frontier, in *Advances in Dermatology,* 6th ed., Callen, J. P., Dahl, M. V., Golitz, L. E., Greenway, H. T., and Schachner, L. A., Eds., Mosby, St. Louis, 1991, 73.

99. Life Sciences Research Office, Research opportunities on immunocompetence in space, Fed. Am. Soc. Exp. Biol., Bethesda, MD, 1985.

100. **Moorthy, A. V. and Zimmerman, S. W.,** Human leukocyte response to an endurance race, *Eur. J. Appl. Physiol.,* 38, 271, 1978.

101. **Fischer, C. L., Daniels, J. C., Levin, W. C., Kimzey, S. L., Cobb, E. B., and Ritzman, S. E.,** Effects of space flight environment on man's immune system. II. Lymphocyte counts and reactivity, *Aerospace Med.,* 43, 1122, 1972.

102. **Konstantinova, I. and Antropova, E.,** Effect of space cabin environmental parameters and space flight factors on certain mechanisms underlying immunological reactivity, *Rev. Med. Spac.,* 46, 383, 1973.

103. **Mandel, A. D. and Balish, E.,** Effect of space flight on cell-mediated immunity, *Aviat. Space Environ. Med.,* 48, 1051, 1977.

104. **Cogoli, A. and Tschopp, A.,** Lymphocyte reactivity during space flight, *Immunol. Today,* 6, 1, 1985.

105. **Taylor, G. R., Neale, L. S., and Dardano, J. R.,** Immunological analyses of U.S. Space Shuttle crewmembers, *Aviat. Space Environ. Med.,* 57, 213, 1986.

106. **Cogoli, A., Tschopp, A., and Fuchs-Bislin, P.,** Cell sensitivity to gravity, *Science,* 225, 228, 1984.

107. **Bechler, B., Cogoli, A, and Mesland, D.,** Lymphocytes in spaceflight, *Naturwissen,* 73, 400, 1986.

108. **Gmünder, F. K., Lorenzi, G., Bechler, B., Joller, P., Muller, J., Ziegler, W. H., and Cogoli, A.,** Effect of long-term physical exercise on lymphocyte reactivity: similarity to spaceflight reactions, *Aviat. Space Environ. Med.,* 59, 146, 1988.

109. **Grigoriev, A. I., Burgrov, S. A., Bogomolov, V. V., Egorov, A. D., Kozlovskaya, I. B., Pestov, I. D., Polyakov, V. V., and Tarasov, I. K.,** Medical results of the MIR year-long mission, *The Physiologist,* 34 (No. 1 Suppl.), S44, 1991.

110. **Konstantinova, I. V., Sonnenfeld, G., Lesnyak, A. T., Shaffar, L., Mandel, A., Rykova, M. P., Antropova, E. N., and Ferrua, B.,** Cellular immunity and lymphokine production during spaceflights, *The Physiologist,* 34 (No. 1 Suppl.), S52, 1991.

111. **Manie, S., Konstantinova, I., Breittmayer, J.-P., Ferrua, B., and Schaffar, L.,** Effects of long duration spaceflight on human T lymphocyte and monocyte activity, *Aviat. Space Environ. Med.,* 62, 1153, 1991.

112. **Rose, A., Steffen, J. M., Musacchia, X. J., and Mandel, A. D.,** Effect of antiorthostatic suspension on interferon-α/β production by the mouse, *Proc. Soc. Exp. Biol. Med.,* 177, 253, 1984.

113. **Sonnenfeld, G., Morey, E. R., Williams, J. A., and Mandel, A. D.,** Effect of a simulated weightlessness model on the production of rat interferon, *J. Interferon Res.,* 2, 467, 1982.

114. **Gould, C. L., Lyte, M., Williams, J., Mandel, A. D., and Sonnenfeld, G.,** Inhibited interferon-γ but normal interleukin-3 production from rats flown on the space shuttle, *Aviat. Space Environ. Med.,* 58, 983, 1987.

115. **Kimzey, S. L., Johnson, P. C., Ritzmann, S. E., and Mengel, C. E.,** Hematology and immunology studies: the second manned Skylab mission, *Aviat. Space Environ. Med.,* 47, 383, 1976.

116. **Benton, E. V., Almasi, J., Cassou, R., Frank, A., Henke, R. P., and Rowe, V.,** Radiation measurements aboard Spacelab 1, *Science,* 225, 224, 1984.

117. **Cogoli, A., Valluchi-Morf, M., Mueller, M., and Briegleb, W.,** Effect of hypogravity on human lymphocyte activation, *Aviat. Space Environ. Med.,* 51, 29, 1980.

118. **Guanghua, Y., Shuqing, W., and Jin, N.,** Influences of simulated microgravity and hypergravity on the immune functions of animals,. *The Physiologist,* 34 (No. 1 Suppl.), S96, 1991.

119. **Ritzmann, S. E. and Levin, W. C.,** Investigation of man's immune system (M 122), part B. Skylab medical experiments altitude test, NASA, Johnson Space Center, 1973.

120. **Mikhaylovskiy, G. P., Dobronravova, N. N., Kozar, M. I., Korotayev, M. M., Tsiganova, N. I., Shilov, V. M., and Yakovleva, I. Ya.,** Variation in overall body tolerance during a 62-day exposure to hypokinesia and acceleration, *Space Biol. Med. (Transl. Kosmicheskaya Biologiya i Aviakosmicheskaya Meditsina),* 1, 101, 1967.

121. **Gmünder, F. X., Kiess, M., Sonnefeld, G., Lee, J., and Cogoli, A.,** A ground-based model to study the effects of weightlessness on lymphocytes, *Biol. Cell,* 70, 33, 1990.

122. **Vacek, A., Bueverova, E. I., Michurina, T. V., Rotkovska, D., Serova, L. V., and Bartonickova, A.,** Decrease in the number of progenitors of fibroblasts (CFUf) in bone marrow of rats after a 14-day flight onboard the Cosmos-2044 biosatellite, *Folia Biol. (Praha),* 36, 194, 1990.

123. **Sonnenfeld, G., Mandel, A. D., Konstantinova, I. V., Taylor, G. R., Berry, W. D., Wellhausen, S. R., Lesnyak, A. T., and Fuchs, B. B.,** Effects of spaceflight on levels and activity of immune cells, *Aviat. Space Environ. Med.,* 61, 648, 1990.

124. **Galbo, H.,** *Hormonal and Metabolic Adaptation to Exercise,* Thieme-Stratton, New York, 1983.

125. **Bunt, J. C.,** Hormonal alterations due to exercise, *Sports Med.,* 3, 331, 1986.

126. **Kjær, M.,** Regulation of hormonal and metabolic responses during exercise in humans, *Exerc. Sport Sci. Rev.,* 20, 161, 1992.

127. **Blalock, J. E.,** A molecular basis for bidirectional communication between the immune and neuroendocrine systems, *Physiol. Rev.,* 69, 1, 1989.

128. **Ader, R., Felten, D. L., and Cohen, N.,** *Psychoneuroimmunology,* 2nd ed., Ader, R., Felten, D. L., and Cohen, N., Eds., Academic Press, San Diego, 1991.

129. **White, J. A., Ismail, A. H., and Bottoms, G. D.,** Effect of physical fitness on the adrenocortical response to exercise stress, *Med. Sci. Sports Exerc.,* 8, 113, 1976.

130. **Davies, C. T. M. and Few, J. D.,** Effects of exercise on adrenocortical function, *J. Appl. Physiol.,* 35, 887, 1973.

131. **MacNeil, B. and Hoffman-Goetz, L.,** Chronic exercise enhances *in vivo* and *in vitro* cytotoxic mechanisms of natural immunity in mice, *J. Appl. Physiol.,* 74, 388, 1993.

132. **Cupps, T. R. and Fauci, A. S.,** Corticosteroid-mediated immunoregulation in man, *Immunol. Rev.,* 65, 133, 1982.

133. **Goodwin, J. S., Messner, R. P., and Williams, R. C.,** Inhibitors of T-cell mitogenesis: effect of mitogen dose, *Cell. Immunol.,* 45, 303, 1979.

134. **Gillis, S., Crabtree, G. R., and Smith, K. A.,** Glucocorticoid-induced inhibition of T cell growth factor production. I. The effect of mitogen-induced lymphocyte proliferation, *J. Immunol.,* 123, 1624, 1979.

135. **Munck, A., Guyre, P. M., and Holbrook, N. J.,** Physiological functions of glucocorticoids in stress and their relation to pharmacological actions, *Endocrine Rev.,* 5, 25, 1984.

136. **Munck, A. and Guyre, P. M.,** Glucocorticoids and immune function, in *Psychoneuroimmunology,* 2nd ed., Ader, R., Felten, D. L., and Cohen, N., Eds., Academic Press, San Diego, 1991, 447.

137. **Johnson, H. M., Torres, B. A., Smith, E. M., Dion, L. D., and Blalock, J. E.,** Regulation of lymphokine (interferon-γ) production by corticotropin, *J. Immunol.,* 132, 246, 1984.

138. **Koff, W. C. and Dunegan, M. A.,** Modulation of macrophage-mediated tumoricidal activity by neuro-peptides and neurohormones, *J. Immunol.,* 135, 350, 1985.

139. **Smith, E. M. and Blalock, J. E.,** Human lymphocyte production of ACTH and endorphin-like substances. Association with leukocyte interferon, *Proc. Acad. Sci. U.S.A.,* 78, 7530, 1981.

140. **Smith, E. M., Brosnan, P., Meyer III, W. J., and Blalock, J. E.,** An ACTH receptor on human mononuclear leukocytes, *New Engl. J. Med.,* 317, 1266, 1987.

141. **Lolait, S. J., Lim, A. T. W., Toh, B. H., and Funder, J. W.,** Immunoreactive B-endorphin in a subpopulation of mouse spleen macrophages, *J. Clin. Invest.,* 73, 277, 1984.

142. **Besedovsky, H. O., del Rey, A., Sorkin, E., and Dinarello, Ch. A.,** Immunoregulatory feedback between interleukin-1 and glucocorticoid hormones, *Science,* 233, 652, 1986.

143. **Lehmann, M., Kapp, R., Himmelsbach, M., and Keul, J.,** Time and intensity dependent catecholamine responses during graded exercise as an indicator of fatigue and exhaustion, in *Biochemistry of Exercise,* Knuttgen, H. G., Vogel, J. A., and Poortmans, J., Eds., Human Kinetics Publishers, Champaign, 1983, 738.

144. **Brooks, S., Burrin, J., Cheetham, M. E., Hall, G. M., Yeo, T., and Williams, C.,** The responses of the catecholamines and β-endorphin to brief maximal exercise in man, *Eur. J. Appl. Physiol.,* 57, 230, 1988.

145. **Kjær, M., Christensen, N. J., Sonne, B., Richter, E. A., and Galbo, H.,** The effect of exercise on epinephrine turnover in trained and untrained subjects, *J. Appl. Physiol.,* 59, 1061, 1985.

146. **Kjær, M. and Galbo, H.,** Effect of physical training on the capacity to secrete epinephrine, *J. Appl. Physiol.,* 64, 11, 1988.

147. **Watson, J.,** The influence of intracellular levels of cyclic nucleotides on cell proliferation and the induction of antibody synthesis, *J. Exp. Med.,* 141, 97, 1975.

148. **Carlson, S. L., Brooks, W. H., and Roszman, T. L.,** Neurotransmitter-lymphocyte interaction: dual receptor modulation of lymphocyte proliferation and cAMP production, *J. Neuroimmunol.,* 24, 155, 1989.

149. **Madden, K. S. and Livnat, S.,** Catecholamine action and immunologic reactivity, in *Psychoneuroimmunology,* 2nd ed., Ader, R., Felten, D. L., and Cohen, N., Eds., Academic Press, San Diego, 1991, 283.

150. **Hadden, J. W., Hadden, E. M., and Middleton, E., Jr.,** Lymphocyte blast transformation. I. Demonstration of adrenergic receptors in human peripheral lymphocytes, *Cell. Immunol.,* 1, 583, 1970.

151. **Hellstrand, K., Hermodsson, S., and Strannegård, Ö.,** Evidence for a β-adrenoceptor-mediated regulation of human natural killer cells, *J. Immunol.,* 134, 4095, 1985.

152. **Beckner, S. K. and Farrar, W. L.,** Potentiation of lymphokine-activated killer cell differentiation and lymphocyte proliferation by stimulation of protein kinase C or inhibition of adenylate cyclase, *J. Immunol.,* 140, 208, 1988.

153. **Tønnesen, E., Christensen, N. J., and Brinklov, M. M.,** Natural killer cell activity during cortisol infusion and adrenaline infusion in healthy volunteers, *Eur. J. Clin. Invest.,* 17, 497, 1987.

154. **Kraut, R. P. and Greenberg, A. H.,** Effects of endogenous and exogenous opioids on splenic natural killer cell activity, *Nat. Immun. Cell Growth Regul.,* 5, 28, 1986.

155. **Shavit, Y., Terman, G. W., Martin, F. C., Lewis, J. W., Liebsekind, J. C., and Gale, R. P.,** Stress, opioid peptides, the immune system, and cancer, *J. Immunol.,* 135, 834s, 1985.

156. **Shavit, Y., Martin, F. C., Yirmiya, R., Ben-Eliyahu, S., Terman, G. W., Weiner, H., Gale, R. P., and Liebeskind, J. C.,** Effects of a single administration of morphine or footshock stress on natural killer cell cytotoxicity, *Brain Behav. Immun.,* 1, 318, 1987.

157. **Goldfarb, A. H., Hatfield, B. D., Sforzo, G. A., and Flynn, M. G.,** Serum β-endorphin levels during a graded exercise test to exhaustion, *Med. Sci. Sports Exerc.,* 19, 78, 1987.

158. **McMurray, R. G., Forsythe, W. A., Mar, M. H., and Hardy, C. J.,** Exercise intensity-related responses of β-endorphin and catecholamines, *Med. Sci. Sports Exerc.,* 19, 570, 1987.

159. **Howlett, T. A., Tomlin, S., Ngahfoong, L., Rees, L. H., Bullen, B. A., Skrinar, G. S., and McArthur, J. W.,** Release of β endorphin and met-enkephalin during exercise in normal women: response to training, *Br. Med. J.,* 288, 1950, 1984.

160. **Farrell, P. A.,** Exercise and endorphins — male responses, *Med. Sci. Sports Exerc.,* 17, 89, 1985.

161. **Sibinga, N. E. S., and Goldstein, A.,** Opioid peptides and opioid receptors in cells of the immune system, *Ann. Rev. Immunol.,* 6, 219, 1988.

162. **Matthews, P. M., Froelich, C. J., Sibbitt, W. L., Jr., and Bankhurst, A. D.,** Enhancement of natural cytotoxicity by β-endorphin, *J. Immunol.,* 130, 1658, 1983.

163. **Wiik, P.,** VIP inhibition of monocyte respiratory burst *ex vivo* during prolonged strain and energy deficiency, *Intern. J. Neurosci.,* 51, 195, 1990.

164. **Gerhardsson DeVerdier, M., Steineck, G., Hagman, U., Rieger, A., and Norell, S. E.,** Physical activity and colon cancer: a case referent study in Stockholm, *Int. J. Cancer,* 46, 985, 1990.

165. **Whittemore, A. S., Wu-Williams, A. H., Lee, M., Shu, Z., Gallagher, R. P., Deng-ao, J., Lun, Z., Xianghui, W., Kun, C., Jung, D., Teh, C.-Z., Chengde, L., Yao, X. J., Paffenberger, R. S., and Henderson, B. E.,** Diet, physical activity, and colorectal cancer among Chinese in North America and China, *J. Nat. Cancer Inst.,* 82, 915, 1990.

166. **Severson, R. K., Nomura, A. M. Y., Grove, J. S., and Stemmermann, G. N.,** A prospective analysis of physical activity and cancer, *Am. J. Epidemiol.,* 130, 522, 1989.

167. **Frisch, R. E., Wyshak, G., Albright, N. L., Albright, T. E., Schiff, I., Jones, K. P., Witschi, J., Shiang, E., Koff, E., and Marguglio, M.,** Lower prevalence of breast cancer and cancers of the reproductive system among former college athletes compared to non-athletes, *Br. J. Cancer,* 52, 885, 1985.

168. **Blair, S. N., Kohl, H. W., Paffenberger, R. S., Clark, D. G., Cooper, K. H., and Gibbons, L. W.,** Physical fitness and all-cause mortality: a prospective study of healthy men and women, *JAMA,* 262, 2395, 1989.

169. **Paffenberger, R. S., Hyde, R. T., and Wing, A. L.,** Physical activity and incidence of cancer in diverse populations: a preliminary report, *Am. J. Clin. Nutr.,* 45, 312, 1987.

170. **Adrianopoulos, G., Nelson, R. L., Bombeck, C. T., and Souza, G.,** The influence of physical activity in 1,2-dimethylhydrazine induced colon carcinogenesis in the rat, *Anticancer Res.,* 7, 849, 1987.

171. **Klurfeld, D. M., Welch, C. B., Einhorn, E., and Kritchevsky, D.,** Inhibition of colon tumor promotion by caloric restriction or exercise in rats, *FASEB J.,* 2, A433, 1988.

172. **Vena, J. E., Graham, S., Zielezny, M., Brasure, J., and Swanson, M. K.,** Occupational exercise and risk of cancer, *Am. J. Clin. Nutr.,* 45, 318, 1987.

173. **Vena, J. E., Graham, S., Zielezny, M., Swanson, M. K., Barnes, R. E., and Nolan, J.,** Lifetime occupational exercise and colon cancer, *Am. J. Epidemiol.,* 122, 357, 1985.

174. **Hoffman-Goetz, L., MacNeil, B., Arumugam, Y., and Randall Simpson, J.,** Differential effects of exercise and housing condition on murine natural killer cell activity and tumor growth, *Int. J. Sports Med.,* 2, 167, 1992.

175. **Reynolds, H. Y.,** Immunologic system in the respiratory tract, *Physiol. Rev.,* 71, 1117, 1991.

176. **Reyes, M. P., Smith, F. E., and Lerner, A. M.,** An enterovirus-induced murine model of an acute dilated-type cardiomyopathy, *Intervirology,* 22, 146, 1984.

177. **Ilbäck, N.-G., Fohlman, J., and Friman, G.,** Exercise in coxsackie B3 myocarditis: effects on heart lymphocyte subpopulations and inflammatory reaction, *Am. Heart J.,* 117, 1298, 189.

178. **Simon, H. B.,** Exercise and human immune function, in *Psychoneuroimmunology,* 2nd ed., Ader, R., Felten, D. L., and Cohen, N., Eds., Academic Press, San Diego, 1991, 869.

179. **Peters, E. M. and Bateman, E. D.,** Ultramarathon running and upper respiratory tract infections, *S. A. Med. J.,* 64, 582, 1983.

180. **Berglund, B. and Hemmingsson, P.,** Infectious disease in elite cross-country skiers: a one-year incidence study, *Clin. Sports Med.,* 2, 19, 1990.